vitamin C until after 8 to 11 days. This shows that the mentally ill had a "deficit of about 2,400 to 3,000 milligrams of vitamin C. A deficit of 1,000 milligrams or at the most 1,500 milligrams may be regarded as pathological (disease-causing)," says the author. The need for vitamin C in preserving mental health is obvious from this research—it is down to actual figures.

A Precise Example

The value of B vitamins for mental health was emphasized by a piece in the *British Medical Journal* (May 10, 1958). It told of a 71-year-old man who was suffering from an arthritic condition that required medical care, although mentally the man had always been sound. The attending doctor, who knew the patient well, was astounded one day to find sudden mental deterioration in the man, which resulted in confusion, incoherent speech and even inability to find the lavatory in his own house or to put on his clothes.

The doctor instituted a treatment consisting of 50-milligram tablets of niacin (a B vitamin) 3 times a day. The patient improved steadily, and in a month, was wholly recovered. He discontinued the treatment without consulting the doctor and he suffered a relapse. Once again the vitamin was prescribed, and the patient recovered in a week.

These are only a few of many examples of nutrition as a factor in regaining mental health. We are anxious to see further, more concentrated exploration of this theory.

Sight and Hearing Problems

The individuals who have sight and hearing difficulties are certainly more likely than the average person to have an accident. Both of these difficulties are involved with deficiencies of vitamin A. Night blindness for example, is an absolute symptom of vitamin A deficiency. The *Lancet* (May, 1958) says a lack of animal protein is a factor in near sightedness. The *American Journal of Ophthalmology* (May, 1950) blamed a lack of vitamin A and calcium for near sightedness. *Medical Press* (June 4, 1952) said that a shortage of thiamin (a B vitamin) could cause amblyopia (an unexplained dimness of vision). Conjunctivitis (a painful inflammation of the membranes of the eyelids) is due in many cases to a lack of vitamin A (*American Journal of the Diseases of Childhood*, July, 1941).

Many hearing problems are also attributable to lack of vitamin A. In the *Archives of Otolaryngology* (May, 1951), Dr. M. Joseph Lobel covered the subject in detail. He quotes Barlow as saying that a deficiency in vitamin A, which causes changes in the mucous membranes of the throat, might produce changes in the middle ear which could become permanent. Cody, another researcher, tells of impaired hearing in laboratory rats made deficient in vitamin A. In 1933, Rosenfield gave cod liver oil (rich in vitamin A) to patients with otosclerosis and improved the hearing of many of them. Here again the evidence is abundant and cannot be included entirely in this space.

We think we have proven that nutrition has a place in the scheme of accident prevention. It is intimately bound up with mentality, emotions, sight and hearing. Legislation for new highways, seat belts, clear markings for danger spots, safer construction of cars and dozens of other anti-accident gimmicks are fine, but without a driver who can see and hear well, and who knows what he is doing, they are useless. Let our highway safety programs stress nutrition first if they intend to remedy the basic cause of accidents.

What Has Advanced Age to do with Accidents?

Are you a bad accident risk because you're over 65? The Travelers Insurance Companies' booklet, *Deadly Reckoning,* says no. In 1960, they say, only 6.5 per cent of the drivers in fatal accidents were over 65. Contrast this rosy picture with the deadliest group, 25 to 64 years, who figured in 65.9 per cent of the fatal accidents that year. The number of drivers in this group is, of course, much greater.

As a rule, over-65 drivers, if they are physically well, are likely to be safer than any others. They are mature, experienced and patient, in comparison with youngsters, or even those of middle age. That explains, somewhat, the reason for this good driving record. As with all statistics and generalities, these do not hold good for everybody. There are drivers over 65 who have automobile accidents as well as accidents in the home. What makes them different from the safe majority? We believe that diet plays a great part in accident proneness. We think that it might be the deciding factor in an older person's accident. Remember, good food makes for good nerves, alertness, good bones, quick reflexes, etc. That many over-65 citizens fall short in this requirement is evident from an article in the *New York Times* (March 12, 1961) by Howard Rusk, M.D.

Broken Bones in Older People

Dr. Rusk tells us that persons over 65 make up 9 per cent of the population in the United States. This small percentage accounts for 28 per cent of all accidental deaths and 20 per cent of all serious disabling injuries. Once an older person is injured seriously enough to be hospitalized, his stay is usually a longer one. In 1957, Dr. Rusk tells us, the average stay for accidents of older people was a week longer than that of the total population.

One of the main reasons for the increased time in the hospital is that older people often break bones in accidents. (Commonest among the accidents in older people is fracture of the hip.) These fractures, even with modern orthopedic techniques, such as pinning and nailing the bones together, heal slowly, if at all. When they do not heal, the patient is confined to bed or wheelchair for the rest of his life. Such broken bone injuries, along with strokes, fill more hospital beds than any other type of disability.

The reason for this reluctance of older bones to heal is the brittleness that seems to set in with age. Research has shown the miracle bone meal preparations can perform in forestalling such brittleness, in the bone of individuals of any age. The value of this calcium-rich food in uniting broken bones that had shown no sign of knitting together in spite of months, and even years, of standard treatments has often been proven. The strength of bones is in calcium and other minerals. Using a supplement which supplies them in good measure seems like common sense to us, especially when age is in the picture. If brittle bones are a part of the problem of later years, we say, fight the problem before it puts you in the hospital. You don't have to break a bone if you should fall, provided bone meal makes up part of your diet.

Pedestrians Have Faith

Dr. Rusk writes that older persons are involved in a large number of accidents as pedestrians. There are several reasons for that. Their hearing and vision are often impaired. And sometimes elderly pedestrians exhibit a flattering, but misplaced faith in the power of the driver. The reason may lie in the fact that older people who, as pedestrians, are involved in an accident with a car, have never driven a car. These people do not realize the limitations in stopping or maneuvering a vehicle.

What about the older people who are still driving? When should they stop? Should they be stopped by law, once they have reached a certain age? Here again we say the individual must be considered. Some drivers in their eighties drive beautifully, while some drivers in their fifties are a menace, as are some 20 year olds.

Weeding Out Unsafe Drivers

The answer for weeding out unsafe drivers seems to lie, in part, in the system of periodic physical examinations when certain ages are reached. Such tests of eyesight and reflexes cannot tell the state everything it should know about a driver's ability, but it is a help.

There was once some talk about asking family doctors to pass judgment on the fitness of their patients as drivers. There were several drawbacks. For one thing, doctors were reluctant to take on the responsibility of deciding for a patient whether or not he could drive.

For another, personal considerations often tend to influence doctors to make allowances which would permit unsafe drivers to drive anyway.

We would like to emphasize one important factor concerning elderly drivers which is generally left unmentioned—that is, their use of drugs. Those arriving in the upper age brackets without the plague of one chronic disease or the other are quite rare. Arthritis and heart disease are practically universal complaints among these people. The drugs given to combat the symptoms can often effectively interfere with driving ability. The tranquilizers sometimes given to help keep blood pressure down, also act to soften the intellectual and mechanical reactions of the person using them. Maybe this effect seems inconsequential for the patient who spends the day in an easy chair. But for one who drives or who walks through busy traffic, the extra second it might take to react in an emergency can mean serious injury or death.

The drugs used against arthritis, the hormones especially, are apt to cause undesirable attitudes in drivers. Some of their side effects are mental aberrations, suicidal impulses, excessive irritability, etc. Add any of these to the normal stress of driving on a crowded parkway or on a busy downtown street, or being stuck behind a slow-moving truck on your way to an important appointment, and you can see the makings of an accident.

The matter of diet is important in the safety with which a driver handles a car. Many of our older citizens tend to eat little and seem to concentrate, when they do eat, on the foods that are of least value nutritionally speaking. They budget small incomes by eating plenty of starches and sweets, both of which are cheap and filling. Their diets are notably lacking in B-vitamin foods, such as organ meats, wheat germ and brewer's yeast.

The B vitamins are essential for maintaining a healthy nervous system and, of course, a quick-acting brain. Sweets are quick to deprive the body of these B vitamins, and the casual eating habits which neglect to replenish the body's supply of B vitamins leave the road wide open to absent-mindedness and woolgathering, as well as nervousness and indecision. We have always advocated the use of B-vitamin supplements for everyone every day. For those over 65, who drive, the need is undeniable.

Why Steadiness and Balance Fail

The lack of balance, tendency to fall, slower mental processes, uncertain control of posture and gait in older people are explained somewhat by Dr. J. H. Sheldon in the *British Medical Journal* (December 10, 1960). "It is well known that aging is accompanied by a loss of nerve cells from the brain. . . . It is suggested, therefore, that the fundamental factor underlying the senile liability to fall is a decrease in the number of healthy nerve cells available. . . . Certain difficulties of movement which are common in old age become easier to understand on this basis. . . . The adverse effects of this cellular poverty will inevitably be accentuated by the interference with the blood supply to the region. . . ."

Careful diet and use of food supplements can help in two ways, if Dr. Sheldon is correct. The B vitamins will strengthen the nerve cells, making those which remain healthier and less likely to deteriorate. This means more nerve cells to do the necessary work, and more efficiency in them, too. Vitamin E will help in making the curtailed blood supply which Dr. Sheldon mentions, count for a good deal more than it normally would. The vitamin E holds a generous supply of oxygen in the blood, which means less blood will do more work —less strain on the heart, less problems when the blood supply to the brain is curtailed.

Lack of nutrition and tendency toward accidents cannot be divorced. A healthy, well-nourished individual of 16 or 65 is still a better accident risk than one who pays no attention to the way he eats. For older folks, especially, good diet is cheap insurance against accidents of all kinds.

Accidents and the Holiday Season

People often remark, with relief, that they're glad the days of flaming candles on the Christmas tree are past. Who could enjoy Christmas with the threat of a tragedy hovering so closely? Well, today's electric bulbs are certainly an improvement, and although hot bulbs, dried trees and faulty wiring still present a hazardous combination, we no longer chance the slight draft that could tip a flaming candle into the draperies or the Christmas tree, or the chance of a gauzy Christmas dress exploding into flame upon brushing by a candle.

Old dangers have been replaced by new ones, however, and the parent who wants his family to enjoy the holidays instead of merely surviving through them can take a few simple precautions that will set him at ease. There are ornaments and toys that can be avoided with no lessening of Christmas gaiety and much increased peace of mind.

Bubbling Lights

For example, the candle-shaped bubbling lights which are a common sight at Christmas time, offer a great curiosity attraction for children. They can't seem to resist touching the lights, even pulling them from the tree. The *New England Journal of Medicine,* in one of its early winter issues of 1960, mentioned that children sometimes break the bulbs and drink the intriguing contents—generally methylene chloride. The result of drinking this liquid can show itself in mild depression of the central nervous system, followed or preceded by excitement of the system. If large amounts are drunk, there is danger of liver or kidney damage. Is it far-fetched to concern oneself over the possibility of a child actually doing such a thing as to break one of these candles and drink the contents? Any parent of young children knows that they are quite capable of just this type of experiment.

And what about youngsters eating the "icicles" and the "angel hair?" Small children do it. Luckily, the icicles are poorly absorbed in the intestinal tract, so frank poisoning is unlikely, but intestinal obstruction and choking when the attempt is made to swallow a wad of the stuff is a possibility. The misty-looking "angel hair" is actually spun glass. Children are attracted by its cotton-candy appearance, and are likely to try swallowing some. The glass can cause serious internal irritations.

Red Berries and Dancing Mothballs

Kids love the look of red holly berries, and they are quite likely to presume that they can be eaten. The holly berries contain a toxic compound which causes severe vomiting, diarrhea and depression of the central nervous system. The white mistletoe berry is also toxic, though the exact source of toxicity has not been defined.

The Abbot publication *What's New* (winter, 1960) tells of a new holiday wrinkle called "dancing moth balls." The stunt consists of placing moth balls in a colored solution of vinegar and water and then adding baking soda which releases carbon dioxide at the surface, causing the moth balls to "dance." The toxic properties of moth balls, eaten or even inhaled, makes this a risky form of amusement.

"Snow" sprays just had to come as a logical extension of our preoccupation with aerosol containers. Everything is sprayed with the "snow"— windows, Christmas trees, mirrors, packages, toys— and kids love doing it. The "snow" is a plastic material, and the propellant, or gas which shoots it from the can probably consists of halogenated hydrocarbons—methylene chloride and freons. These are toxic, and can easily be breathed in by the children nearby as the spraying goes on. It must be borne in mind that these droplets are light enough to be sprayed, to float through the air, and this means that they can be inhaled, too. Spray cans of "snow" should not be handled by children; even for grownups they present a hazard. Wear a mask if you must use one of these things.

Colorful Fires

Fireplaces always get a workout during the holidays. In recent years it has become popular to use so-called "fire salts" which produce multicolored flames on the yule log. This product can cause severe metal poisoning if swallowed. The colors result from burning salts of copper, barium-selenium, lead, thallium, arsenic and antimony. Intestinal irritation and subsequent vomiting are the usual results, if a child should swallow such salts. Milk, raw egg white, flour or starch should be given at once, and a physician called. The container should be kept so that the physician can know exactly what poison was ingested, as this allows for the most effective prescription of an antidote if one exists.

Model trains are the central attraction of most Christmas displays where boys are concerned. Truly the models of today do everything a real train does and then some. One of the newer attractions is the smoking engine. The smoke is the result of a chemical reaction in cartridges, which contain metaterphenyl or kerosene and cedar wood oil. These are poisonous substances, and one is not hard-put to imagine an intense little boy working at the tracks or one of the model houses while the smoke is rising from the engine right into his face. And again, cartridges such as those used here are almost irresistible to the tot who explores by putting everything into his mouth that will fit there.

Do you make your own Christmas cards? Your own decorations for the house? We think this is an admirable custom, and a reflection of the true spirit of Christmas. We would only caution that the work should be done in a room that has plenty of ventilation. Some of the poster paints used have a poisonous base that escapes into the air. In a closed room these toxic fumes can accumulate and cause headache, nausea and vomiting. This possibility is accented by the closeness of the work and the likelihood that several containers might be open at the same time, as the artist uses one color after the other.

If poisoning of any type should occur (except for caustic alkaloids or kerosene), dilution and evacuation of the substance is the first aim. Household materials such as table salt, powdered mustard or soap, dissolved in water usually will induce vomiting. With a child who is already frightened, trying to force these distasteful preparations down his throat is often a waste of time and patience. It is better sometimes to induce vomiting by placing the child in a face-down position with his head low and tickling the back of his throat with a finger or a spoon handle. Biting can be prevented by placing a wedge between the child's teeth. Afterward the child is kept quiet and warm until the doctor arrives.

Dangerous Toys

Of course, to the child, Christmas means, mainly, toys. Parents should be on the lookout for bad design in toys which might lead to serious accidents as children play with them. In the *British Medical Journal* (May 2, 1959), we read of a Junior Chamber of Commerce Committee which carried out an inquiry on the hazards of toys. Members of the committee filled in questionnaires to record information about children they knew. They gathered data about 336 children in this way. It was found that 138 of the children (41 per cent) had had accidents caused by toys. Some of the children had figured in more than one accident for the total number of accidents was 209. Of these, 33 were classed as serious, and two more were fatal.

The causes of the accidents were predictable, all due to bad design: mechanical toys with knife-sharp edges to the metal, highly inflammable celluloid, teddy-bear's eyes on sharp pins, lead in the paint on the top, or in the material of which it was made. Many of the toys had parts which could be too easily detached and swallowed. Then there were knives and air guns. Neither of these should find its way into the hands of a child. Both can be fatal weapons.

The Problems of Holiday Eating

Eating at Christmastime presents a real problem to the health-conscious parent. Hard candy and gift boxes of chocolates are everywhere. Visiting is frequent and meals are all off schedule. Everybody has gooey, sugary homemade cookies and hot chocolate and soda is the only thing offered to the children at many of the homes they visit.

What can one do? For one thing, avoid having such things around your own house. Have *your* sweets consist of dates, figs, fruits and nuts. Most of the children who visit you will probably welcome the change from the junk they've been eating! For a drink, offer fruit juice or cider—adults and children will enjoy them.

If you go visiting, ask your friends in your beforehand phone conversations to forego serving sweets to you and your children. Tell them that a piece of fruit would be appreciated if they care to serve something. True friends will respect your wishes in such matters.

It is difficult to insist that your children be omitted when sweets are served. The young child who is the only one forced to sit out an ice cream party is indeed an unhappy soul. We believe that such denial may be almost as harmful in some cases as to eat the ice cream with everyone else for that one time. If a hostess is so unthinking as to put you in such a position, and you know your child will be upset at being excluded, allow him to participate, but supervise the helping so as to keep it minimal, and vow to avoid future visits. Hostesses who think they are doing the "poor child" a favor by using such tactics must be informed as emphatically as necessary, that they definitely are not!

With the traditional partying, close quarters in large gatherings and stepped up activities, food supplementation should be advanced to meet additional needs. Vitamin C especially should be employed to keep colds, grippe and other holiday infections at a safe distance.

Diet and Safe Driving

By J. I. Rodale

A talk given at the Fall Safety Forum of the Ohio and Pennsylvania Motor Truck Association Council of Safety Supervisors and Cooperative Safety Patrol, October 26, 1960.

I don't think I would be here this morning were it not for an experiment conducted by John W. Jacobson, Director of the Accident Control Division of the F. J. Boutell Driveaway Company of Flint, Michigan.

In this experiment, which began in 1947, 18 drivers were chosen to whom a vitamin diet supplementation was made available at cost.

What was the result? On the basis of a 5-year fleet average, these 18 men had a combined accident frequency of .28 or 357,143 miles per accident as against .38 or 263,158 miles per accident for the rest of the company's drivers. This was a 35 per cent reduction for the 18 men who had supplemented their diet.

There are people who are alive today and still walking around because of what these 18 men did, and it was all done by nutrition. There is medical evidence that the health of the nerves, the amount of mental energy one possesses, the action of one's mind and even one's personality are directly connected with the adequacy of one's diet.

As veteran students of accident prevention on the streets and highways, you know the term accident proneness. There are people who are accident-prone.

There are whole *families* who are accident-prone. Some of them make comfortable livings from this tendency of theirs. All kinds of theories are held for this, and psychiatrists and other medical men devote a lot of time to this problem. But I wonder if any of them has ever questioned the fact that poor nutrition runs in this kind of family, usually of a lower grade—a sort of submarginal group. Their minds are not nourished properly. They cannot make split-second decisions. Many of these accident-prone individuals drive cars.

Our Declining Mental Power

In 1955, I wrote a little 64-page book entitled Is OUR INTELLIGENCE DECLINING? because I saw a general deterioration in the average level of intelligence.

We picture ourselves as a race of geniuses, but an organization in England which has studied the collective intelligence of Americans and Britons has come up with the startling finding that the general mental power is declining about 2 per cent per generation.

Our educational level rises, but our intelligence is going down. Being able to memorize textbooks and pass college examinations does not necessarily give either shrewdness of intellect or the ability to get quickly out of the path of a fast-moving truck.

In my little book there is this statement: "Arnold A. Hutschnecker, M.D., in his book *The Will to Live,* says that 80 per cent of the population needs the help of a psychiatrist." From what I have seen, 80 per cent of the population needs the help of a dietician.

Walter Dobson, of Manchester University, England, recently said that we are living in "The Age of Inattention." We are developing a great mass of indifferent people who cannot concentrate on anything.

Accident Proneness and the Food We Eat

This inattention, this drugged mental sense, this confused, fuzzy state of mind is national disease number one. It is the main contribution to accident proneness, and few doctors and experts have thought of incriminating the national malnutrition as the basic cause of it. They overlook the progressive devitalization of our foods, the increase in its chemicalization in the factories.

Each year, new and more powerful chemicals are perfected which are toxic, in order to do this and that to food, to make more profits for the food producers, to make food more salable or easier to manufacture. Today, over 1000 of these poisonous chemicals are on the market. What effect do they have on our health? Very few worry about that! What effect do they have on our nerves and our ability to handle ourselves mentally?

The Effect of Vitamin B on Mental Ability

Coming back to my little book, I describe in it a work called *Effect of Added Thiamin on Learning.* (Thiamin is another name for vitamin B_1.) The book was written by Dr. Ruth Flinn Harrell.

The author describes a 6-week experiment with orphans at the Presbyterian Orphans Home at Lynchburg, Virginia. It involved 104 children, from 9 to 19 years of age. Half of the children were given a vitamin B_1 pill each day. The other half received what is called a placebo, which contained merely some filled material. But both kinds of pills looked and tasted alike, so that the power of suggestion would not enter into the experiment.

At the end of the 6-week period, it was found by a series of tests that the group that was given the vitamin gained about one-fourth more in learning ability than the other group.

Then Miss Harrell experimented with a group of children who had never learned to speak and who were considered so mentally handicapped that language was beyond their capacity. These children learned much more rapidly when vitamin B complex was added to their diet and in two instances, developed speech and were able to live as normal children.

Many truck drivers are fearfully deficient in vitamin B. Incidentally, every swallow of an alcoholic beverage uses up some of the body's store of vitamin B. Your ideal truck driver should be on the *wagon.*

Mental Illness in Animals

In my little book I quoted a statement from the *New York Times* of February 19, 1954, as follows:

"Ottawa, February 16—Canadian biologists are studying herds of mentally sick Nova Scotia moose in the hope of learning something about the treatment of human madness. About half of the moose in the province are believed to be out of their minds as the result, it is thought, of the physical deterioration of their brains, caused by malnutrition."

What made the Canadian biologists believe that? According to the *New York Times,* it is the climatic changes that have taken place in Canada during the last few hundred years. . . . As the climate grew warmer, certain types of plant food on which the moose depended for a balanced diet, disappeared.

The motor and sensory nerves of the animals are out of order and they crash into fences and bushes. Crash into fences—doesn't that come close to our subject?

A truck driver's motor and sensory nerves must have a sharp edge . . . an edge which unfortunately can easily be dulled by an unbalanced diet.

The Rebuilding Cycle of the Body

Some people conceive the brain as a finished thing, but at no time of life is this true. The blood is continually nourishing it. All cells in the body, wherever they may be, are in a cycle of destruction and rebirth. Old cells die—new ones take their place.

The popular conception that the body changes every 7 years is not true. Recent research by atomic scientists has revealed that over 98 per cent of the body is renewed *every year,* including the brain. And the quality and potency of our diet can be a tremendous factor in the building up or tearing down of that brain.

I will give you an example. In a healthy blood stream there should be a certain relationship between the calcium and the phosphorous. It should be 2½ times as much calcium as phosphorus. This has been ascertained through the examinations of hundreds of thousands of specimens of blood from healthy and sick persons. A good blood functions best when the calcium to phosphorus ratio is 2½ to 1.

But the consumption of sugar products and a devitalized refined diet low in vitamins and minerals reduces the calcium in this ratio. It might become 2 to 1 or 1½ to 1. This means trouble of various kinds, especially to the nervous system and the brain. This defective blood cannot feed the brain properly.

How many truck drivers do not have the proper ratio of 2½ to 1 of the calcium to phosphorus in their blood stream? Until this ratio is rectified, is it safe to let them handle fast-moving trucks?

A Lesson from My Play

Several seasons ago, my play *The Goose* ran for 4 weeks in a small off-Broadway theatre in New York City. Its premise was that the jitterbug diet of youngsters today is one of the major causes of juvenile delinquency, and it proved that a poor diet can cause confusion in thinking and a distortion in one's sense of values. These are some of the factors at the bottom of delinquency.

Delinquency in life and irresponsibility at the wheel of a truck are practically handmaidens.

Here is an astounding fact that I brought out in my play: in a recent survey of the eating habits of 3,000 juvenile delinquents, it was found that on the average they ate only 3 meals a week at home —only 3 meals out of 21. The rest of the time, they ate in cheap candy stores and hot dog-hamburger luncheonettes, with their accent on sugar and refined starches, soda pop, ice cream, cakes, pies and white bread with so much of the nourishment removed.

What do you suppose is the calcium-phosphorous relationship in the blood of these hoodlums? And your truck drivers on long distance routes—don't they patronize more or less this kind of eating place?

PREVENTION System Stresses Vitamins

In the system advocated by PREVENTION magazine, the taking of vitamins assumes an important place. Why? Because man seems to be doing everything he can think of to destroy the vitamins in his food. He cooks it, he stores it too long, he cuts such things as carrots into strips and exposes them to the air, he does many other things in factory processes, all of which destroy vitamins. So we must restore these vitamins or we will be undernourished.

In this system we take vitamins with vengeance, and in the last 10 years, this has produced spectacular results.

Vitamin A

Let's talk about these vitamins, beginning with vitamin A. In the popular imagination, when this vitamin is mentioned, one immediately thinks of the eyes. In other words, vitamin A is good against night blindness and sensitivity to glare. But don't let anyone fool you—*all* the vitamins are needed for good eye health, not only vitamin A.

I discussed this in an article I wrote for *Pageant* magazine, September, 1959. It was titled "Will the Right Diet Improve Your Sight?" and it showed that not only vitamins, but also good diet, with special attention to the quality of protein, are important for the health of the eyes.

I don't have to tell you that healthy eyes are important to truck drivers. The eyes are continually standing guard as the truck moves along. But actually it is not the eyes—it is the mind behind the eyes that is important. As an example, a weary truck driver told Harvard scientists how he was hurt when he saw a calf in the path of his moving truck. He swerved and overturned his truck. It was found later that there had been no calf there at all—it was just a "dream image," common to many persons who drive when they are too tired.

Sunflower Seeds for the Eyes

As far as the eyes are concerned, 10 years ago I made the discovery that there is something in *sunflower seeds* that is extremely potent for eye health and that enables them to withstand glare. Thousands of people have found greater eye comfort since they have been eating these seeds.

I used to be terribly sensitive to snow. If I walked a half hour in the snow, I would see pink. Then, for a certain reason, I added sunflower seeds to my diet and two weeks later, when my car broke down in a snowstorm, I was able to walk two miles with no eye trouble at all. I used to have to wear dark glasses at the beach, but today I never have to. I used to have to wear dark glasses when driving long distances. . . . Now I don't have to. But the effect is not cumulative. If I stop eating sunflower seeds for about a week, I cannot do these things.

Now, if what I have found is true, can you imagine how important it can be for every truck driver to eat a liberal amount of sunflower seeds every day? Sunflower seeds are available with their shells off at health food stores and are a delicious tidbit.

How to Get Your Vitamin A

Coming back to vitamin A, we believe in taking some of it in vitamin form every day. We suggest halibut liver oil perles, which contain both vitamins A and D.

This is because when you eat a fish, you eat only the bland meat part. You don't eat the liver, or the eyes, or other obscure, but nutritionally potent organs.

So, because we don't eat primitively anymore, we must supplement our diet with the parts that are missing. The Chinese eat lamb's eyes, because by experience they have found that their health thrives upon it. On a fishing pier in Palm Beach, I noticed sandpipers beginning to eat fish that were left lying about. They would always start with the eyes. Eyes are extremely rich in all vitamins, and are made up of the highest class protein.

I don't ask truck drivers to eat fish eyes, but they can get the equivalent through sunflower seeds, halibut oil perles and other items which I am about to discuss.

Vitamin A is important for skin health and for fighting colds and general infections.

Vitamin B

We will now go on to vitamin B, which we have already mentioned.

Vitamin B_1 is needed for the health of the nerves. Poor nerves can contribute to almost any condition of trouble in the body. When a person becomes irritable and angry very easily, he is usually vitamin B_1-deficient.

A research at Harvard, which comprised a survey in 11 northeastern states, revealed that auto drivers are "getting progressively more irritable in the squeeze of mounting traffic congestion." And it is going to get worse.

Airplane pilots in World War II suffered blackouts in the air on account of vitamin B_1 deficiencies. Lack of vitamin B_1 also makes people jittery, restless and tense, and unable to stand noise.

Three Los Angeles doctors recently proved that if one gets angry enough, he can suffer a stroke. A person who has a full supply of all of the vitamin B complex is more stabilized and does not get angry as easily.

There was an experiment performed at the State Hospital in Elgin, Illinois, some time ago. By creating vitamin B_1 deficiencies in some of the patients, the researchers caused their characters to change. One old man who had been quite amiable threatened to break up the furniture. A young man went into blind rages, screaming at the top of his lungs.

But as soon as these patients' diets were supplemented with yeast extract, which is very rich in vitamin B, they became normal again.

We suggest 3 natural food supplements to give a person vitamin B: brewer's yeast, wheat germ and a de-fatted liver tablet called *desiccated liver*.

Vitamin C

We will now take up vitamin C. Vitamin C is of the utmost importance to a driver of a truck, because it plays such a big part in the make-up of the skin. Vitamin C helps to form a substance called collagen, which is the glue that holds the body's cells together. A skin that contains enough vitamin C will heal more rapidly. It is a stronger skin. It will not bruise as easily.

Vitamin C is also an anti-infection agent. So your truck driver who is not vitamin C-deficient will not bruise as easily, and if he does get bruised, there will be less likelihood of an infection developing. Vitamin C, in combination with vitamin A, is a powerful factor in preventing colds. Thousands of folks have proven this and written us about their experiences.

Vitamin C is also of terrific value in excreting poisons from the body. In an experiment with house painters, those who were given vitamin C did not get lead poisoning. This could be important for the health of truck drivers, who are continually breathing in the fumes of lead-containing gasolines. Vitamin C is essential for people living and working in conditions of atmospheric smog. Smoking uses up vitamin C. Every puff destroys some of the body's store of this vitamin.

The vitamin C we recommend comes from the fruit of the rose plant, called rose hips, which contains 40 times the vitamin C of citrus fruits.

Vitamin D

Vitamin D is associated with vitamin A in halibut liver oil, which we have already discussed. Vitamin D is very important in connection with the body's use of calcium and phosphorus.

You have all heard, no doubt, that man can get vitamin D from the sun's ultraviolet rays. But don't depend on it, what with so much smog in our cities and how little sun the average modern man gets!

No—take those few capsules of halibut liver oil every day for vitamins A and D.

Vitamin E

Now we come to a terribly important vitamin for truck drivers —vitamin E. It is made from vegetable oils and its function is to oxygenate the arteries, veins and capillaries of the body.

Vitamin E is the answer to the troubles caused by our sedentary way of life in this twentieth century. It is a miracle vitamin, and is saving the lives of thousands of heart patients.

Credit for the discovery of what vitamin E can do to hold heart disease in control goes to Evan Shute, an M.D. of London, Ontario, Canada, whose work on it began 20 years ago.

I have been a heart case since a boy 8 years old. My father died of a heart attack at age 51. Three brothers died of heart attacks, aged 51, 56 and 62, respectively. A sister died of a heart attack at age 64.

I have been taking vitamin E since Dr. Shute's work was announced 20 years ago. I am going on 63, and should live to 100, unless run down by some truck driver who is suffering from malnutrition. I walk an hour a day. I go for 5 hour hikes across mountains. And 7 years ago, I was turned down for life insurance on account of my heart!

Benefits Derived from Vitamin E

Vitamin E oxygenates the arteries. It prevents other valuable substances in the body from being consumed by oxygen. Vitamin E dilates the blood vessels. Vitamin E is an anti-clotting agent. This means that it will prevent thrombus, the blood clot that kills so many people today, including truck drivers. There are hundreds of researches showing the value of vitamin E for heart disease, pregnancy, diabetes, diseases that might involve amputation of limbs and many other conditions.

A heart attack or a stroke at the wheel of a fast-moving huge piece of automotive equipment . . . one shudders to think about it! And vitamin E can often prevent it.

Take the case of a stroke. . . . It is a paralysis caused by lack of blood in part of the brain. . . . But vitamin E, through its oxygenating action, aids in forcing the blood into all the body's extremities. Can you imagine what this can mean to a driver of trucks?

In Italy recently, there was a symposium on vitamin E, to which doctors came from all over the world, testifying as to the wonderful results obtained with it. But our U.S. doctors say, "There is no evidence," and rarely use this vitamin in heart cases.

I believe vitamin E to be so important in the question of accident prevention on the roads that your organization ought to form a committee to investigate it and report back to you one year from now. So much for vitamin E.

The Value of Desiccated Liver

I would like now to talk about a food supplement that can help drivers to stay awake at the wheel. It goes by the strange name of desiccated liver, and is available in tablet form to be swallowed with water. It is animal liver with the fat, fibre and moisture removed. Its value is also heightened by the fact that it is a raw product. Cooking kills out all of the enzymes in food and a good portion of the vitamins.

The value of desiccated liver as a conserver of energy was proven by B. H. Ershoff, M.D., and written up in the *Proceedings of the Society of Experimental Biology and Medicine* for July, 1951. His findings were based on an experiment Dr. Ershoff performed with mice. Two groups of mice were given the same diet, except that one of the group had the benefit of added desiccated liver. Then the mice were set to swimming in tanks. The group that did not have the liver swam on average about 13 minutes before they drowned. In the desiccated liver group, 3 mice swam for 63, 83 and 87 minutes. The other 9 mice of this group were swimming vigorously at the end of two hours when the test was terminated.

We published an article about desiccated liver, and it created a sensational interest in this food supplement. Thousands of people began to take it, and hundreds of letters began to stream in as to its miraculous effects on people. A man who formerly could last for only one set of tennis could now play 3 sets with ease. People could stay up later, etc., etc.

Can you picture what this one food supplement could mean to truck drivers? I understand some of them are taking very questionable drugs to be able to stay awake at the wheel—drugs which have dangerous side effects.

The Importance of Bone Meal

Now we come to another food supplement that is specific for truck drivers, called bone meal; it is available in tablet and powder form.

Gardeners have used bone meal as an organic fertilizer with wonderful results. It has been standard in dog feeding for many decades. When pigs get a disease called the scours, bone meal clears it up almost instantly.

Bone meal can practically stop the formation of tooth cavities in young and old. It's so much better and so much more scientifically feasible than trying to prevent cavities by fluoridating our drinking water. But the most important thing to truckers is that bone meal knits the bones into a strength that does not permit easy fracture. This has been proved with dogs. Poor dogs! Some of them had to suffer fractures to prove the point.

My Family's Experiences with Bone Meal

There have been some striking examples of the value of taking bone meal in my own family. We have been taking it now for about 10 years.

About 5 years ago my eldest daughter Ruth was returning from a trip. She left very early in the morning and was traveling alone. It was so foggy that she couldn't see in front of her very well.

Suddenly in going around a curve, she went over a steep bank, the car turning over several times, she was thrown against the front door to her right, which opened, and then she was propelled 20 feet into a frozen field. Do you know that she did not suffer even a scratch in a bone?

Several years ago, coming downstairs in the middle of the night, while half asleep, I fell down a whole flight of stairs. Not a bone scratch!

My youngest daughter, Nina, about 21, fell down a flight of stairs and did not suffer a bone scratch. It looks as if we're an accident-prone family, doesn't it? But we all have good alibis and strong bones.

Another example—this daughter, Nina, of whom I have just spoken, had plastic surgery done on her nose about 5 years ago. I told the surgeon to sharpen his knives because Nina was a bone meal taker, but the doctor thought I was joking. He told me afterwards that hers was the hardest human bone he had ever encountered. He had a lot of trouble, and the operation took much longer than usual.

Milk Drinking

Now how does the milk-drinking, non-bone meal taking population compare?

A few years ago, a man in Louisville, Kentucky, stood on his head to amuse his children, and broke his neck. When a man whom I know just lifted his arm and hit it against an overhead open cupboard door, he broke a bone. While an artist friend was walking to put some litter in a can in his garden, he merely tripped and broke an ankle bone. It will be a year before he will be as good as before. An actress in walking backstage tripped over some ropes and suffered a bone fracture.

There is a general calcium deficiency in the population. This means more than just a calcium deficiency. . . . It means a distortion in the 2½ to 1 calcium-phosphorus ratio in the blood. . . . It means that the organs of the body are not getting the benefit of the right kind of blood.

Our family, consisting of my wife and me, 3 children and their spouses, and 5 grandchildren—13 persons in all—represent an island in a sea of malnourishment—a ready made experiment in the value of bone meal. The total number of tooth cavities in this group is less than 10 per cent of what it averages in the rest of the population.

Disadvantages of Milk

Now, you might say, "Can't we get our calcium from milk?" There are people who have drunk quarts of milk a day, and who are forced to wear dentures at an early age.

Bone meal is made from the selected bones of calves. The product is as fine as talcum powder, and is compressed into tablet form. The formula of bone meal is pretty close to that of human bone and the dentine of teeth.

Milk, on the other hand, lacks certain mineral elements. Not only that, but cows have been artificially bred to become milk factories. Milk today is not the same as it was formerly. Today the dairyman is paid a premium for extra fat content of the milk . . . and extra fat is suspected as a cause of heart attacks. Dairymen are not worried about the mineral content of the milk at all.

But I say to you safety men who are concerned with the health of truck drivers, see to it that eventually, every driver under your jurisdiction gets a daily ration of bone meal.

Advice Concerning the General Diet

I have not said much about the general diet and its contribution to safe driving. It has been proven that it is important to start the day off with a good breakfast. In the case of truck drivers, this should be extra-heavy, with the emphasis on protein. I would include eggs and meat in the breakfast of a truck driver. There should be the barest minimum of bread, cereals and such starches. If I were a truck driver, I would eat none of these. I would also recommend two medium sized bananas as part of the breakfast. That bananas are fattening is a fallacy. Bread is about the most fattening food there is.

Another rule: Eat a minimum of foods processed in a factory, for these processes remove essential elements and add dangerous chemicals. This still leaves meat, fish, eggs, fresh fruit and vegetables. Huge meals can come from these 5 categories. Eliminate all packaged goods, all processed meats, such as bologna, frankfurters, etc. Order a hamburger rather than the hot dog if you are in that kind of an eating place. The hot dog is quite chemicalized compared to the hamburger.

Drivers Must Avoid Artificial White Sugar

The concluding item I'd like to talk about is artificial white sugar. Every truck driver should shun it as the plague. This means no pies, cakes, ice cream, candy or soda pop. Now what is wrong with sugar? Primitive peoples eat sugar cane and are perfectly healthy. But when so-called civilized people bring white sugar products to them, then all the white man's ills fall upon them. Why should this be?

Nature likes wholeness. Man can thrive upon wholeness in his diet. But begin to fragmentize, to refine, and you are not eating a food. You're eating a chemical.

If you were ever in a sugar refinery, you would have seen the multiplicity of vats in which everything is removed from the raw brown sugar. All the vitamins, all the minerals, all the enzymes, all the protein and other valuable nutrients are removed.

What remains behind is a bleached carbon compound—practically nothing more than carbon, hydrogen and oxygen—a chemical.

And in the process of digestion, it has to steal thiamin, one of the most important of the B vitamins in the body.

Sugar eaters are highly deficient in thiamin, which I have shown to be so important to the proper functioning of the nerves and the mind. Sugar eaters have a fuzzy intellect. They cannot make quick decisions. An oversugared individual behind 15 tons of moving equipment is not my idea of good truck management.

Cause and Effect of Low Blood Sugar

There is a book called *Body, Mind and Sugar*, by E. M. Abrahamson, M.D., and A. W. Pezet, which gives masses of medical evidence against sugar. The main theme of the book is that overconsumption of sugar causes low blood sugar. I am sure that your average truck driver is going around with a low blood sugar.

You see, diabetes is not caused by overeating sugar. It is caused by a defective pancreatic gland, which cannot produce enough insulin to counteract the effect of sugar. *Then,* the diabetic has to cut out sugar.

But in the case of the average person with a normal pancreatic gland, when sugar is consumed, the pancreas produces the insulin to break it down properly. When the normal person takes in *too much* sugar, the pancreas goes haywire in its desire to protect the body, and too much insulin is produced, thus causing low blood sugar.

Dr. Abrahamson's book is full of the mental and emotional symptoms of low blood sugar. No driver with a low blood sugar should be permitted to drive a truck. He is a menace on the highways, and there are thousands of them on the highways. Some of them see imaginary calves. Such a condition is caused by low blood sugar plus fatigue.

People have the idea they need sugar for energy. This sort of energy lasts about 10 minutes—the blood sugar goes up, then comes the body's insulin, and the blood sugar plunges downward, whereupon the person becomes starved for more sugar. Thus, one bottle of soda pop leads to another—a vicious cycle.

The best thing for sugar and energy is natural fruit—plus desiccated liver.

Summary

Now for a quick review. *Halibut oil* pills (vitamin A) and *sunflower seeds* for the eyes.

Vitamin B—Brewer's yeast, wheat germ and desiccated liver . . . for the mind, its alertness and its ability not to go haywire in an emergency.

Vitamin C—Prevents colds and promotes quick healing of wounds. It contributes to a healthy skin.

Vitamin E—For the heart and circulation of the blood. Can prevent heart attacks behind the wheel.

Desiccated liver—For greater energy.

Bone meal—To prevent fractures of bones, not only in accidents, but in the active movements of a truck driver in and round his truck.

A good general diet—A minimum of factory-produced food. And *finally,* no artificial sugar.

Special Restaurants for Truckers

Now, I would like to make a suggestion. As I understand it, trucking management indicates eating spots where the drivers are supposed to stop for their meals. Why not work with the owners of these restaurants? Have them make available fresh fruits in season. In fact, they should have a liberal array of fruits for sale for truck drivers to take along so as to alleviate the rigors of the road.

But please! No eating while driving. I wonder if there are any statistics of truck accidents caused by drivers who are eating at the wheel.

At these truck drivers' stops there should be a full array of desserts made without sugar. Most any dessert that is made with sugar can be made with honey. Honey is a whole product. It is not refined. It is healthful. My wife makes a wonderful gelatin as a substitute for jello. She uses honey in it instead of sugar and it is delicious. As flavorings, grape juice and other non-sugared products can be used. A delightful gelatin can be made with prune whip— just prunes and gelatin—nothing else.

In such restaurants shelled sunflower seeds can be sold. Also, such things as brewer's yeast and wheat germ. Incidentally, wheat germ flakes mixed with non-sugared applesauce makes a terrific dessert. And a delicious ice cream can be made with honey instead of sugar.

The truckers can almost dictate to these restaurants. The latter would not want to lose their patronage. People are creatures of habit. Teach them new habits, and they will hold on to the new habits just as stubbornly.

Another suggestion . . . Why can't your trucking companies establish 3 to 4 of your own restaurants on the road. . . . Here you can really experiment, and you can even allow civilians to eat there. If you would do such a thing, I would love to help.

One more suggestion . . . For a limited time, in order to help drivers develop the fruit-eating habit, give them a present of a paper box kit packed full of fruit. Give it to them as a token of Godspeed on the road. Not good speed . . . Godspeed, a token of good will and friendship.

And who knows? If a truck driver's diet becomes really tops, his whole character might change. As a member of a union, he might become a more rational person to negotiate with. But you will have to feed the organizers and top union officials, too.

Well, I wish I had more time. I have hardly scratched the surface of the subject. But I hope I have given you something to think about, something out of which a beginning can be made in this undeveloped field of promoting safer driving through better nutrition.

Acne

You Don't Have to Outgrow Acne to Cure It

As far back as medical history goes, there are records of people being afflicted with acne. The ailment is mentioned in classical Greek literature under the name *ionthoi.* To the ancient Romans, it was *varus.* It was known to the Egyptians and plagued the Babylonians. Yet right up to the present day, medical science is not certain about either the cause or causes of acne, or how to treat it.

Acne is a minor illness. It has never been known to kill anyone, nor, in the usual sense of the word, does it incapacitate the person afflicted with it. Nevertheless, it can have serious consequences and must be taken seriously. Occurring most often in adolescence, it can cause or intensify personality disorders and the acute emotional disturbances to which many youngsters are prey. The *British Journal of Dermatology,* October, 1961, expresses the opinion that there is a definite relationship between "the more disfiguring dermatoses, such as acne," and antisocial behavior. It also points out that medical attention resulting in alleviation or cure of the cosmetic ailment, is of great assistance in achieving a reform of juvenile delinquents.

Although acne usually clears up with advancing age, it will frequently leave pock mark scars that, to a woman, at least, can seem tragic. Certainly there is nothing pleasant or desirable about this common affliction of adolescence. So far as we are concerned, it is time the medical profession took this problem more seriously and stopped treating it as a "normal" manifestation of adolescence. With the vast research resources at their disposal, our doctors surely have a responsibility to learn how to heal acne and spare our young people its possible consequences.

There is also a responsibility to learn how to prevent acne, a matter we cannot claim to understand as fully as we'd like to, or as we hope to understand it in the future. However, even though there seems to be practically no knowledge about acne that is established

beyond doubt, there are a good many promising and partially successful results of experiments, that are worth reviewing for clues as to
what we can encourage our young people to do, in the effort to
prevent, get rid of or, at least, alleviate acne.

The Prevalent Theory

"Acne, one of the most common of skin diseases, is associated
with overactivity of the oil glands of the face, chest and back," says
Bruce Bairstow, M.D., in *Today's Health* for November, 1961. In a
carefully written, lay-language exposition of the dominant belief of
American doctors, he goes on to say: "This overactivity is due to
hormones produced by endocrine glands that begin functioning at
puberty. The hair canals, into which the oil glands open, become
plugged and the oily mass stagnates in them. Darkening of the
surface of the plugs by oxidation leads to formation of the familiar
blackhead. Inflammation around these minor plugs causes pimples
and pustules."

This may sound as though Dr. Bairstow were very certain that
the changing function of the endocrine glands in adolescence is the
cause of acne. However, in the same article he goes on to point out
other facts quite contradictory:

"Acne can occur later and some of the most difficult cases come
during adult life."

". . . certain foods will make it worse. Some physicians believe
too much fat and carbohydrates may contribute to acne . . .

"Some soft drinks, those with high sugar content (Are there any
that *don't* have a high sugar content?—our comment), have a
tendency to cause acne to flare up . . .

"Some think that a blackhead goes on to a systic or a pustular
lesion because of an allergic factor."

To further complicate the matter, Louis A Brunsting, M.D., in
the *Journal of the American Medical Association* (December 16,
1961) points out: ". . . the exact mechanism is not understood. To
say that acne results from an imbalanced estrogen-androgen (female
and male hormone) ratio, is to repeat an unproven oversimpli-
fication, . . ."

Treatments Disappointing and Dangerous

With a few exceptions, practically all medical authorities seem
to agree that, while it may not be a cause, an excessively high proportion of male to female hormones (androgen to estrogen) is at
least associated with typical adolescent acne. However, attempts at
cures through hormone treatment have proven both disappointing
and dangerous. "At present there is no good endocrine treatment
for acne," says Dr. Brunsting, who explains: "In young men, a dose
large enough to be effective will be feminizing." He adds that there

may be *some* beneficial effect in young women in whom acne is associated with menstrual irregularities. The danger of cancer, always a possibility when estrogen is artificially added to the system, is not mentioned by Dr. Brunsting.

Another treatment used with apparent irresponsibility by *some* doctors is a course of X-ray exposure. The stated purpose is to dry up the sebaceous glands, which is to say, to damage them and inhibit the production of oil. It is peculiar that this treatment continues, even though no one has claimed any great success with it, and there is the obvious danger of overexposure, if not immediately at the time of the acne treatment, then later with dental or other facial X-rays. It should always be remembered that X-ray has a cumulative effect, and should, therefore, be avoided except in case of extreme necessity.

Some doctors are also prone to use tetracycline, a broad spectrum antibiotic, to treat acne, even though it seems to be well established that the presence of staphylococci in acne infections is not a cause of acne, but a result of it. To us, this resembles the use of penicillin for the common cold, on which penicillin is known to have no effect. It is just asking for trouble by doctors who have forgotten how to practice any kind of medicine but the shooting of "magic bullets."

Many other treatments have been tried, with such disagreements on results and varying reports of success that to quote all the authorities involved, would require more space than is available here. Doctors in the Southwest seem to agree that excessive exposure to sunlight will induce or aggravate acne. In other parts of the country, doctors recommend sunlight. One authority, answering a question in the *Journal of the American Medical Association* feels that enough sunlight to cause peeling, thus unblocking the pores, will be beneficial, but that any excessive exposure will induce greater activity of the oil glands, and thus aggravate the acne.

Sulfur, incorporated in an emulsion or paste, has also been used with some success to induce peeling of the outer layer of the skin. Dr. P. F. Borrie of St. Bartholomew's Hospital, London, warns, however, that "Care must be taken not to cause too drastic a reaction and this is especially likely to occur in fair-skinned individuals."

What About Foods?

Where there is so much disagreement and confusion about a common affliction, we are accustomed to expect that the answer may be found in the neglected field of nutrition. In this case, there are some nutritional clues that we expect may become increasingly helpful and important as study of acne goes on.

Practically all practicing dermatologists seem to agree that chocolate, iodine and bromine will stimulate acne, and the avoidance of these substances is generally recommended. The bromine is found in certain bromidic headache and indigestion patent remedies which are easily avoided. Iodine, of course, occurs principally in shellfish and iodized salt, and chocolate is practically everywhere in the diet of our young people today. These substances are prohibited as a matter of course by all doctors attempting to treat acne. Other foods usually banned, according to the *Journal of the American Medical Association,* are "roasted" (fried, that is) nuts, ice cream, cheese, butter, pork fat and gravy.

Health-conscious folks will note immediately that the foods doctors have found it helpful to prohibit in acne cases are all foods that promote the formation of saturated, fatty acids within the system.

Investigating this clue further, we find that there are at least a few researchers—Urbach and LeWinn, in their book *Skin Diseases, Nutrition and Metabolism,* and G. Proserpio, Ph.D., and M. Capra, Ph.D., writing in *Drug and Cosmetic Industry,* November, 1960— who have postulated that *acne may be a kind of diabetes of the skin.*

A Lipid Metabolism Disorder

As a hypothesis worth further investigation, we might go a step further and guess that acne may ultimately turn out to be a disorder of the lipid metabolism (fat utilizing), which may be caused by an excess of androgens, such as is typical of most adolescent boys and many girls, but may also be brought about by a variety of other causes, such as too much exposure to strong sunlight.

In possible corroboration, we find that in India, where there are fewer fatty foods available to stimulate acne, but the sun is hotter and more malevolent, vitamin A has been used with outstanding success in acne treatment (*Journal of the Indian Medical Association,* March, 1954). Vitamin A, of course, is stored in the fat and is essential to a proper lipid metabolism in the body. We might reason from this that overstimulation of the sebaceous glands, caused by the strong and ever-present sunlight of India, demands greater amounts of vitamin A to maintain a healthy lipid metabolism than the diet will normally provide.

In the United States, attempts to treat acne by the addition of vitamin A in therapeutic quantities to the diet has had some success, but it has been less than spectacular. This, testing our theory, we might have expected, for in a diet over-rich in animal and hydrogenated fats, vitamin A is not enough to maintain proper lipid metabolism. The only answer we know for that, is to eliminate the solid hydrogenated fats and substitute the unsaturated fatty acid-rich vegetable oils. For this, we recommend such foods as sunflower seeds, corn oil, fish liver oil supplements, safflower and soy oils and egg yolk.

Not knowing for certain, we do not venture to predict. But if any of our readers, or their families and friends, who may be troubled with persistent acne, care to experiment in the elimination from their diets of all animal fats, hydrogenated (solid) oils and cooked oils, and the use of the above-mentioned foods rich in both vitamin A and unsaturated fatty acids, we should be most interested in hearing from them and learning what results they have gotten. Eventually, *we* hope to learn something from our readers.

In conclusion, let us quote from an article on the subject by Paul de Kruif, in *Today's Health* (March, 1957). "The affliction may be perpetuated by an upset chemistry . . . of the entire human being. Persistent acne often clears up after treatment of infected sinuses, tonsils or teeth. A regimen of plenty of sleep, outdoor exercise and a well-balanced diet often may speed the action of skin care . . . It seems as if a sick skin can be healed only by a healthy body."

Deflating a Headline on Acne Treatment

In *Drug Trade News* (March 20, 1961), we came across a headline which sounded as though it should have been reserved for a cancer cure or a new form of heart surgery: "Lauds Estrogen-Chlorothiazide Combination in Treating Acne." This potent combination of drugs is being used against a disease which, W. W. Bauer, M.D., in *This Week* magazine (March 12, 1961), says ". ... is usually outgrown in two or three years without damage to the complexion. The self-consciousness produced by the appearance of the skin is often more serious than the actual disease . . . greasy foods and excessive sweets are restricted or omitted from the diet . . . Try to remember that practically all boys and girls have the experience of acne . . ."

We called these drugs potent, and we wish to emphasize that point. Any hormone drug used at any time in life and for any reason, creates serious problems for the body to cope with. Sometimes an illness is so severe and the need for a supplement to the hormone supply so obvious, that the use of hormones is justified as a calculated risk. A risk it is, too. The effects can include abnormal sexual characteristics and tendencies, mental aberrations, grotesque swellings of the face and extremities, etc. The danger that lurks in the unguarded use of tranquilizers such as chlorothiazide is even better known. The most alarming results are severe illness in the form of genito-urinary distress and a possible upset in the electrolyte balance of the body fluids. Redness and itching of the skin, also numbness, may occur as a result of using this tranquilizer.

These are just a few of the objections to these two drugs being used to remedy a situation which admittedly remedies itself if left alone. The results in 72 per cent of 55 patients (all of whom had been previously treated with standard anti-acne therapy) were that "premenstrual flareups of acne were moderately or completely suppressed." The combination of the hormone and the tranquilizer used concurrently on 6 patients (that was the total number on which the combination was tried) was superior to the use of either drug alone. The drugs are, says the physician, "moderately effective." This is lauding the combination?

The Treatment's Merit

What have we then? We have one researcher who tested two drugs on 55 patients saying that the drugs used individually affected a premenstrual acne condition in about 38 of the subjects. Of these, some were moderately affected (we don't know if "some" means 37 or 15 or 5 persons) and some were completely cured. The combination of both drugs used on only 6 persons, merely showed that using both drugs together was more effective than either used alone— meaning only a greater percentage of 6 subjects were "moderately" or "completely" relieved. Rather a flimsy structure upon which to "laud" the effect of a combination of drugs.

But wait—these far-from-conclusive results were achieved on patients "also treated with standard anti-acne therapy." (Cut down on sodas, candy and fried foods and wash frequently.) "Concurrent X-ray therapy was given to 4 patients." This is the kind of science we are to accept: no controls, concurrent therapies given along with the experimental substances, and inconclusive results based on subjective observations and a much-too-small number of subjects. *Drug Trade News* took its report from the AMA *Archives of Dermatology* (82:821, 1960). Maybe they are trying to make it sound better than it was in the hope of stimulating sales of chlorothiazide and estrogen. As they report it, Dr. Frank E. Coria's experiment sounds useless. Perhaps he was less sensational and more honest in his formal report.

Even if it had all been as good as the headline, we must protest the use of such radical therapy for such a minor condition. Acne is basically a nutritional phenomenon and is best treated by a change in diet. Such treatment is perfectly safe, and will be effective if properly carried out. Why fool around then with "500 milligrams daily for 10 days" of a tranquilizer dosage, and estrogens "given in doses of 1.25 milligrams to 2.5 milligrams daily for 8 to 13 days before the period"? These are dangerous drugs in potent doses. Who wants to risk his future health or his life to get rid of acne when there's no guarantee of the result and when there is a safer, more effective alternative?

Vegetable Oils for Acne

The distressing teen age problem of acne may have met its match in unhydrogenated vegetable oils. In the *Archives of Dermatology* (June, 1959), Dr. W. R. Hubler said that even patients who suffered from acne in its worst form "improved with remarkable rapidity" with oral use of corn oil.

It is common practice for doctors treating acne to prescribe a low-fat diet; however, such a diet often results in unintended weight loss and fatigue. The unsaturated fats in the vegetable oil help to maintain weight and vigor in the patient. The oil also relieves the unpalatable dryness of a low-fat diet.

We think Dr. Hubler's treatment is an excellent one, for it provides an excellent means of acquiring the unsaturated fatty acids so vital to the body's well-being and helps to create the habit of using unhydrogenated oils instead of the common and unhealthful hydrogenated ones. Though Dr. Hubler used corn oil in treating his patients, other vegetable oils are equally acceptable. Among them are peanut, safflower, sunflower, wheat germ and others. Even if you have no skin problem, unhydrogenated vegetable oils should be included in your daily diet—at least several tablespoonfuls with your regular green salad.

Alcoholism

Alcoholics Short on Vitamin C

If alcoholics, as is often claimed, have personal problems that lead to drink, the problems are multiplied by the nutritional deficiencies common to one who has been drinking heavily. We know, for example, that an alcoholic is invariably short on vitamin B_1 as well as others of the B complex. The *Journal of Nutrition* (no date) prints an article by David Lester and others (submitted for publication July 21, 1959) which shows that alcoholics also sustain a grave loss of vitamin C. For this experiment, 85 alcoholic patients in a hospital ward were tested for vitamin C supply in the blood upon admission. A group of 23 non-alcoholic patients were used as controls.

It was found that 500 milligrams of vitamin C daily for a week was required to bring the alcoholic's blood level of this vitamin to a normal reading. A dosage of 250 milligrams per day was tried, and found inadequate to do the job.

Small wonder at the number of people who die of alcoholism. The body's most needed nutrients are casually flushed away as a result of the habit and are seldom replaced. Nutrients are the fuel and lubrication of the body, in the way that gas and oil are used in an engine. If they are missing, the engine soon stops working and is often ruined beyond repair. The body is no different; it must have proper operating supplies.

Why take a chance on alcoholism? Don't drink any alcoholic beverages at all (even one drink robs you of important nutrients), and be certain that your nutritional needs are well taken care of, so that no craving can develop.

Alcoholism—A New Clue

We have made several attempts to interest the medical fraternity in the nutritional aspects of alcoholism. We have quoted recognized experts in the field of science who relate these two undeniably. The results are the same: the problem of alcoholism is treated with drugs, confinements in hospitals and nursing homes for the so-called "drying-out period" (where no effort is made to improve the basic nutrition), sad conferences with long-suffering relatives who are urged to "try to understand" and pep talks from members of worthy organizations such as Alcoholics Anonymous. This last, especially, has done much good in alleviating the terrible situation in which these people find themselves. But none of these measures tackles the basic problem: what makes these people compulsive drinkers? Why can't they take it or leave it alone, as most people can? We believe the answer lies in a nutritional deficiency, a craving by the body for some nutrient, which is somehow temporarily relieved by alcohol.

In spite of the lack of success we have had in getting our medical and social organizations to investigate the nutritional aspect of alcoholism, we keep trying. When we come across some new indication, from a reputable source, that supports our view, we print it, hoping that this time the research grants will go to someone who is willing to explore the field of nutrition and alcoholism thoroughly and objectively.

In a UPI dispatch, carried by the *Milwaukee Sentinel* (January 11, 1961) we read of the work of 3 University of Pittsburgh researchers (Olson, Gursey and Vester) who claim that alcoholism is due to an upset in the body chemistry. In their view, the source of the trouble is a mishandling of tryptophan. This amino acid is an essential raw material for building the body's own rejuvenating proteins. It is used by the body to make compounds necessary to the body's proper operation. Tryptophan is vital in the manufacture of serotonin, which is an operating compound of the brain. It can be assumed that the alcoholic compulsion originates in this organ; the question is, is it due to psychological or organic inadequacies.

Fifty Given Group Test

In their test, the Pittsburgh scientists used the individual body chemistries of 16 apparently normal "social drinkers" and of 34 confirmed alcoholics in isolating a common organic defect in the alcoholic group. They all showed trouble in converting tryptophan into serotonin.

The two groups, after fasting, were given orange juice containing precisely the same amounts of pure tryptophan. The amount was considered sufficient, theoretically, to increase available serotonin in the brain. All the non-alcoholics responded immediately with a light-headed, wonderful glow. None of the alcoholics felt differently.

For more scientific evaluation, the end results of the 3 pathways tryptophan takes in the body were measured. One of these pathways results in the manufacture of serotonin. In the alcoholics, it was observed, through measurement of excreted waste, that this end product was deficient by 40 per cent. The indication was, of course, that alcoholics have a defect which cuts down on the body's manufacture of serotonin.

It should be borne in mind that the body needs the raw material which contains the necessary tryptophan—protein foods. Without a sufficient supply the vital serotonin cannot be manufactured by even a normal person. Perhaps this is the answer to how alcoholism develops in persons who seem to be casual drinkers at the start, and eventually find their craving for alcohol uncontrollable.

We wish to emphasize here that this and other researches show nutrition to be a major, if not *the* major cause of alcoholism. Until the work is done to pin down the nutritional, organic essence of the problem, we will have drives for the treatment of alcoholics and pleas for understanding their problem. Psychiatrists and psychologists will have their appointment calendars filled with hopeful alcoholics who think they can be talked out of their illness. The evidence that the chemical make-up of alcoholics is different has been presented. The answer obviously lies in finding out exactly why, and then correcting the problem.

Algae

Misunderstood Friends of the Waters

Most things in nature have a purpose for existing—even some things which at first seem undesirable, or even harmful. The green, scummy algae which sometimes form on tops of lakes and ponds is a good example of one of nature's misunderstood methods of preservation. In order to flourish, algae need nutrients, which are often supplied by industrial wastes or sewage from any number of sources. Were it not for the algae consuming these nutrients, the ponds would soon become foul with the wastes of civilization. This is one reason why algae-covered lakes are usually found in populated areas, while far-off mountain streams are often "clear as a bell." So the next time you look at an algae-covered lake, remember—it's just another one of nature's misunderstood ways.

Aluminum

A Science Fair Experiment on Aluminum

Antonia Martin and Gerre Grenolds of Montgomery Junior High School did an experiment on the toxicity of aluminum, which was chosen as one of the two from their school to be displayed at the Greater San Diego Science Fair held in April, 1961.

Their project was called "Does Aluminum Affect Living Things?" The conclusion of their experiment was that it does. And this led them to a new problem "Does Using Aluminum in Cooking Affect Man?" Their conclusion was that they believed there is a very good chance of this being true.

Here is the experiment as they carried it out, observed the results and wrote it up in the best scientific manner. And won the prize—second in their division.

General Information

The problem: Does Aluminum affect living things?

Hypothesis: Aluminum does affect life.

The experiment: To test our hypothesis, we used measured amounts of dirt and water in which we placed earthworms and guppies to test the effects of aluminum on these two kinds of living things. We used 6 containers: two of aluminum, two of glass and two of tin-coated steel, and placed guppies in one set, worms in the other. We carefully checked that all containers were under the same conditions (light, heat, etc.) and carefully recorded our findings.

Observations: (a) All fish in aluminum containers died. (b) All worms in aluminum very weak.

Conclusion: Aluminum does affect life.

New problem: Does using aluminum cooking utensils and aluminum foil affect man?

The Experiment

After getting the containers, we were ready to set up the experiment. We arranged the guppies first.

We meticulously measured out 236.5 milliliters of water in a graduated cylinder, to put into each of the containers: one a glass beaker, one a tin-covered steel dog food can (cleaned) and the other a pure aluminum beaker.

The next step was to put in the DeChlor (a prepared dechlorinating mixture). We carefully put half a drop in each container to get rid of the chlorine instantly.

We then took the temperature of each of the guppy containers. They were: glass—76°F., tin—74.5° F., aluminum—74° F.

After that, we sorted the fish according to size and put 7 fish in each container. We set the fish in a place where they would receive approximately the same amount of light and proceeded on to the worm setup.

We dumped the worms into a pie dish to sort them by size and count them. The next step was to put a thin layer of dirt on the bottom of the containers, add 26 worms and fill with dirt to nearly the top.

Results and Conclusions

After doing this experiment carefully 3 times, these have been the results common to all experiments: (a) all the fish in aluminum containers died in from 24 to 36 hours; (b) the earthworms in aluminum containers were very weak after about 36 hours.

From these facts, we concluded that something in the aluminum containers affected the animals. We got several ideas as to the cause of this effect from people that were skeptical about our findings, and we decided to try each one for its validity.

One person said that the fish were blinded by the reflected light of the sun hitting the aluminum. We disproved this by using a dull surfaced aluminum beaker in the third experiment that could reflect little light.

Another stated that possibly the water in the aluminum container absorbed so much heat that the fish were literally cooked to death. We showed the fallacy of this idea by taking the water temperature of each of the containers, and found them to be within one or two degrees of each other at all times.

Therefore, ruling out all other possibilities, we concluded that *aluminum does affect living things,* and that our hypothesis was correct.

This led us to our new problem, *does using aluminum in cooking affect man?,* which we leave for the scientists to find out, but we, at least, know that there is a very good chance of this being true.

Table 1: Observations and Results of Experiments Using Aluminum

Scale of Health: I—excellent   II—normal   III—poor   IV—dead

Experiment No. 1

	GUPPIES		WORMS	
Date	*Container*	*Health*	*Container*	*Health*
3/10/61	Aluminum	II	Aluminum	II
	Glass	II	Glass	II
	Tin	II	Tin	II
3/11/61	Aluminum	III	Aluminum	II
	Glass	I	Glass	II
	Tin	I	Tin	II
3/12/61	Aluminum	IV	Aluminum	III
	Glass	I	Glass	II
	Tin	I	Tin	II

Experiment No. 2

	GUPPIES		WORMS	
Date	*Container*	*Health*	*Container*	*Health*
3/12/61	Aluminum	II	Aluminum	II
	Glass	II	Glass	II
	Tin	II	Tin	II
3/13/61	Aluminum	IV	Aluminum	III
	Glass	I	Glass	II
	Tin	I	Tin	II

Experiment No. 3

GUPPIES

Time	*Date*	*Container*	*Temperature*	*Health*
2 p.m.	4/8/61	Aluminum	74°F.	II
		Glass	76°F.	II
		Tin	74.5°F.	II
2 p.m.	4/9/61	Aluminum	72°F.	IV
		Glass	72°F.	I
		Tin	72°F.	I

EARTHWORMS

Time	*Date*	*Container*	*Health*
2 p.m.	4/8/61	Aluminum	II
		Glass	II
		Tin	II
2 p.m.	4/9/61	Aluminum	II
		Glass	II
		Tin	II
9 p.m.	4/10/61	Aluminum	III
		Glass	II
		Tin	II

Anemia

You Can Take Steps against Anemia

When we read that one out of every 8 prospective female blood donors was rejected during World War II because of anemia, and that a study of this by the Florida State Health Department revealed 42 per cent of the school children in one town as suffering with some degree of anemia, we are reminded again that Americans aren't as healthy as they should be—and could be. The anemia these people suffered from was largely of the type that is completely curable by proper diet.

Anemia (literally, "lacking in blood") comes in many forms, some very serious, some so mild that the victim is not even aware that he has any ailment at all. He is vaguely tired and weak and appears to be pale. Ask him and he will tell you he is well. Many people do not realize that they have a right to feel vigorously healthy. They consider themselves healthy if they can get through the day. Many anemia victims have felt sluggish almost all their lives, and expect no more than this in the way of vigor.

A Matter of Quantity and Quality

Anemia is due either to a shortage in the quality or quantity of red blood cells. For example, simple blood loss from a cut or wound can cause anemia. This occurs when the body tries to restore the normal volume of blood by diverting other body fluids into the blood stream. The fluids can be transferred rapidly enough, but the vital ingredients of the blood take longer to manufacture. Hence, for some period, the value of the blood is limited and below par. The victim is anemic.

An insufficient number of red cells, or a shortage of iron in the red cells can also cause anemia. This is a case in which the actual amount of blood is not affected, but the quality is lacking. That is, the basic problem in all anemias—a decline in the quality of blood. We believe then that the way to prevent anemia is to know what the blood needs and see that there is plenty of what is needed available.

Severe forms of anemia which can cause death are not the ones which occur most commonly. These anemias are the result of the body's inability to make good blood, due to some basic disorder in the bone marrow, spleen or liver. Aplastic anemia is one of these. Then there is pernicious anemia, once fatal to most victims, merely because it had not yet been discovered that a lack of vitamin B_{12} in the system is the cause. However, we intend to discuss only those anemias which are known to respond to nutrients, pure and simple. These anemias can be avoided and can be corrected.

What Iron-Deficiency Anemia Is

In the United States, we have what might be designated as our own national anemia, iron-deficiency anemia. This occurs when the body's intake of iron is wanting or when absorption of iron is poor. The iron is necessary to build strong red blood cells. These cells have a major function—to carry oxygen from the lungs to other parts of the body and to transport waste products back to the lungs to be exhaled. The "redness" of these cells is due almost entirely to a chemical known as hemoglobin. This vital chemical is rich in iron, so it is obvious that, when there is little iron, hemoglobin's quality is poor. From this proceed the consequences of poor oxygen supply in the blood for nourishing the tissues, and an inefficient system for getting rid of the waste thrown off by the cells.

The iron so vital to all of this is in high demand at all times. Over half of the body's supply at any one time is in motion in the blood stream. The rest is stored for emergency purposes in the blood-making organs. The system sounds quite efficient, and one cannot readily imagine the body's being completely out of iron. But there are serious thieves of iron which can cause depletion almost before one can guard against it.

Men Less Vulnerable

Men have been endowed by nature with an advantage in their ability to retain iron. Women, children and elderly persons on the other hand are constantly threatened with a loss of iron stores. In adult women's menstrual periods, blood cells and iron are lost, and if the blood flow is very heavy, iron reserves are severely taxed. Adolescent girls have the added disadvantage of continuous body growth making demands on the body's iron supply, aside from the menstrual loss.

Pregnant women sacrifice iron to their expected baby. As it grows within the womb, it requires iron for its developing organs as well as for its blood supply. If the pregnant woman is accustomed to great blood loss in her menstrual periods, she is likely to have begun her pregnancy with a low iron supply, which she has never really had a chance to replenish. Women who are aware that such a situation could occur in their own case, should be sure to reinforce their iron supply through iron-rich foods and food supplements. They will remain healthier throughout pregnancy and are more likely to deliver a healthy baby.

The problem with older people is multifold. Many older people do not have an appetite for food of any kind. This includes the foods they need for their iron supply. Other oldsters rely on cheap and easy-to-prepare foods which have little nutritional value. Finally, the intestinal action of aging people is not always as efficient as it was designed to be. Even when they eat a diet sufficiently high in iron, these people might have such poor absorption of this element in the intestinal tract that they still fall short of the amount they need to have an efficient blood supply.

The *British Medical Journal* (November 28, 1959) carried a report on anemia in the elderly, which told of tests on 256 men and women over 65. The 101 men tested showed 5 per cent who were below par in hemoglobin levels, and 13 per cent of the women were also anemic. The authors pointed out the fact that anemia in men is always considered more serious, and in this series, the assumption proved to be correct. In two of the men, anemia appeared to be the result of a cancerous condition; in one, leukemia; in one, Addisonian (pernicious) anemia; and in the last, a bleeding duodenal ulcer.

Concerning the women, 10 of the 20 cases of anemia were due entirely to nutritional deficiencies, and in two others, poor nutrition was a contributing factor. All of these responded to oral iron supplements and had not relapsed after one year of observation.

In the *Lancet* (May 31, 1958), another factor concerning anemia in the elderly was brought to the attention of British physicians. It was shown that anemia in older persons is often the result of some unsuspected internal bleeding. Of 156 unselected hospital patients, 61 (41 per cent) were found to be anemic. The anemia in most of the cases was of the iron-deficiency type.

On testing, it was discovered that occult (intestinal) bleeding was more than twice as common in anemic patients than in non-anemic. The authors concluded that this established a causal relationship between anemia and intestinal bleeding in older people, and that physicians who diagnose anemia in the elderly should check carefully for this bleeding in them as well.

Anemia in Infants Common

Anemic states in infancy are considered commonplace, according to the experience of Beryl D. Corner, M.D., which she discussed in *Medical Press* (August 27, 1958). Basically, says Dr. Corner, the child's blood formation does not reach a definite, adult pattern until after the first 10 years of life, due to the rapid bodily changes occurring during those years. However, in spite of these expected fluctuations, a diagnosis of clinical anemia is not uncommon in children during their early years. Alterations in diet and minor infections are labeled as possible causes of profound changes in blood formation.

If the mother has insufficient stores of iron in her own body while carrying the child, infant iron-deficiency anemia is likely to result. Other causes might be prematurity, multiple births or excessive blood loss during delivery. Normally, the iron store should be adequate to provide for red cell formation during the first 3 months of life, and iron-deficiency anemia, if it occurs after that time, is due to inadequate dietary intake of iron. One researcher, Mackay, found this type of anemia so prevalent in his experience that he believed "nearly 50 per cent of full term infants in the East End of London were suffering from iron deficiency" after 6 months of age. A diet confined to milk is one cause, he suggested. Human breast milk has some iron, but cows' and goats' milks have negligible quantities.

B and C Vitamins Necessary

Dr. Corner offered some other interesting possibilities as causes of infant anemia. Chronic diarrhea from any cause might reduce iron absorption. Failure of vitamin B absorption can also be responsible for anemia. The disease, kwashiorkor, associated with severe protein deficiency is rated a common cause of anemia.

Interesting to us is Dr. Corner's assertion that vitamin C, aside from its effect as a general stimulant to red cell formation, also helps to create a proper climate for the absorption of iron from the intestinal tract. Anemia is sometimes the only absolute indication of subclinical scurvy. In such cases, administration of 500 milligrams daily of vitamin C for 10 days, then 50 milligrams per day as a maintenance dose, produces a rapid favorable response, with neither iron nor liver supplements needed.

Underexcretion of the thyroid hormone, thyroxin, can result in severe anemia, since this hormone is an essential stimulant to bone marrow activity. Nephritis, rheumatism, syphilis, rickets, long-standing round worm infestation and chronic infection are all to be investigated as possible causes of anemia in children.

A summary of the basic causes of anemia in early childhood, as given in the *Journal of the American Medical Association* (January 5, 1952), might act as a guide for mothers who are anxious to avoid the problem in their own children:

1. Overemphasis on milk—many children will not eat other foods required for growth and development, if they drink large quantities of milk.

2. Failure to wean baby from breast or bottle during the last months of the first year.

3. Failure to teach the child to feed himself, holding a spoon and drinking from a cup.

4. Failure to continue administering supplementary vitamins after the first few months.

5. Parents' poor understanding of what constitutes a satisfactory diet.

6. Lack of periodic physical examinations.

Epileptic patients whose attacks are held in check by anti-convulsant drugs are mentioned in the *Lancet* (May, 1958) as possible candidates for anemia. It was deemed wise by the author that the blood of epileptic patients receiving such drugs be examined regularly for signs of anemia. Successful treatment of anemia, if it should be present, is said to have a remarkable effect on the improvement of epilepsy. Folic acid is mentioned as particularly effective in the treatment of anemia.

What Anemia Does to the Heart

It is logical to expect that interference with the blood's capacity to retain and carry oxygen to the tissues, as happens when the oxygen-rich hemoglobin is reduced in anemic blood cells, will have some effect on the heart. The heart's normal efforts are not sufficient to deliver the amount of oxygen they were meant to deliver. The heart, therefore, must work harder than it normally would to supply even the minimal quantity of oxygen.

In the *Medical Journal of Australia* (October 3, 1953), an article on this very subject remarked on the fact that the heart is the one organ which shows physical change in chronic anemia. The body compensates for the added burden the heart must carry by increasing the heart's size. This was found to be universally true among one series of anemic patients studied. Changes in the electro-cardiogram (graphic measurement of heart activity) readings of anemic persons occur in some 20 per cent of the cases. The authors concluded that, since chronic anemia does cause heart enlargement and abnormal heart action, it must be considered formally, as a cause of heart disease.

It is apparent that the assimilation of iron is a basic factor in most cases of anemia. The question is how one can be sure that the body will absorb the maximum of the iron one gets in one's diet? In the *Lancet* (March 26, 1955), an editorial told of experiments using radioactive iron isotopes which could be measured in food before it was eaten, and traced in the body for measurement after the food was eaten. It was shown that only 10 per cent, or less, of the iron contained in food is normally absorbed by humans.

The experiment uncovered this important fact: The combination of foods is of great importance in regulating the amount of iron the body will absorb from iron-rich foods. ". . . the only two persons who absorbed more than 10 per cent had been given chicken muscle. Iron-deficient patients only sometimes absorbed more than 10 per cent from eggs, but they more often exceeded this level if chicken liver, vegetables and yeast were given. *An important finding was that ascorbic acid (vitamin C) usually increases the assimilation of iron from food . . .*" (Italics are ours.)

So it is evident that the foods we eat in company with other foods have a definite effect on each other. Without the food values of one, the value of another might be lost to the body. Forestall this possibility by eating only those foods rich in nutrients whenever possible. The *American Journal of Clinical Nutrition* (January-February, 1955) printed the findings of J. F. Mueller and J. J. Will which were that vitamin B_{12}, folic acid (another B vitamin) and ascorbic acid are intimately involved in problems of anemia. Each was shown to be an active therapeutic agent when applied in the proper type of anemia case.

Why Protein Affects Anemia

Protein deficiencies were cited by the *Canadian Medical Association Journal* (March, 1955) as possible causes of anemia. There are 4 globin molecules in one molecule of hemoglobin. Each globin molecule contains all the essential amino acids and some nonessential ones. Of course, we depend on our foods for amino acids, and the more complete the protein food, the more likely we are to achieve the full complement of amino acids we need for proper richness of hemoglobin. Due to the complexity of the globin molecules, however, no single amino acid deficiency can be shown to be responsible for anemia. Consequently, the administration of single amino acids to patients with anemia has little effect, yet full attention to protein in the diet is obviously very important.

Getting the Elements You Need

Do iron and other dietary elements that are factors in anemia occur freely in the foods you eat? In June, 1940, the Mississippi Agricultural Experiment Station put out *Technical Bulletin No. 26,* which analyzed the anti-anemic potency of some commonly-used southern foods—turnips, greens, mustard, collards, lettuce, spinach and tender greens, cowpeas, soybeans, lima beans, pinto beans, sorghum and sugar cane syrups and blackstrap molasses. These vegetables were tested and found to be effective in varying degrees for hemoglobin regeneration. The legumes were much more effective than the leafy vegetables when fed at the same level as the vegetables. Blackstrap molasses appears, also, to be an excellent source of the minerals that affect anemia.

The vitamin C which was named as an effective therapeutic agent in treating anemia is, of course, abundantly present in fresh fruits and vegetables, and in rose hips, available as a food supplement. Vitamin B_{12} and folic acid are plentifully contained in wheat germ and brewer's yeast. They are also present in all the organ meats. These meats are also high in iron and protein and should be on everyone's menu several times a week. Desiccated liver is an excellent food supplement which supplies many of these much-needed nutritional elements which offer protection against, and can often cure, many types of anemia.

Anemia in a Junior High School Class

Experience and research have taught us to expect the worst in evaluating the health of our nation's youngsters. Though this view might seem cynical and pessimistic, experiments and reports by serious researchers all over the United States only serve to reinforce our attitude. One of the most unusual, and convincing, of these reports came to us from a junior high school science instructor in Ohio.

A class of junior high school pupils chose as its annual group science project a study of blood, blood types, the Rh factor and anemia. Each student was required, with his parents' consent, to give a few drops of blood for study and analysis. A drop was needed for finding the hemoglobin (oxygen-carrying cells) content, a drop to determine the presence or absence of the Rh factor and a few more drops were used to determine the actual blood type.

The results of these tests and observations certainly made an interesting and worthwhile project. The children came away knowing their respective blood types, a very useful bit of information, and aware of their Rh-factor status. But most important of all, they found that most of the class was frankly anemic or bordering on anemia.

Teen-Agers Are Anemic

According to the Tallquist Hemoglobin Chart, a standard for such measurement, hemoglobin readings of 70 or below are considered anemic for either sex. In the class, 2 per cent of the students had a hemoglobin content of 50; 48 per cent had a content of 60; 35 per cent had a content of 70; 13 per cent had a content of 80; 2 per cent had a content of 90. A reading of 85 to 100 is considered normal for men and 80 to 100 is considered normal for women. For men, 70 to 85 is suggestive of anemia, and for women, 70 to 80.

According to the study carried out by the class, then, 54 per cent of the girls were anemic, 38 per cent borderline anemia and 8 per cent normal. Among the boys, 47 per cent were anemic, 50 per cent borderline anemia and 3 per cent normal. This was a group of average teen-agers, not a sanitarium class. These are the kids that are shown devouring sugar-coated dry cereals, drinking pop and munching chocolate bars in television commercials. These are our healthy kids. Next time the papers or magazines carry notices that tell you our country's population is too well fed and healthy to bother with health foods and vitamins, think back to this class and the results of its experiment. How much better do the junior high and high school pupils in your town eat than the ones in Ohio? You'd probably find the similarity of general diets astounding. Are your children getting the iron, calcium, protein and other blood-building food elements they need to keep them healthy?

Anticoagulants

They're Too Free with Anticoagulants

Your circulatory system operates under a constant strain. Every time you move, you rupture many of your capillaries, the tiniest blood vessels in your body. You could bleed to death as a result of climbing up a flight of stairs if it weren't for the fact that your blood possesses the ability to clot or coagulate. When there is a break in the wall of a vessel, certain factors are released by the breakdown of blood platelets. An interaction among the components of the blood quickly produces a sticky net across the break which traps the larger blood cells and forms a clot. Clots are formed, too, in vessels in which the flow of blood has been reduced to a trickle, as happens when we wear tight or restricting clothing or cross our legs and ankles or sit on them.

Persons of 50 or 60 years of age tend to have more blood clots than younger people. More clots seem to occur in obese people and people who live under conditions of constant stress and strain than in people who are of normal weight and who live uncomplicated, unharried lives. There are also people whose blood contains more than the average amount of clotting substances and these persons develop clots easily.

An enzyme in the blood generally dissolves clots which have been formed, but sometimes it cannot and the clots are trapped in the capillaries, or they break loose and float about in the blood stream until they lodge in the lungs or other vital organs. A stroke is the result of a major blood clot which has lodged in the heart. Serious complications and even death can be caused by a floating clot. The unfortunate truth is that a person who has been hospitalized from one blood clot will usually experience trouble with more clots. Doctors often prescribe regular dosage with drugs which can keep the blood from clotting. These drugs are called anticoagulants.

Anticoagulants Stop Chemical Changes in Blood

Anticoagulants are able to prevent the blood from clotting by interfering with the chemical changes occurring in the clotting blood. Many of the drugs can keep the clotting process from starting at all while others can stop the process at any one of its phases. Only a few of the drugs can dissolve clots which are already in existence. Fibrinolysin, for example, is an enzyme ordinarily circulating in the blood. Its job is to dissolve clots by acting against the clot former, fibron, and in this respect, it is superior to another enzyme manufactured by the body, trypsin. Trypsin dissolves other proteins in the blood plasma and thus reduces the amount of the ingredients necessary to coagulate the blood. As a consequence, hemorrhaging is more likely to occur in patients treated with trypsin than with patients treated with fibrinolysin.

The third type of anticoagulant native to the human body is a fast-acting and complex blood sugar called heparin. Heparin is powerful, but its effectiveness is lost within a few hours. Therefore, heparin is usually given to a patient in combination with another anticoagulant which produces longer-lasting effects. Heparin must be used with caution because average or large doses may cause hemorrhaging.

There are many synthetic anticoagulants and drugs. Most of these drugs belong to the family of chemicals known as coumarins. The coumarins made their appearance in 1931 when hundreds of sheep and cattle in the midwest died from a strange malady called the "sweet clover" disease. The animals were being destroyed by a substance which prevented their blood from clotting and caused the animals to die from violent internal hemorrhaging. Six years later, Doctor Karl P. Link and his group of chemists succeeded in isolating the substance, coumarin.

The potential toxicity of anticoagulants is increased by their accumulation in the body's cells. Manufacturers of the anticoagulants warn that the drugs must not be administered if there is any evidence of renal or hepatic disease. Any lowering of kidney or liver function hinders the breakdown and excretion of blood.

Proper Dosage Varies Daily

This would mean that the danger of hemorrhaging is increased. We have already pointed out that an average dose of some of the anticoagulants may cause hemorrhaging and so the exact individual dosage is important. A minor change in diet or in the patient's general health may completely reverse the clotting ability of the blood. Many doctors require that their patients submit to weekly blood sampling tests to determine the blood's clotting time. The dosage is then adjusted accordingly, because an overdose of any anticoagulant can make healthy blood vessels bleed and a person in good general health is in danger of bleeding to death.

Hemorrhaging is the greatest single drawback to the use of anticoagulants. The *Dental Digest,* May, 1957, warns that persons who use anticoagulants run the risk of serious hemorrhaging when they undergo oral surgery for tooth extraction. Two cases of persistent and serious hemorrhage have been reported by the New York Veterans Administration Hospital. The blood loss during some dental operations is equal to that encountered in major surgical procedures. The Veterans Hospital and the *Digest* would encourage patients who must submit to dental surgery and who also are under anticoagulant therapy to withhold the drugs prior to surgery and take them again only when danger of hemorrhage has passed.

Hemopericardium

Dr. John Tziniolis in the *Medical Journal of Australia,* August 26, 1961, recalls the discovery of Wright and his associates, who found in 1954 that 4.1 per cent of 589 patients treated with anticoagulants died from heart rupture or hemopericardium (flooding of the sac which contains the heart), while only 2.4 per cent of 442 untreated patients died from the same cause.

There were 3 times as many cases of hemopericardium in a group treated with anticoagulants as in the group that was not treated, found Waldron and his associates. Lang and Aarseth, in 1959, found that incidence of hemopericardium or cardiac rupture in the treated group was twice the number of the untreated group. A year earlier, the same two doctors had reported that, out of 89 cases who came to autopsy, 8 showed an excessive anticoagulant effect before death. Two other patients had had an overdose of anticoagulants at some stage of their treatment. They decided that treatment with anticoagulants increases the risk of hemopericardium.

Serious hemorrhaging in their unborn children may be the result of the taking of anticoagulants by pregnant women. The *British Medical Journal* (2: 719, 1955) records the work of Gordon and Dean who had as a patient a woman who was receiving anticoagulants for a blood clot deep in her femur. Although tests showed that the clotting time for her blood was adequately under control and although the drug was discontinued before she went into labor, the first twin was stillborn and the second twin died within two weeks. There had been no reason to suspect that anything had gone wrong during the pregnancy. An autopsy showed that both twins had died from multiple hemorrhages attributed to anticoagulants which the mother had taken. Gordon and Dean warn against the taking of the drugs routinely by pregnant women unless their condition is very serious, and they advocate no anticoagulants at all in the last 4 weeks of the pregnancy.

Gangrene of the Breast

Anticoagulants seem to present special problems to their women users. In the *New England Journal of Medicine* (263: 909, 1960), Charles S. Kipen writes on another complication of anticoagulant therapy: gangrene of the breast. This is a very rare condition with only a few cases having been reported and these as a result of such diseases as diabetes, plastic surgical procedures, infectious organisms and toxic agents, and certain types of strokes.

Dr. Kipen's report is based on two cases of women who developed gangrene of the breast after they were given anticoagulant drugs. In the first case, a 65-year-old woman was admitted to the hospital for treatment of a congestive heart failure. Earlier, she had been a patient at another hospital and while there, she had fallen out of bed and bruised her breast. Within 5 days, her breast was swollen and tender and entirely covered with ecchymosis (a condition which occurs when fluid leaves its normal cavity, characterized by purplish skin). At this point, the anticoagulation therapy was discontinued and vitamin K was given to the patient. The doctors diagnosed the condition as massive hemorrhage of the breast induced by the anticoagulant. Nine days later the woman was dead.

Vitamin K Is the Antidote

It is interesting to note that the antidote for hemorrhaging induced by anticoagulants is vitamin K. As little as 5 to 15 milligrams are all that is necessary to restore the clotting properties of the blood. In severe cases, repeated doses may be given either by injection or orally.

To us, it is important not only that vitamin K can help the blood to clot faster, but the research has shown that it can help to stabilize the blood. That is, it helps to maintain an equilibrium in the blood, so that it does not clot excessively or too slowly. It helps to keep blood pressure at an even keel, and there are no dangerous side effects from its use. Another vitamin, vitamin E, also has the tendency to normalize blood and blood pressure levels.

Appendix

Keep Your Appendix as Long as You Can

It is fairly well accepted medical practice these days to remove the appendix whenever the occasion presents itself. If one is operated on for gallstones, ulcers or intestinal adhesions, it is quite probable that the surgeon will remove the appendix, "while I'm in there." There is no need for the organ to be diseased. The reasoning is that sometime it might become diseased and have to be removed anyway, so why not now? Besides, it's not really doing any good in the body.

This last assumption has been contradicted in recent years by the interesting results of research on the appendix. One of the most important findings, in the light of our increased exposure to radiation, is that of Dr. Dieter H. Sussdorf of the California Institute of Technology, Pasadena. *MD* magazine (August, 1960) reported on Dr. Sussdorf's finding that the appendix apparently helps the body to muster its forces in fighting the effects of postradiation infection. This condition occurs when the body's ability to manufacture antibodies is impaired. Any infections can run rampant then before the body can fight back. If the patient dies, it is not from radiation, but from infection.

In studying the effects of whole body radiation used as a treatment for cancer, Dr. Sussdorf systematically covered one organ after the other with a protective lead shield. He observed that shielding the appendix gave greater protection against postradiation infection than did shielding any other organ. The reason for this was obscured by the fact that the appendix is not directly involved in the formation of antibodies. It was concluded, then, that the appendix somehow increases the ability of the spleen (seat of the formation of antibodies) to recover from radiation damage. When such damage is severe, the spleen is temporarily paralyzed, as it were, and its antibody function greatly impaired. Lymphoid cells from the shielded appendix fill the need by migrating to the damaged spleen to manufacture antibodies there until the spleen can recover enough to take over once more.

Without an appendix to perform this supplementary function, the danger of exposure to fall-out or even to prolonged therapeutic X-ray is increased. Well enough if the organ were diseased and had to be removed to save a life, but, if it were removed only because a surgeon had the abdomen open anyway, the needless loss of the added protection it could have given is indeed tragic.

Weakened Abdominal Wall

Another unfortunate result of appendectomies is the suspected predisposition to inguinal hernia caused by them. This was discussed in the *Illinois Medical Journal* (May, 1960). While the author was cautious about making a definite cause and effect pronouncement, he (James Scott, M.D.) quotes the suggested principle that any abdominal incision weakens the structure of the abdominal wall. He mentioned several surveys of groups of appendectomy patients who later suffered hernias. One of these, which concerned 196 male patients with inguinal hernias at a Veterans Hospital in Illinois, disclosed that 16.3 per cent developed postappendectomy inguinal hernias.

We hope you will mention this to your surgeon if he should suggest a two-in-one operation that will needlessly deprive you of your appendix. The human body is not so haphazardly constructed that parts of it exist for no useful purpose. Because one can exist without tonsils or appendix, it does not follow that these organs are useless when left in the body. As we have seen, the appendix performs a vital function under the stress of radiation poisoning, and its value in other difficulties yet to be encountered in our changing world, cannot be measured. The value of tonsils as a filter for infectious organisms has been shown again and again. Obviously, we are better off with such a protective device than without it, even though its removal is hardly likely to be fatal. We agree that an infected organ should be removed when it creates a serious danger for the rest of the body, but we believe that such a situation should be a requirement in considering removal.

Removal of the Prostate

The prostate gland is another favorite for unnecessary removal. Here again, it is not our intention to say that there is no case in which the prostate should be removed. Certainly if the gland is diseased to a point at which no recovery is possible, removal may be the only answer. But oftentimes, prostate swelling is a benign condition that can be relieved or completely cured by diet or massage of the gland. We object to the quick conclusion that an operation is the only answer before other things have been tried. The *Journal of the Maine Medical Association* (March, 1958) reported an experiment in which the use of 3 amino acids (glycine, alanine and glutamic acid) in capsule form benefited 92 per cent of the subjects who suffered from a prostate condition. Unsaturated fats, richly contained in vegetable oils have also shown themselves to be useful in these cases. A German doctor, W. Devrient, found the use of pumpkin seeds to be a beneficial treatment for prostate gland enlargement. The prostate gland secretes the fluid which acts as a vehicle for the male sperm cells. Without this fluid, there is no way for the sperm to travel through the male urethra and through the female vaginal canal to the uterus to fertilize the eggs. In other words, sterility is a result of prostate removal.

There is a purpose for every part of the body, either for the physiological function of it, or as an aid in adjusting itself to its environment. Hold on to every part you can. If the tonsils are not creating a health problem, keep them; if the appendix is giving you no trouble, don't let anyone remove it; if your prostate is giving you trouble, be sure you've tried diet and massage before allowing it to be removed; keep your teeth as long as you can, unless they are infecting your system. Your body comes equipped for efficient operation—don't interfere with it unless you have no other choice.

Arsenic

A Poisoning Epidemic with Arsenic

From July to November of 1900, the people of Manchester and Liverpool in England were terrified by one of the most mysterious epidemics ever recorded. Over 6,000 people became seriously, sometimes fatally, ill in those few months. The symptoms were similar, but the victims were from all walks of life, from all social classes. There was little to tie them together. Only one thing—it was discovered, eventually, that they all drank beer.

This little remembered epidemic among beer drinkers remains one of the historic instances of mass poisoning due to a part of the manufacturing process. It was found, at last, that the commercial glucose used in making beer by a local brewery contained arsenic. Also, a less noted circumstance was the fact that the malted barley, essential to the brew, was dried in the fumes of arsenic-containing malting fuels. The procedure was a time-honored British custom, for it was held to impart a characteristic smoky flavor to English ales, as distinguished from the German and Austrian beers. There the malted barley was dried by radiant heat without coming into contact with smoke and fumes.

The Symptoms

The reasoning that opened the obscure possibility that beer might be responsible for this wholesale poisoning is interesting. The victims were considered, at first, to be suffering from lead poisoning, because of some of the symptoms, but the tell-tale lead line usually found on the gums of such victims was missing. A visiting medical officer, on inspection, was told of the frequent occurrence of shingles (herpes zoster) among these patients. The officer must have been inspired to come up with the answer: there must have been arsenic in the beer these people drank, because only arsenic, of all known drugs, causes shingles. Tests indicated that the hunch was correct. The situation compared with a similar epidemic in Paris in 1828, when arsenic had been mistakenly added to wine in place of gypsum, then commonly used as a clearing agent for wines.

The complications which arise in processing are well illustrated by this beer epidemic. The 5 breweries involved were all supplied with glucose by the same company. When samples of everything used by this company in making glucose were analyzed, it was discovered that the sulfuric acid contained a very large amount of arsenic. This acid came from still another firm, which had, for many years, shipped dearsenicated acid, but suddenly changed its practice and sent crude acid which contained large quantities of arsenic. Of course, there had been no systematic analysis of the sulfuric acid by the breweries to test its quality, so they went on using the poisoned acid for years. The result was a greatly increased death rate from peripheral neuritis, alcoholic neuritis and chronic alcoholism in the area supplied by these breweries during that time.

Of Current Interest

The article which told the story above appeared in the *New England Journal of Medicine* (October 6, 1960). What followed was of even greater interest to us. The author, Dr. Henry S. Satterlee, expressed concern over the fact that little attention has been paid to the finding that incriminated the arsenic rising in the fumes from the malting fuels. Even without the dangerous sulfuric acid in the glucose used to make the beer, the arsenic in the fuel would be seriously objectionable from a health viewpoint. Arsenic is a deadly poison, no matter what its origin. Dr. Satterlee quotes the *British Medical Journal* in 1955 as saying that arsenic is in first place among the recognized cancer-causing elements that are present "in the smoke of chimneys and the fumes of cars." The mention of arsenic as an air pollutant is not frequent enough, yet in these days of engines and industry, our exposure to such dangers in the air is very real.

The arsenic concentration in the air we breathe indoors (called expired air) is 110 micrograms per cubic meter. This reading is 3 times the tolerance limit set in 1943 for "background arsenic" under controlled conditions in crowded buses, theaters, subways during rush hours or in crowded dormitories!

For a long time, the presence of arsenic in meats (as a fattener), in fruits and vegetables (as an insecticide) and in tobacco, has been recognized as a potent cancer-causing factor, but this business of arsenic in the atmosphere has had short shrift from science. Dr. Satterlee says the true significance of the poisonous effect of arsenic in the atmosphere has yet to be measured by realistic methods of air sampling. Until this is done, the problem will continue to be minimized and ignored by industrial toxicologists and public health authorities in the United States. In England, this question is gettting more attention in relation to its part in the rise of the cancer rate.

Arsenic from Underground

The increasing role of petroleum fuels in our way of life also concerns Dr. Satterlee, for arsenic is closely bound up with these fuels. He writes, " . . . it is clear that the ever-increasing combustion of vast quantities of petroleum fuels, mined and piped from subterranean and submarine depths is at the same time exhuming a "trace element," arsenic, from safe burial within the fossilized strata of a whole geologic epoch, and foisting it upon the modern biosphere. Such vitiation of the human environment with a chemical element possessing catalytic and anticatalytic potentialities, and also capable of forming pyrolytic conjugates with phenols and polycyclic hydrocarbons in smokes and tars, is sure to alter normal biologic cycles of animal and plant metabolism in an unpredictable manner." This is a complex way of saying that modern living and modern technological advancements have led to the liberation of vast amounts of arsenic into the atmosphere. No one seems interested in determining the effect of this added poison on the humans who breathe it. Nor is anyone doing anything to determine what effect the presence of added arsenic in the atmosphere will have on other elements naturally present. It is known to accelerate some reactions in the laboratory, and to slow down others, as well as to merge with carbons in smokes and tars to form strong carcinogens. We're breathing at least 3 times the maximum of this kind of air under the best conditions. When we live near smoke-belching factories or exhaust-ridden highways—to name just two aggravated conditions—we are getting far, far more than 3 times the accepted safe maximum of atmospheric arsenic.

Another Unknown Emerges

As an aside to the cigarette smokers who aren't worried by tobacco tars and arsenic, may we point to the work of the Drs. Sunderman of Jefferson Medical College, Philadelphia. *Science News Letter* (October 8, 1960) reported on their findings, which showed the strong possibility of heavy smokers getting cancer by long-time inhalation of the trace amounts of nickel in cigarette tobacco. The doctors experimented with rats of a species especially resistant to lung cancer. The rats were subjected to 30-minute inhalations of nickel carbonyl, in concentrations of 4 parts per million, 3 times a week for one year. Two or more years after the first exposure, cancerous lung tumors were observed.

Who gets such concentrated amounts of nickel carbonyl? Estimates of the amount of nickel that might be inhaled by heavy smokers (2 packs a day) of cigarettes, the researchers say, are similar to that proved cancer-producing in the rats. Industrial workers who are exposed to nickel carbonyl or nickel dust are also known to have a high percentage of lung cancer.

Here are two fresh factors which have not been considered by most of us, nor by most researchers, in connection with cancer cause. Who knows how many more elements we use every day which are just as dangerous? Who knows what the next year's research will uncover? Who knows what food we are eating now that will be discovered to contain a dangerous poison? Only avoidance of foods that have been tampered with can guarantee freedom from dangerous chemical additives. Eat natural, organically grown foods whenever you can.

Aspirin

Is Aspirin Dangerous? You Bet It Is!

"N. Y. PHARMACISTS' AD WARNS ASPIRIN IS 'NOT HARMLESS' "

This is a headline which appeared in *Advertising Age* (July 20, 1959), a trade paper which calls itself "The National Newspaper of Marketing," that must have startled many of its readers and alarmed a good many aspirin manufacturers. Health-conscious readers would not be so shocked, since the problems with aspirin are really an old story to them. But to the makers of aspirin, who have built millions of dollars worth of business on the fiction that one can always use aspirin for safe and dependable relief, this was unwelcome publicity. What was even a worse blow was the source of the warning about aspirin, an organization which represents retail druggists. When even this group—the main salesmen for aspirin—comes out against aspirin, that's bad.

The ad which this organization paid for, was a quarter of a newspaper page and was sent to various pharmaceutical associations for placement in their local papers. The headline read, "So You Think Aspirin Is Harmless," and the copy went on to warn the public about the "growing number of accidental poisonings involving aspirin." It tells of 7,247 accidental poisonings reported by the New York City Health Department, of which 11 per cent (about 800) were caused by aspirin. In Arizona in May, 1959, the ad says, there were 30 aspirin poisonings out of a total of 88 from all sources. The ad didn't detail all of the incidences of aspirin poisonings—it couldn't. Just about every health department in the country has had similar reports. The *Chattanooga* (Tennessee) *Times* (April 18, 1960) carried a short piece about conditions in Knoxville, Tennessee. A poison control center official there reported between 40 and 50 cases of aspirin poisoning in 8 weeks. Half of these, he said, were brought on by overdoses given children by parents.

Aspirin and Infants

The *Canadian Medical Association Journal* (November 26, 1960) went into the trouble with aspirin in detail in an article by Crichton and Elliott. The authors analyzed 58 cases of aspirin poisoning, 41 of them in children, which had come to their hospital, Calgary General Hospital, within 4½ years. Their first observation is that, ". . . the majority of serious salicylate (aspirin) poisonings in children were therapeutic in origin and therefore largely preventable . . ." The report went on to say that the aspirin given to children as part of a treatment (not the aspirin taken by them accidentally) is the real problem. Aspirin, given for colds or fever, sometimes

58

brings on symptoms of extremely serious illnesses and can cause great confusion among diagnosticians when the children are examined. Many of the aspirin-poisoned children discussed in the article appeared to be suffering from pneumonia, meningitis, epileptic-like seizures and the type of high fever that usually indicates acute infection. So many cases of aspirin poisoning in children are diagnosed as pneumonia, that the authors believe that "air hunger (panting and gasping) in young infants should be taught as primarily due to salicylate poisoning until proved otherwise." In two of the cases the authors saw, which had pneumonia symptoms due to poisoning with aspirin, the examining doctors diagnosed pneumonia and prescribed —imagine!—more aspirin.

The authors of this paper gave this final word on aspirin for babies, which, we think, should be committed to memory by every parent and physician:

"The majority of serious cases of salicylate poisoning admitted to this hospital were infants in the therapeutically induced group. The severity of the illness, the diagnostic pitfalls, the complexities of recommended treatment remove any margin of safety, especially in infants in whom the electrolyte patterns can change rapidly. It is clear that these cases have happened largely owing to lack of knowledge of the dangers in the use of salicylates, especially in the adult tablets, by both physicians and parents. These cases continue to appear in spite of the information from governmental agencies (Canadian), safety councils and other public bodies."

New Material Appears Continually

Our files are crammed with new material on aspirin poisoning, or as *MD* magazine (December, 1960) calls it, "a treacherous, complex and most common danger." This periodical, too, mentions the special danger aspirin holds for children under 3. It mentions the respiratory difficulties that mark aspirin poisoning, or salicylism, the acidosis that also occurs due to an interference with a cycle of carbohydrate metabolism.

The literature on aspirin comes from everywhere. *Dental Abstracts* (October, 1960) carried "no" to aspirin when they printed an evaluation by a Swiss doctor which said, ". . . acetylsalicylic acid (aspirin), even when taken in comparatively small amounts (from 300 to 600 milligrams) . . . stimulates the anterior lobe of the pituitary gland in its secretion of adrenocorticotropic hormone, thereby causing a premature release of cortisone by irritation of the adrenal cortex. . . . In dental practice, neither buffered nor unbuffered forms of aspirin or aspiric combinations should be used for alleviation of intense pain. Various more effective analgesic agents are available."

The *British Medical Journal* (May 7, 1960) carried a letter from two doctors who called attention to the anticoagulant powers of aspirin. The letter matter-of-factly recognized that aspirin can cause vomiting of blood, due to its irritation of the gastric mucosa (stomach lining), but it warned too that persons whose blood is already slow to coagulate take a serious risk in using aspirin, for it lowers even more the amount of the element in the blood, prothrombin, largely responsible for coagulation. They report on a patient who hemorrhaged from the external ear and the renal (kidney) tract after oral administration of aspirin. He was 56 years old and had been having long term treatment with anticoagulants. Bleeding from the sites mentioned occurred within 24 hours after two doses of an aspirin compound. The authors stated that such a patient is one more and more frequently met in general practice.

Thyroid Is Slowed Down

Work on aspirin and its effect on the thyroid was reported in the *Lancet* (April 30, 1960). The observers found that, while there was no direct effect on the thyroid, salicylates interfered with the production of a hormone which stimulates the thyroid into activity. The net effect is, of course, that thyroxin, the vital secretion of the thyroid gland, is diminished. In cases in which the thyroid is already underactive, salicylates could be an extremely dangerous drug, especially if used over a long period of time.

A large amount of research has been done on the damaging effect of aspirin compounds on the lining of the intestines. The aspirin companies, of course, dispute that there is such an effect and emphasize in their advertisements, the mildness of their product. These interests were no doubt gratified by the appearance of a report from the *British Medical Journal* (Vol. 1, p. 1106, 1960) which asserted that the dangers of aspirin are exaggerated. In their report, the authors stated that the incidence of ulcers and upset stomach in chronic users of aspirin is no more frequent than that of normal persons who do not use aspirin.

This view is a rare one, however, and we find it hard to reconcile with information, for example, which appeared in the *AMA News* (November 14, 1960). Two physicians from Louisiana State University School of Medicine reported that aspirin is especially dangerous for patients with ulcers or a history of ulcers. "Bleeding ulcers or bleeding of intestinal tract where there is a history of ulcers, have been attributed to overdoses of aspirin."

How the Buffers Work

The manufacturers of aspirin compounds sought to counteract the bad impression created by such findings in announcing buffered preparations, which are supposed to dissolve faster than regular aspirin. (Irritation of the stomach wall is attributed to bits of aspirin that refuse to dissolve quickly.) In the *New York Times* (June 3, 1960), we read that two researchers at the University of Buffalo School of Pharmacy discovered that, while the dissolving time of buffered aspirins is less than 5 minutes, the disintegration time, during which the pill falls apart into little pieces, but does not dissolve, is longer for buffered aspirin than plain aspirin. So, actually, there is no advantage to one type over the other. Buffering is what the advertising trade would call a "sales gimmick."

The gastric difficulties brought on by aspirin preparations appear to be nearly universal. Two French doctors, whose report was carried in *Presse Medicale* (December 10, 1958), believe that "aspirin provokes isolated digestive hemorrhages and is the drug most frequently responsible for ulcerous hemorrhages." Their work, based on observations of 52 patients, showed that digestive disturbance usually took place a few hours after the absorption of aspirin, usually within 24 hours.

In the *New York Times* (March 15, 1959), the undesirable gastric effect of aspirin was emphasized by an article which said, "Serious qualms over possible danger from the use of aspirin have been expressed recently in several scientific reports from Britain, the Netherlands and Canada. All present strong evidence that aspirin probably causes minor gastrointestinal bleeding in a high proportion of heavy users, may be responsible for massive bleeding in many ulcer cases and is a possible cause of 'severe iron-deficiency anemia' of uncertain origin. At least 7 such scientific reports have been published in foreign medical journals since 1952. . . ." The anemia was thought to have been caused in one patient by as few as 8 to 10 aspirins a week.

In a report on the subject of aspirin and intestinal irritation, to the *Lancet* (March, 1959), the authors said that, of 106 patients admitted to their hospital with bleeding ulcers, 57 (over 50 per cent) admitted having taken aspirin within 48 hours of their initial bleeding. Of 106 patients admitted without bleeding ulcers, only 17 per cent had taken aspirin in the previous 48 hours. An interesting point made in this report: "Of the people whose hemorrhage followed ingestion of aspirin, half knew that aspirin gave them indigestion." These people were sick and actually knew that the aspirin would make them sicker —possibly fatally so in the case of ulcer patients—and they took it anyway!

Some Suggested Action

It is estimated that, in Britain, four billion aspirins a year are consumed. The count for the aspirin eaters of the United States is surely much higher. The danger of aspirin has been made abundantly clear, not only in cases of ulcer, but in other physiological processes described here. If doctors are influenced at all by what they read in their professional journals, they should be warning every patient they see against having aspirin in the house.

We like the suggestions for the government's dealing with aspirin —especially in the case of children—which were offered in the afore-mentioned article by Crichton and Elliott:

1. Alert the public to the fact that salicylates, particularly adult salicylates, "are potentially fatal poisons for young children. It is not unreasonable to expect that manufacturers should help and guide in this regard."

2. More emphatic labeling of salicylate compounds containing adult doses, for example, " 'contains salicylate—dangerous to babies. DO NOT GIVE TO CHILDREN UNDER 5 YEARS OF AGE.' In this connection, it is worth noting that 'tamper-proof' bottles are not always tamper-proof."

The authors also had some suggestions for the medical pro-fession:

1. "More emphasis, especially from departments of therapeutics at undergraduate level and in postgraduate refresher courses, on the doses of salicylates which will produce intoxication at various body weights.

2. "Education of the nursing profession along similar lines. When we took histories from patients, it was not uncommon to find that adult salicylates had been given to infants for minor febrile illness or colds on the advice of a nurse, and then repeated frequently in blind faith by the parents."

If your doctor should prescribe aspirin for you or your child, he may have good reason for doing so, but ask him to be sure. Let him know that you would prefer doing without it if he does not feel it is absolutely necessary. Show him this information and ask him if he is familiar with the material quoted here, written by his colleagues. Surely he should believe the researchers in his own profession.

"America's Best-Loved Pill"

The aspirin is an American institution which ranks with Mother, Baseball and the Lincoln Memorial. Not only is it considered almost un-American to say anything unflattering about any of these, but if you did, no one would believe you were serious. Now we have nothing but praise for the latter 3 of these institutions, but about aspirin, "America's best-loved pill," we have other feelings.

Columnist Delos Smith in a column printed in the *New Britain Herald* (October 9, 1961), told of experiments which showed that aspirin "can cause internal bleeding, but the amounts of blood lost internally are not nearly enough to be threatening—provided the aspirin taking is moderate." Moderate—what does that mean? Moderate for whom? Are 8 aspirins in a day moderate for a secretary with chronic headache or menstrual cramps? Is that amount moderate for a chronic arthritic whose doctor has told him to take aspirin for the pain as often as he feels it is necessary? Are 8 aspirins in a day a moderate dose for a mother with a headache, and 3 small children on her hands? How about for a high school boy with a cold and a high fever? What is moderate for one is excessive for another and minimal for a third. But one can safely bet that the person who takes aspirin at all will be more likely to take too much than not enough. He's convinced that the aspirin won't do him any harm, why shouldn't he take a good dose?

Proof That Aspirin Is Dangerous

Mr. Smith reported on an experiment in which the subjects were given two aspirin tablets 4 times a day, and this dose was found to cause some internal bleeding, "but not nearly enough to be threatening." He noted that the experiment called for more aspirin than the average person ever takes. We strongly dispute the proposition that 8 aspirins a day consitute an unusual dose—"A couple of aspirin every two hours " is a fairly common prescription. We believe that many people bleed internally from aspirin intake without ever suspecting it. "But it's not dangerous." Not dangerous to whom? Patients taking anticoagulants are forbidden aspirin by discerning doctors. What about people with ulcers, people who are anemic, hemophiliacs (those whose blood has difficulty in clotting normally) and dozens of others who may have special problems when internal bleeding occurs? Some of these people don't even know what disease they have! And if 8 aspirins will cause some internal bleeding, many Americans must have their insides awash with blood, because of the number of aspirins they use per day.

More Trouble with Aspirin

The impression still persists, even among medical men, that aspirin is utterly harmless and can be given to relieve pain from almost any cause in almost any person. We have always campaigned against this faulty appraisal of aspirin's safety. We have repeated the warnings carried in the medical journals about aspirin's ability to mask symptoms of serious diseases, and thereby cause misdiagnosis, and of its causing disease on its own. While this material has come from experts in their fields, doctors still appear to be ignorant of the danger in aspirin, or prefer to ignore it.

In *Science News Letter* (July 8, 1961), the problems presented by treatment with aspirin were added to by a report from the American Rheumatism Association's annual meeting. Three scientists from the National Institute of Arthritis and Metabolic Diseases described two cases of rheumatoid arthritis that were mistakingly diagnosed as gout, because of high levels of uric acid in the patients' blood, a characteristic criterion of gout. Their doctors treated them with colchicine, a standard gout remedy, and got no results. It was found, upon further investigation, that the high uric acid levels had been caused by low doses of aspirin taken to relieve joint pain, not by gout at all.

Researchers Suggest Aspirin Substitute

On analysis of why this phenomenon should occur, it was suggested that low doses of aspirin probably act by blocking the normal secretion of urate by the kidneys. The urate backs up and accumulates in the blood in abnormally high levels. Large doses of aspirin have the opposite effect. One wonders what measure of high or low aspirin dosage will hold true for everyone. What is "high" for one patient could be "low" for another. The research team wisely suggested that a substitute for aspirin should be used as a pain reducer for gout patients.

So much for gout and arthritis patients. What about the rest of the population? What about those who pop an aspirin in their mouths every hour for relief of their daily headaches, or the cold sufferers who rely on aspirin, or the children who take aspirin for slight fevers and upset stomachs, at their mother's insistence? Are their doses high or low? What happens to their elimination of uric acid? Is this the only bodily function that is altered or interfered with by aspirin? How will we ever find out?

Safety with the use of aspirin has too many loopholes. Why use it? Vitamins C and A are much more effective in treating colds, and the B vitamins have been shown to be most effective in curing chronic headaches. Good diet and proper food supplementation will take care of anything that aspirin will—without its dangers.

Athletics

Poor Sportsmanship in Hypnotized Athletes

The devious means being devised for athletes to win their competitions are slowly replacing the old spirit of fair play. The ability of the athlete is only incidental these days to how many fast breaths of pure oxygen he can take before going back into the game, or how quickly he can lose weight on a crash diet to get himself into a lower, easier division in wrestling. The latest wrinkle in this barely ethical kind of athletics is the use of hypnosis. The athlete is hypnotized and bidden to do almost superhuman work on the field.

In the *American Medical Association News Release* (July 22, 1960), this practice was condemned on the grounds that hypnosis might aggravate physical impairments of which the athlete is not aware. He might also exceed his own physical limits and become exhausted to the point of serious harm. He might, in this state, expose himself to injury by concentrating so intently on his performance that he ignores previously learned safety measures.

Oh yes, the AMA adds—"It's not good sportsmanship."

Avocado

Avocado Is Something Special

A salad with greens and tomato is a popular and wonderfully healthful addition to a meal, but add an avocado and you have something really special. This delightful tropical fruit has become well-known in the past 30 years, because modern transportation methods have made it possible to ship avocado anywhere in the United States. It has a great many assets to recommend it and if you haven't made avocado a part of your diet yet, you really should.

You will find that avocado is unlike any other fruit you have ever tasted. It is roughly shaped like a large pear, and when properly ripened, its dark green skin covers a meaty, melon-like pulp that has about the consistency of a ripe Bartlett pear, but oily. The avocado should have a "give" to it, as you hold it, when it is ripe. The flavor is neither sweet, like a pear, nor tart like an orange; it is subtle and rather bland, nut-like. It is a flavor that might take a little getting used to—not because it is unpleasant, but because the flavor is hard to define in the light of our experience with other fruits. Sometimes it takes several "eatings" of avocado to catch that delightful quality in taste that has made it such a favorite throughout the world. Once you become an avocado fan, you will look forward to the season each year with eager anticipation.

The avocado is a fruit that is native to our Western Hemisphere, and grows on a broad-leafed evergreen that requires tropical or semi-tropical temperatures. The Spanish explorers brought the fruit to the attention of the civilized world, but its use was confined to the immediate areas in which it was grown, since its perishability did not allow for long distance shipping. The populations of California, Florida and Cuba were the only people who could enjoy the avocado.

Naturally Dormant and No Spray Danger

Today, refrigerated carriers have made the shipping of avocados possible to any place in the world. The fruit is allowed to mature on the tree, but it is still firm at this point. It is brought to packing houses, cleaned and graded as to size and quality, and packed in protective excelsior. The fruit is then cooled to 42° F., a temperature at which it lapses into a sort of dormant state. This cooling does not change the avocado in any way, it just delays the natural softening of the fruit until a grovelike temperataure (room temperature) is restored. This happens on the grocer's shelf or in your kitchen.

One of the most attractive things about avocados is that they do not require processing of any kind. There is no dyeing or waxing or gassing needed. If the temperature is controlled properly, the avocado will delay its ripening until needed. And unlike other fruits, one cannot eat the skin of the avocado. It is thick, much like an eggplant's skin, so that poison sprays, if they are used, present no hazard to the consumer.

Nutritious and a Cholesterol Reducer

Good taste and versatility, plus safety from spray poisons would be enough to recommend the frequent use of such a fruit, even if its nutritional values were limited. Avocados, however, are very rich in nutrients. Their main asset is an abundance of unsaturated fatty acids, so necessary for maintaining the good health of the circulatory system. Aside from this, the average portion contains some protein, an appreciable amount of vitamins A and C—about one-tenth of the minimum daily requirement—and about a third of the official vitamin E requirement. The B vitamins are well represented, especially thiamin and riboflavin. Calcium, phosphorus and iron are present in worthwhile amounts, and 11 other minerals also have been found in varying trace amounts. None of these values is destroyed, nor significantly altered by refrigeration storage.

Dr. Wilson C. Grant, of the Veterans Administration Hospital, Coral Gables, Florida, and the University of Miami School of Medicine, set out to discover if avocados, because of their high content of unsaturated fatty acids, would reduce the cholesterol in the blood in selected patients. The study comprised 16 male patients, ranging in age from 27 to 72. They were put on control diets to determine as accurately as possible, the normal cholesterol level of their blood. Then they were given ½ to 1½ avocados per day as a substitute for part of their dietary fat consumption. Measurements of the blood were taken twice a week. Of the 16 patients, 8 showed significant decreases in total serum cholesterol ranging from 8.7 to 42.8 per cent. Of the 8 who experienced no change, 3 were diabetic and one was extremely prone to high cholesterol content in the blood. In none of those who participated did the cholesterol level increase. It either stayed the same or went down. For those readers anxious to reduce the cholesterol level in their blood, there seems to be every reason for trying avocado as a means to this end.

How to Serve Avocado

How does one eat avocado? It can be served perfectly plain in the shell, merely by cutting the fruit in half, tip to tip, removing the round pit, and sprinkling the cut surface lightly with lime or lemon juice to keep it from turning brown. If you are adding the avocado to a salad, cut it in two, remove the pit and peel the skin from the fruit. Then slice it lengthwise or in crescents, or dice it and toss it with the greens and your own dressing. A favorite recipe for avocado salad calls for two peeled avocados cut into crescent-shaped slices (the end pieces cubed) alternately arranged with the thin wedges of two large tomatoes and placed on a bed of two quarts of torn salad greens. The arrangement makes an attractive picture. Just before serving the course, toss it in a dressing of ⅓ cup salad oil, 1½ tablespoonfuls of vinegar, ¼ teaspoonful of dry mustard, ½ teaspoonful of black pepper and a dash of tobasco sauce.

Avocado blends as well or better with fresh fruits of all kinds, and adds a new sensation to fruit salads that can include apple wedges, peach and pear halves, pineapple chunks and berries or grapes.

As a main course, a half of a large avocado, unpeeled, makes an unusual and delicious container for your favorite tuna or chicken salad recipes.

Most super markets carry avocados as do fruit specialty shops. They are available year-round in the West, Southwest and the Florida area of the United States. Elsewhere, they are most plentiful from January through May. Keep asking your grocer about them to make sure you get a taste of his very first shipment.

By the way, don't discard the pit. Stick two toothpicks into it, directly opposite each other, so that they will rest on the edges of a kitchen water glass filled with water so that the pit rests partly in the water. In a few months, the pit will sprout and eventually become a small tree which will bring additional pleasure from your avocado.

Bacteria

Bacteria Can Be Buddies

Doctors love to label other people as "faddists," but as far as we can see, our doctors themselves are demonstrably the greatest faddists of all times. Even such plagues of temporary madness as hula hoops and the Twist dwindle to insignificance before the monumental proportions of fashionable cures that have ultimately turned out to be menaces to the nation's health. Millions of our children have fallen victim to the frenzy of surgeons to remove their tonsils, first line of defense of the respiratory system. Millions more still suffer painful burning, blisters, allergic reactions and even skin cancer because of old, now discredited, medical propaganda urging maximum exposure to summer sunlight.

But of all the danger-fraught medical fads ever perpetrated on the world-wide association of willing guinea pigs, one of the most foolish and lacking in perception has been the frenzied crusade of our healers to eradicate bacteria. Ignoring the cautions of the more sagacious researchers, ever since Pasteur, doctors have tried to cure everything by exploding veritable atom bombs to wreak indiscriminate slaughter among the bacterial populations of our bodies. Reasoning so simply one might almost call it simple-mindedly, they have calculated that, since some bacteria cause illness, the way to eliminate illness is to eliminate all bacteria. Fortunately for all of us, their disinfectants and antibiotics have not been as effective as expected and the bacteria have survived the onslaught.

Without bacteria, human life would probably come to an end.

Lawrence Galton, scientific writer of the *New York Times* magazine, pointed out on December 3, 1961, that bacteria are indispensable for the fertility of our fields, that the benign bacteria in our bodies fight the malignant ones and preserve our health, that they are vital to the digestive processes, and that we are only at the very beginning of understanding of the many ways bacteria are and can be useful.

Among many other things, Galton reports that, "Bacteria also are being employed now to treat common intestinal upsets and even to repair some undesirable side effects of mold antibiotics. The fact is that the healthy human gut normally is full of bacteria; their bulk exceeds that of food and food wastes by a ratio of two to one. And most numerous among them is the *Lactobacillus acidophilus.*

"These friendly bacteria are credited with curbing the growth of harmful organisms. As long as there is a beneficent dominance of them, others are kept in proper place as harmless minorities. . . ."

Galton goes on to point out that antibiotics kill off these needed *lactobacilli,* and that investigators at Michael Reese Hospital in Chicago are now feeding high concentrations of these bacilli to patients with intestinal disorders. "The results, they report, have been excellent: 'extraordinarily rapid' relief."

Yogurt, a Protective Food

What we find especially remarkable about this development is that it comes after many years of hurling the epithet "faddist" at those of us who have advocated that people eat yogurt as an aid to health. And what is yogurt? It is defatted milk soured with *Lactobacillus acidophilus* and containing a high concentration of those bacteria which are vitally necessary for the health of the intestines.

As long ago as 1954, we pointed out that researches had shown that yogurt would help protect us against the bacteria causing dysentery, typhoid, pneumonia and numerous other diseases, and that antibiotics, inescapably present in our foods, were robbing us of the benign intestinal flora we need.

This is truer today than it was then. Nothing has been done to curb the use of antibiotics in animal feeds. It has been encouraged and has increased, despite the evidence of penicillin and other antibiotic residues in practically all animal products that we eat. In terms of individual sensitization and the possible creation of new diseases by bringing about hardier mutant strains of malignant bacteria, the possible results of these residues are well known. But a subtler and no less dangerous possible result is the destruction or weakening of the benign bacteria our bodies contain.

Banting, Sir Frederick

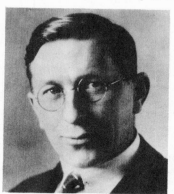

Sir Frederick Banting, the Canadian physician and scientist who discovered insulin was born at Alliston, Ontario, Canada, November 14, 1891. Upon completion of his preparatory studies in the Alliston schools, Banting entered the University of Toronto in 1912 to begin studies toward his medical degree. He achieved this honor in 1916, and then entered the Canadian Army Medical Corps, winning the Military Cross for valor. The following years were taken up with various endeavors— practice as an orthopedic surgeon, research assistant in physiology at the University of Western Ontario and professor of medical research at the University of Toronto. It was in this last position that Banting together with J. J. R. MacLeod and Dr. C. Best, began research work on the internal secretions of the pancreas gland which was to lead to the discovery of the hormone, insulin. Banting's discovery can best be evaluated in light of the normal life diabetics can now lead due to their use of insulin. For this great contribution to medicine, Banting shared with MacLeod the Nobel Prize for physiology and medicine awarded in 1923.

Bacteria Maintain Our Health

We depend on these bacteria to maintain the internal balance we call health. Dr. Rene Dubos, head of the Rockefeller Institute and one of the world's leading research scientists, once told the National Institute of Health scientists that the supposedly deadly microbes are not nearly as dangerous as generally believed. He was quoted by the *North American Newspaper Alliance* as pointing out that bacteria and viruses become dangerous only when the body's natural balance is disturbed, but that "Otherwise, even the most virulent of them are harmless."

In the same talk, Dr. Dubos pointed out that, "it is practically impossible to infect volunteers picked at random with some supposedly highly infectious diseases if the experimenters do not know how to upset the internal environment so as to produce the right conditions." He named the common cold and bacillary dysentery as two diseases that experiments had found it practically impossible to communicate by contact alone, but that are easily contracted when the internal balance has been disturbed. He then warned that the antibiotics could, in curing one illness, leave a person far more susceptible to others.

Hospitals Are a Case in Point

Hospital experiences with the use of disinfectants have pointed to similar conclusions. All hospitals, today, use very powerful disinfectants in washing their floors and walls, sterilizing, etc. Yet time after time, it has been noted that hospital patients are particularly prone to contracting diseases while hospitalized. The hospitals have tried to solve the problem by using still more powerful disinfectants, but without success. Can it be because the disinfectants indiscriminately destroy *all* bacteria, including the benign ones that would normally fight and check the disease bacteria?

Editor Rodale once said: "It seems to us, that all of us rely too much on drugs of one kind or another for everything. Given a healthy baby, brought up on a sound nutrition program, and a nursery kept clean according to ordinary standards, we need not worry about germs or reach constantly for a disinfectant."

Dr. Rene Dubos, in the speech previously quoted, said the same thing a little differently: "Long before anybody knew anything about germs, many physicians were very successful in treating patients. They had no sulfa drugs, no antibiotics, no immunity serums. The secret of their success probably lay in a highly developed, and perhaps instinctive, skill in treating the patient as a whole, rather than looking, as does the modern doctor, for one cause of a condition and treating only that."

Our actual relationship with the bacteria in our bodies seems to be of the type known as symbiosis—an alliance based on mutual dependence. If we take care of them, they take care of us. Even the disease bacteria can exist within us in limited numbers doing no harm and possibly even doing some good, so long as they do not become too many. Dr. W. B. Coley, a New York physician, is one of those who have experimented with disease bacteria in the treatment of cancer, with apparently promising results. The all-important problem for control and utilization of bacteria would seem to be the maintaining of a healthy balance in the body.

Important Work Performed

Not being faddists, we believe that people should eat naturally and avoid the drugs and germ killers of medical fads. In this natural way, our systems keep down the numbers of possibly malignant bacteria. Our intestinal flora, in a healthily functioning condition, manufacture a good part of the vitamin supply we need. They prevent putrefaction of food in our intestines by destroying the bacteria that would ordinarily cause it, thus protecting us against toxic conditions such as putrefaction would cause. They digest our pectin for us, as we could not digest it without them.

In the world outside our bodies, it is the bacteria that are responsible for decomposing all dead organic matter and returning it, in its original chemical constituents, to the earth. Without bacteria, we would lose our topsoil and be unable to grow food. Our cattle could not digest the grasses they eat. And now, Galton tells us in the *New York Times* magazine, bacteria can be used to cleanse our water of poisonous industrial wastes, and even to cleanse the air of pollutants.

Isn't it time we let up on the indiscriminate destruction of these microscopic organisms that are our indispensable partners in life?

Baldness

Women Are Balding

Women can curl their hair if it's straight, they can dye it if the color doesn't suit them, but they can't seem to do anything about hair that is falling out. The part begins to widen and the scalp becomes more visible; the hairbrush has a bush of dead hair in it after each brushing—the lady is actually becoming bald!

In *McCall's* magazine (July, 1960), we read that one New York dermatologist had a record of 28 such cases within a year. This doctor, with several others, found that in 5 years, this problem had advanced so much that the number of all the patients in the first 4 years added up to the number in the fifth year. This was 9 times as many cases as in the first year. And the majority of the women were under 40 years of age, and many were under 30.

A questionnaire was sent to members of the American Dermatological Association concerning this problem. More than half of those who responded had also seen an increase in this type of balding. There was, unfortunately, no uniformity in their suggestions concerning the cause or a cure. One doctor said nylon brushes with harsh, square-cut bristles tear hair out by the roots. Another doctor noticed 24 pony-tailed young women who were losing their hair. He suggested the tight pull-back of the hair as the cause. Another dermatologist blamed tight hair rollers.

We, too, have warned against pulling the hair too tight in setting it and against nylon-bristled brushes. Several investigations have found the lack of one mineral or another to seem to influence baldness, but no conclusive proof has been presented. One researcher made a good case for salt as a cause of baldness.

We do know that baldness is unnatural, and must be caused by a lack in the body or the use of an unhealthful food. We think the safest, most effective step one can take to avoid baldness is to eat a diet high in the essential proteins, vitamins and minerals. Give your body what it needs to make hair and the hair will always be there.

Lack of Protein May Cause Falling Hair

Changes in hair are almost constantly present in protein malnutrition. Alterations in the color, texture, straightness, denseness and "pluckability" have been described. In children who live in the environment of tropical areas, where sunshine, dust and lack of hygiene are prevalent, it is difficult to establish when the color and texture are abnormal. These factors, however, will not alter "pluckability," and easily plucked and detachable hair has been suggested by Guatemalan workers as an additional indicator of protein malnutrition. The sign is investigated as follows: "A group of 20 to 30 hairs from the anterior half of the head is taken between the thumb and index finger and pulled firmly and steadily. In an undernourished child, 10 or more hairs will be plucked easily and without pain." (J. M. Bengoa, M.D., D. B. Jelliffe, M.D. and C. Perez, M.D., MPH., in an article in the *American Journal of Clinical Nutrition,* November-December, 1959.)

Bioflavonoids

The Precious Bioflavonoids

Capillary fragility is the term applied to a condition in which the tiny blood vessels that carry blood to every cell of the body become so fragile that they may break under increased pressure or if a tiny clot should clog them. The importance of keeping the walls of the capillaries strong and healthy is immediately apparent when one considers the incidence of "strokes." A "little stroke" is a hemorrhage from one of these small blood vessels. The term "stroke" is usually applied to a hemorrhage in a brain artery, resulting in paralysis and unconsciousness. Sometimes the word is applied to hemorrhages in other parts of the body.

While hardening of the arteries is apparently the commonest cause of strokes, it seems evident that protecting the welfare of the smallest arteries—the capillaries—will prevent these small vessels from bursting and hemorrhaging. Bruises are the result of capillaries bursting, allowing the small amount of blood they contain to spill out into the tissues. "Pink toothbrush" is the result of hemorrhages from the small blood vessels or capillaries of the gums.

The capillaries, like the nerves, service every cell of the body. Carrying their precious fluids, they spread in a fine and almost endless network throughout the body. They enter each cell and fluids pass through their walls into the cell tissue. The only reason we do not suffer serious consequences when one of them ruptures is that they are so tiny that another capillary can take up the work and provide blood until the broken one is repaired. But when the break comes in an artery wall in an important spot like the heart or the brain, there is a much larger hemorrhage. Permanent and very serious damage may result.

Here is a list of diseases in which we know that capillary fragility is one symptom: hypertension (high blood pressure), arteriosclerosis (hardening of the arteries), diabetes, rheumatoid arthritis, allergy, asthma, obesity and the complications of the menopause. Quite a list, isn't it?

A group of doctors at a Trenton, New Jersey, hospital experimented by giving a certain food substance, a bioflavonoid plus vitamin C, to a group of patients suffering from these diseases, whose capillaries were definitely fragile. They reported on their results in the *American Practitioner and Digest of Treatment* (June, 1955). Thirty-seven patients were given hesperidin, the food substance; another 37, with similar symptoms, were not.

73

Results of Experiment

At the end of 5 years, here were the results:

Of the group of patients who did not receive the bioflavonoid plus vitamin C, 4 died as a result of hemorrhages, one suffered a stroke and remained bedridden, only 32.4 per cent showed normal capillary fragility and 54 per cent showed no change.

Of those getting the bioflavonoids, two died of diseases completely unrelated (pneumonia and a prostate operation). There were no deaths from causes related to blood vessels. Of these patients, 63.1 per cent had normal capillaries, 19.3 per cent had borderline measurement and in 17.6 per cent, there was no change.

In a later article in the *International Record of Medicine* (January, 1960), two physicians, George J. Boines and Steven Horoschak, tell of relieving muscle cramps in postparalytic polio with the same bioflavonoid-vitamin C preparation. They treated 19 patients. They tell us that polio patients who were started on the vitamin substance and who continued to take it throughout their convalescence and rehabilitation program, did not, at any time, complain of muscle cramps, while patients who interrupted the treatment prematurely did complain of moderate to severe muscle cramps. The 15 patients who continued with the treatment were, these physicians tell us, "successfully relieved and fully controlled."

Bioflavonoids Are Part of the Vitamin C Complex

Their explanation is that the bioflavonoids are essential for the body to absorb and use vitamin C. Since vitamin C is necessary for the manufacture of the cementing substance between cells, the bioflavonoids are also necessary.

Dr. Carl T. Javert of Cornell Medical College has used bioflavonoids to great advantage in treating women who could not have children because of habitual miscarriage. Giving the would-be mothers a diet high in foods rich in these substances and food supplements containing them, as well, he set a record of perfect babies with full-term delivery for 91 mothers out of a group of 100.

Dr. Robert B. Greenblatt of the Medical College of Georgia treated 20 women who had had from 2 to 8 miscarriages. Fifteen of them had normal babies. As you can see from these records, not all miscarriages are the result of weakened capillary walls. But many admittedly are.

Bioflavonoids aid in recovery from radiation wounds and injuries. *Science News Letter,* as early as 1948, reported that "a substance in lemon peel" protected animals against X-ray doses which would otherwise have been lethal. Hemorrhages are one symptom of the illness, which comes from too much radiation. The discovery was important for cancer sufferers who are taking X-ray treatments.

One other noteworthy use of the bioflavonoids was discovered by a doctor at Baylor University's Department of Obstetrics and Gynecology. Dr. Warren M. Jacobs stated in the August, 1956, issue of the *Journal of Surgery, Gynecology and Obstetrics* that a bioflavonoid compound controls the complications resulting from the Rh factor in the blood of a prospective mother.

Women who have a certain factor in their blood called the Rh negative factor may marry men who have an Rh positive factor, which is antagonistic to the negative factor. In such a marriage, when the mother becomes pregnant, antibodies may develop in her blood to fight the antagonistic blood cells being produced by the baby. These antibodies may destroy the baby's red blood cells and the only way of saving the baby may be a complete transfusion of all the baby's blood, removing it and replacing it with blood from a donor. Accord-

---

Barton, Clarissa Harlowe

The founder of the American Red Cross, Clarissa Harlowe Barton, began her outstanding career in the field of philanthropic services as a teacher and later as a clerk in the patent office at 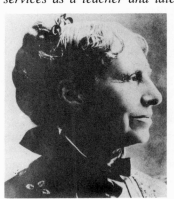 *Washington, D. C. The outbreak of the Civil War marked the advent of her list of distinguished ventures and accomplishments causing her as a lay person to take a prominent position beside the professional pioneers of medicine. Clara Barton became a volunteer nurse in the army hospitals during the war, working so untiringly and efficiently that President Lincoln, in 1865, placed her in charge of locating the missing men of the Union armies. Her devotion to duty led her next to the aid of the Grand Duchess of Baden in the preparation of military hospitals during the Franco-Prussian War. While in this role, she also assisted the Red Cross Society. When, in 1881, the American Red Cross was organized, Clara Barton was rightfully chosen as its president. From this point on her life was molded in the pattern of one possessed with an almost fanatical zeal to help others. The list of her benevolent services stretches out almost endlessly, until, in 1904, Miss Barton broke down physically and resigned her post in the Red Cross.*

ing to Dr. Jacobs, the bioflavonoid compound controls this condition without the need for transfusion. We have not seen any further information along these lines in medical journals, which seems strange to us. This is a serious problem for many married couples and it seems that much more research should be done.

Other Uses for Bioflavonoids

Here are some other conditions for which the bioflavonoids have proved to be successful:

1. Bruising which is inevitable in certain occupations. Sportsmen such as football players, boxers, etc., have found that the bioflavonoids minimize the effects of rough treatment.

2. Rheumatism and rheumatic fever. These two conditions appear to be related to a deficiency in vitamin C and the flavonoids. Taking vitamin C alone seems to help. But taking it with the flavonoids appears to accomplish much more.

3. One researcher reported good results in psoriasis patients who took the flavonoids and vitamin C.

4. The blood vessel disorder of the eye which afflicts diabetics seemed, in some cases, to show improvement with bioflavonoid-vitamin C treatment.

5. One researcher reported excellent results in treating asthma with the compound.

6. Eye doctors using the flavonoid compound have reported good results in cases of hemorrhages into the eye.

7. In many cases, colds and other infections can be controlled by taking, at the first sign of a sniffle, large quantities of natural vitamin C, which contains the bioflavonoids.

What Are the Bioflavonoids?

The bioflavonoids are brightly colored substances that occur in foods along with vitamin C. They are called by various names, since there are several parts to the flavonoid complex—hesperidin, rutin, vitamin P, flavones, flavonols, etc. Officially the bioflavonoids cannot be designated as a vitamin. However, it seems obvious that their place is established in human nutrition and it is only a matter of time until we will have discovered many new things about them, including the fact that they are essential to human nutrition and have the other qualifications for vitamins

Where can you get bioflavonoids? The food substance from which the researchers got their product was citrus fruit. It is contained in the white skin and segment part of the fruit, not in the juice. It seems that you lose large amounts of bioflavonoids when you juice oranges and strain the juice. A freshly peeled orange may contain as much as 1,000 milligrams of them, whereas strained juice from that orange may contain as little as 100 milligrams. Don't juice citrus.

Lemons, grapes, plums, black currants, grapefruit, apricots, cherries and blackberries also contain bioflavonoids. We have no facts on what percentage of this valuable substance may be destroyed when fruits are cooked or canned. Until we do, it seems wisest to depend on fresh fruits only for your supply. We know that a considerable quantity of vitamin C is destroyed by heating and processing.

The natural food supplements contain the bioflavonoids along with vitamin C. The reason for this is simply that all natural vitamin C products are made from foods—they are not put together synthetically in laboratories. So, whatever naturally accompanies the vitamin C in foods, is present in these supplements. There may be, and probably are, many other valuable things that accompany the vitamin which no one has discovered as yet. If you take the natural supplement, you get all these. A synthetic vitamin C tablet cannot, of course, contain them, since scientists do not know what they are.

We recommend getting your vitamin C and bioflavonoids in a product made from rose hips, green peppers or some other natural foods. Rutin, which comes from buckwheat leaves, is a good food supplement for bioflavonoids.

Russia Interested in the Bioflavonoids

The U.S.S.R. has taken the role of vitamin P (the bioflavonoids) in maintaining good health most seriously. In *Food Field Reporter* (April 25, 1960), a column is devoted to the remarks of Dr. Boris Sokoloff, Director of the Southern Bio-Research Institute at Florida Southern College, in which he tells of a 282-page book, *Vitamin P— Its Properties and Its Application,* consisting of 31 papers written by leading Russian scientists.

The research was carried on in Moscow, Leningrad and Kiev institutions, and the scope is such that it is apparent that the U.S.S.R. considered it to be of national importance. A large vitamin P plant was constructed in Russia in 1954.

Dr. Sokoloff cited some of the findings which appeared in the book: Vitamin P is in wide use as a preventive for colds and influenza, as well as in various conditions where capillary injury is present. It increases tolerances of animals to high altitude flying—probably the human animal as well. It increases the number of red blood cells. (Have we done anything on this score to counteract leukemia?)

When used with vitamin C, it is beneficial in the treatment of muscular dystrophy, decreases blood pressure moderately, has a protective influence against radiation injury and decreases high cholesterol blood content in rabbits. It is completely nontoxic, even given in large doses.

Take advantage of vitamin P—the Russians have pointed the way toward using its full potential.

Blackstrap Molasses

Blackstrap Molasses—A Nutritious Sweetener

In the United States, molasses has long been one of the stand-bys of folk medicine. Many of our ancestors, finding themselves toward the end of winter to be in a condition that they described as "peaked," swore by molasses as a vital ingredient of the "spring tonic" they believed restored their energy, and sense of well-being.

We have no belief whatsoever in a remedy just because it was used in folk medicine. Neither do we scoff, however. If people have believed something for a long while, there *may* be something to it. We are willing to take it seriously, to investigate it as well as we can, and to try to understand whether it may still be of value.

Accordingly, when there was a "fad" for blackstrap molasses several years ago, Editor Rodale investigated and concluded that, among sweeteners, blackstrap ranks high in nutritive value, but that there is no reliable evidence of its being any kind of wonder food or having any of the miraculous powers attributed to it. His opinion was that blackstrap, as a food with a high sugar content, is one that a person is better off without. However, if you *must* use a sweetener, blackstrap has a high vitamin and mineral content that makes it far better for the purpose than refined sugar.

We can deduce that our forefathers, lacking modern storage and distribution methods, experienced a shortage of the mineral-rich green vegetables and of fresh meat each winter. A couple of months of such restricted diets, and many of them probably suffered from mild anemias as spring came on. Molasses, which is rich in both iron and the B-complex vitamins, would have had a curative effect on such a condition if taken in large enough quantities.

Today, however, when we have available at all times such valuable iron- and vitamin B-rich additives as desiccated liver and brewer's yeast, there is little excuse for ever developing the run-down condition that is a mild anemia, and we can guard against it or overcome it without taking into our systems the dangerous sugar content of molasses.

What It Contains

This sugar content, according to a study conducted by L R. Richardson, Professor of Biochemistry and Nutrition at Texas A. and M. College, and reported in *Agricultural Marketing* for April, 1959, varied from 44 to 66 per cent in samples tested under the supervision of the Agricultural Marketing Service of the Department of Agriculture. This sugar is not as injurious as the crystals of refined white sugar which are extracted from the sap of the sugar cane, leaving the

78

blackstrap molasses as the "waste" end product when no more crystalline sugar can be removed. Refined sugar causes abnormally low levels of blood sugar, excessive hunger, fatigue, tooth decay and probably many other functional disturbances as well. Fruit sugar, which is taken into the system accompanied by a natural balance of vitamins and minerals in the fruit, is utilized far better without disordering the system as crystalline white sugar does. The same is true of honey, and while we cannot find any conclusive studies that have been made, in all probability, it is true of blackstrap molasses as well.

Here is a list of the minerals and vitamins to be found in 100 grams (5 tablespoonfuls) of blackstrap molasses, and the approximate amounts of each:

CALCIUM—*258 milligrams*	THIAMIN—*245 micrograms*
PHOSPHORUS—*30 milligrams*	RIBOFLAVIN—*240 micrograms*
IRON—*7.97 milligrams*	NIACIN—*4 milligrams*
COPPER—*1.93 milligrams*	PYRIDOXINE—*270 micrograms*
POTASSIUM—*1500 milligrams*	PANTOTHENIC ACID—*260 micrograms*
INOSITOL—*150 milligrams*	BIOTIN—*16 micrograms*

From the above list, it is readily seen that blackstrap molasses is particularly rich in calcium (nearly twice as much as milk in the same amount), iron, potassium and the B vitamins, especially inositol. It, therefore, is worth serious consideration as a food.

As a matter of fact, some 100,000,000 gallons a year are used as livestock feed, both in pure liquid form and as an ingredient of manufactured feeds. As such, blackstrap joins company with wheat germ, rice polishings, and other highly nutritious "waste products" of which human beings are deprived by manufacturing processes, but which farm animals get in abundance.

We have no objection to providing the very best nutrition for farm animals, which is why they are given these "waste products" to eat. We simply think it's time it was generally recognized that people —most people, anyway—are as good as cattle and deserve as good food.

Our Recommendations

To recapitulate: blackstrap molasses is recognizably a highly nutritious food; it is not a medicine and we see no reason to believe, aside from the somewhat laxative effect it is said to have, that it is of any particular therapeutic value in the quantities in which it would normally be consumed. If you must use a sweetener in any food, we consider molasses or honey highly preferable to refined sugar. Since blackstrap has more than 50 per cent sugar content, usually, it would be unwise, in our opinion, to consume it in large quantities for the possible therapeutic value of its vitamins and minerals. One can easily get the same nutrients in other foods, without the sugar, and in food supplements.

The stories about blackstrap being "dirty" or "unfit for human consumption" are obviously nothing but slanders. Were such stories true, blackstrap would not be permitted to be sold. The Food and Drug Administration has full authority to seize and prevent the sale of contaminated or inedible foods.

Blood

The Blood Protects Health and Life

Without a constant blood supply, there is not a single cell of our bodies that could live for more than a short while, measurable in minutes. Spreading itself through every organ, tissue and fiber of our beings, nourishing, cleaning, repairing, maintaining health and life itself, the blood stream and its way of working is surely one of the greatest miracles of Creation!

We think of blood, and see it, as a fluid. But within that fluid, there are trillions of organisms too small to be seen, except with a powerful microscope, all of them performing functions essential to survival and health with unerring efficiency and precision. According to an article in *Today's Health* ("Your Amazing Circulatory System" by J. D. Ratcliff, January, 1957), the blood has an estimated 60,000 to 100,000 miles of route that it travels in a single grown person. It provides the exact food and services required by each of several trillion body cells, with unerring precision, in a healthy body. So complex that, after hundreds of years of scientific study, it is still not fully understood—so vital that our lives and well-being are utterly dependent on its health—surely the blood deserves all the care and assistance we can give it as it performs its fabulous tasks.

What are these tasks and how does the blood perform them?

How the Blood Functions

There are perhaps a dozen logical starting points for a description of how the blood does its work. Let's arbitrarily pick one: how the blood distributes the food we eat to the parts of the body that need it.

Our food, in the main, is digested (if we eat digestible food) in the stomach and small intestine. This means that it reacts chemically with the digestive enzymes that glands pour into the tract. The nature of the chemical reaction is a change of the food substance into some other substance made up of smaller molecules. Sometimes it takes several digestive steps to break the molecules down into other molecules small enough to pass through the walls of tiny blood vessels and into the blood stream. Meats are transformed into amino acids, oils into fatty acids and so on. These have such small molecules, they float right through the 5 million or so tiny protuberances in the small intestine, called *villi,* each of which contains a tiny blood vessel. Dissolved into the plasma, the watery portion that makes up about 60 per cent of the blood, these tiny molecules of digestive matter float through a network of capillaries into the portal vein, whence the blood flow carries them into the liver.

The liver does its own remarkable job of permitting only enough of each type of food to pass it to maintain the proper proportion of that food in the blood stream. The rest is either stored in the liver for future use, or destroyed.

If there is a deficit of any type of food, the liver makes it up out of its stored surplus. It is largely because of this regulatory function of the liver that the blood plasma carries a constant supply of amino acids, blood sugar, fatty acids and vitamins and minerals. As pointed out by J. D. Ratcliff in his *Today's Health* article, the plasma is like one of those endless belts they have in certain cafeterias. The selection of available foods keeps flowing by, with each cell of the body taking what it requires at any particular moment, and the liver replacing each food as it is extracted from the plasma.

The only thing the liver does not put into the plasma is the water that the plasma basically is. Water, without any chemical change, is easily absorbed through the membranes of the digestive tract and becomes part of the plasma. Too much water is easily filtered out by the kidneys, which use it in their work of purifying the blood stream. But for too little water, the body has no answer. That is why one can die of thirst very fast, in just a few days, if there is no water supply at all, while it is possible to live for as long as a month or longer without food, on the reserve supplies of the liver. Some water is supplied in the foods we eat, but it is extremely important that we all drink enough to be sure of an adequate water supply.

It is also easy to see how important it is that we keep our water, and hence our blood plasma, free of such poisons as fluorine and chlorine. Drink pure water from springs or deep wells if you possibly can. If you are compelled to drink city water, boil it first.

The Red Blood Cells

The blood has been studied intensively for hundreds of years. Most of its work has been long known. In recent years, however, there have been marked advances in knowledge of the blood in the way of determining just *how* the blood performs its miraculous work. These new additions to our knowledge, have all come through the comparatively new science of biochemistry. Accordingly, for the most modern and accurate descriptions of the functioning of the blood, we turn to the work of a prominent biochemist, Dr. Isaac Asimov, Ph.D., who teaches the subject at the Boston University School of Medicine.

Dr. Asimov, in his book *The Living River* (Abelard-Schuman, 1958), points out that the red cells of the blood, which number 17 to 25 trillion, have no nucleus and are unable to reproduce themselves, which is why they must constantly be produced by the marrow in our bones. For this reason, some authorities deny that they are true cells and prefer to call them corpuscles. There is no difference except in the name.

The red cell, according to Dr. Asimov, is made up largely of a protein called hemoglobin and water. The function of this cell is to serve as an incredibly efficient means of transporting oxygen throughout the body, from the lungs. It is able to do this because the hemoglobin molecule contains 4 iron atoms. Each iron atom, by its chemical nature, is able to combine with an atom of oxygen. A single red cell contains about 270,000,000 hemoglobin molecules, and is able to carry up to 4 times that many atoms of oxygen, because of the iron atoms contained in the hemoglobin.

Now we begin to see the chemical tragedy of what is commonly called iron-deficiency anemia. The body lacking in iron is unable to form enough hemoglobin, and as a consequence, there are not enough red cells in the blood. This makes the blood unable to draw enough oxygen from the lungs, and tissues all over the body become oxygen starved. This is a terrible thing to happen to anyone, yet a common affliction among people who neglect their diets.

Don't you be one of them. Make certain you get enough liver, our best source of iron, every day, and make sure your system can absorb and utilize the iron by taking the B-complex vitamins with it. Desiccated liver has been highly recommended by J. I. Rodale for years, with additional brewer's yeast or other B-complex source supplements for added certainty.

Interestingly, a shortage of oxygen in the air we breathe is not nearly so perilous as a shortage of iron to carry the oxygen to our cells. Over a period of time, in an oxygen-poor environment such as the high altitudes of tall mountains like the Andes and the Himalayas, a person with enough iron and B vitamins in his diet may develop up to 3 times the normal amount of red cells in his blood. These additional cells seize a much larger proportion of the oxygen in the air, and thus supply the tissues with as much as they require. This is the reason why, if you move from a place near sea level to a high altitude location like Denver or Mexico City, for the first week or so you find yourself sleeping more and lacking energy. It takes that long until your blood accumulates enough additional red corpuscles to supply you with all the oxygen you need.

The White Blood Cells

Far more complicated in structure and purpose than the red cells, the white blood cells are fewer in number, yet still remarkably many. The blood stream of the average man contains about 75 billion of them.

These white cells are true cells, larger than the red corpuscles and possessing nuclei, which enables them to reproduce themselves. There are a number of varieties of them in the blood, according to Dr. Asimov, differing as to size and the shape of the nucleus. The most prominent type, the polymorphonuclear leucocyte, making up about three-fifths of all the white cells in the blood, is not absolutely dependent on the flow of blood for its motion, but is able to move itself by expanding and contracting.

Being whole creatures in themselves—like amoebas—these cells have to eat. What they eat is foreign bacteria. In some way that no one has yet determined, these white cells can sense the presence of hostile bacteria in the body. Those nearby are attracted to any site of infection almost as soon as the invading bacteria enters the tissue. Joining other white cells carried there by the normal flow of the blood stream, they all choose to remain in the infected area, attacking and eating the germ invaders. This is what causes the swelling, inflammation and pressure pain around an infection, which is a kind of battleground.

The leucocytes do not always win the battle, and they practically always have some casualties that are killed by the invaders. Pus is a collection of millions of destroyed white blood cells. "Swollen glands" are enlarged and made painful by unusual accretions of white corpuscles, which gather at the lymph nodes to filter infectious bacteria out of the blood stream. Such a glandular swelling is a sign of an infection in the area, though usually not in the gland itself.

Other leucocytes than the polymorphonuclear perform the same infection-fighting function, but are not able to control their own motion.

Antibodies

The bone marrow and lymph nodes, which ordinarily produce white cells, can be stimulated by a dangerous invasion to produce other protein substances that serve as major allies of the white cells in the battle of the blood. In a sense, the antibodies are designed specifically to the mold of a particular invader. They combine chemically with the invading germs, either killing them outright or so seriously hampering their ability to function that they fall easy prey to the white cells. Sometimes it is not the germ itself that makes the trouble, but rather the toxin it produces. In such a case, the antibody will neutralize the toxin or carry it out of the blood stream.

Dr. Asimov states that, once antibodies are formed, they often maintain themselves in the blood stream for an indefinite period of time. This is what gives us immunity to many diseases.

"Such an immunity is usually a sign of the continuous presence of the antigen (bacterium or virus) in the body, in quantity sufficient to present molds for antibody formation, but not enough to make anyone sick. If the bacterium or virus were to leave us completely, the antibody would gradually be eliminated (no blood protein lives forever) and, without the stimulation of the antigen serving to produce more, our immunity would be lost.

"So the presence of some germs in our body (even disease germs) is a good thing."

So says Dr. Asimov in *The Living River*. If our doctors actually succeeded in their efforts to make our blood streams sterile tracts in which nothing can live, via antibiotics and disinfectants, they would only leave us prey to new and more virulent illnesses.

Platelets and Clotting

In addition to the red and white cells, there is a third type of formed body in the blood. These are much smaller than the other cells, and their only apparent function is to protect the blood itself —by promoting clotting when that is necessary, and not, otherwise.

A blood clot is a mass of blood cells tangled in a network of protein fiber, called fibrin. Fibrin is very useful stuff to close a wound, but obviously there cannot be any in the blood stream itself, or it would stop the circulation. What there is in the blood stream is fibrinogen, a free-flowing protein that can be quickly changed into fibrin when necessary. The change is brought about by an enzyme, thrombin, which is contained in the blood embryonically as prothrombin.

If we go a couple of conversion steps further, we finally come to the platelets. Tiny, sealed containers, they break when they come in contact with the open air, as in a wound. Substances they release convert thromboplastinogen to thromboplastin, which combines with calcium ions to form prothrombin and finally, the enzyme thrombin, which changes fibrinogen to fibrin and closes the wound, sealing in the blood.

This is a complicated and technical proceeding that we ordinarily should abstain from describing. We have detailed it here to illustrate how many safeguards or intermediate steps the blood has, to protect itself against internal clotting.

Being so delicate in structure, platelets probably rupture internally at times, especially when smashed by high blood pressure against hardened arterial walls. The fast action of the spleen in removing damaged and badly formed platelets from the blood helps prevent serious consequences, and so does the complicated, 10-step series of reactions by which a broken platelet finally leads to the formation of fibrin.

Dietarily, our best protection against the possibility of internal blood clotting is vitamin E, the wonder vitamin found in sunflower seeds and in wheat germ supplements. Or to put it even more simply, even if we don't always know why, following a program of natural foods and supplements is our best protection against a host of possible difficulties, because it supplies all the body's needs for good health.

Bone Meal

Importance of the Natural Minerals in Bone Meal

Use it as it occurs in nature. This has always been our rule for using nutrients. We've recommended that one use rose hips as a source of vitamin C because it occurs there in large concentrations, and is surrounded with valuable elements which help the body to use it most profitably. We say use brewer's yeast or desiccated liver for B vitamins because they occur in quantity in these foods and are again accompanied with the other elements best suited to their use in the body. For calcium supplementation, Editor Rodale has been a pioneer in the introduction of bone meal because of its richness in calcium and other mineral factors which the body must have for proper use of calcium. Here again, the calcium alone cannot be used to full advantage without the presence of other nutrients.

Research Vindicates Us

Vindication of our viewpoint has come through the researches of many scientists who have found greater success in the use of naturally occurring nutrients than in the use of artificial or synthetically prepared ones. Recently, we found records of several experiments with a bone meal preparation used in Europe, and prepared by a Swiss laboratory. As with the bone meal used in the United States, the preparation is made from the long bones of young animals (calves, in the U.S.). The bones are freed of fat and are hollowed, but are processed in no other way before grinding. Several European scientists have used this preparation, with astonishing results, in the treatment of varying types of disorders of calcium metabolism of the bone. Most interesting, among the reports made is that of Martin Frank and Fritz Heppner, published in the German journal, *Langenbecks Archiv und Deutsche Zeitschrift für Chirurgie* (Vol. 274, p. 159, 1953).

These men discovered that incomplete calcium preparations are unsatisfactory in treating a number of hard-to-heal fractures and mineral-absorption problems. It was seen that an intake of calcium presupposes a simultaneous and corresponding supply of phosphorus. If one or the other is in short supply, a calcium- or phosphorus-deficient osteoporosis results. That is, for a lack of one or the other, the bones become porous and lose their strength.

If the calcium supply is much greater than the phosphorus intake, the body must match the calcium by taking away from its own phosphate deposits to maintain the calcium-phosphorus balance. The phosphorus comes from the bones, and the result of its loss is a honeycombing of the bones, osteoporosis, which weakens them in spite of a large calcium intake.

Balance Easily Upset

The relationship of calcium-phosphorus is a shaky one under the best conditions. The hormonal system (pituitary, parathyroids, thyroid gland, etc.) can throw it off, as can the influence of vitamin D. Vitamins C and A can also have an adverse effect on the balance. It is easy to understand, then, the clinician's preoccupation with getting proper amounts of calcium and phosphorus in a supplement. Unless they are used in the right way, they do more harm than good. As they occur in the bones of animals, they are perfectly suited to humans. The bones of animals also meet another requirement. They contain carbon and it is necessary, for the absorption of calcium, that carbonic acid and phosphoric acid be present. It is this inter-relationship that allows for normal callus formation which soon turns to bone. However, if all 3 elements are not present, the callus simply doesn't turn into bone.

As can be seen from just these few examples, the body's use of calcium is based upon a complex series of "if's." A doctor who wants to treat a slow-healing fracture cannot hope to cover all possibilities by using one mineral as a treatment. He cannot be sure that one mineral, say calcium, is the only one lacking. There might be a shortage of phosphorus or carbon, or one of a dozen other minerals the body uses to build strong bones. A supplement made of the bones themselves is the only sure way to know that all the necessary elements are present. Drs. Frank and Heppner used such a preparation on a number of cases of poor fracture healing and calcium metabolism. We will print here several of their case histories and let the reader draw his own conclusions as to the merits of a full bone supplement.

A 24-year-old man sustained a fracture of the shank as a result of an accident on October 21, 1951. His leg was put into traction on the same day and remained there until November 8, 1951— about 4 weeks. Then, for a whole year, until November 5, 1952, no callus formation was evident. The cast was not removed because the leg could stand no walking pressure. The bone supplement was given, a total of 20 tablets, for about 2½ months. The cast was removed and the callus showed complete hardening as a weight-bearing bone.

Leg Fracture

A 47-year-old woman suffered a fracture of the right leg with marked displacement. She, too, had the leg in traction from the day of the accident, August 23, 1951, to September 1, 1951. After that, the lady wore a cast and used a cane until January 4, 1952. There was almost no callus formation. The bone supplement was given for 3 weeks (201 tablets), after which time an X-ray showed a distinct increase in callus formation and bony progression. The fracture was soon completely healed.

An unusually responsive situation occurred in a 57-year-old woman who fractured a leg in September, 1950. In January, 1951, she formed a false joint (pseudarthrosis). Usual treatment was not helpful and a bone graft was done in March, 1951. By January of the following year, the fracture was not yet healed and the patient could not walk without a cast. Bone meal therapy was then begun —one tablet 3 times a day for a little over two months. At the end of that time, the leg was completely healed and the patient was walking on it with no difficulty.

Mineral Deficiency in Pregnancy

A pregnant woman of 26 experienced violent pains in the left wrist during the last few months of pregnancy and during lactation. A plaster splint and calcium medication were to no avail, and the pain stopped only with the cessation of lactation. About a year later, in the final months of another pregnancy, the trouble began again. Along with the other problems came recurrent dental caries, which would not yield to treatment. The bone supplement was employed as a treatment for 3 months—one tablet 3 times a day. Twelve days after this treatment was begun, X-rays showed a return to normalcy in the wrist. The pain disappeared with the complete use of the hand restored, and the caries problem defeated.

In all, the authors tell us that the bone meal preparation was used on 14 patients with success in all cases. They recommend its use in all types of fractures and other mineral-deficiency cases and feel that the attending physician should not wait until other possibilities to promote healing have been exhausted. If the course of treatment is begun two, three or four weeks after the accident, the time of healing will be shortened, and the resultant bone formation firmer and more lasting.

We applaud the use of such a treatment as natural bone for

promotion of healing in fractures, but we would go one step further. Why not use such a preparation to prevent fractures? Since the main function of any bone meal supplement is to restore a proper mineral balance in the bones, why not maintain such a balance at all times? Why not include a few of these tablets in the regular daily diet, so that one is assured of all of the elements one needs to keep the bones firm? This is the way to avoid fractures and other manifestations of ill health that can occur through lack of minerals in the body. Bone meal is probably the least expensive of the food supplements, and one of the most valuable. Don't cheat yourself of the insurance it offers.

Scientific Background for Bone Meal

You may have found, as we have, when you are talking to someone about bone meal as a food supplement, that they demand to know whether or not you have any scientific background for your statements. You may be asked, can you prove what you say? What scientists back you up? How do I know you aren't just saying this on your own?

Because we, too, are almost always challenged in this way, we are especially glad when we find new scientific evidence of the effectiveness of bone meal as a food supplement. We have published a book, BONE MEAL FOR GOOD TEETH, which contains much of the scientific proof that we have dug out of medical and scientific journals and books. Now we have happened upon more fine medical evidence about bone meal and its worth as a food supplement.

A Spanish medical journal, *Medicina clinika,* was the source of our information. The article was entitled "Pure Powdered Bones from Young Animals for the Treatment of Certain Rheumatic Diseases," by R. Cirera-Volta. Dr. Cirera-Volta, at the time he wrote the article, was on the *Journal of the Faculty of Medicine, Medical Hospital and Society of Barcelona,* Spain.

Our author believes that people suffering from various types of rheumatic diseases should be taking calcium and phosphorus—two important minerals. (Of these two, calcium is the one most often found lacking in American diets.) Powdered bone seemed to him to be the best source of calcium and phosphorus because the two minerals exist in bone naturally and in proper proportion. That is, their proportion is the same as that of human bones. So, in giving bone meal, you could not make the mistake of giving too much or too little of one of the minerals. A certain relationship between the two is important.

We like to eat bones, Professor Cirera-Volta believes, as dogs do. This indicates the need for the minerals they contain. He thinks that we show our nutritional needs in other ways, too. Manual workers at hard labor prefer to eat carbohydrates; those doing hard mental work crave proteins. We have never met with this observation before, nor are we entirely sure that Dr. Cirera-Volta is correct. Certainly protein foods are extremely important for people doing hard manual work, even though it is true that they can probably use more carbohydrate foods without suffering from too many calories.

Once he began to study bone meal, our author tells us, he found that considerable research and experimentation had been done in Europe.

Bone Meal Protects Cells

He quotes Professor Julius Von Reis of a clinic in Berne, Switzerland, who gives patients calcium in many diseases: tuberculosis, bone diseases, chronic infections, allergies. Its effectiveness comes partly from the fact that it makes the cell membrane less permeable. That is, harmful substances cannot so easily enter into individual cells of the body to do them harm.

Dr. Von Reis says, too, that the small fibers and cartilages which make up the bones are the places where minerals are stored. So he believes that giving whole bone meal is a good idea because all of this valuable material is present in the bone meal.

Professor Leuthardt of the University of Geneva, Switzerland, has reached the following conclusions about bone meal: The minerals in it are best dissolved in an acid solution like the digestive juice in our stomachs. The calcium content of the bones of animals who have not been fed bone meal is much less than that of animals which have been eating bones. One can assume that the same might be true of human beings. Then, too, human beings who eat bone meal excrete less calcium than those who do not take bone meal, thus showing that the calcium has been absorbed by the body—at least 53 to 70 per cent of it, according to experiments he has done.

Testing these ideas, Professor H. L. Kung of the Pediatric Clinic at Basel, Switzerland, gave bone meal as a daily supplement to a number of children, testing the amount of calcium they retained—that is, the amount of calcium that actually went into their bones and teeth. He gave some of the children bone meal, and others the kind of calcium preparation you would get at a drug store—calcium gluconate and calcium phosphate. He found, day by day, that the children retained more calcium on the days when they were taking bone meal. He also found that, even after they had stopped taking the bone meal, they still retained more calcium than the other children who had not had bone meal. So apparently, the bone meal conditioned them in some way so that their bodies could make better use of calcium, even after they had stopped taking the food supplement.

Bone Meal for Healthy Bones

Professors Demos Gatti and Pietro Nicol of the University of Bologna experimented with giving bone meal to 20 children, 5 to 13 years old. The "reserve" of stored calcium increased in all of them while they were taking bone meal. This is much the same thing as Dr. Kung proved—calcium from bone meal is not lost to the body by being excreted. It goes into bones, blood and teeth where it is needed. These same investigators in Bologna also found that nursing mothers, who got bone meal as a food supplement daily, had considerably more calcium in their milk than those who got no bone meal.

Here is some evidence of the importance of bone meal for healing bone fractures. Kurt Hohl of the Cantonal Hospital of Zurich, Switzerland, describes a woman cancer patient who had a fractured hip which would not heal. She was given bone meal everyday for two months, along with massive doses of vitamin D, which helps the body to assimilate calcium. The bone healed and she could leave her bed for the first time.

Drs. D. Gatti and P. Nicoloj, in the *Pediatric Clinic* (1951), tell of giving bone meal to under-par children. The weight gain which followed made these authors believe that bone meal contains substances which act as hormones and enzymes capable of stimulating growth. O. Bucher and J. Th. Weil commented in the review *Experentia* in 1951 on their experiments showing the influence of bone meal on broken bones in a laboratory test tube. Bone meal stimulates the formation of a callus on the broken bone within 8 days, they report.

Professor J. Eschler of the University Clinic, Freiburg (Germany), studying both animal and human patients, came to the conclusion that bone meal given for broken bones is effective because it stimulates the formation of the substances that actually form the bone —the calcium, phosphorus, iron and other minerals.

A. J. Held and Fred Piquet, writing in the Swiss journal *Praxis* speak of tooth decay in relation to bone meal. Working with children of 5 and 6 years of age for 3 years, they found that regular giving of bone meal decreased tooth decay, even in children whose treatment began after the age of 5.

Dr. O. Popp of the Orthopedic Hospital in Vienna describes results he got from giving bone meal to 35 patients suffering from orthopedic diseases of the bones. The bone meal was highly beneficial in 26 cases, good in 5 and not effective in 4. Some of the patients most benefited were suffering from retarded bone knitting, from osteomyelitis, from tuberculosis of the bone and Pott's disease (a disorder of the spine). Cases of osteoporosis were also greatly benefited. This is the softening of the bone so often found in older people.

We believe that Dr. Popp's findings certainly indicate that all older folks should be taking bone meal to assure the health of their bones.

Dr. Cirera-Volta, the author who collected all this miscellaneous material, believes that bone meal should be used in treating arthritis and diseases of this kind. He points out that one of the first symptoms of such diseases is that the bones become "demineralized" near the small joints. That is, the minerals waste away from the bone structure leaving the bone porous. These minerals should, of course, be replaced, and bone meal may be the answer. He reminds us that the calcium in the bone meal also strengthens the heart and muscles.

He points out, too, that hormones often given for relief of the pain of arthritis (we suppose he means ACTH and cortisone, two hormone drugs) may demineralize the bones so effectively that there are many cases among arthritis patients of bones that break without any pressure or accident—simply from general weakness. So, in any case of arthritis where he is giving hormone drugs, Dr. Cirera-Volta also gives bone meal.

This Spanish researcher believes that bone meal, taken as a food supplement, will accomplish the following improvements in arthritis patients: (1) remineralize bone; (2) lessen inflammation; (3) make it easier to get rid of swelling and (4) improve the activity of the muscles and the heart.

He believes, too, that bone meal should be used in cases of osteoporosis, osteomalacia and osseous atrophy, because, in these diseases, he says, the tissues that hold the bone together have lost the capacity to hang on to the minerals. Bone meal brings to such tissues not just the minerals, but also the bone tissue which stimulates the bones to build new structures and cement the minerals firmly to it. Dr. Cirera-Volta speaks in terms of building. He says, "We might say that this medication brings not only the bricks and the mortar, but also the material which forms the framework of the skeletal parts, the proper disposition of which imitates the art of construction with reinforced concrete."

How much bone meal should one take, according to Dr. Cirera-Volta? He does not give exact doses, but he believes that the doses should be "very strong," because he has never seen any ill effects in patients taking bone meal.

Bone Meal Answers Many Needs

We have long expressed the opinion that bone meal would be the answer to tooth decay in America if it were given half the push fluoridation has received. Unfortunately, bone meal does not have the commercial possibilities that sodium fluoride has, as a by-product of the aluminum industry, and the result has been almost no publicity from organized medicine or industry and government. Those who have found the tooth-saving value of bone meal have had to do so in the face of hoots and snickers from friends who are uninformed, and even from doctors and dentists who should make it their business to be better informed. Aside from the undeniable fact that bone meal is a proven deterrent to tooth decay in children and adults, it is also guaranteed to be safe, even beneficial for the rest of the body. Neither of these claims can be made for fluoridation.

In all of the talk about bone meal's effect on the teeth, we sometimes neglect the other equally important values offered in bone meal. It is, after all, a stronghold of calcium, phosphorus and other minerals which are vital to every function of the body, not just the health of the teeth. We have always tried to emphasize this point, for we feel that it is a supplement everyone should be using, regardless of the state of their teeth. Here are several examples of what we mean.

An Experiment with Children

Dr. C. Cornet-Jacquemoud, writing in the Swiss journal *Modern Problems in Pediatrics* (Vol. 1, 1954), reported on his observations in the use of a bone meal product. His opinions are based upon the treatment of 123 children: 60 cases were in poor general health, but without definite pathological symptoms, 26 were children convalescing after acute illness, 22 were cases of tuberculosis, 15 were cases of delayed dentition.

The first group had poor appetite, didn't sleep well, weight and growth curve below normal, prone to chills and infections and skeletal and dental development was unsatisfactory. The ages ranged from 6 months to 10 years, 10 months. They were given powdered bone for from ½ to 3 months. (Five of the subjects could not be counted in the final appraisal: 4 cases could not be followed up accurately, and one girl, aged 21 months, refused to take the powder.) Thirty-nine of the 55 remaining cases responded very well to the treatment; 9 had satisfactory results; 7 had shown no response at the end of 3 months. That means 80 per cent of the children had a favorable response.

Many U.S. Children Afflicted

This general kind of rundown condition is one which afflicts many of our children in this age group. Anxious parents drag the children from one doctor to another trying to cure this very thing— that indefinable aspect of a child which shows him to be under par. Certainly it would be a small investment to try bone meal in such a case, especially since it presents an 80 per cent chance for a cure, and the cost is minimal. Obviously, in such cases, there is a lack of nutrients which appear to be supplied, in most cases, by bone meal.

Of the 26 children convalescing from acute infectious diseases, 18 were reported as having been successfully treated with the bone meal preparation and 6 as satisfactorily treated. In one case, the treatment was termed ineffective, and in another, a 19-month-old girl refused to take the supplement.

Concerning the tuberculosis cases which figured in this experiment, the author admits that a greater number and more time to work with them would have given a better picture of the value of the bone meal preparation, but the results as he saw them were presented. He divided the 22 patients into two groups: those with positive tuberculin reaction, but no visible symptoms and those with symptoms. Dr. Cornet-Jacquemoud's evaluation was based upon improvement of general condition, of appetite, sleep and body weight. The group with no visible lung damage, but definitely possessed of the infection, ranged in age from 2½ to 14 years, and the treatment lasted from two weeks to two months. Two cases were ruled out because of the author's inability to follow up in one instance and refusal to take the supplement in another. The results in the remaining 11 were these: 4 cases very good, 4 cases good and 3 cases no change.

Group II, the group with observable lung damage, consisted of 9 patients—16 months to 14 years. The treatment lasted for from 16 days to 7 weeks. Five cases showed "very good" response; in 2 cases, the result was "good"; in one, it was unsuccessful. The remaining case showed improvement, but the author concluded that a change of surroundings might have been responsible and so it was not included.

In the 15 cases of delayed appearance of teeth in children of 8 to 15 months, the treatment lasted for from 15 days to 12 months. Six cases showed very good results, 4 cases had good results, 3 cases did not respond to treatment and 2, suspected of irregularity in taking the powder, were disqualified.

Very Well Tolerated

Dr. Cornet-Jacquemoud remarked that the bone meal preparation was very well tolerated, and that severe side reactions have never been observed. Though he could give no definite figures as to duration of treatment, it could be assumed that, the more recent the disability, the more rapid the effect of the supplement. In any case, overdosage need not be feared, even in treatments of long duration. Of course, this is true because bone meal is a natural food, and an overdose of it would be as likely as an overdose of roast beef or lima beans.

In Europe, the value of bone meal is recognized by everyone. In the United States, it is considered a fad food. However, the Europeans are improving their health by using bone meal, and we, because we think we are so much more intelligent, are losing that opportunity.

The Safety Factor in Bone Meal
By Robert Rodale

The knowledge that bone meal contains more strontium 90 than some of the processed calcium supplements—such as calcium phosphate and calcium lactate—has raised the question in some people's minds as to whether bone meal is still a safe food supplement. Keeping in mind our policy of supplying accurate information about the food supplements we recommend, we have made a thorough study of the question of the strontium 90 content of bone meal. Later, J. I. Rodale takes up some of the general aspects of this question. However, we have found that the method with which the body metabolizes calcium and strontium 90 is of particular importance in evaluating the safety of bone meal, and warrants detailed discussion.

. First, let us look at the question of how much radiation we are now being subjected to. As we all know, the earth itself is radioactive, and has been so since the beginning of time. The amount of radiation given off by the bricks in the wall of your house and the rocks in the ground varies from 7 to 15 rads. That is called "background radiation." The amount of radiation we are receiving now from strontium 90 varies from 0.2 to 0.4 rads, or 1/17th to 1/75th of background radiation. Tolerance levels for radioactivity have been set by various scientific groups. These levels vary from 10 to 100 times background radiation. However, even the scientists who set these levels admit they are vague guides and should conceivably be set lower or higher.

Strontium 90 in Food

Now, let's proceed to the matter of how much strontium 90 is in the food that we eat. The figures I present to you will be in the form of "strontium units." A strontium unit is one micromicrocurie of strontium 90 per gram of calcium in the item of food. Note that strontium is only measured in terms of calcium. That is a clue to the very close relationship between strontium and calcium that I will discuss later. Actually, strontium and calcium are known as "sister" elements and strontium 90 associates quickly with calcium.

Bone meal, according to our tests and tests made by others, contains about 5 to 20 strontium units. Here are figures for other foods, as reported in the issue of *Science* magazine for July, 1958:

PEAS	21.3	BROCCOLI	8.5
BEANS, CUT GREEN	18.4	OKRA	18.0
BEANS, CUT GREEN	8.6	BRUSSELS SPROUTS	12.0
BEANS, WAX	11.3	CAULIFLOWER	22.5
CORN	28.4	WHEAT (N.Y.)	22.8
SWEET POTATOES	13.3	WHEAT (UNKNOWN)	37.5
LIMA BEANS	8.4		

Note that bone meal has a considerably lower amount of strontium 90 per gram of calcium than any of the common vegetables and grains noted in the above list. Milk is currently running about 10 strontium units and meat about 20 units.

Confusion about bone meal and its strontium 90 content has arisen from the fact that some people have assumed that total strontium 90 *intake* is related to total strontium 90 *retention* by the body. Even though bone meal does contain smaller amounts of strontium 90 than other foods, these people say, the fact that bone meal is so rich in calcium means that the body takes in a lot of strontium, too. However, that is not a correct assumption. It has been demonstrated conclusively that the human body discriminates against strontium in favor of calcium. There are two reasons for this favoring of calcium over strontium. First, calcium passes through the walls of the gastrointestinal tract faster than strontium. Second, a larger proportion of strontium than calcium is excreted in the urine.

Experts' Opinions on Bone Meal

Therefore, in evaluating the effect that a certain food will have on the actual *retention* of strontium 90 by the human body, it is far more important to consider the ratio of strontium to calcium in that food than it is to try to add up the total amount of strontium that will be consumed. A man who has done much pioneer work in uncovering this preference by the human and animal body for calcium over strontium is Professor Robert H. Wasserman of the Department of Physical Biology, New York State Veterinary College, Cornell University. In order to help clarify this concept in your mind, I will quote from a letter from him replying to my inquiry about his work:

"There are processes in the mammalian system that distinguish between these elements (calcium and strontium) such that the overall effect is to reduce the strontium 90 concentration in the body. Observations have led to the conclusion that the retention of strontium 90 is more related to the strontium 90 to calcium ratio in the diet than to the absolute amount of strontium 90. In other words, the degree of strontium 90 deposition is better assessed by thinking in terms of the strontium units per gram of calcium rather than the strontium units per gram of diet. Thus, although bone meal may be relatively high in strontium 90, it is also high in calcium content; therefore, the strontium 90 calcium ratio in bone meal may actually be lower than in other foods, especially plant sources of calcium. For example, the current levels of strontium 90 in milk (Public Health Service report, July, 1961) are running about 10 strontium units. From our own data on the comparative metabolism of calcium and strontium, it can be calculated that the strontium 90 concentration in bone would then be roughly 20 units. Meat from these same animals would then contain roughly 20 strontium units also. In the same report, I see that Canadian wheat averaged about 90 strontium units. Since the deposition of strontium 90 (in the body) is related to the strontium to calcium ratio, the addition of strontium 90 in the form of bone meal may not appreciably change the strontium to calcium ratio of diet and, therefore, the amount of strontium 90 deposited per unit of bone mass would be essentially unchanged."

Another scientist who has done work on the metabolism of calcium and strontium in the human body is Professor George K. Davis, Director of Nuclear Activities at the University of Florida in Gainesville. Here is an excerpt from a letter from him dated September 13, 1961: "It is true that much of the strontium in bone meal will not be deposited in the bones of a human, because of the high level of calcium present in the bone meal and the selective action which the body has against strontium 90. I would recommend bone meal as a source of calcium and phosphorus in the diet."

Whole Wheat High in Strontium 90

One food which is likely to cause the most strontium 90 to be retained by the human body is whole wheat. As you saw from the list of foods presented above, wheat rates among the highest foods in strontium content. And some wheat contains even higher amounts —such as the Canadian wheat with 90 strontium units reported by Dr. Wasserman. But the significant thing about wheat is that it does not have the high calcium value of a food like bone meal, so therefore, does not offer the body as good a chance to select the calcium and reject the strontium. It is interesting that white flour contains less strontium than whole wheat flour, because the wheat husks which are exposed to air-borne strontium are removed when grain is processed into white flour.

Analyses of normal diets for strontium value have been made by different organizations, and the relatively high strontium content of wheat has been noted. However, even those values have not been considered worrisome at this time—for two reasons: (1) the strontium 90 content of wheat is still low in comparison with background radiation; (2) the average person gets only about 3 per cent of his diet from whole wheat products. Although we do not recommend wheat products, there are many health-minded people who consider whole wheat to be one of the healthiest of all foods and whole wheat accounts for far more than 3 per cent of their diet. If strontium 90 ever becomes more of a factor in our diet, these people should perhaps consider reducing the amount of whole wheat products they consume.

There has been a lot of talk about the use of strontium 90-free calcium pills to protect yourself against strontium 90 retention. Linus

Pauling, the famed atomic scientist, has been the primary advocate of that method. Since limestone provides abundant supplies of calcium below the surface of the earth and hence, free of strontium 90 contamination, it is possible to make strontium 90-free calcium pills— either by using raw ground limestone itself or processed forms of limestone, such as calcium phosphate.

Another material with interesting possibilities as a calcium source low in strontium 90 is fish bone meal. While it is true that the oceans do contain measurable amounts of strontium 90, the calcium content of sea water provides fish with the means to reject from their bodily systems much of the strontium 90 they do take in. One sample of fish bone meal we had analyzed showed a content of less than one third of a strontium unit. Therefore, it contained 1/15th as much strontium as animal bone meal rated at 5 strontium units. However, we do not feel that anything definite can be assumed based on this one analysis, and are now proceeding with a program of analyzing more samples of the bones of different types of ocean fish.

In summary, bone meal is still a safe source of calcium and phosphorus. Its ratio of strontium 90 to calcium is lower than that for most other foods, and according to the most commonly accepted scientific thought, it is that ratio which is significant in determining how much strontium 90 is actually retained in the human system.

Is the Strontium 90 (Fall-Out) in Bone Meal Dangerous?

By J. I. Rodale

In the August, 1961, issue of Consumer Reports, published at Mount Vernon, New York, there appeared an article entitled "Calcium Tablets and Strontium 90" which discussed the quantities of strontium 90 in various forms of calcium products. Strontium 90 is the fall-out from atomic explosions, and some scientists predict that, in the future, it may become a factor in causing leukemia, or cancer of the blood, and mutations or stillbirths in the human race.

This Consumer Reports project chose bone meal as a sort of whipping boy and compared it with 3 straight calcium products from the point of view of strontium 90 content, and this is what they found:

DICALCIUM PHOSPHATE	0.1	CALCIUM LACTATE	0.2
CALCIUM GLUCONATE	0.3	BONE MEAL	4.9

The bone meal showed, on the average, 20 times more strontium 90 than the 3 other products. The question now arises, on the basis of this Consumer Reports test, shall we discontinue taking bone meal?

We cannot substitute either or all the other 3 products for bone meal. It would be like taking refined white sugar rather than the whole sugar cane. Bone meal contains rare mineral elements and other substances that science has as yet not discovered. Bone meal will reduce the number of cavities in the teeth to the vanishing point; it will strengthen all the bones of the body; it will make the work of the heart easier by regulating the pulse; it will do many other things.

This *Consumer Reports* article has been read by some people taking bone meal who have written us that they are worried. I say, don't worry! Don't forego taking one of the most valuable food supplements just because *Consumer Reports* says so.

Let us take a look at this *Consumer Reports* organization!

Two Magazines

There are two *consumer* types of magazine. One is the *Consumer Reports,* that we are discussing, published at Mount Vernon, New York. The other is the *Consumer Bulletin,* published at Washington, New Jersey. The one we are dealing with, *Consumer Reports,* has consistently fought us, while the *Consumer Bulletin* has been very friendly to our cause. For example, the latter, in its August, 1961, issue, said, "Especially objectionable is the close tie between the food trades and researchers in nutritional science." Doesn't this sound like something we would say? The Washington, New Jersey, outfit has also been fighting the use of chemical additives in foods.

But the Mount Vernon organization has been practically always in line with our opposition—the scientists and food companies—and intimated that anyone who follows a system such as ours is a food faddist or even worse. A typical giveaway, right in the very article we are attacking, is their statement, "Indeed CU (*Consumer Reports*) believes that, since bone-derived tablets have no advantage over those derived from minerals, manufacturers probably should not use bone at all." This is the most unscientific statement I have heard in a long time. It completely disregards many medical researches done specifically with bone meal which show its superiority over straight calcium products.

For example, in the *Canadian Medical Association Journal* of June, 1944, there is reported a case of a child complaining of growing pains who was given dicalcium phosphate, one of the products tested by *Consumer Reports,* and it gave no results. Then they gave him bone meal and in one week, he was playing as hard as any of his schoolmates. Another item, reported in the *Canadian Medical Association Journal* (June, 1944), concerns an experiment with pregnant women, some given bone meal, others a regular calcium product (dicalcium phosphate). The bone meal women suffered no dental neuralgia, nor had aching legs nor leg cramps at night, nor on delivery, and had practically no cavities, but not so the women on the dicalcium phosphate.

Any Danger in Added Calcium?

The *Consumer Reports* publication takes another vicious swing at us when it says, "Some scientists point out that added calcium may upset the body's nutritional balance and even bring on such ailments as kidney stones." Actually, the average American is calcium-deficient and is excreting calcium all the time. Any excess would be excreted.

But Dr. Henry C. Sherman of Columbia University has done many experiments in his laboratory showing that amounts of calcium far above the generally accepted minimum not only do no harm, but actually make for a longer and healthier life. He says: "Extended pathological investigation has shown that doubling a normal food calcium intake did not increase the incidence of abnormal calcification in the body, as of arterial walls or other tissues."

Dr. Clive McCay of Cornell University takes up the question of whether or not hardening of the arteries and calcium deposits in the kidneys can be caused by too much calcium in the diet. Readers have asked us this question and we are glad to repeat here exactly what Dr. McCay has to say on the subject (and remember, please that Dr. McCay is one of the world's outstanding authorities on nutrition): "In the course of two decades of research with rats, we have seen groups at the time of death with heavily calcified arteries and kidneys while parallel groups were relatively free. This calcification of soft tissues was due to unknown variables in the diet and could never be related to dietary calcium."

Here is an excerpt from the *American Journal of Clinical Nutrition* (September, 1961), by Dr. D. Mark Hegsted: "It seems to me that calcium intake cannot be the only etiologic (causative) factor in renal stones. There are many areas in the world where calcium intake is low but renal stones are common."

Yet *Consumer Reports* says that an excess of calcium can cause kidney stones. This is a common fallacy and can be forgiven in the common man, but not in an organization that so many persons look to for correct scientific information. We must consider this when we analyze supposedly scientific statements made by *Consumer Reports*.

Tolerance Levels Unknown

Its statements are so shaky and uncertain. For example, it says, "No one knows for certain at what level the accumulation of strontium 90 in food and bone becomes a danger." The article states that even the *Journal of the American Medical Association* begged the question regarding the use of calcium as an antidote to strontium. It says, "There remain many unknowns concerning the possible dangers of radioactive fall-out . . ." Finally no one seems to be certain what effect the accumulation of strontium 90 may have over many years.

In a second article on the subject (October, 1961), *Consumer Reports* said, "It is feared that strontium 90 held for years in the bones may possibly cause bone cancer and leukemia, although there is no proof as yet that such is the case . . . this radioactive substance has not been with us long enough for anyone to evaluate the long-range effects in terms of the human life span." It also says, "As with most other aspects of fall-out hazard, the many gaps in scientific knowledge make anything more than educated guesses impossible."

I have gone through much so-called scientific data, and one nuclear scientist says one thing while another says completely the opposite. Nobody knows! I never saw so much misinformation and conflict on any one subject I have ever investigated.

The general effects of strontium 90 were studied at a meeting at Colorado State University in September, 1961, at which were present most of the authorities in this field, and I think that Dr. P. S. Henshaw, an Atomic Energy Commission biophysicist, reflected what I think is the best generalization on the subject. He said that it is not known whether the suggested tolerance levels of radiation are too conservative, too liberal or *"even whether they may be beneficial to life."* Wouldn't that be something—a condition that one thinks is harmful could turn out to be beneficial?

Dr. Henshaw speaks about background radiation levels—the radiation that is in the atmosphere and that we are breathing in all the time. He said, "Tolerance levels have been set in the range of 10 to 100 times background radiation levels. Based on observations of animals' manifest vigor, it is believed that lasting injury is produced by daily exposures substantially more than 1,000 times background level."

Here is the statement of Dr. John N. Wolfe, head of the Atomic Energy Commission's Environmental Science Branch, made at this Colorado meeting: "At the radiation levels thus far measured, we can find no biological effects on man or the plant and animal life on which his existence depends."

Here is a third statement, made by Dr. Francis J. Weber, chief of the service's radiological health division: "The amount of radioactivity found in food, water and the air has been running well under the safe levels."

The Hiroshima Effect

I think what confuses the situation is the effect of the original atom bomb blast at Hiroshima. I will call this the Hiroshima effect. For example, studies recently made at Hiroshima and Nagasaki show that there have been significant changes in the sex ratio of children born to the survivors. There may have been increases in other undesirable mutations in the newly born, but this is caused by exposure to hundreds of thousands of times the safe exposure levels—not the insignificant amounts of fall-out that we find in our food and water.

A scientist exposes daphnia (a type of very small fresh-water animal) to excessive amounts of radiation, which affects the birth rate. They subject trees to excessive amounts of radiation and they drop their leaves earlier. The public reads about these experiments and becomes frightened, but these experiments in no wise parallel the conditions under which we consume strontium 90 in our food and drinking water and in the air we breathe. They are the Hiroshima type of effect.

In Nevada in 1945, during atomic tests, the effects on cattle were studied. Of a herd of 100 cattle, 60 were subjected to varying amounts of radiation; 40 were not. At the end of 4 years, the 60 exposed to radiation weighed 100 pounds less (about 16 per cent) than the 40 that were not exposed, and there were more deaths among them. But this is in the Hiroshima category. It doesn't approach anywhere near our problem.

It is like the toxic effect of taking vitamin A. Consume it up to about 100,000 units a day and you are safe. Take 400,000 units a day and it will have toxic effects, although with regard to strontium 90, the gap between danger and no danger is infinitely greater.

Russia's Tests

Many persons became worried by the resumption of Russian nuclear tests, many of them made inside Russia, one of them in the Novaya Zembla region. The fall-out from one of them was wafted by the winds to eastern Finland and such Soviet cities as Murmansk and Leningrad. A U.S. Weather Bureau top expert on fall-out said that the Russians timed the shots in complete disregard of wind conditions.

Here's an item from the *Journal of the American Medical Association* (175/9, 821, March, 1961) to the effect that grain imported from the Soviet Union into England had at least 5 times more strontium 90 than grain which is imported from the United States.

Now is Russia crazy? Are they deliberately trying to destroy their own people? The answer must be that Russia knows much more about fall-out than our scientists know. They are ahead of us in space science, and this has probably led to research in radiation and fall-out, which has led to advanced knowledge in the effects of strontium 90 on people. It is interesting to note that one of the latest defectees from Russia was a scientist who said he was not free in Russia to work out a method for removing strontium 90 from the human body. Perhaps, the Russians feel such a method is not necessary. Of course, this is my own personal opinion, and you are entitled to yours. And I do not suggest that atomic tests should continue.

Experiments on Dogs

This question of strontium 90 in bone meal is not new to me. It has been constantly on my mind for several years. But what made me confident that we needn't worry about its effect on people, was its effect on dogs. Here, I thought, is the perfect experiment with exact results. Dogs breed at least once a year. Thus, since Hiroshima, there have been about 20 generations of dogs. Have they been affected? This question is significant, especially since, according to Dr. Clive McCay of Cornell, most dogs consume one to five per cent by weight of bone meal in their diet and have not been affected. Dr. McCay has one to two hundred dogs under observation at all times.

But there is another factor that is affecting dogs—which we must not confuse with strontium 90—and that is the artificiality of breeding pedigreed dogs. Increasing numbers of pedigreed dogs are suffering from hereditary abnormalities, but "much of this trouble," says Mr. S. F. J. Hodgman, of the Canine Health Center, London, "has been caused by man's deliberate and persistent breeding of animals of unnatural shapes and sizes merely to satisfy the whims of fashion." But you will not find this condition prevailing in mongrel dogs, or in decently bred pedigreed dogs.

In connection with the symposium of radio-ecology recently held at Colorado State University, marine biologists stated that no genetic abnormalities had been noted in fish examined during the studies, and they breed every year. I haven't heard of genetic difficulties in the breeding of chinchillas and the prolific rabbit. In my walks in the country, I see hundreds of rabbits, but never one who limps or who has 5 legs.

The French are great users of bones. There is the witticism, "Lend a Frenchman a bone for an hour and he will make a soup out of it; lend it to him for 3 hours and he will create a banquet; *give* it to him and he will open a restaurant." According to some opinions of fall-out dangers, the French should be dying of cancer and leukemia like flies.

Amounts of Strontium 90 in Foods

Now let us go back to *Consumer Reports'* comparison of the amounts of strontium 90 in the 4 products, in which the bone meal had 20 times more strontium 90 than the straight calcium products. That is a lot of strontium 90 if you measure it per gram of calcium in the product, but when you measure it against the fact that the bone meal tablets are so tiny, while the foods we eat are so bulky, then the presence of the percentage of strontium 90 in bone meal doesn't mean much. For example, think of 6 tiny tablets of bone meal against the amount of milk some persons drink a day (and they get it also in bread, ice cream, cheese and many other food products as well), and you can see that we must look at it objectively.

In an article in *Science* (July, 1958), there were printed some charts listing the strontium 90 contained in various foods. Bear in mind that the *Consumer Reports* of Mount Vernon gave the average strontium 90 of bone meal as 4.9. For ease of reference, let us call this 5. But look at the comparisons with other food covered in the *Science* article:

PEAS	21.3	BROCCOLI	8.5
BEANS CUT GREEN	18.4	OKRA	18.0
BEANS CUT GREEN	8.6	BRUSSELS SPROUTS	12.0
BEANS, WAX	11.3	CAULIFLOWER	22.5
CORN	28.4	WHEAT (N.Y.)	22.8
SWEET POTATOES	13.3	WHEAT (UNKNOWN)	37.5
LIMA BEANS	8.4		

Of course, an adjustment must be made for the amounts of calcium in each of these foods, for it is in the calcium that the strontium 90 is contained. But, considering everything, according to my calculations, one gets 9 to 10 times more strontium from sources other than bone meal. We get a lot of it from the air, not only in breathing it in, but through our skin. This occurs 24 hours a day.

I gave this mathematical problem to two persons—one who is against bone meal, and one who is for it. The one who is against it figured it that way, and came up with a bad set of statistics. The other one's calculations turned out well for our side. These figures are so tricky that they require a professional atomic physicist-mathematician to come up with correct figures, and I'm sure that even then, some other scientists will knock holes in them. You would imagine that 2 + 2 = 4, but not in reference to strontium 90.

We had the same trouble with the amount of fluoride in bone meal. They put only one part per million of fluoride in water in an attempt to reduce dental caries, but in bone meal there is 200 to 300 parts per million of fluoride. But aside from the fact that, in bone meal, the fluoride is in the safer form of calcium fluoride, whereas in the water they use the highly soluble sodium fluoride, when we figured the large amounts of water a person drinks and the small volume of 6 tiny bone meal tablets he takes a day, the amount turned out to be the same in both cases—but with the safety factor that, in the bone meal, it was calcium, not sodium, fluoride.

Eliminating Foods High in Strontium 90

Let us look at another factor. If one follows our system, he naturally eliminates most of the foods that are extremely high in strontium 90. The system completely rules out all milk and dairy products of every kind. It also says "no" to all wheat, rye and barley grains in whatever form they come—bread, cereals, noodles, etc.

According to the second *Consumer Reports* article (October, 1961), "In the 1959 study, CU learned through separate analyses of milk from 8 cities that this food was contributing slightly more than half of the total strontium intake." This statement is backed up by one in *Science,* for September, 1957: "In the U.S., it is estimated that 70 to 80 per cent of the dietary calcium comes from dairy products," and it is in the calcium that strontium 90 is found.

Wheat, we know, also looms large in the human diet, varying widely between individuals, and you can see from the figures already given that it is extremely high in strontium 90, but being low in calcium, it provides only about 3 per cent of the total diet of strontium 90. This is a figure given by *Consumer Reports,* and I would like to see it checked. It looks too low for my money.

Here is another reduction-factor effect of our system. We are against the use of table salt, and yet salt picks up radioactive fall-out in large quantity. We have been taught that strontium 90 is found only tied in with calcium, and yet table salt *has* no calcium. It is sodium chloride. But here is a quotation from the Swiss magazine *Wendepunkt* (August, 1961) which will muddy the issue for us: "In the case of mankind, textbooks and tables teach that he needs about 10 grams of table salt daily. Since natural foods contribute hardly more than two grams a day, salt is therefore an indispensable necessity. However, since salt picks up radioactive fall-out *in large quantity,* L. K. Dahl, M.D., was commissioned by the Atomic Energy Commission of the United States several years ago to investigate thoroughly the salt needs of men. Atomic warfare could easily make the salt supply impossible for any long period of time. Dahl was amazed to find that the question had hardly ever been investigated." The Dahl study showed that man needed no more than ½ gram of salt a day, instead of 10, and that natural foodstuffs per day of diet contain about two grams. So, salt attracts a goodly amount of fall-out material, and we do not use it.

Still another item—eggs! We have always recommended them highly, even to heart cases. Dr. George K. Davis of the University of Florida claims that the strontium 90 of the egg goes to the shell, and the egg itself is pretty low in this substance.

So, in the health sytem we recommend, we consume no dairy products, eat no bread, take no salt and eat eggs, all of which are important factors in substantially lowering strontium 90 in the diet.

Protection through Proper Foods

Now let's discuss another aspect of our problem. As the *Consumer Reports* article said, some person can·be affected by strontium 90, while others will be affected far less, or not at all. This is where a system of good diet comes in.

The fact that, through the diet, people can protect themselves even from the worst diseases, is demonstrated by the work of Kinusita, the Japanese pathologist, working at the Memorial Hospital, New York, who has shown that, when rats are fed an adequate, well-balanced diet, the ingestion of a cancer-producing substance known as "butter yellow" is innocuous. However, when the rats are maintained upon an inadequate diet, especially lacking in vitamins, the ingestion of this chemical causes inflammatory changes in the liver followed by cancer of this organ.

The best protection against all cantaminants, whether chemical additives in food, chlorine in drinking water, pollution in the air or strontium 90, is to follow a healthful diet. If you say, "Mr. Rodale, I don't see eye to eye with you on everything," then don't hold me responsible if something unexpected happens. This means walking at least an hour every day. If you take one-a-day capsules and don't supplement them with the vitamins and minerals needed in larger quantities, then you are not seeing eye to eye with me. But first you will have to prove to me, with conclusive clinical evidence, that the strontium 90 in bone meal is dangerous. It has not been proven.

I would like to discuss another factor about bone meal. If you will check the amount of strontium 90 per milligram of calcium, you will find that in bone meal, it is far less than in the average food. However, bone meal has much more calcium. But the fact that in bread, the calcium attracts far more strontium 90 than the same amount of calcium in bone meal would seem to indicate, perhaps, that there is something about the calcium in bone meal, possibly the kind of compound that it is a part of, that has some significance. I would like to have *Consumer Reports* explain this to my untutored mind.

Another thought: Is it possible that it is a good thing that strontium 90 is held locked in the calcium? This may be a method the body uses to prevent it from going into other compounds where it could do immediate harm. This should be investigated, but it would probably require a complex and expensive series of experiments.

Magnesium in Bone Meal

I have purposely withheld my most potent ammunition to the end, and that is the large amount of magnesium in bone meal. Bone meal is very rich in magnesium, whereas milk is not. Bone meal has about ¾ of one per cent of magnesium, which is an enormous amount as far as magnesium goes. It is 73/10,000 of the bone, whereas the magnesium in milk is only 14/100,000, or a minuscule amount in comparison.

Magnesium is a terribly neglected item in nutrition . . . I have accumulated a large amount of clinical information to show how valuable it is in heart disease, polio, cancer and many other diseases. Right now, I wish to speak of magnesium's effect in cancer. Since bone meal carries this valuable antidote (magnesium) against cancer in such a liberal amount, it must be considered as an item of the utmost importance in our daily diet. At the same time, I refute completely any possibility that bone meal in any way can be a leukemia or a general cancer causer.

The evidence I submit is from my booklet entitled CANCER: CAN IT BE PREVENTED?, published in 1950. Here is the pertinent information about cancer:

"We will talk about the researches of Professor P. Schrumpf-Pierron, whose work is written up in the *Bulletin de l'Institut d'Egypte,* Vol. XIV, 1932, and February 15, 1932, and others. He talks about the rarity of cancer in Egypt where malignant cases are only about one-tenth that of Europe. What is the cause? After exhaustive studies and research, the Professor came to the conclusion that it was due to too much potassium and too little magnesium in the food of Europeans. On the other hand, in the soils of Egypt the conditions are reversed; that is, more magnesium in relation to the potassium.

"There seems to be a definite relationship between magnesium and potash wherever it is found, whether in the soils, rocks or other places. Where there is an oversupply of potash there is always an undersupply of magnesium and vice versa. Schrumpf-Pierron studied the cancer statistics for France in relation to the rock structure underlying its soils. It worked most uncannily. Wherever he found an excess of potash, there he discovered less magnesium and more human cancer cases. Wherever he observed a minimum of potash, he found a maximum of magnesium and fewer cancer cases. This means that people who eat food raised in certain soils that obtained their nutriments from the rocks which underlie them, get certain elements into their foods because of this. Such a condition would apply more to France than to the United States, because in a country like France, there would be more of a tendency to consume food near the point where it is raised. But in the United States, with our more advanced industrial conditions, where even the poorer peoples will eat winter vegetables raised in California, Florida and elsewhere, and a great deal of citrus foods, etc., and meats that are shipped long distances, local deficiencies and unbalancings of nutritional elements may tend to be corrected to a certain extent.

"When Schrumpf-Pierron found that an excess of potassium in the rocks of a region tied in with an excess of cancer in that section, we should note that excess potassium means excess carbohydrates in plants grown there and, therefore, reduced protein in the foods. Farmers should know that it is best, therefore, to use dolomitic limestone when they apply lime, because it is rich in magnesium and acts as a safety factor in relation to the potash in the soil."

In connection with this information, let me stress that potassium is not a factor in cancer. On the contrary, potash compounds have been given as a medication in cancer. But evidently, the reason Schrumpf-Pierron found more cancer in regions where the soil abounded in potassium was because of the low magnesium in such soils.

Other Researchers See Magnesium-Cancer Correlation

Schrumpf-Pierron was not the only one who found a correlation between a deficiency of magnesium and an increase of cancer. I will quote from *Cancer and Diet,* by F. L. Hoffman, of the Biochemical Research Foundation of the Franklin Institute, Philadelphia, 1937): "The question is raised with regard to the deficiency of magnesium in the soil in regions subject to a high cancer death rate which cannot be disposed of without evidence to the contrary. I feel strongly that the suggestions made to this effect are deserving of being followed up, particularly the work of Robinet (1930) in the Rhine districts, as published in the Bulletin of the French Association for the Study of Cancer. Also, corresponding studies made by him in Italy are indicative of a correlation too pronounced to be ignored. For example, he shows that in the province of Ravenna, with . . . no magnesium in the soil, the proportion of deaths from cancer in one thousand deaths from all causes was 96.77. In the province of Rome, with a magnesium content of 0.08, the proportion of cancer deaths was 46.90. In the province of Cagliari, with a magnesium content of 0.25 the cancer proportion was 14.0."

In reference to Robinet's study of cancer in England and Wales there was a discussion by Dukes in the April, 1932, issue of the *Cancer Review,* in which the following appeared: "There appears to be marked association between a low cancer mortality and the presence of magnesium in the soil."

Hoffman in *Cancer and Diet* writes further: "In 1932, the *Journal of Cancer* published a brief note on the treatment of cancer with magnesium chloride, by Henri Dufour, according to which the course of the neoplasm (cancer) was retarded considerably as the result of magnesium treatment, but the observation was based on only two patients."

Incidentally, at this period, in which many medical workers were getting results in cancer with magnesium, the whole magnesium idea was being ridiculed and fought by "orthodox" members of the medical profession, which is probably the reason why it is not used today in cancer research. Here is a scandal if I ever smelled one.

Hoffman mentions 4 or 5 other physicians who obtained results in cancer with magnesium, but always he cites other doctors who find this or that wrong with the experiments, just as they do today with Krebiozen, Koch, Droznes-Lazenby and others who have records of curing cancer.

I am not through with the subject of magnesium, but so much for this time. And please remember that bone meal is extremely rich in it.

Opinions of Scientists

I now would like to present the opinions of a few scientists on the subject of strontium 90 in bone meal. I wrote to Dr. Alfred Aslander, head of the Division of Agriculture of the Royal Institute of Technology in Stockholm, Sweden. He was the one who introduced the idea of bone meal for human consumption into Sweden. Here is his reply, dated August 18, 1961:

"Our Scientists over here have declared that the content of strontium 90 in bone meal is too small to be dangerous. Our Royal Medical Board recommends bone meal for children. An analysis of January 4, 1961, shows that one liter of milk (a little more than ¼ of a gallon) contains as much strontium 90 as 3 grammes of bone meal (1/10 troy ounce of bone meal). The daily dose of bone meal is about one gramme, so we are getting more strontium 90 in our milk consumption than in bone meal. And then we must consider all our other foods. All foods contain strontium 90.

"The real trouble is that our analytical methods are so sensitive. It is possible to determine such minute doses of strontium 90 and other radioactive matter that some people get nervous. At present, there is—according to our scientists—no danger. I, my children and their children are going to continue to take bone meal. We trust our scientists!

"Water is very dangerous if it is 10 feet deep, but you may without risk walk in the dew, even with bare feet!!!!!

"As far as I understand the situation, the hysteria about strontium 90 was started by the anti-atomic-bomb association. And it would be a good thing if it would be possible to stop the manufacturing of atomic bombs. But it would be still better if the bombs were stopped by sound arguments, not by hysteria."

"One of the Finest Foods"

I wrote also to Dr. Melvin E. Page, who conducts one of the most unusual laboratories in the world, dealing with the chemistry of the human body. It is located in St. Petersburg, Florida. He replied, "I think probably the only way not to get any strontium 90 is not to eat, but, as it is generally accepted that calcium in a way nullifies the action of strontium 90, and some even recommend calcium as an antidote for strontium 90, then I would think that bone meal possibly is one of the finest foods we have . . .

"You and I both know that bone meal is far ahead of dicalcium phosphate. I like the statement in your letter that bone meal, consisting of about 30 per cent calcium, would seem to carry its own medicine for the elimination of strontium 90.

". . . the more efficient the person's body chemistry, the greater his ability to defend himself. The less efficient his body chemistry, the less ability he has to defend himself against anything. This should apply to strontium as well as almost anything else."

Will Continue to Take Bone Meal

My wife and I have taken bone meal since about 1945, and we're going to continue to take it. The 11 other persons in our family, our 3 children, their spouses and their children have been taking bone meal and will continue to take it. *Consumer Reports* should worry more about the more than 100 chemical additives that are put in our food every day, that are the cancer-causers, and not put the dust into the public eyes with this red herring scare bugaboo of bone meal.

Bone meal has been a miracle in my life. It has practically stopped the formation of all tooth cavities. It has helped to regulate my pulse, and therefore is of extreme importance to my heart condition. It has strengthened my bones against fracture as proven by two serious accidents which did not even result in the tiniest scratch in any bone. When I asked my daughter Nina what her attitude was on the subject, she said, "Stop bone meal? Never. Whenever I have done so, my nails started to go to pieces." And when nails start to go to pieces, it is not just the nails. This is merely one symptom, and shows that there is something seriously at fault generally in the body.

In conclusion, think of Dr. McCay's Cornell dogs, some of whose diet is 5 per cent by weight of bone meal per day. My daily diet weighs about 3¼ pounds and my 6 bone meal tablets weigh about a gram; 1/1500 of *my* diet per day is bone meal. The way I figure it is that those 5 per cent dogs are eating about 80 times more bone meal per day than I am, with no ill effects.

Breast Feeding

New Help for Nursing Mothers

By Niles Newton, Ph.D.

EDITOR'S NOTE: *The following is an article which appeared in* Child-Family Digest *(October, 1960) written by a distinguished author* (Family Book of Child Care), *teacher, mother and pioneer in the field of educating the modern American mother to the physical and psychological advantages of breast feeding. We believe that mother's milk is the safest and most desirable food for an infant, and we hope that Dr. Newton's brief recapitulation of the functions involved and the results to be expected will lead new or expectant mothers to investigate further the aptly termed "art" of breast feeding.*

"We never try to convert anybody," said Mary White as she cuddled 4-month-old little Mary to her breast. "We started our League to help mothers who *want* to learn about the womanly art of breast feeding.

"And what a lot of mothers there are looking for the kind of help and encouragement we give them!"

The La Leche League of Franklin Park near Chicago was founded less than 4 years ago, yet now League mothers are getting from 3 to 4 thousand letters a year and countless phone calls for help. At present, La Leche groups offer instruction for mothers at 19 different locations with new ones being added regularly.

It all started with a conversation between two nursing mothers at a picnic for families. Tall, slim Mary White with flashing dark eyes was talking to Marian Tompson, a petite, pretty woman with auburn hair. They report the conversation went something like this:

"How easy to take a nursing baby on a picnic!"

"No bottles, no fuss and bother. Isn't it too bad more mothers can't nurse their babies?"

"So many of the girls have said they envy us for the easy way we feed our babies and for the way we seem to enjoy it."

"Some of them have tried and failed. Why can't somebody do something to help them?"

"Why can't we . . .?"

And so the idea of the League was born.

Both Mary White and Marian Tompson knew from experience how much help and encouragement can mean to a mother struggling to breast feed her baby. Mary got her help from her husband, Gregory. Greg was away in service when Mary tried to feed Joe, their first baby. Joe was put on both breast and bottle.

"You know what that means," said Mary. "You start out with a little bit of formula in the bottle and pretty soon you are putting more and more formula in it."

When Bill, the White's second son, was born, Greg was home.

"Breast feeding to me just seems like the natural thing to do," explained Greg. Through his constant praise and encouragement, Mary learned the art of successful breast feeding so that their Bill, Peggy, Katie, Anne, Regina, Mike and now Mary have been fed without the need for bottles.

Marian had her breast feeding troubles another way. She managed to breast feed her first little girl, Melanie, for several months. When Deborah arrived, however, she was told with great finality, "Your milk will go away if you have another little one at home." So, of course, it did after 6 weeks, because her confidence in breast feeding had been lost.

By the time Allison came along Marian nursed her only a week and then went through weeks of formula troubles.

But when Marian's fourth little girl, Laurel, was born, she had happily found a doctor who encouraged breast feeding and a good friend, Mary White, whom she could phone anytime her old doubts and fears came back again. She no longer felt alone in her struggle to feed her babies naturally. Laurel and then later, Sheila and Brian were fed without bottles.

Marian and Mary, together with 5 other mothers, Edwina Froehlich, Betty Wagner, Mary Ann Cahill, Viola Lennon and Mary Ann Kerwin formed the first La Leche League. Altogether, these 7 mothers had breast fed babies for a total of 287 months or almost 24 years. They know from practical experience the problems a mother faces when she tries to breast feed, and how to overcome them.

At first, the League confined itself to studying research on breast feeding, reading aloud to each other all the medical information they could find. They brought friends interested in breast feeding to the meetings.

As their experience grew, they developed a series of meetings open to anybody in the community who was interested. The series of 5 meetings with lectures covers all aspects of breast feeding, touch on pregnancy, childbirth, family nutrition and emphasize the need for a new philosophy of mothering.

"Resign yourself to a more easy-going kind of life," League mothers explain. "When your baby is in your womb, he knows only YOU. Then he is born and suddenly loses YOU. No doubt his early crying is more from this sense of loss of YOU than from hunger. When you hold him close and nurse him, you give him what he needs most. You mean much more to your baby than a clean white bed, snug warm covers or the right temperature for the room. YOU are your baby's whole world the first few months of life."

The last meeting of the series is a "Fathers Only" night. A physician who is a well-known speaker on marriage and family life leads a discussion on "Fathering." "Fathering" is very important from the League's point of view in creating the type of home where breast feeding flourishes.

"That doesn't mean being an assistant housekeeper, however!" the League hastens to explain. "Fathers can help most by giving praise and moral support and by being dependable protectors and providers. We have seen mothers overcome terrific obstacles including extreme lack of confidence in themselves because of a sympathetic and encouraging husband."

There is, however, much more to these League meetings than just the topics covered.

I attended a meeting of the Franklin Park group at LaVerne Bollig's smart new home. Chairs were arranged in a big circle. I could hardly believe my eyes when I saw nine babies snuggling in their mother's arms. Most of the other women in the room were pregnant.

We went around the room introducing ourselves and telling about our breast feeding experiences. One tall girl, who looked like a model, told how she had bottle fed her first 3. Then she saw her neighbor, helped by the League, breast feeding her baby happily. She decided to give it a try and here she was, her 3-week-old breast fed baby on her lap, eager to learn more about the various aspects of breast feeding.

Some other mothers present were nursing their first baby, or expecting their first baby, but a good number were mothers of 3, 4, 6 and even 9 children who had had trouble breast feeding and wanted to have a better experience this time.

Young breast fed babies are in need of frequent comforting sucking, so that during the course of the evening most of the babies were unobtrusively nursed. Thus, the mothers attending the meeting had a little practical demonstration of what their great grandmothers saw all around them throughout their growing-up years. Example is a potent teaching tool.

"The meetings were so successful they multiplied like an amoeba," explained Betty Wagner. The League prefers to have groups of no more than 12 to 15 mothers. This way they can keep the personal touch as well as serve delicious refreshments. When the groups get too large, they split into two. Half the experienced mothers meet with each group.

Meanwhile, others, mothers in other cities, began to hear of the League and intensified their activities. For instance, in Cleveland, Martha Pugacz, a breast feeding mother of 5, had been helping other mothers on an individual basis for years. She began writing letters to the editors when the newspapers published material on breast feeding and similar subjects. Each time a letter by her was published, she received calls from women who needed help with breast feeding. When she learned of the La Leche League of Franklin Park, she organized a Cleveland group in their footsteps. This group also multiplied, holding meetings in different sections of Cleveland. Other groups started in Brooklyn, Buffalo, Dayton, Denver and in smaller cities in several states.

But the main burden of mail still falls on the original group at Franklin Park.

"It's a real problem," explained Edwina Froehlich whose home at 3332 Rose Street, Franklin Park, Illinois, serves as the official address of the League.

"We want to preserve the personal touch. We have written a breast feeding manual called the *Womanly Art of Breast Feeding* that gives the information we have found most helpful to breast feeding mothers. However, with every manual we send to a mother, we try to write a personal letter asking about the mother's individual problems."

Each mother who helps with the League correspondence has her own style, but all are women who know the art of successful breast feeding from personal experience. The keynote of each letter is encouragement and sympathy.

For instance, this is the answer to a letter from a mother who had not nursed her first two and managed to nurse her third, only after spending the first month crying "because I was so unsure of myself."

"I still lack confidence, as everyone thinks it is foolish," she wrote in the letter appealing for help.

The League mother who answered this letter wrote:

"Bless you for nursing your third baby after having failed the first two times. You certainly are succeeding beautifully and should have no cause for worry this time. However, I certainly know how you feel about lack of confidence and encouragement. There are a lot of 'helpful people' around all the time trying to tell us we can't or shouldn't be nursing our babies for all sorts of reasons. But try to remember that these same people in all likelihood have never successfully breast fed a baby of their own. I am currently nursing our 3-month-old eighth baby and we are both loving it."

The League finds the problem of relatives comes up time and time again. Particularly difficult are mothers and mothers-in-law if they have not breast fed their children. Somehow it is very hard for them to see the younger generation do what they did not do. Their constant "That baby is fussing again," or "Is the baby really getting enough to eat?" wears down many a new mother.

Mothers who have breast fed their children are more likely to encourage their daughters and daughters-in-law, except for a few who are very poor, or who have just come from rural areas. To such grandmothers, bottle feeding may be a symbol of a new higher status in life for the young family.

They do not realize that, actually, breast feeding is popular with women who have had the advantages in life. For instance, a recent study at Harvard found that women who had attended college more frequently tried to nurse their first babies than women who had not attended college. When both father and mother had college training, 8 out of 10 couples tried to breast feed their first babies.

The Harvard breast feeding study also singles out doctors' attitudes as a real problem in the area of breast feeding today. Summarizing the findings of the study in the *New England Journal of Medicine,* the report comments:

". . . Certainly medical and nursing students are getting very little practical training in breast feeding technics."

Differences in breast feeding management can be seen in the different numbers of women trying to breast feed their babies in different states. A nation-wide study showed that, out of every 100 mothers leaving the hospital, 62 in Arizona were breast feeding as compared with 18 in Massachusetts. The Harvard study comments, "The attitude of medical practitioners, who are responsible for most of the ante-natal supervision in the United States, probably accounts both for the regional variation in amount of breast feeding and its general low prevalence."

The League itself has had wonderful cooperation from a few doctors. Patients are referred to it to learn the "housewifely aspects of breast feeding." In contrast to this, the daily mail and phone calls bring requests for help from many women, heartbroken because doctors have ordered premature weaning for a happy nursing couple.

The case of one mother of a two-month-old baby is typical. Her baby developed a rash on the front part of its abdomen. Her doctor prescribed an ointment *and* prompt weaning. She called the League in tears. The League urged her to get another medical opinion from a doctor familiar with breast fed babies. The second physician prescribed the same ointment for the simple case of diaper rash, but no weaning. The rash cleared promptly.

The physicians working with the League are quick to defend the behavior of their colleagues. They point out that physicians are very responsive to patient pressure. When they begin to realize that many of their patients really want to breast feed, they will learn to do more to help them.

"Most doctors have been taught in medical school that breast feeding is the best way," one commented, "but they haven't been taught just how to help a mother who wants to breast feed. So naturally, the first phone call from a distraught mother saying 'My baby is fussing. What shall I do?' results in a formula prescription.

"I have noticed, though, that doctors whose own children were bottle fed are naturally more likely to propose bottle feeding than those doctors who have seen successful, happy breast feeding in their own homes."

Fortunately, organized medicine is becoming aware of the problem. The *Journal of the American Medical Association* editorialized as follows:

". . . many women who do not nurse their babies could do so successfully if a positive attitude toward this function were fostered early in pregnancy and adequate instructions were given."

G. P., published by the American Academy of General Practice, comments:

". . . there is a growing and militant campaign for the promotion of the womanly art. Our ladies know what they are talking about and what they are doing, and it is high time for physicians to give them full support."

Most doctors, however, no matter how much they want to encourage breast feeding, are so rushed, they find it difficult to have time for the day to day support a mother needs while she is learning to breast feed. Here is where the League can be particularly helpful.

"It takes a long time to get over doubt," Gloria Watson explains. "Sometimes mothers don't phone us because they hate to bother us. Then we try to remember to phone them to see how they are getting along. It's a type of personal encouragement that means so much."

Rose Mary Schultz agrees. "The greatest help I got from the League was the second day I got home from the hospital. It was a life-saving call."

Gail Kaberlein's help from the League, on the other hand, came from being able to attend their meetings.

"I came to the League meetings for 6 months before my first baby was born, and by that time I was so *confident,* nothing could go wrong."

Her confidence was bolstered by getting to know women like Mary Jane Brizzolara, comfortable, relaxed leader of another Chicago La Leche League group who is at present nursing her sixth baby.

"I just assumed that the good Lord gave me breasts for this reason," she commented to me as she held her newest baby in her arms.

"I felt I was just too high-strung and nervous to nurse," exclaimed Ray Rachford calling attention to her pretty doll-like face and bright blue eyes.

"I had trouble feeding my first, so I bottle fed my next 3. Then I came to a League meeting to scoff. But they had a logical sensible answer to every question. Through their help, I was able to breast feed my fifth child."

The League puts emphasis on being able to give sensible answers to each question, in addition to building a general feeling of confidence. Medical references are given and research is cited. Here are the questions often asked by mothers and answers as they might be given by a League mother.

"What do I do when I want to go out?"

"What will you be doing when you go out? Most times you will be going some place where you can easily take the baby along. A baby is usually the 'Belle of the Ball' at a meeting or party. Nursing can be so slyly done that people just don't realize what you are doing."

Mary White recently attended a dinner party taking her baby with her as usual. Her amused host later reported that, after she left, the other guests had quite a discussion. Had she nursed the baby or had she merely cuddled the baby?

She had, of course, nursed the baby, but with help of a two piece outfit over a half slip and a nursing brassiere, the whole process was so discreet one could not be sure.

"If you feel you really can't take the baby along, express your milk after feeding in a bottle 24 hours ahead of time," the League advises. "Then this can be used as a bottle in case the baby needs you while you are out. It will be the same type of milk he is used to. However, very often it's not so much for food that the baby is fussing as for HIS MOTHER. As a mother of a young baby, you will want to stay near him as much as possible."

"What about the other children?"

"Giving attention to older children is easy if you are a breast feeding mother. Instead of using your second hand to hold the bottle you have it free to cuddle your toddler or to hold a book to read to your pre-school child.

"Then, too, it's a wonderful 'facts of life' education program. Such a natural way to learn! As a matter of fact, one of the League mothers reports that her neighbors are beginning to send over their young children to her saying. 'Go see what Mrs. Wagner is doing!' "

"How will I know if my baby is getting milk?"

"I know just how you feel. That was my constant worry with my first baby. The first question to ask yourself is 'Do I change diapers?' If your baby is wetting and soiling himself, he must be getting something at the other end.

"If you are feeding your **new** baby every 2 to 3 hours during the day and once or twice at night, you are almost sure to have plenty of milk. This is the natural feeding rhythm most babies prefer."

The notion that babies don't have to be fed except every 4 hours became common along with slow-digesting cow's milk formulas. In the days when doctors saw mostly breast fed babies, they recommended more frequent feedings.

For instance, Dr. Southworth, in Carr's *Practice of Pediatrics,* published in 1906, recommends the following pattern of feeding:

first day—4 nursings
second day—6 nursings
rest of first month—10 nursings a day
second and third month—8 nursings a day
fourth and fifth month—7 nursings a day
sixth to eleventh month—6 nursings a day

Dr. Southworth also approved of night feeding up through the fifth month.

"How disgusting!" is often the reaction of people who are familiar only with the current ideal of a-few-big-meals-as-young-as-possible.

"How wonderful!" is the reaction of many women who have successfully and abundantly breast fed their babies on self-demand.

"That's the way breast feeding often works. How comforting to hear of someone who understands!" they add.

Modern psychiatrists may be particularly interested in hearing the "old-fashioned" number of feedings a day. For many of them have been emphasizing that frequent cuddling and holding during feedings can build a baby's feeling of security.

"How will I get time to nurse my baby so much?"

"Do you spend a lot of time washing and putting sterilizing ointments on your nipples? It isn't necessary, you know. A research study published in the *Journal of Pediatrics* actually recommends *against* the use of soap, tincture of benzoin, alcohol or other similar substances because they may cause nipple pain.

"Nursing is so simple and easy. No bottles to heat up or formulas to prepare or bottles to wash! Then, too, night feedings are a whiz. No lights to turn on. No long trips to the refrigerator. No screaming baby while you prepare the food. So naturally you and the baby don't get so wide awake. Most of our League mothers just pop the baby into bed with them to nurse. They curl their arm around the baby to protect him as they snooze.

"Of course, babies *do* take time. Both bottle and breast fed babies need a lot of attention. There is less time to do things when you have a new baby in the house. We in the League know just how you feel. Most of us have big families and busy husbands and no cleaning women or other help. We have learned to housekeep more simply.

" 'PEOPLE are more important than THINGS,' we tell each other."

"My milk has left me, what shall I do?"

"Why do you think so?" asks the League advisor.

"I just know, my baby is screaming."

"Well, milk just doesn't flip in and out like that. If you stopped nursing now, you would have a hard time getting rid of it. Nature wants you to nurse. Perhaps you are overtired. Have you been doing anything extra the last few days?"

When the baby is several weeks old, the League has found, many mothers begin to overdo. Often, as they question, they hear about week-end guests or a special rush about something.

The resulting fatigue is enough to bring back the mother's old doubts about her milk supply. The League urges the mother to get rested up for a few days.

"The baby is more important than dust bunnies," they say. Soon things are usually going smoothly again.

Another crisis time is at about 3 months. At this time, babies normally begin to stay awake more between feedings. The inexperienced mother often mistakenly thinks this is due to her lack of milk, rather than to the baby's normally increasing wakefulness.

Whenever doubts about breast milk occur, the League emphasizes the need for rest and a sensible diet, along with plenty of frequent sucking using both breasts at each feeding.

"My baby's bowel movements are so loose, what's wrong?"

"Is this the first baby you have breast fed? No wonder you are surprised. Bottle fed babies often have hard formed movements, but breast fed babies have easy soft movements. They are yellow in color and about as thick as cream sauce. Sometimes, when the baby is small, they come as frequently as 6 or more times a day. Later, the baby may have just one enormous soft movement every 3 or 4 days. This is perfectly normal for a breast fed baby.

"Of course, even breast fed babies do very occasionally get tummy upsets. Their movements then will contain pus, mucus or blood, or are excessively loose or frequent. Call your doctor in this case."

"Is there something wrong with my milk?"

"Are you expecting human milk to be like cow's milk? Actually human milk usually looks thinner and bluer than cow's milk. It's a lot sweeter, too, and, of course, human milk is just right for babies, the way cow's milk is just right for calves. That is why allergies like eczema are much more common in babies fed cow's milk than in babies fed human milk.

"Or perhaps you notice that the color of your milk has changed. Early milk does look thicker and richer. It is called colostrum. It is perfectly normal for it to become thinner in a few days."

"My baby is a slow gainer, does this mean he is getting too little milk?"

"We are so used to the bottle as the normal way of feeding that we are apt to blame breast milk when anything seems out of line.

"One of our mothers had an interesting experience. She had a petite baby who was gaining at a slow rate. Naturally, she and her doctor suspected undersupply of breast milk, until they looked up the records of the rest of her babies. One of the previous babies, also the petite type, had had just the same type of weight gain, but that time she and the doctor were not worried because it was a bottle baby!

"Of course, there are some babies who don't get enough milk. We warn mothers who are feeding their babies only every 4 hours in the daytime that they need to watch their babies carefully to see that they are getting enough milk. In our experience, too little milk is seldom the real problem when young babies are fed in the natural rhythm of every 2 to 3 hours during the waking hours of the day, along with night feedings as long as the baby wants them."

Breast fed babies do gain less and weigh less beginning about four months of age. But heavier weight does not always mean better health any more than it does in adults. As a matter of fact, one extensive study showed quite the opposite. The older bottle fed babies weighed more but had more sickness.

"I have less milk since I started giving my baby solid foods. What's wrong?"

"We have heard that question over and over again—so much in fact that we began to wonder whether the current fashion of starting solid foods in the first month or two didn't actually harm breast feeding. So we carefully studied the scientific literature on the subject.

"We learned that the famous Doctor Arnold Gesell, after devoting his life to studying how babies and children develop, wrote as follows:

" '. . . a premature attempt to introduce solids during the first 4 months sometimes invites regrettable results. The baby's neuromuscular system is not mature enough to handle solids competently. . . . Moreover, if supplementary food is added too early, the mother's milk balance is upset. A premature administration of solids may result either in marked reduction or overproduction of mother's milk supply, for the baby consumes less at the breast.'

"We also found a surprising statement in a recent report by the Committee on Nutrition of the American Academy of Pediatrics. It reads in part, 'Lacking is proof obtained from controlled observations that feeding of solid foods at ages earlier than 4 to 6 months of life is nutritionally or psychologically beneficial . . . Consideration should be given to the possibility that it is the adults responsible for administering the solid food who are emotionally satisfied rather than the baby.'

"We also found that Dr. Frank Howard Richardson and Dr. Paul Gyorgy, who are well-known for their work in breast feeding, have cautioned against the early introduction of solids. Our own medical advisors agreed. Because of this, we have told mothers that early heavy use of solid foods may interfere with breast feeding."

Far more convincing than verbal statements, however, to mothers who attend the La Leche meeting, is the sight of active, beautiful babies of 2, 3 and 4 months of age whose mothers have never had the bother and mess of feeding them "solid foods." Instead, they have used the time for more frequent breast feeding.

"I never knew a baby could look so well without solid food," they are likely to exclaim."

"My breast is infected. Do I have to wean my baby?"

This question comes up tragically often because many mothers and babies bring home resistant staphylococcal infections from the hospital.

The League answers the question this way.

"As with any abnormality, call your doctor. If you notice a reddened area on the breast or nipple, a very tender or sore spot or lump in the breast and especially if you have a fever, call him promptly.

"But tell your doctor you would like to continue to nurse the baby so he will understand your point of view," the League cautions.

Actually, infections may become worse if nursing is stopped. Research published in *Surgery, Gynecology and Obstetrics* found that many breast abscesses formed only *after* active attempts to stop nursing had been made. The overfull, engorged breast is more likely to have serious infection.

"Let your baby nurse as much as possible on the infected breast," is the advice of Dr. E. Robbins Kimball, a leading midwestern pediatrician. Dr. Kimball has had considerable experience with breast feeding, since 8 out of 10 of the babies he cares for are still breast feeding at 3 months.

"I have treated more than 100 patients with breast infections with the frequent suckling method," he explained on the phone to me. "Only part of the breast is affected by the infection, so that the baby continues to get plenty of food. In not a single case, did there appear to be any harm to the baby from suckling from an infected breast."

The mother, too, seems to gain from this type of treatment. Most of the mothers recovered in 3 days, although a few continued a number of days longer. In contrast to this, a group of 30 mothers who had been ordered to stop nursing, continued to have breast infection for an average of two months. Half of them needed surgery to drain one or more abscesses.

"My treatment is not new," emphasized Dr. Kimball. "I am following the recommendations of Dr. Charlotte Naish, the famous British pediatrician. She suggested keeping the baby on the breast, in addition to hot packs and bed rest for the mother. We use antibiotics as well, of course."

Dr. Kimball's research has given a new note of hope to breast feeding mothers who want to continue to nurse in spite of breast infections. The La Leche League tells mothers about his research.

"When should I wean my baby?"

"Breast feeding can continue as long as you and your baby enjoy it!" the League advises. "It is important for babies to have a variety of other foods after they are 5 or 6 months old, but that doesn't mean that breast feeding has to stop altogether. In fact, many of our mothers enjoy nursing some months longer to continue that wonderful feeling of closeness."

One hundred years ago, American mothers usually fed their babies from 12 to 24 months or even longer. In many parts of the world today, breast feeding continues throughout the second year. The idea that weaning should take place early in the first year became popular only after bottle feeding became popular.

No matter when weaning is done, however, it should be done so slowly that the mother feels no pain from an over-full breast and that the baby shows no signs of being upset.

"We don't want to end a wonderful experience with a baby screaming or pining for what it can no longer have, nor with a mother's breasts painful with unused milk. If weaning is done slowly enough, that just does not happen," the League explains. "Our favorite phrase as far as weaning goes is 'Let the baby set the pace.' "

"Do you think everyone should breast feed her baby?"

"There are some real obstacles to breast feeding. If the mother has tuberculosis or whooping cough at the time the baby is born, she would have to be separated from her baby until she was noninfectious. Other rare physical conditions may also rule out breast feeding.

"Then, too, there are psychological obstacles. Probably about one out of five mothers is actively opposed to breast feeding.

"Our aim is to help the other mothers, the large majority of mothers, who can get satisfaction from breast feeding if they have the chance to really learn the art. For them, the chief obstacles are lack of knowledge and encouragement from relatives, friends, doctors and hospitals. Many of us did not breast feed some of our babies because of these pressures. We know it is hard. We are trying to help mothers who have similar problems."

There is one thing about the advice the League gives that stands out above all. *Here* is the voice of practical experience. The mothers themselves know how a sore nipple or over-full breast feels, and what it's like to be haunted by fear of not enough milk. They also know the closeness and love of the breast feeding couple, the deep feeling that what they are doing is in tune with their womanly nature.

"It's not just breast feeding we are interested in," Mary Ann Cahill explains, "but a different way of mothering. Because of this, we have been interested in other ways of promoting closeness between mothers and babies.

"For instance, when Dr. Grantly Dick-Read was here in 1957, we sponsored a lecture by him on natural childbirth. There were just 7 of us in the Franklin Park League and you can imagine how our husbands felt when they learned we wanted to guarantee a lecture fee of $700.00! Fortunately, the Dick-Read lecture was very popular and we were able to add a bit to our treasury.

"Our financial needs have been modest because the real thing we have to offer is the neighborly interest of an experienced mother. We never charge for help. We do sell our manual, *The Womanly Art of Breast Feeding,* for two dollars and also a child-care book we particularly like because it tells of easy ways of toilet training and short cuts to housekeeping. These have brought us some income. Now that we are incorporated as a nonprofit institution, La Leche League of Franklin Park, Incorporated, we are getting some charitable gifts.

"The name, La Leche League, by the way, comes from the name of the Spanish Madonna, known as 'Our Lady of Happy Delivery and Plentiful Milk.' However, we are a nonsectarian organization and welcome everybody of all races and religions who is interested in breast feeding.

"Our organization has been simple as well. One of the original 7 has moved away, but the rest of us continue as officers of the board. We don't have 'members' the way some clubs do, but our board has expanded to 25 mothers from all over the Chicago area who sponsor classes in their own localities. Experienced mothers in other states, who are interested in helping, organize their own League meetings. They usually also sell our manual. However, because of publicity, we get the heavy load of mail. Just 15 of the most experienced of us answer these letters."

I was amazed when I learned how small a group of women founded and carry on the work of La Leche League of Franklin Park, for they have started something that has given help to mothers all over the country. Nor are these women free to give all of their time. They are wives and mothers, usually with several children. Most of them were either pregnant or nursing a baby at the time I visited them. They made me realize more than ever before how much busy mothers can accomplish when they work together to help others.

References to Quotations and Papers Directly Mentioned in This Article

"Breast Feeding," *Journal of the American Medical Association*, 161: 1569, 1956.

DOUGLAS, J. W. B. "The Extent of Breast Feeding in Great Britain in 1946 with Special Reference to the Health and Survival of Children," *Journal of Obstetrics and Gynecology of the British Empire*, 57: 335, 1950.

GESELL, ARNOLD and ILG, F. L. *Infant and Child in the Culture Today.* New York: Harper & Brothers, 1943 (18th edition), p. 89.

GYORGY, PAUL. "Trends and Advances in Infant Nutrition," *West Virginia Medical Journal*, 53: 131, 1957.

MEYER, H. F. "Breast Feeding in the United States: Extent and Possible Trend. A survey of 1,904 hospitals with 2¼ million births in 1956," *Pediatrics*, 22: 116, 1958.

NEWTON, MICHAEL, and NEWTON, MILES. "Breast Abscess: A Result of Lactation Failure," *Surgery, Gynecology and Obstetrics*, 91: 651, 1960.

NEWTON, NILES. "Nipple Pain and Nipple Damage," *Journal of Pediatrics*, 41: 411, 1952.

REPORT COMMITTEE ON NUTRITION. "On the Feeding of Solid Foods to Infants," *Pediatrics*, 21: 685, 1958.

RICHARDSON, FRANK HOWARD. *The Nursing Mother.* New York: David McKay & Company.

SALBER, E. J., STITT, P. G., and BABBOT, J. G. "Patterns of Breast Feeding Factors Affecting the Frequency of Breast Feeding in the Newborn Period," *New England Medical Journal*, 259: 707, 1958.

SOUTHWORTH, DR. "Maternal Feeding," *The Practice of Pediatrics* (Philadelphia: Lea Brothers & Company, 1906), pages 89-107.

"The Womanly Art," *G. P.*, 19: 83, 1959.

Burns

A New First Aid Treatment for Burns

Burns are a common household hazard and the first aid remedies seem to vary from house to house and doctor to doctor. Most people use some kind of grease over the burn, some do nothing and "let the air get at it," while still others wrap it deep in gauze and rags. Instinct, however, tells us to plunge the burn into cold water to take the heat away, but that procedure has been frowned upon by medical men until now.

In the *Journal of the American Medical Association* (August 27, 1960), ice water was recommended as the best first aid measure for burns covering up to 20 per cent of the body. Dr. Alex G. Shulman tells us that his experiments with burns and cold water were begun as a result of a burn with boiling grease received by himself. He plunged the hand into a tub of cold water, and found the pain alleviated and that the burn healed more rapidly than expected. He decided to use the same therapy on his patients.

The Cold Water Treatment

The method is to place the burned area immediately into a basin containing tap water, ice cubes and the disinfectant, hexachlorophene. For burns of the head, neck, chest, etc., where immersion is impractical, he applied towels chilled in a bucket of ice water. The cold treatment is continued until it can be stopped without return of pain—usually within 30 minutes to 5 hours.

Dr. Shulman has treated 150 patients in this manner, including some chemical and electrical burns. Whereas the pain usually lasts 24 hours or more on a first degree burn, relief for these patients was immediate and the pain was almost totally absent by the time the patient left the office two or three hours later. ". . . although the primary injurious effect of the burn has taken place, the usual inflammatory process secondary to the burn can be reduced in degree and indeed, at times reversed by ice-water therapy," says Dr. Shulman. "The time factor between injury and treatment determines the result. This treatment should be initiated by the patient or first aid attendant at once. This would be far more effective first aid treatment than applying butter or grease which will only have to be painfully removed by the attending physician."

We think Dr. Shulman's treatment is well worth a try, because the pain of a burn, with or without grease on it, is intense and his treatment sounds like a simple, sensible way to cut down on suffering, and to promote a quicker healing.

Cancer

Cancer: Can It Be Prevented?

By J. I. Rodale

First let us look at our problem. How prevalent is cancer? Here are figures showing how many persons per 100,000 population in the United States died of cancer from 1900 to 1959:

1900	64	1935	108
1910	76	1940	120
1920	83	1945	127
1925	92	1947	132
1930	97	1959	147

An analysis of these figures should make one question the oft-repeated statements one encounters in newspapers, magazines, books and the radio, that the mortality figures show that we are getting healthier. Every year shows a small but persistent increase over the preceding one. It is an increasing tendency that shows no desire to let up. When I bring these figures to the attention of physicians or to some laymen, the invariable answer is that these cancer statistics are misleading. They say that, due to better diagnostic techniques, more and more cases show up in the statistics which were formerly attributed to other diseases. Therefore, it must be expected that the figures *will* show an increase and that we must not be alarmed about it. However, *that* excuse has now been worked threadbare. I have heard that argument for the last 30 years, but anyone who will investigate will find that, while that may have been true in 1910 or even in 1920, since then diagnosis has made so much progress that around 1930 to 1935, it had become more or less perfect and the medical profession became proud of their brilliant achievements in this field. So for all practical purposes, we reached a point, let us say, 20 or 30 years ago when diagnosis improved to such an extent that any further improvement would show up only in tiny, fractional decimal points.

Is Life Expectancy Increasing?

Another reason is given, that since more persons are attaining to a higher age, and that since cancer is a disease affecting older persons, naturally it would be expected that there would be a gradual increase in cancer deaths per 100,000 population. There are two parts to this assumption and both are incorrect. First, are there really more older persons? The mortality figures are only figures and sometimes figures can be misleading. Do we really have a greater life expectancy? *Time* magazine of December 4, 1944, said: "In the past 44 years, past-65 life expectancy has increased only slightly. Women (white) of 65 can now expect to live a year longer than they could have in 1900; male expectancy has increased only half a year." This apparent discrepancy between the actual and what the public thinks is so, has to do with babies that used to die due to poor hygiene. It is due also to other conditions that do not affect *you*. You are not a baby that died in childbirth or in the first few years of life.

Cancer Is Not Caused by Old Age

The second error is the supposition that cancer is a disease of old age. Then why did the Metropolitan Life Insurance Company say the following in a release to the press, February 18, 1949? "With the virtual conquest of the common childhood diseases, cancer now ranks high among the causes of death of youngsters, according to the statisticians of the Metropolitan Life Insurance Company. In the company's experience, cancer recently has accounted for one out of every 9 deaths from disease at ages 1 to 14 years, while as late as 1930, the ratio was only one out of every 50. Since that year, the death rate from cancer among children insured in the Industrial Department has increased about 40 per cent." And now it is sky-rocketing.

Professor Hoffman, who is mentioned later on, said in the book there quoted: "After many years' thoughtful consideration and exhaustive statistical study, I am fully convinced that the apparent increase in cancer is real, and not to be explained away by changes in the age or constitution, or improvement in diagnoses." Nothing will be gained by arguing. Let's tackle the problem and argue afterward. We must realize that, in the civilized world today, we are in the midst of a dread curse and American brains must do something about it. When we are faced with figures which show that from Pearl Harbor to V-J Day, 294,476 American soldiers and sailors were killed, but that during the same period 607,193 Americans died of cancer, we can better visualize what the cold cancer statistics mean, and that it is an emergency situation, a crisis, which demands bold, aggressive treatment. A statistician studying the trend of these cancer increases must come to the conclusion that if the tendency is not curbed, half the population will be killed off by cancer in the next 50 to 150 years.

Prevention or Cure?

I would like to mention the work of the late Dr. Frederick L. Hoffman who was connected with the Prudential Insurance Company of America and with the Biochemical Research Foundation of the Franklin Institute of Philadelphia. He was a medical man of high repute who traveled all over the world studying cancer to see if he could obtain a clue to its causation. He devoted his life to it. In 1915, the Prudential Press published his book of 826 pages entitled *The Mortality from Cancer throughout the World.* In 1937, the Williams and Wilkins Company, conservative medical publishers of Baltimore, Maryland, published his 767-page book called *Cancer and Diet,* in which he quotes much evidence and the work of many physicians who hold that diet is an important element in cancer.

Artificial Chemicals and Artificial Foods

Very early in the book, Dr. Hoffman becomes suspicious of commercial fertilizers. I am going to quote from his work:

"The food supply for this population (alluding to urban communities) is therefore naturally becoming more and more artificial and modified by a wide range of processes, some of which unquestionably react injuriously on the human organism. There is another factor involved to which hardly any attention has been called and that is the nature of the food supply itself, which is being altered as the result of alterations in the nature of the soil in which the food is raised. This applies particularly to the composition of the mineral constituents of the soil which, to an increasing extent, are being modified by the addition of artificial fertilizers, which also are becoming more and more chemical and artificial in contrast to the use of natural manures in the earlier days, when the soil retained most of its original fertility and growth producing capacity. In other words, any one of the principal food products consumed at the present time does not by any means represent the same natural mineral composition of, say, 50 years ago . . .

"Granting that the prevention of soil exhaustion, is the function of fertilizers, its effect on human consumption has attracted little attention. Since our body is precisely what it feeds upon, chemical alterations must have affected human development and biological activities to an extent well deserving of more thoughtful consideration. The composition of foodstuffs now raised for farm animals has for many years received close attention, but the chemical composition of human foodstuffs has been treated with indifference. We are still of the belief that it is immaterial from what soil or sources our foodstuff is derived, although the evidence is overwhelmingly to the effect that measurable differences occur which may have serious consequences when the process is extended over a lifetime.

"As the result of the introduction of chemical fertilizers, there has been a marked increase in the crop production. The average amount of wheat in bushels per acre has increased from 9.9 in 1886 to 27.3 in 1958. The relative yield per acre varies, of course, widely for different sections of the country, having been as high as 28 bushels in Arizona and as low as 5.3 bushels in North Dakota. These figures are for 1931. It is a reasonable inference that the nutritional qualities, particularly mineral content, must vary proportionately to the use of chemical fertilizers in different sections, but I am not aware of any data to substantiate this conclusion at the present time. What is true of wheat is true of other grains or vegetables that enter into the food consumption of the American people. Everywhere efforts are made to increase the yield per acre, but what the effect of this hazard is on the mineral or vitamin content of the food is not revealed.

"The foregoing conclusion can also be applied to animal husbandry and dairying. It is, to my mind, an open question if there is not a substantial difference in milk supplied by cows artificially stimulated to a milk yield far above the average. Again the same conclusion may be applied to artificially fed steers and pigs."

All of the above shows independent, creative thinking, for it was written long before Sir Albert Howard's writings on the organic method were available to the public. Dr. Hoffman quotes from the

Yearbook of Agriculture for 1932 to show that, in the earlier days of the use of commercial fertilizers, the fertilizer was not as concentrated and soluble as it later became, but was mixed with waste or by-products of industry, so that equal tonnages by weight would mean more chemical potency in the commercial product of the last 20 or 30 years. He then quotes from the 1932 *Yearbook:*

"The American farmer, in his agricultural operations, applies 8,000,000 tons of fertilizers annually. It is frequently pointed out that this is an average application of 40 pounds for each acre of land under cultivation in this country, as contrasted with 500 pounds for The Netherlands, where intensive farming is generally followed."

Artificial Chemicals and Incidence of Cancer

Dr. Hoffman did not attempt to discuss the effect of so much commercial fertilizers on the health of the people of The Netherlands, so I looked up the comparative cancer statistics for the United States and that country taken from Hoffman's book, *The Mortality from Cancer throughout the World.* Here are figures for 1900, 1910 and 1955:

	U.S.	Holland	Italy
1900	64	91	52
1910	76	106	65
1955	146.5	159.8	128

Note the higher rates for Holland. Observe the lower cancer rate for Italy where extremely small amounts of artificial fertilizers were used.

The late Dr. Max Gerson of New York City, a cancer specialist, had this to say at a hearing in Washington relating to Bill No. S. 1875 held on July 1, 2 and 3, 1946, to authorize the government to sponsor cancer research, which was not passed:

"The fundamental damage starts with the use of artificial fertilizer for vegetables and fruits as well as for fodder. Thus, the chemically transformed vegetarian and meat nourishment, increasing through generations, transforms the organs and functions of the human body in the wrong direction.

"Another basic defect lies in the waste of excrements of the cities. Instead of returning the natural manure to the fruit-bearing soil, it is led into the rivers, killing underwater life. The natural cycle is interrupted and mankind has to suffer dearly for the violation. Life in forest and wilderness should teach us the lesson.

"But we can regain the lost defense and healing power if we return as close as possible to the laws of nature as they are created."

Dr. George Miley of the Gotham Hospital, New York City, who worked with Dr. Gerson on some of these cases, testified at the hearing as follows:

"We do know experimentally that diet definitely does influence cancer. There is a lot of experimental work done, very good work, done to substantiate that . . . It is reasonable to assume that the closer one's diet is to nature and the soil, with fresh fruit from the trees and fresh vegetables directly from the garden, the nearer one is to normal health."

I want to quote also the *New York Times* of December, 1940. (I do not have the record of the particular day.) It said:

"According to Dr. Alexander Brunschwig of the University of Chicago, in the current national bulletin of the American Society for the Control of Cancer, there is experimental evidence to suggest that in animals, at least, inadequate diets may serve as adjuvants to the action of certain cancer-producing compounds.

"An illustration of this point is the recent work of Kinosita, the Japanese pathologist, working at the Memorial Hospital, New York, who has shown that, when rats are fed an adequate, well-balanced diet, the ingestion of a cancer-producing substance known as 'butter yellow' is innocuous. However, when the rats are maintained upon an inadequate diet, especially lacking in vitamins, the ingestion of this chemical causes inflammatory changes in the liver followed by cancer of this organ.

"Such experiments, if they can at all apply to man" states Dr. Brunschwig, "would suggest that, while an adequate, well-balanced diet does not in any way insure against the development of cancer, it does contribute to the maintenance of a general normal body economy and in this way, might tend to obviate the progress of other diseases or pathologic conditions which might themselves favor the development of cancer.

"It is perhaps not too far-fetched to state that, when a better understanding of the mechanism of cancer development in man is obtained, the factor of diet may assume greater importance in attempts at prophylaxis (prevention) and control of the disease than can now, in our present state of knowledge, be the case."

Quotes from Researchers

Take the case of the late Dr. John R. Davidson, of Winnipeg, Manitoba, who, during his entire professional life, specialized in cancer work. Let me quote Dyson Carter, who wrote in *Saturday Night*, a newspaper published in Toronto:

"The story is straightforward. We take it up at the time when Dr. Davidson abandoned his practice and professorship to give all his energies to research. That was 12 years ago. Davidson was convinced then that cancer was caused by changes within the body resulting from improper eating. 'Cancer is a nutritional deficiency disease,' he declared.

"This conclusion was derived from experiments on mice. Davidson found that the regular experimental forms of cancer could be produced easier in mice that had been raised on food lacking in vitamins. The opposite was also true. Mice fed special vitamin-rich diets were very resistant to cancer. Furthermore, after generations of mice were raised on vitamin-deficient diets, the offspring became more and more liable to cancer. In this, Dr. Davidson believed that he had a clue to the puzzling fact that there are 'cancer susceptible' families, although the disease is definitely not hereditary.

"Linking the Davidson research with the virus theory, it could be said that the cancer virus, existing in bodies, passes over to the active, virulent form under certain definite chemical conditions brought about by prolonged lack of sufficient vitamins.

"Dr. Davidson was able to produce mice families susceptible to cancer. In 5 generations, by feeding with 'excess' vitamins and minerals, he bred from those susceptible mice a new generation quite free from any abnormal tendency toward cancer. This type of evidence —the reversible demonstration—is among the most powerful that can be provided by experimental science.

"What are the vitamins used in the Davidson research? Mainly those associated with chicken embryos and with wheat germ. Why? Because the doctor's work convinced him that the disease of cancer is related in some way to normal cell multiplication that takes place so rapidly in developing embryos, such as that of the fertilized hen's egg. Here again there is nothing that is scientifically unsound.

"But it is from his clinical work that Dr. Davidson has collected most convincing evidence. He has stopped human cancer from spreading. He has completely cured some cases. A child suffering from lymphosarcoma and given only a few months to live was gradually restored to health without surgery or radium. After 3 years, the affected glands were cured and normal.

"In this case, the treatment consisted of special feeding. The Davidson diet is adjusted to individual patients, but in general, includes large amounts of fresh vegetable juice (carrot and lettuce), raw vegetables (carrots, spinach, lettuce, peas, beans), wheat germ and rare beef. In addition, the patient gets massive doses of vitamins in the form of cod liver oil, wheat germ oil and brewer's yeast. Finally, there is a preparation made from chick embryos."

Dr. J. Ernest Ayre and Dr. W. A. G. Bould, of the Royal Victoria Hospital and McGill University, in April, 1946, announced that they had discovered many cases of cancer that were due to vitamin deficiencies in the diet. They stated that there is "excellent circumstantial evidence to suggest that the nutritional deficiencies may have been a primary factor leading to the malignancy."

Dr. Arthur L. Wallace, a practicing physician for 45 years in

Nashua, New Hampshire, appeared before the State Agricultural Advisory Board at Concord, New Hampshire, on August 31, 1947, and said that, "If foodstuffs contained more nutrition, people would not be so susceptible to diseases such as cancer, heart ailments and other organic disorders. There appears to me to be too much seeking after disease-carrying germs these days, and then searching for wonder drugs to kill them off. It would be more beneficial if we corrected the nutritional deficiencies of the earth, and made people so healthy that they would not be susceptible to these same germs." He stated that "Nutritional deficiency in the soil is the chief cause of increased diseases among people."

Sir Arbuthnot Lane, a famous English surgeon, has said: "Long surgical experience has proved to me conclusively that there is something radically and fundamentally wrong with the civilized mode of life, and I believe that unless the present dietetic and health customs of the white nations are reorganized, social decay and race deterioration are inevitable."

I was amazed to read that the late Dr. Alexis Carrel in his classic *Man the Unknown* was aware of the dangers of using artificial fertilizers. In this book, he said: "Man is literally made from the dust of the earth. For this reason, his physiological and mental activities are profoundly influenced by the geological constitution of the country where he lives, by the nature of the animals and plants on which he generally feeds. His structure and his functions depend also on the selections he makes of certain elements among the vegetal and animal foods at his disposal. The chiefs always had a diet quite different from that of their slaves. Those who fought, commanded and conquered used chiefly meats and fermented drinks, whereas the peaceful, the weak and the submissive were satisfied with milk, vegetables, fruits and cereals. Our aptitudes and our destiny come, in some measure, from the nature of the chemical substances that construct our tissues. It seems as though human beings, like animals, could be artifically given certain bodily and mental characteristics, if subjected from childhood to appropriate diets."

Carrel also remarks: "It (the organism) is also affected by the deficiencies of the essential physiological and mental functions. The staple foods may not contain the same nutritive substances as in former times. Mass production has modified the composition of wheat, eggs, milk, fruit and butter, although these articles have retained their familiar appearance. Chemical fertilizers, by increasing the abundance of the crops without replacing all the exhausted elements of the soil, have indirectly contributed to change the nutritive value of cereal grains and of vegetables. Hens have been compelled by artificial diet and mode of living, to enter the ranks of mass producers. Has not the quality of their eggs been modified? The same question may be asked about milk, because cows are now confined to the stable all the year round, and are fed on manufactured provender. Hygienists have not paid sufficient attention to the genesis of diseases. Their studies of conditions of life and diet, and of their effects on the physiological and mental state of modern man, are superficial, incomplete and of too short duration . . ."

Dr. Carrel was also aware of the danger in placing too much confidence in the mortality statistics as a measure of our health. In this regard he said: "All diseases of bacterial origin have decreased in a striking manner . . . But we still must die in a much larger proportion from degenerative diseases. In spite of the triumphs of medical science, the problem of disease is far from solved. Modern man is delicate, 1,100,000 persons have to attend the medical needs of 120,000,000 other persons. Every year, of this population in the United States, there are about 100,000,000 illnesses, serious or slight. In the hospitals, 700,000 beds are occupied every day of the year . . . Medical care under all its forms, costs about $3,500,000,000 yearly . . . The organism seems to have become more susceptible to degenerative diseases."

Now comes another physician of high standing, Dr. James Asa Shield, who, at a convention of the Southern Medical Association on November 8, 1946, at Miami, Florida, attacked the use of chemical fertilizers in no uncertain terms. Let us quote from the *Associated Press* dispatch which was sent across the wires of the country and which was printed in dozens of newspapers: "Dr. James Asa Shield, assistant professor of neuropsychiatry of the Medical College of Virginia, said, in an address before the Southern Medical Association convention here today, that food produced from soil fertilized with chemicals has caused an increase of degenerative diseases throughout the United States.

"Shield charged that agriculture's attempt to correct soil exhaustion with chemicals has not been successful.

" 'The doctor must demand that the agriculturist produce a food that will meet the multiple cell needs for best growth, development and function,' he said.

"Dr. Shield said one degenerative disease, multiple sclerosis, is virtually unknown in the Orient, where natural manures and plant refuse are used as fertilizers.

"He said the death rate from the disease in the United States is almost as high as the infantile paralysis death rate.

"Inorganic chemical fertilizers 'at times disturb the chemical balance of the soil and in turn affect the health of the animals that feed on the crops,' the doctor reported.

"Despite deficiencies in vitamins, proteins and fats in the Chinese diet, they have no sclerosis of their nerves, their blood vessels, blockage of their veins or hypertension.

"He said several European countries that use chemical fertilizers have a high incidence of sclerosis and other degenerative diseases.

" 'The incomplete fertilization program carried on in Europe and the United States is contributing largely to the inadequacy of the quality of the diet, with deficiency of minor minerals and unknown factors of this diet contributing to and being largely responsible for the presence of multiple sclerosis.' "

A Nutritionist Speaks

One of the greatest nutritionists of our time, Dr. E. V. McCollum of Johns Hopkins University, said, "When it comes to getting out of the soil and into the plant elements which may be there already but which the plant cannot now secure, the advocates of what is called the organic school of soil improvement have a good many persuasive arguments to present for their side of the case. Organic ferment may well stir up and release trace elements and other elements which commercial fertilizers alone can never provide." This quotation was given in the *Land* magazine.

The *American Journal of Digestive Diseases,* in its June, 1948, issue, referring to a book by N. Philip Norman, M.D., and James Rorty, called *Tomorrow's Food,* said:

"A careful study of the English authors who recommended natural compost for fertilizing purposes, particularly McCarrison and Howard, and of the experimental work of Maynard, Albrecht, Brody and others in this country, leaves one convinced of several facts. One fact is that, until proper soil fertilization is practiced, we shall not be able to obtain from food (nor from artificial vitamins) the strongest known impetus to health. A second fact is that, where 'pedigreed' food products have been eaten under proper conditions of cooking, a most *amazing* degree of health has been obtained both clinically and in experimental animals. It is not too much to say that such nutrition has been proved capable of *banishing disease of all kinds and of conferring a vigorous old age.* As Minot has recently indicated, the most important research today is nutritional research. Nobody knows the breadth, depth or extent of the benefits in store for mankind as a result of the patient, laborious efforts of our nutritional experts."

The *American Journal of Digestive Diseases* says further:

"Norman undoubtedly believes that 'proper' nutrition is capable of conferring upon an individual or a group, in due time, a superlative degree of fitness capable of relative immunity to infections and to the terrible degenerative changes so common now among older persons . . . I think the best efforts of us all should be dedicated to what Norman has in mind. There are countless hurdles in the path. Vested interests will fold up only on public demand. Education alone can create a suitable public reaction. The *ideal of perfect nutrition* is the most dynamic concept before the profession today."

Dr. Norman was consulting nutritionist for the New York City Departments of Health and Hospitals.

I have to stop somewhere with these quotations from the thoughts of physicians. There are available dozens more. They show clearly that many physicians believe that there is some connection between the use of artificial fertilizers and the increasing incidence of cancer. Yet, when one springs this concept upon a doctor who has not studied the subject, he thinks you are crazy to think such a thing. Doctors must be made to think along the lines of good health coming from a soil rich in humus. They must set up experimental projects in which cancer cases, in the early stages, are fed on an exclusive diet of foods raised organically.

Organically Grown Foods, a Preventive of Cancer

By J. I. Rodale

In the February, 1961, issue of the *American Journal of Proctology,* an extraordinary piece of research has been reported, which could revolutionize and simplify the whole concept of cancer. But before I comment on it, I should like to reproduce the entire article, called "Anti-Malignancy Factors Apparently Present in Organically Grown Foods," by Donald C. Collins, M.D., F.I.A.P.

"This clinical note is written with considerable hesitancy, and yet on 5 different occasions during the past 36 years of practice, I have seen a marvelous phenomenon occur.

"Five patients have been observed with extensive malignancies, proven by biopsies, of either the gastrointestinal tract, or blood (leukemias), or sarcomas. Strangely, these 5 individuals all died many years later from diseases unrelated to these former malignant processes. It was shown in all 5 instances, following most thorough and painstaking autopsies, performed by highly competent pathologists, that no discernible pathologic evidence could be found then that such patients had ever previously had the various malignant diseases, proven by adequate biopsies to have been present in the past.

"The only constant factor in the lives of these 5 persons was the fact that they all ate home-raised, organically grown foods that were free from various chemical preservatives and insect-repellent sprays. Unfortunately, here in Los Angeles we have learned, to our dismay, that smog apparently destroys these beneficial factors in organically grown foodstuffs. Possibly, such optimum foods possess unidentified antibiotic factors that are antagonistic to malignant growths in some humans. Some recent evidence attributes such beneficial actions to certain antibiotics studied so far.

"This brief clinical note is written with the hope that it may prove of possible benefit to other coloproctologists dealing with apparently hopeless malignant disease in their own patients. Surely, this recommended adjuvant therapy is innocuous and might prove life-prolonging or even arrest the further progress of malignant disease. This is certainly worth trying and remembering for possible future use."

This article appeared in February, 1961, and its contents should have been blared forth in the press. Yet not a word about it has been published in newspapers, magazines or medical journals, other than where the original article was published. *Time* and *Newsweek,* which regularly comb medical journals for news on the medical front, failed to pick up this item. Perhaps this is due to the fact that orthodox medicine and the U. S. Government, as an official attitude, have characterized followers of the organic method as crackpots, cultists and food faddists.

The orthodox cancer-cure structure is such an elaborate setup with its billion dollar plant of hospitals, fancy treatment, X-ray machines and other equipment, physicians, research men, technicians, etc., that it won't readily accept such a simple medicine—organically grown food—as a substitute. They will not stand by and see their impressive cancer edifice, with its millions of cancer fund income, collapse. They would lose face.

In the meantime, hundreds of thousands of people all over the world are dying and suffering from this dreadful disease, and no one bats an eyelash. In this respect, I must recall the amazing words of Dr. A. I. Lansing, the outgoing president of the Gerontological Society, who said on November 8, 1958, that finding a cure for cancer and heart disease would be a major financial disaster which would bankrupt the social security system and the big insurance companies. Is this why Dr. Collins' cancer cure results were not publicized?

We had a similar experience when there was published in November, 1949, the results of a feeding experiment with mice, sponsored by the Soil and Health Foundation, of which I am president. The experiment was performed by Dr. Ehrenfried Pfeiffer at his Spring Valley, New York, laboratory. The results clearly showed that mice fed organically grown food suffered far less from cancer. Copies of the bulletin were sent to hundreds of medical journals and to the press, but none of them took any notice of it.

A doctor once said that cancer is Nature's revenge on man for living artificially. Eating organically grown food is living naturally. Eating chemically grown food full of chemical additives is living artificially and carries with it the possibility of getting cancer.

Anyone who has the smallest plot of soil should grow the vegetables for his family without using chemical fertilizers or poison sprays. Only composts and organic fertilizers and certain kinds of powdered rock should be used. It is not only insurance towards good health, but furnishes better-tasting food. And it is amazing how much food can be grown in a small plot. Besides, you will see creation before your very own eyes.

How Effective Is Krebiozen?

The question of the value of Krebiozen in the treatment of cancer has aroused hopefulness, curiosity and indignation among many Americans. No cancer drug has ever been the center of such a storm of controversy, and unorthodox cancer drugs are notoriously controversial. Universities, state and federal courts, even Congress, have become involved. Law suits featuring well-known scientists, pathologists, the American Medical Association have also been in the picture. At least 3 books have been written purporting to tell the Krebiozen story.

We are frequently questioned as to the value of Krebiozen. We are asked if it will cure this or that type of cancer, where it can be obtained, how much it costs, how soon it will take effect, etc. We are not qualified to answer most of these questions. They can be answered by the Krebiozen Research Foundation, 105 West Adams Street, Chicago, Illinois.

National Cancer Institute Sponsoring Objective Test

For the final word on just how good Krebiozen really is, an objective test by the National Cancer Institute is being undertaken. It is felt that, if the experiment is set up properly, the final results will speak for themselves. Salutary effects on the terminal patients involved will vindicate Krebiozen's claims; lack of beneficial change in them will silence, for once and for all, Krebiozen's promoters who claim an unfair and biased evaluation of the drug by the American Medical Association.

While the results of this test are being awaited, cancer cases are constantly cropping up and victims are wondering what Krebiozen would do for their own case. They write and call to ask us what we have heard from patients who have tried using Krebiozen. The reports we get are varied. Some people say they are helped, others say they are not. We have no way of knowing what the circumstances of each individual were at the time of the treatment. We can't tell how far the cancer had gone, how faithfully the treatment was followed, how encouraging the doctor was about using Krebiozen for the specific type of cancer, etc.

Letter Gives Personal Experience with Drug

We were pleased, therefore, to come across this letter to the editor of the Buffalo (New York) *Courier Express,* printed in the October 18, 1961, edition of the paper. The letter is valuable because it gives a personal experience with the drug in a completely understandable manner. It follows in full:

STATES KREBIOZEN HELPED ILL SISTER

EDITOR: Sally Zirmba requested information regarding Krebiozen in your column on October 3. May I offer my first-hand experience? On June 2, 1961, my sister underwent surgery for a brain tumor. The biopsy proved it malignant and further study found it to be a metastasis from the kidney.

Three weeks after surgery, the symptoms all returned. Cobalt therapy was started. Results were frightening. Her eyesight went; left side became paralyzed; her hair fell out. She was given narcotics and kept in a semi-stupor. On September 1, we secured her release from her cancer specialist who stated she was not responding to the cobalt. He told me, in answer to a direct question and in the presence of my father and my husband: "Your sister has 4 months to live at the outside. She can go at any time."

She was recorded as a terminal case. We located a doctor who would administer Krebiozen. On September 4, all narcotic intake ceased. On September 5, she received her first injection of Krebiozen and one each week thereafter. On September 26, she returned home to her husband and son and does light housekeeping. The paralysis is now resolved; hair growth progressing; eyesight 80 per cent restored. Temperature, blood count, pressure, reflexes and weight gain all restored to normal.

We have no doubt in our minds that, with continued use of Krebiozen, she will live a completely normal life with less difficulty than diabetics taking insulin. Every week she and her husband travel 600 miles to receive Krebiozen and will continue this schedule until another doctor can be found (in their area) who will administer the drug. M. L.

After reading this letter, there is a basis, we believe, from the layman's point of view, for deciding whether or not Krebiozen is worth a try.

Miscellaneous Facts on Cancer

We Gave Cancer a Head Start

In the *Wall Street Journal* (March 8, 1961), an article describing a new approach to the cancer problem was printed. It told of the concept of using the body's own powers of immunity for fighting the invasion of cancer cells. The theory here is that, in cancer patients, the body's natural ability to defend itself might somehow have been impaired, and the artificial stimulation of this ability could be the best means of combating cancer. The theory is bolstered by the fact that, in many cancer patients, skin grafts from another person take hold and grow for unusually long periods of time. In a healthy person, it is almost universally true that a skin graft from a source other than the person's own body rarely lasts more than 10 or 12 days. The healthy body rejects the foreign substance through its immunity mechanism, and acts to destroy the graft. These defense mechanisms are apparently defective in cancer patients.

In tests, transplants of normal adult skin were made in numerous patients with various types of cancer. Over a third of the cancer patients held the grafts 30 days or more, some indefinitely. Even baby pigskin grafts survived unusually long. Normally, animal skin grafts are cast off even earlier than human skin. It is presumed that the normal body throws off the "foreign" cancer cells in the same way. Further evidence is provided in the fact that cancer cells cannot survive in a healthy person, as shown in tests with healthy volunteer inmates at an Ohio penitentiary. The men allowed live cancer cells to be implanted under their skin. Nodules or lumps appeared at first, but within 3 weeks, all signs of cancer had disappeared. The reaction closely resembled a normal person's reaction to skin grafts.

Scientists have found at least two substances in the blood which, with white cells, seem to be involved with immunity. One of these, present in high quantity in the penitentiary inmates, is properdin, a substance in which some cancer patients appear to be deficient. Of course, properdin alone cannot be considered entirely responsible for the defense of a normal body against cancer.

This whole idea of a body's natural immunity being used against cancer was formally proposed at least 10 years ago in the theory behind Krebiozen. Krebiozen is distilled from the blood of horses which have successfully defended themselves against a sometimes fatal animal disease known as "lumpy jaw." It was presumed that something in the blood chemistry of the horses which had been responsible for this factor could be identified as conquering the disease, and that, if isolated, it might have the same reaction against cancer if injected into a human. The results were gratifying to those who originated the theory and others who have since worked with this substance. Even the most skeptical observer would have to admit, upon examining the records of the patients treated with Krebiozen, that it is worth further study. Due to some unfortunate and extraneous difficulties, the American Medical Association has seen fit to mark the treatment as useless on the basis of its provably fraudulent investigation. Agitation for a fair test of Krebiozen still goes on as of this writing. Doctors are uninformed about it, or simply refuse to use Krebiozen because of the pronouncements against it by organized medicine.

Now we have the Sloan-Kettering Institute for Cancer Research coming up with a similar idea, based on the principle of using natural immunity. The progress will probably be rapid in investigating this proposed solution since its origin was in such orthodox surroundings. One must wonder, however, what a complete and friendly investigation of Krebiozen would have uncovered by now. What number of cancer victims would have been helped by the new knowledge gained by pursuit of the original theory? We are now 10 years behind due to the fact that we ignored an opportunity to investigate.

A Different Theory on Cancer Causes

Dr. E. Haslett Frazer made an interesting comment on the cancer question in the July 25, 1959, issue of the *Medical Journal of Australia*. He says, "It would seem that the repeated application or ingestion of irritants—*the latter including devitalized and preserved foods* (italics ours)—might have some bearing on the health of the particular cell structure involved." He then quotes Dr. Llewellin Davey as saying, in the May 30, 1959, issue of the same magazine, that "chronic irritation, long continued, whether mechanical, chemical or bactericidal seems to be the only cause of cancer yet agreed to." The unusual part of the letter is Dr. Frazer's suggestion that the sites chosen for this pathological change might be governed by a psychological disturbance. In plainer words, one's mental state might determine the type of cancer by which one is attacked.

This idea is an interesting one, and certainly has its possibilities. Illness brought on, and/or prolonged, by mental attitude is a well-recognized fact. Could the mental agitation so characteristic of our time, caused largely by the diet we eat, be expressing itself in the increased cancer rate that we are experiencing?

Cancer from the Open Fire

The charcoal barbecue pit is a new fixture on the American scene. In the past 10 years, we have come to love the taste of charcoal. Outdoor and indoor pits are a status symbol. The highway beaneries feature charcoal-broiled hot dogs, hamburgers, steaks, etc., and do a big business.

In the *Eugene* (Oregon) *Registar Guard* (November 8, 1961), a *United Press International* release tells of Dr. Charles Huggens, cancer surgeon and researcher, and his remark that highly smoked foods have been found to contain cancer-inducing substances. Since barbecued foods over charcoal flame are indeed highly smoked, the item took on great significance in our eyes.

Dr. Huggens said the "coal tar created by the decomposition of wood or coal is the problem, just as it is in cigarettes." He told a news conference that "coal tar deposits were found in products smoked in barbecues, charcoal broilers and even those roasted over open fires."

The American Indian ate plenty of food cooked over an open fire, did he get cancer from it? We certainly don't have any way of checking on that question. However, we do know that his exposure to other cancer causers was more limited than ours. He had no food contaminated with other chemical compounds to preserve freshness, softness, hardness, etc. He did not breathe exhaust fumes and industrial smoke. In other words, he was not exposed to the atmospheric hazards and food processing problems we meet each day. He had no choice but to risk the consequences of open fire cooking; we have. Why expose yourself to yet another health hazard by eating charcoal broiled or barbecued foods? You can cook meats and vegetables with a safe source of heat, such as electricity or gas, with no inconvenience at all.

Of course, an occasional cook-out won't do any real harm. But many citizens have made a fetish of foods cooked over an open fire and eat them several times a week. This is repeated exposure to a known danger. Why take the chance?

Cereals

Good Nutrition with Brown Rice

Nutritionists are still wondering when the American people will get the sense and courage to demand unpolished rice, exclusively, from their grocers. As in the case of white bread, the rice manufacturers simply decided that white rice is easier to handle and store than brown, and we, like sheep, have followed their lead. We eat polished rice, not because we don't like brown rice, but because many of us don't even know what brown rice is or that it is readily available.

What is the difference between white and brown rice? One word says it all: nutrition. The "brown" which is processed out of most rice is the part which contains 10 per cent of the protein, 85 per cent of the fat and 70 per cent of the minerals you could be getting. It also contains 400 per cent more thiamin, 300 per cent more riboflavin and 300 per cent more niacin than white rice. These are major B vitamins, vitamins which researchers find sadly lacking in the diets of most Americans.

Other vitamins are robbed in the processing of brown rice, but in the *Indian Journal of Medical Research* (March, 1960), a report appeared on the importance of choline, one of the B-complex vitamins, which makes an appreciable appearance in rice polishings, that is, in the "brown" which is removed in making white rice. It has long been established that choline is effective in preventing fatty livers, an early step in working up to the dangerous condition, cirrhosis of the liver. Fatty livers have also been known to respond to therapeutic doses of choline. The authors of this paper determined to discover whether the amount of choline contained in rice polishings alone would be enough to counteract or prevent the development of fatty livers.

Five groups of rats were used: one group had all choline removed from its basal diet; two groups had .04 gram and 12 grams added respectively; the final two groups ate the basal diet plus .04 gram and 30 cubic centimeters of rice polishings, respectively, per 100 grams of diet.

Choline in Rice Polishings Protective

The animals were sacrificed periodically, and the livers removed from them for examination. Data showed clearly that the rice polishings concentrate in the greater amount (30 cubic centimeters per 100 grams of basal choline-containing diet) leads to the prevention of fatty livers in rats. A lesser concentrate (15 cubic centimeters per 100 grams) could not be depended upon for such prevention, and the diets became less effective in this area as the choline count decreased. Choline in sufficient amounts, then, can forestall fatty liver in rats and presumably in humans. The choline content of rice polishings concentrate is 122 milligrams per 100 grams.

The average American diet is not so rich in choline that one can afford to pass up rice polishings as an easy, economical source of this precious nutrient. The foods rich in B vitamins are largely neglected by modern eaters. With bun-and-coffee breakfasts, hot-dog-and-soda lunches and frozen-pizza-and-coffee dinners, the choline intake is pitifully low. The organ meats (liver, kidney, lungs and heart) are the best sources, and almost nobody these days eats them unless forced to do so. Turnip greens, barley, soybeans and spinach, aside from eggs, are by far the richest choline foods and rarely appear on the average menu. Rice is a food most people like to eat, and one which goes well with an endless variety of foods. Imagine yourself preparing a food for your family which they not only will enjoy, but which could be their best source of nutrition out of an entire day's eating. Serving brown rice instead of white would accomplish this. And brown rice is not a great hardship for the tastebuds. It is very close to white rice both in appearance and taste. The best way to prove this to yourself is to try a box of brown rice—it's very inexpensive—and make your own judgment on its merits. Your family might not even know the difference.

Many health-conscious persons use wheat germ and rice polishings as part of their daily diet as well. And why not? What better concentrated source of B vitamins can one find? These supplements are easy enough to add to one's other foods—salads, meatloaves, casseroles, etc. and can hardly be noticed, except as an unusual flavor improver.

Fights Disease

While you're improving the flavor of your meals and your general health, you are getting nutrients which have been proven helpful in cases of high blood pressure and ulcers. The aforementioned choline has proven its value, in animal experiments, against cancer, anemia and edema. Choline is found to be plentiful in human breast milk, and calves fed on choline-deficient milk have shown alarming symptoms leading to death. Some of the sick animals were saved, however, by adding nothing more than choline to their diets. Again we caution against the use of B vitamins, such as choline, separately, unless administered under a doctor's supervision. Best results are obtained when choline is ingested as it occurs naturally, as in the case of brown rice or rice polishings. While we have concentrated upon choline in these pages, we do not wish to discount the other values in brown rice. The B vitamins, some of which were mentioned, are all present, including the rarer biotin, para-amino-benzoic acid and pyridoxine. Good amounts of phosphorus, protein and fat are part of the brown rice kernel, too.

Wild Rice

Wild rice should be mentioned here because it is often confused with brown rice. Wild rice is usually used in very expensive restaurants to set off fowl or other roasted meats. Actually, it is not rice at all, but a food of completely different botanical origin. Wild rice grows almost entirely in Minnesota in relatively small amounts, and the scarcity of it (no more than 500,000 pounds a year) makes this food prohibitively expensive, about $1.00 a pound. If you can afford it, you will be eating the finest of nutritious foods, as rich in most ways as brown rice. Either one of these will be an important aid to you in maintaining good health.

Cheese

Artificial Holes in Swiss Cheese

For hundreds of years, the holes in Swiss cheese have been occurring on their own due to the natural gas formed within the cheese itself as it matures. Now, commercial cheese manufacturers have found a way to imitate nature with the job of perforating the cheese by using a gaseous form of hydrogen peroxide (actually a powerful antibiotic, according to Andre Voisin in *Soil, Grass and Cancer*). The gas will be pumped into the cheese and the holes will be sort of "burped" out. Why is this new process suggested? Because the cheese can be turned out cheaper and quicker. Who will benefit? Not the consumer, for cheesemakers feel that cheese produced in this way will not be as tasty as the natural product.

Wisconsin, "The Dairy State" and capital of our cheese producing industry, currently has statutes against cheese produced in this way, and it looks as though the state will fight to maintain them. In the *Milwaukee Journal* (March 6, 1960), the Wisconsin State Attorney General said that peroxide-produced cheese was not Swiss cheese. Labeling it so would be contrary to federal and state laws. However, in spite of this logical view, the federal Food and Drug Administration has recently announced its intention to approve the use of the chemical. The tentative way out seems to be labeling such cheese as something other than Swiss cheese. It will probably be called "Swiss-like" cheese, or some other misleading name, and be buttressed with advertising that will make the true product seem inferior.

We are not in favor of the use of milk or milk products by adults, but many persons do use them, and it is insupportable that they should be compelled to buy a product that has an added chemical for which there is no excuse. The natural Swiss cheese keeps as well and tastes better than the hydrogen peroxide product. As to the health hazard of this chemical in our food, no one has done any work on that. We think that a letter to the FDA asking why they intend to allow such unwarranted contamination of this food would not be amiss.

Chemicals in Food

A History of Food Additives

That there is nothing new under the sun is as evident in the study of the history of food additives, as it is with most other tried and true tricks. Actually, the addition to food of any foreign substance is, technically, food adulteration. In its crudest form, it is as old as commerce itself. During this century, it has developed into a branch of applied science, necessitating laws to be passed, government agencies and laboratories to be maintained for the purpose of detecting impurities and protecting the general public. With advanced learning, the world has progressed from the simple practice of weighting bread with a stone, to the use of aniline dyes, antiseptic chemicals, substitutions and synthetics of all description in almost all foods. The main reason for finagling with food is exactly the same today as it was in its earliest inception: more profit for the food peddler. The main reason has been masked by such excuses as preservation, refrigeration, eye appeal, processing, refining. All this adds up to progress. This so-called progress instituted more flagrant abuses of existing food laws, more legislation sorely needed, more watchdogs to track down the abuses and abusers, more poison and less nutrition for the consumer, but with it all, more gain for the food suppliers.

Food Laws through the Ages

Now, back to history! Ancient Rome and Athens actually had to appoint food inspectors, because certain classic gentlemen were using color and flavoring agents. Back in 1203, in Merrie Olde England, King John issued a proclamation throughout the kingdom against additives in bread. Henry III, following him, issued a statute to protect the public from the "dishonest dealings of bakers, vintners, brewers, butchers and others." This was the first statute known to prohibit tampering with human food and was enforced until 1709, when it was repealed.

Germany's method of punishing unscrupulous food dealers was swift and sure. From 1390 to 1482, records exist verifying that such offenders were dragged out of town, branded or pilloried and their products destroyed. One wine seller was made to drink 6 quarts of his own impure wine, after which he died.

In France, successive food ordinances appear from the years 1330 to 1672. The chief penalties carried large fines and confiscation. From 1725 to 1847, England passed legislation against specific foods —tea, coffee, cocoa, sugar—that were altered or colored. At about this time the public became concerned about some of the outrages

144

aimed at their food. In 1850, Dr. Arthur H. Hassall's microscopic examination of coffee (chicory enriched) led him on to other food examinations. He pursued this work for 4 years, under the auspices of the "Lancet Analytical Sanitary Commission." His findings, published regularly and universally accepted, contained these appalling statistics: 3 of 34 brands of coffee were pure. Foreign substances ranged from chicory, roasted corn, beans, potato flour or acorns; of 49 breads, all contained alum; of 56 cocoa samples, 8 were pure; of 26 milks, 14 were impure; of 28 cayenne peppers, only 4 were genuine and red lead and vermillion were found in the remaining samples. The most startling finding concerns sweets. Tests of over 100 samples of candies showed that 59 contained chromate of lead, 11 gamboge, 12 red lead, 6 vermillion, 9 arsenate of copper and 4 white lead. Although most of the foods mentioned are not essential for good nutrition, Dr. Hassell's exposé led to public pressure for protection. The passage of England's "Sale of Food and Drug Act, 1875," still in effect, but much amended, was Britain's answer.

The Work of Dr. Harvey Wiley

While Britain's battle was being waged, our champion, the tireless warrior for pure foods, Dr. Harvey W. Wiley, emerged on the American scene. To survey the entire field of Dr. Wiley's efforts, which led to the enactment of the Pure Food and Drug Act, 1906, would be a herculean task. Suffice it to say that, as state chemist of Indiana from 1874-1883 and subsequently, as Chief of the Bureau of Chemistry in the United States Department of Agriculture from 1883 to his resignation in 1912, until his death in 1930, he devoted his life to the cause of pure food.

His earliest battles were against such preservatives as boric acid, borax, formaldehyde (embalming fluid), salicylic acid or ortho-hydroxybenzoic acid (produced from oil of wintergreen or synthetically, large doses of which can produce deafness, headache, delirium, vomiting, hemorrhage or heart failure), sulfurous acid (which can cause nephritis), sodium fluoride (which interferes with digestion). Another terrifying target was one of the chief coloring agents willfully added to canned green vegetables, sulfate of copper. Green vegetables, under these conditions, were definitely injurious to health. The Pure Food and Drug Act forbade the use of this metallic coloring agent, along with antimony, arsenic, cadmium, chromium, mercury, lead and zinc. Forbidden, too, was the vegetable coloring, gamboge and all coal tars. Sulfur dioxide and benzoic acid still were permitted, however.

The foresighted Dr. Wiley had conducted experiments from 1902 to 1907 with his 12-man volunteer "Poison Squad." He dealt with 7 specific food additives: boric acid and borax; salicylic acid and salicylates; sulfurous acid and sulfites; sulfate of copper; saltpeter. For 5 years the courageous men of the "Poison Squad" were fed these poisons in food under scientific conditions. The findings were published as parts of *Bulletin 84, Bureau of Chemistry,* comprising 7 parts. Parts VI and VII, dealing with sulfate of copper and saltpeter, were never published. Three years later, the Remsen Board banned copper and saltpeter (previously used in coloring cured meats). For 3 years longer than necessary, these dangerous additives were permitted to be used. Who will ever know at what price?

In 1904, Dr. Wiley stated, "It appears . . . that both boric acid and borax, when continuously administered in small doses for a long period or when given in large quantities for a short period, create disturbances of appetite, of digestion and of health." This report was adversely criticized. Both these agents are used as preservatives and medications today. However, it is most interesting to note that approximately two years ago, the Department of Health of New York City sent a bulletin to all city dentists and doctors stating that boric acid is a toxic agent: not permissible as an eyewash or for bathing wounds, etc. Even though Dr. Wiley recognized its disturbing qualities over 55 years ago, even though it has been proved to be unsafe for external use, reputable drug companies still manufacture boric acid, doctors still prescribe it and the nation still consumes it and uses it as a disinfectant.

History repeats itself. The Pure Food and Drug Act, so valiantly fought for, left much to be desired. Through no fault of its instigators, the auspicious beginning has not been a conclusive victory. There are many loopholes in spite of many amendments. Amendments that were offered for consideration 50 years ago by Wiley are still being fought for in Congress. The average uninformed consumer has been given a false sense of security in thinking that every well-packaged item, labeled as to contents, is safe to eat, because there are protective food laws.

Power of the Food Industry

The lords of the food industry obviously believe they can give or take away. They take away the staples of the nation's nutrition in grain, meat, fruits, vegetables. They strip them, bleach them, refine them, freeze them, cure them and all but turn them into sawdust, and after all this energy and waste is expended, they, in turn, enrich, color and add more chemicals to the massacred substances that remain.

What is the tolerance of the individual to the accumulation of all so-called safe amounts of extraneous matter in our foods? Who can tell?

It seems that the country is at last waking up to the danger of sprayed and processed foods, and therein lies our salvation. Up to now, food manufacturers have used our ignorance as their main selling point. They added whatever they chose, took out whatever was expedient and added any coloring they thought would appeal to the consumer. The product appeared on the grocer's shelf and, because it had gotten that far, we assumed it was safe to eat. Independent research has proven this to be untrue. The laws under which the Food and Drug Administration must operate, offer plenty of opportunity for manipulation by unscrupulous individuals, and Big Business is full of such individuals. Consumers are beginning to discover that this is true, and with the publicity about cancer incidence, have become more concerned about what is contained in what they eat.

What Can Be Done?

There are several things to be done to improve the situation. First, write to the manufacturer and tell him that you are opposed to his use of food additives—any food additives—and that you will discontinue buying his products so long as such objectionable material is contained in them. Next, tell your grocer that you would appreciate his stocking foods which do not contain dangerous food additives, or you will shop at a store where such items are available. Both of these are excellent means of forcing a change, for they both hit in the most vulnerable spot—the cash register. If enough such complaints are registered, a change will soon be made; these men are in business to sell. They need you!

Finally, write to your Congressman, assuring him that you are interested in pure food and that you will support him in any effort he makes to tighten the food laws. Keep your eye on the newspapers and write again each time you see that a law pertaining to the food industry is up for a vote. With enough support of this kind, Congress can pass legislation which will really protect us, the kind we really need.

What We Know about Our Food Supply

Why do you have such trouble convincing friends and neighbors of the seriousness of the situation where present-day foods are concerned? One of the reasons, of course, is that they never run across any information of this kind in the books and magazines they read or in the radio and TV programs to which they are exposed. They reason that these things can't be true or they would be mentioned in some of these various avenues of communication.

We have known for a long time that programs on radio and TV, as well as magazine and newspaper articles, are rather closely censored by the advertisers whose money supports these various media. We were not aware of just how closely regulated these things are until we happened across some revealing information along these lines.

Advertisers Dictate What Can Be Said

Variety, the newspaper of the entertainment industry, carried an article in its issue of October 26, 1960, discussing the orders sent out by advertisers concerning what may and may not be said on programs they sponsor.

Federal Communications Commission examiners, questioning the producers of various TV shows, have uncovered the restrictions laid down by some on shows they sponsor. Liggett and Myers (tobacco company) specify in their directions to the producer that "while we do not want to create an impression of one continual smoke-filled room, from time to time in the shows, we feel 'natural' smoking action is a requisite. . . . There are many incidental ways the show can help. For instance, background shot of cigarette machine in restaurant, train or bus station—a poster or display piece in a drug store—the end of a carton sticking out of a shopping bag . . . Obviously a 12-year-old should not be shown smoking. College men and women can be pictured smoking without any fear of criticism. . . We don't want public criticism in encouraging the too young or 'too young looking' to smoke. On the other hand, the high school and college market is extremely important to Liggett and Myers as future longtime customers."

Children, teen-agers and adults will, we assume, watch the Liggett and Myers sponsored shows. Regardless of the dramatic content, all viewers will be treated to as much subtle suggestion as possible, indicating that it is desirable, acceptable and commonplace to smoke and to buy cigarettes. The special note about high school students indicates that this is not considered "too young" to be dragging on a cigarette, while toiling over homework. Understandably, it is difficult for parents to persuade their high school age youngsters not to smoke when accepted TV programs, perhaps featuring teen-age idols, present teen-age smoking as desirable.

Some European countries have laws which forbid the advertising of cigarettes entirely.

You Are Encouraged Not to Think

General Mills, whose food products range from flour to many other types of processed food, present the producer of TV shows which they sponsor with a lengthy list of prohibitions. The dramatic content of the show is hedged around with so many forbidden items that we wonder how any writer worthy of the name could possibly create anything worthwhile, from the dramatic viewpoint. No controversy of any kind is allowed. "Where it seems fitting, the characters should reflect recognition and acceptance of the world situation in their thoughts and actions, although in dealing with war our writers should minimize the 'horror' aspects."

To continue, "There will be no material on any of our programs which could in any way further the concept of business as cold, ruthless and lacking all sentiment or spiritual motivation."

And "Special attention shall be given to any mention, however innocuous, of the baking business . . . Food subjects commercially treated cannot be presented with a program content that is unappetizing or tends to affect nausea upon the listener or viewer. If there is any question whatever about such material, it should be deleted." (The instructions go on to forbid mention of any other cowboy or "competitive" horse—Trigger or Silver, for instance.)

Miles Laboratories who sponsor Nervine and One-a-Day Brand Multiple Vitamins specify: "There should be no reference to headache, upset stomach or the taking of remedies to relieve same. There should be no statement or situation in conflict with One-a-Day Brand Multiple Vitamins. There should be no taking of bromides or sedatives for which Nervine might be used. There should be no representation of doctors, dentists, druggists or drug remedies in a derogatory manner or in situations embarrassing to them as a group."

The makers of Coca-Cola specify exactly which words actors must use in inviting other actors to have a drink of Coke. They outline the way the drink must be served, how the label must be displayed while pouring the drink; no half-consumed bottles are ever to be left to suggest a disinterest on the part of the drinker. And, strangely enough, "Children under 13 years of age should not be shown with Coca-Cola." According to the TV advertiser's code, apparently, it's all right to smoke if you're over 12, but you mustn't drink Cokes until after 13. It seems rather strange to us that such a rule should be laid down for Cokes. The American Medical Association carries ads in *Today's Health* for Coca-Cola!

Mars Candy runs into another kind of difficulty. On children's programs, the reward for good behavior is usually a sweet. "Go and buy yourself all the ice cream and cookies you want," chuckled a character in the program called Buffalo Bill Junior, much to the distress of the sponsors. Mars Candy wants children to buy nothing in the way of sweets but Mars Candy.

"TV is not intended to be a moral or cultural uplift," said the national chairman of the Writers Guild of America, writing in the official publication of the Screen Actors Guild. "It is devoted entirely to a specific form of advertising, namely brainwashing. The sole object is to condition the reflexes of all potential customers as if they were Pavlov's dogs.

"It is *all commercial*," he went on. "The so-called entertainment portion has the single function of associating the product with the common good. The formal commercial specifies the product brand label."

Movies Are "Advised" by Commercial Interests

That movies are rapidly coming in for the same brainwashing treatment is apparent from a release that recently came to our office. On the stationery of the National Confectioners Association appears a memo to Motion Pictures Producers from the Chairman of the Board of the Association, Victor A. Bonomo, stating that the movies have to help the candy business dispel a lot of untrue and unsavory notions that have been going around about the healthfulness of candy. Is candy a primary cause of overweight? Nonsense, says the Confectioners Association, "candy is no more caloric than many other food products and its nutritive values are considerable. Yet many of the negative statements emanate from the medical profession."

Mr. Bonomo goes on to say that, in the movie *The Bellboy,* there was a scene involving candy and overweight which "disturbed our industry greatly" because it was "extremely damaging to candy." He realizes, he goes on, that movies are the most powerful communications medium in the world, so he hopes sincerely that such a gross misrepresentation of fact will not occur again.

So far as calories are concerned, we must point out that Mr. Bonomo has been misinformed. Ounce for ounce, candy contains more calories than any other food, except for pure sugar and pure fats like butter and oil and some varieties of nuts. We know people who eat a quarter or a half a pound of candy at a sitting.

But, regardless of his understandable bias in favor of his product, Mr. Bonomo is attempting to dictate to a great communications industry so that they will soft pedal, gloss over or omit entirely any situations wherein his product might appear in an unfavorable light, even though, by his own admission, *the medical profession makes "negative" statements about candy.*

Do you understand now why your favorite characters in movies and TV eat any amount of candy and soft drinks and smoke all the cigarettes they want, but never put on weight or suffer from chronic coughs? Do you see how the image of the perfect middle class American family, always well, always happy, is forcefully associated in the mind of the viewer with the products advertised? How can there be anything unhealthful about present-day American food or habits when we never see anything about it on TV or in the movies? And very infrequently in magazines and newspapers!

By their own admission in the FCC testimony, today's advertisers are subtly exercising thought control to compel viewers to buy their products. Because of the peculiar psychological standards by which programs are written to result only in acceptance of products, there can be no such thing as real entertainment for entertainment's sake in this field.

The Unknown Poisons You Eat Every Day

"This is a good and well-documented book. It can be recommended to objective readers who are not likely to be frightened by the possibility of finding 'death in the pot.' " So says the December, 1960, issue of the *Lancet,* a famous British medical journal, referring to *Chemicals in Food and Farm Produce: Their Harmful Effects,* by Franklin Bicknell, M.D.

Dr. Bicknell, who is consulting physician to the French Hospital, London and the co-author of a definitive book *Vitamins in Medicine,* does not pull punches or make statements he cannot prove.

Is the Chemical Carcinogenic?

Speaking of the method used at present to determine whether or not a chemical additive (dye, in this case) is cancer-causing, Dr. Bicknell reminds us that results differ according to the kind of animal tested. If 2-naphthylamine is used on rats, ferrets, rabbits or cats, it is "proved" not to cause cancer; tested on dogs or man, it does cause cancer. "So one is left with the fear that, however many species do not develop cancer from some dye, yet man may—as indeed he does with sodium arsenite, which does not cause cancer in any experimental animal yet used."

Then, how many animals should be used in a test? To test a dye on only two species of animal requires about 1,500 animals if there is some doubt as to whether they may be unusually resistant to cancer. After you have tested the chemical on the animals, you still have no idea as to whether changes in diet, other chemicals added to food, physical accidents, leanness or obesity, illness or pregnancy —any of the circumstances that might occur in a human life—will cause an apparently harmless dye to become cancer-causing.

"Such possibilities are not academic niceties," Dr. Bicknell goes on, "since fat men are more prone than thin to cancer, while in animals and, presumably, in man, both excesses and deficiencies of essential ingredients of food may enhance the susceptibility to cancer —presumably by altering the amount of dye converted in the body to a cancer-causing substance."

Now, how long should the chemical (in this case a dye) be fed to determine whether or not it is cancer-causing to man? If you feed the chemical to an animal throughout its life, will you get the same results you get feeding the same substance to a man during his much longer life? No one knows. It is known that some chemicals fed to the mother during pregnancy can cause lung cancer in the unborn child 6 months after birth, so feeding experiments should be conducted for at least two generations, and preferably three.

Finally, how should the dye be given to the animal? If it is fed and causes no harm, this may indicate only that the animal cannot absorb it, whereas man may absorb it, especially when it is eaten with emulsifying agents, as it may be in the case of confectionery products, cake, etc. So if you test the dye's safety only by injection, this is no proof that man is safe when he eats it.

Cancer-Causing Substances Are All Around Us

"Probably few if any substances added to food are themselves capable of causing cancer," says Dr. Bicknell. "What the body turns them into is the danger." But we actually know very little about such matters, even for a healthy human body, let alone one already disordered by liver trouble, menopause, pregnancy and so forth. *"At present it seems probable that any dye is capable of producing cancer if it is broken down into certain substances by the body,"* says Dr. Bicknell.

"While it is possible to show a dye is dangerous, it is impossible to show it is safe," he goes on. "It is not wise to eat any artificially colored foods, such as jams, iced cakes, sweets, ices, canned peas, margarine, custard powder, etc." The "and so forth" includes (in the United States at least) just about every food that can be bought, even some fresh foods like potatoes, oranges and certain kinds of nuts.

Considering *that any dye may be capable of causing cancer,* depending upon the way the body deals with it, and considering that dyes serve absolutely no purpose in food except to give it a color it does not naturally have, do you see any reason why our Food and Drug Administration should permit any dyes at all in food? If all dyes were forbidden, no food manufacturer could protest that he had to dye the food because his competitor does and he could not sell something that looks drab. Let's campaign for all food to look as it looks naturally!

In succeeding chapters, Dr. Bicknell takes up preservatives, emulsifiers, flavorings, antibiotics, drugs, hormones, insecticides, weed killers in food. Though the *Lancet* believes that such information should be given only to those who do not become frightened by such facts, we believe that any thinking person who reads what Dr. Bicknell presents so clearly and unemotionally will be so disturbed that he will find it almost impossible to eat anything for days.

Cause of Disease

Then, finally, Dr. Bicknell takes up the prevention of disease— the prevention of tooth decay, of congenital abnormalities (that is, deformities at birth), prevention of cancer, diseases of the arteries, heart and kidneys, diseases of the nervous system. Although his description of each disease and its possible causes differs, the same pattern emerges in each chapter: there is no doubt that all of these diseases may be at least partly due to modern food, contaminated with all its many chemicals, and perverted, as Dr. Bicknell says, into something unfamiliar to the body processes by such things as refining and hydrogenation.

Here is the way Dr. Bicknell describes the effects of hydrogenation of fats, to make margarine, or present-day lard or white shortenings used for baking. Abnormal fatty acids are thus produced, having their atoms arranged in such a way that the body is deceived into thinking that this is the normal arrangement, so it proceeds to use them as it uses fats with normal fatty acids.

By the time the reaction has gone too far to be remedied, there is no way to throw them away and begin over again with natural fats. It is like jamming a lock with the wrong key. Not only can the lock not be opened by the wrong key, but one cannot use the right key so long as the wrong key stays jammed in the keyhole.

Other Fantastically Dangerous Chemicals in Foods

Here are some other arresting quotes from Dr. Bicknell's book. On insecticides: "I cannot overstress my belief that in the future, unexpected insidious damage to many organs will be found to be due to protein metabolism, essential amino acid metabolism, being deranged, not only by insecticides, but also by other chemicals, like those used to treat flour, present in our staple foods. There is also the nightmare suggestion that this perversion of protein metabolism might lead to the creation of new viruses.

"Field mushrooms are completely safe, but cultivated mushrooms have recently, in the north and west of England, caused epidemics of diarrhea and vomiting with acute shock and collapse, patients having to remain in hospital for over a week. Apparently, the mushrooms had been sprayed with a 'safe' insecticide, but this had been converted by the mushrooms into an acutely toxic substance. Such unpredictable conversion by plants and by animals of chemicals, themselves reasonably safe, into new and unidentifiable substances of unknown effect, is one of the most dangerous results of agricultural insecticides.

"The daily consumption for many years of such meats (treated with estrogen, a hormone) cannot be regarded with complete equanimity when it is remembered that synthetic estrogens are held to be related to leukemia and cancer; and when, I have been told, the virtually universal estrogenation of meats in the U.S.A. has prevented surgeons from assessing whether the surgical ablation of the estrogen-producing endocrine glands—for the treatment of cancer of the breast —has been successful or whether the pituitary gland must be destroyed, in spite of the inevitable risk and disabilities which follow such destruction." Our understanding of this statement is that doctors, trying to "treat" cancer patients by removing the glands which produce estrogen, cannot tell whether the operation has been successful, since the diet itself contributes so much synthetic estrogen.

Book Helps Fight the Problem

It is difficult to choose passages from *Chemicals in Food* to dwell on, for every sentence is important in our fight against chemicals. And every sentence is carefully documented in a bibliography which includes 291 different scientific references.

It is difficult to understand how any member of the Department of Health, Education and Welfare can read such a book and not take immediate steps toward outlawing many of the thousand or so chemicals now in food—just for the protection of themselves and their own families, even if they care nothing for the welfare of the public in general. No one can challenge Dr. Bicknell's facts.

No one could disagree with his basic premise, except someone with a completely closed mind to any information or someone who has a financial stake in pretending these statements are not true. Dr. Bicknell's basic premise is that there is every reason, scientifically speaking, to believe that many of the substances now in food are terribly harmful. It is impossible to prove that they are not. Since this is so, we should devote every effort to removing them from food, rather than trying to prove that they aren't harmful.

We think you should have a copy of this book to pass around among your friends and relatives, to review before your club or PTA, to quote in your letters to the local newspaper and your Congressman. Better than any other book we have seen, this book demonstrates the terrifying complexity of the problem of chemicals in food and the urgent necessity of its solution if we would avoid widespread and permanent damage to human life.

There's Danger in Food Wrappings and Packages

Let us begin by saying that the booklet *Chemicals and the Food Industry,* Manual 26, of the California Agricultural Experiment Station Extension Service, University of California, lists some 82 chemical substances that are permitted as additives in food packaging materials. It is understood, of course, that many or perhaps all of these chemicals eventually "migrate" into the food. This is the reason why permission to put them into the food packaging had to be obtained. No one cares, of course, what goes into packaging so long as there is no possibility of its contaminating the food.

The word "contaminating" is not used in this connection by most people concerned with food poisoning and packaging, incidentally. They use the pleasanter term "migrating." They speak of tin stearate, for instance, as a "migrant" into food from the packaging. Tin stearate may exist, as a migrant, in food, up to 50 parts per million, in case you are interested.

Why should any foods be wrapped or packaged? Why should

the consumer be exposed to this extra hazard which has nothing to do with food as such, but only with the appearance of the food as it lies on the grocery shelf and the convenience with which it can be transported and stored?

Do you remember the old-time grocery store where sugar was measured into a paper bag directly from the sugar barrel, cheese was cut from a huge wheel, covered against the flies and wrapped by the grocer, rice, candy and spices weighed out into paper bags? Obviously the modern super market cannot be run along these lines.

Self-service, which prevails in most of the grocery business today, necessitates packaging. Packaging is necessary, too, for transportation. Rice packaged on an assembly line where cleanliness is scrupulously maintained is surely preferable to the rice in the old-fashioned paper bag weighed out by the grocer. Cheese packaged at the factory hasn't been breathed on, sneezed on and bent over by every other customer. Packaged spices are fresher and more aromatic than if they have been reposing for goodness knows how long in a jar on the grocer's shelf.

However, the magazines of the grocery trade (a large portion of which is completely taken up with the subject of packaging) indicate that perhaps the main reason for today's packaging of food products is to make them look more attractive to customers. And the resultant frenzy in the packaging industry has begun to take on the dimensions of the women's fashion industry. In many cases, the package seems to be far, far more important than the food it contains. Page after page of text, with glowing pictures in color, are devoted to packaging in the same trade magazine that may grudgingly allow a column or two to news about nutrition or food itself.

But many of the chemicals used in modern packaging are there to treat the food, as well as the eye of the customer. Antioxidants, for example, such as butylated hydroxyanisole, are put into packaging material to help keep the food from becoming rancid. How many foods that you buy have this preservative on the label? How much of it do you suppose you have eaten over a lifetime?

Testing for toxicity the chemicals used in packaging materials seems to us to be a well nigh insurmountable task. It isn't simply a question of laying out one food or another on a piece of packaging material and then testing the food to see whether or not it contains chemicals from the packaging, and, if so, how much and finally whether or not the amount of chemical-from-the-package is harmful.

Nothing is as simple as that. Let us suppose the food tested is dry cereal and we find that exposing the food to the packaging material for a week results in no contamination of the cereal by any chemical in the package. But what if we leave the cereal in the package for a week or a month or a year? What if we store the cereal under conditions of heat or moisture which release more chemical from the packaging material? What if new chemicals added to the cereal cause a change in its susceptibility to absorbing chemicals from the package? What if printing added to the package or string tied around it or wax used to seal it introduce another possible toxic hazard? As you can see, the possibilities for contamination of just this one food are almost endless.

And that's just one food. Let's suppose you want to use this same packaging material for cheese or meat or candy or dehydrated soup or any of the other thousands of packaged foods we buy every day. Different foods have different chemical properties and no one can know how these will react with the chemicals in the packaging material.

What About Wax Cartons for Milk?

A good example of the complexity of the problem is the question of wax cartons used for milk. On June 12, 1959, newspapers throughout the country carried the story that a cancer researcher had discovered that milk cartons contain small amounts of a cancer-causing wax which "migrate" into the milk contained in such cartons. Public concern was instantaneous, widespread and intense. There was not the furor the cranberry incident caused, perhaps because milk is not a seasonal food much in demand at holiday time. However, milk is the basis of the diet of most of our infants and children as well as many ill and old people. Questions poured in to dairies, to newspapers, to the Food and Drug Administration.

Leaders of the milk industry, especially those involved in public relations, must have spent sleepless nights and the milk carton industry was teetering on the brink of certain disaster.

On June 30, 1959, Arthur S. Flemming, then Secretary of Health, Education and Welfare, issued a statement to the press, of which we reproduce the salient facts: "I am informed that both the Food and Drug Administration and the Public Health Service are receiving many inquiries about possible cancer-producing agents in wax used for milk cartons and other food containers.

"I think we should try to clarify the situation with respect to these waxes.

"During the latter part of 1956, Dr. W. C. Hueper of the Public Health Service arranged with the Milk Industry Foundation to collect waxes used by dairies for the impregnation of milk containers. Several months later, the Foundation assembled about 49 waxes for further chemical and biological analysis and sent them to the National Cancer Institute. In June, 1957, 24 of these waxes were sent for study to Dr. Philipe Shubik, of the Division of Chemistry, Chicago Medical School.

"In the fall of 1957, Dr. Hueper received a report from Dr.

Shubik on results of preliminary tests of the 24 waxes. The studies were performed by Dr. William Lijinsky, an associate of Dr. Shubik. It was demonstrated in these studies that one of the waxes contained a known carcinogen (cancer-producing agent) 1,2,5,6-dibenzanthracene. Three additional waxes were suspected, but no carcinogen could be identified. It should be noted that, while this compound has produced cancer in laboratory animals, (it) has not been shown to produce cancer in man."

What happened after that was that the American Petroleum Industry gave 100,000 dollars a year for 5 years for further research. Dr. Shubik promised to publish his findings as he went along. The industry gave him an additional 26 waxes to test. By this time, Dr. Shubik had discovered a new method of testing for the carcinogenic substance, so that he could now detect one part per half-billion parts of wax, rather than the one part per million he could detect before.

Mr. Flemming goes on to say, "Meanwhile, in 1958, samples of the 24 waxes . . . also were sent to Dr. Paul Kotin, Associate Professor of Pathology at the University of Southern California. The major results of this study . . . were published in the April 25, 1959, issue of a British scientific journal, *Nature*.

"The Kotin investigations confirmed the Shubik findings that one wax contained between .5 and one microgram per gram of 1,2,-5,6-dibenzanthracene. The Kotin investigations demonstrated, in addition, that 1,2,5,6-dibenzanthracene added to dairy waxes for experimental purposes was extracted from thin layers of wax by milk."

Scientific Findings Brushed Aside

The last sentence of Mr. Flemming's statement is amazing. He says, "The results of these studies have been reviewed by scientists of both the Public Health Service and the Food and Drug Administration. I am advised that the findings are not final, but no indications of a health hazard have been found."

We can't for the life of us imagine why such a statement should be made, can you? While tests already financed were still being conducted, the head of our health agency had decided, on the basis of incomplete evidence, that there was no health hazard.

What does the milk industry say? *Milk Review and Milk Plant Monthly,* in an "Urgent Bulletin" dated June 19, 1959, points out that the research reported in *Nature* dealt only with a cancer-causing agent which had been put into the wax specifically for their test— not one that naturally occurs in such wax.

True, the release goes on, there was that one part per million of carcinogen that was found in one of the waxes used for milk cartons. But, never mind, the actual cancer-causing substance that was absorbed by the milk from the carton had been put there by the researchers themselves. So the cheerful conclusion is "if carcinogens in dairy wax were the only hazard to human life, we would all live forever."

Unfortunately, they are not the only cancer-causing hazards to human life. And, most important of all, they are not the only cancer-causing hazards to human life which appear pretty regularly in food and items associated with food. If, by ignoring the one part per million of a cancer-causing substance in that one wax, we have added to the already heavy burden of toxic substances leading to cancer, how can we excuse such an action?

And how could the man appointed by the president to watch over our health airily dismiss these waxes as "no health hazard" when the necessary research, bought and paid for by the petroleum industry, had barely begun?

If, as is perfectly possible, Dr. Shubik finds that there is a very definite health hazard involved, who is going to know how many of those condemned to agonized death by cancer were exposed to the final chemical irritation that brought on the cancer through the wax on milk cartons?

We have taken up only one of the many chemicals used in packaging to indicate how complex is the problem and how unlikely it is that it will be treated with the consumer's welfare in mind. The packaging industry is big business. Two billion dollars a year are spent on disposable packaging in this country alone, of which food packaging must be quite an important part. Waxes, incidentally, are used directly on food as well as in cartons.

One further note. The list of chemicals approved for use in the packaging of meat includes synthetic resins, stabilizers, drying oils, colorants and release agents, which are to be used in "rubber or synthetic resins intended for contact with federally inspected meat food products." The list includes 123 chemicals, among them such things as formaldehyde and carbon black which has come under close scrutiny, in another connection, as a possible cancer causer.

Poisons and Poison Pens

One of the most authoritative books on chemical additives is entitled *The Poisons in Your Food*. Its author, William Longgood, is a prize-winning reporter on a great New York newspaper. He has given to the book all the careful attention to fact that a reporter knows is essential for good reporting. He does not call names. He simply states facts, bulwarking them with references from scientific journals, from testimony before Congressional committees, from public statements made by well-qualified public authorities.

Mr. Longgood has no axe to grind. He represents no foundation, no big corporation. He has a conscience, that is all. And he is frightened at the facts he has turned up in his research on chemicals in food.

Some of the Reviews

Take a look at a few of the reviews his book has received. *Science,* the publication of the American Association for the Advancement of Science, calls Mr. Longgood's work "blood-thirsty penpushing." The reviewer goes on to use words like "cultists" and "irresponsible sensationalism." He declares that the few authorities quoted by Mr. Longgood have been quoted out of context, so that the real meaning of their statements has been distorted.

The reviewer for the *New York Times,* we are glad to say, does not resort to name calling—and isn't it strange that his review should be so much more objective and clinical than that in the periodical of the highest scientific body in our land? The *Times* reviewer, Mr. Osmundsen, defends chemicals in food by stating flatly that the population shift from rural to urban areas has diminished the number of food producers and increased the relative number of food consumers. Therefore, we must have chemicals in food, since food must be transported over long distances and stored for greater periods of time.

From Farm to City

Let's examine this seemingly sound proposition for a moment. We'll take our information from a publication of the Food and Drug Administration, *What Consumers Should Know about Additives,* which listed some of the thousand or so additives Mr. Longgood objects to in his book. Emulsifiers. Can anybody not working for a chemical company which sells emulsifiers show us why these substances must now be put in foods because we have moved from the farms into the cities? Stabilizers and thickeners are now necessary, to make smoothness of texture and uniformity of color in foods, according to the FDA. Yet, the *New York Times* would have us believe that Americans would rather starve or be poisoned than to eat a food which does not have a smooth texture and a uniform color! How did the older generation on the farm ever manage to choke down the food grandmother put before them, do you suppose?

Acids, alkalizers, buffers, neutralizing agents are essential says the FDA. They prevent confectioneries from being "grainy," they give taste to soft drinks. How could we possibly get along without these essentials now that we have stopped raising our own food and moved into cities? Bleaching agents are listed by the FDA as necessary as anything yet. Imagine having to eat bread whose flour was "yellowish in color" or English walnuts the same color they had when they fell from the tree!

Of course, the FDA must reveal at the same time that the bleaching agent in flour is not really used because the millers are concerned with our sensibilities about yellow flour, but because bleaching flour saves time and money for the millers. Here are other additives mentioned in the FDA booklet: leavening agents, anticaking agents, hardening agents, clarifying and chillproofing agents, propellants, drying agents and antifoaming agents. Can any sensible person continue to insist that such chemicals as these are necessary because food must be now transported farther and stored for longer periods of time than formerly?

Coal-Tar Dyes

Now, finally, we come to the subject of dyes, coal-tar dyes specifically. Time and again, coal-tar dyes have been shown to be cancer-causing—some of them after they have been certified as completely "safe" for many years. Mr. Osmundsen, will you please tell us just how the removal of many of our citizens from farm to city has made the dyeing of every mouthful of food essential? Mr. Longgood devotes a chapter of his book to dyes. He quotes a cancer expert with the National Cancer Institute, he quotes a scientist from the Food and Drug Administration, he quotes a cancer expert of the University of Florida, he quotes the director of the Melbourne Hospital in Australia on the dangers of dyes and, finally, he quotes the International Union Against Cancer as saying that "not one dye has been proven safe for use in food."

Are such people as these quoted above, quacks and cultists? Or is it only when Mr. Longgood quotes them that they become quacks and cultists?

Dr. Stare's Statement

Now we come to a brief note on Mr. Longgood's book written by Dr. Frederick Stare of the Department of Nutrition at Harvard University. Dr. Stare uses these words in speaking of Mr. Longgood's carefully documented book: "sensation-rousing," "irresponsible stuff," "cultists," "faddists," etc. Dr. Stare points out that we are the best-fed country in the world because you can get lettuce and tomatoes 52 weeks out of the year. The implication is that it doesn't matter if they poison you!

Dr. Stare recommends that you get your information about foods from the National Research Council, the Council on Foods and Nutrition of the AMA (which was publishing assurance of the safety of stilbestrol, even *after* the FDA had forbidden its use in pellets!), the Nutrition Foundation (which was organized and is supported by the large food processing companies). Dr. Stare's department at Harvard also received a grant of one million dollars from General Foods in recognition of his fine work in the field of nutrition.

None of these reviews takes up any of the facts presented in the book. They are unassailable. When a cancer expert, who has devoted his life to this subject, presents evidence that certain substances are very probably going to cause cancer in some people who are exposed to them daily, how can a mere magazine reviewer dare to challenge the validity of such a statement?

Get Mr. Longgood's book and see for yourself the careful and objective way in which he treats this frightening subject of the poisons in our food. Then decide for yourself what value you want to place on reviews that ridicule the book and call the author names. The book is *The Poisons in Your Food* which is published by Simon & Schuster, New York, New York.

Chewing

How Important Is Chewing?

About 50 years ago, health-conscious parents kept an eye out for how carefully their children's food was chewed before it was swallowed. Some books gave it as an absolute rule that 32 chews are necessary to make food fit to swallow. People don't actually worry that much about it anymore, but there are scientific quibbles, still, about the need for chewing food to make it digestible.

The whole process of chewing is an interesting one. Generally, most of us think of chewing as a means of reducing foods to particles that are easy to swallow. That is really only a small part of the process. In *Southern Medicine and Surgery* (February, 1941), we found an absorbing article by J. Van de Erbe, M.D., which gave us a whole new view of this common-place action of chewing. He reminds us that the foods we swallow give us nourishment by the absorption of the nutrients they contain through the stomach wall. Only liquids can be absorbed in this way, so part of the function of chewing is to bring foods closer to the liquid state.

Of the 6 broad categories of foodstuffs we eat, only 3 (vitamins, inorganic salts and water) are ready for absorption into the blood stream without the aid of chewing. The rest (proteins, carbohydrates and fats) must undergo extensive changes before they can be absorbed and metabolized. As for the food, it is affected in 4 ways aside from the obvious mechanical one. A chemical, nervous, hormonal and bacterial change is going on as the chewing progresses.

Taste and Odors Help Digestion

An interesting and immediate effect of any chewing at all is the contact with the taste buds, and the release of appetizing odors which stimulate the nerves of smell and cause the action of the body's digestive organs and juices in the stomach.

In chewing, saliva, of course, plays a vital, often unrecognized, role. Anything put in the mouth causes a flow of saliva, and the saliva has many functions. It causes a chemical reaction; it keeps the mouth clean by excreting certain substances and it liquefies and lubricates the foods which are to be swallowed. Of course, without this last result, we would be unable to swallow our foods.

Saliva suits itself, in an almost miraculous way, to the type of food we eat. For a dry food, the saliva is excessively watery; for acid materials, the saliva is rich in protein for buffering action, etc. Whatever the food, the saliva acts to help in making it more acceptable to the body's intestines. The flow of saliva varies with the individual, causing faster or slower speeds in eating and digestion.

Ptyalin is one of the ingredients in saliva that produces a chemical reaction with food. In this case, only certain carbohydrate foods are affected, but the action is so thorough that it is continued in the stomach. There are other enzymes contained in saliva that work on the other foods to produce chemical reactions which are necessary if food is to be digested properly.

A Cleansing Agent

The saliva, which is activated by chewing, acts as a cleansing flush for the mouth. It washes out food leavings, bacteria and dead cells. When fever comes in illness, the lack of saliva, which is characteristic of feverish persons, is held to be largely responsible for the bad breath one encounters so frequently in such cases.

When poisons are present in the system, saliva often acts as a vehicle for expelling them. Diabetics excrete some excess sugar by this means; in nephritis cases, the saliva is high in urea content; overactive thyroid cases throw off excess calcium by this route. A blue-gray line forms on the gums of lead-poisoning victims, and this is because the lead has been carried there by the saliva; the same is true of sulfur, present in tooth tartar or on decaying teeth. Even polio virus carried in saliva is powerful enough to cause clinical polio if injected into experimental rats or monkeys.

Relaxing

As soon as food is taken into the mouth, the saliva goes to work, whether the food is chewed or not. The true function of chewing is merely to make the food of a size that can be easily swallowed and, in the process, to expose as many surfaces of that food as possible to the work that saliva can do. (Proper occlusion, or meeting, of teeth surfaces is a factor in thoroughness.) A side effect of chewing has been found to be relaxation. In *Psychological Review* (November, 1940), Dr. G. I. Freeman reported on experiments that showed chewing to be restful, provided that it were done in a leisurely fashion. If engaged in strenuously, the tension of the body is actually increased. This probably means that the mandatory chewing engaged in when the rule of 32 times was employed, was actually more harmful than it was helpful.

In the previously quoted *Southern Medicine and Surgery,* Dr. Erbe says that it is futile to chew excessively long. The mouth and tongue have extremely sensitive nerve endings (more sensitive than the finger tips) which do a fine job of letting us know when our food is ready for swallowing. If one chews normally, without any outside pressures hurrying one on or forcing one to slow down, the chewing time is sure to be sufficient.

Dr. Erbe makes one other point. He says that, if more time were spent in the careful selection of food and an adequate diet including all good foods, our digestive systems would not be so outrageously and fatally overworked.

How Much Should You Chew?

Chewing foods dozens of times will not change the fact that they are unhealthful if that is the case. It is much easier for your body to cope with poorly chewed food that is proper to it, than pulverized junk that cannot be digested and used, no matter how carefully it's been chewed.

Editor Rodale has often declared that he chews his food lightly and suffers no ill effect. The point is, however, that he eats healthful foods and does his chewing unconsciously; he does not rush, he just seems to eat faster than others. He swallows when his mouth and tongue nerve endings tell him the food is the proper swallowing size for *him.* He has also suggested that some people have a wider esophagus than others, and that this reduces their need to chew foods finely.

Where your chewing habits fit into this scheme must be determined by yourself. You alone can decide if you chew your food long enough before swallowing it. But whatever you do, be sure that you're eating the proper foods, because if you're not, no amount of care in chewing will save you from the effects of unhealthful foods.

Chewing Gum

The Chewing Gum Question

The *Practitioner* for August, 1959, speculates, rather amusingly, on the possibility that the chewing gum habit in America might well lead to an eventual change in the looks of Americans. By all the laws of science, all of that chewing should have some effect on the size of the muscles of mastication. Big jaws may become our national characteristic, the way the people of the sunny Mediterranean countries generally have swarthy complexions or Englishmen habitually carry umbrellas.

These few chewing gum paragraphs had more sobering data, aside from the basic joke. They told of 306 million dollars spent in America for chewing gum in 1958. Statistically, each of us could have had 200 sticks of the stuff. To mix up a 306 million dollar batch, manufacturers used 150 million pounds of sugar, 50 million pounds of corn syrup, 20 million pounds of dried sapodillo syrup, 24 million pounds of rubber and resin and 6 million pounds of chalk.

From this recipe, we can see that every stick of chewing gum is one-third refined sugar. Not only is sugar known to be a prime cause of tooth decay, but chewing gum keeps the sugar in close proximity to the teeth—the very thing that dental experts say will most surely cause tooth decay. Once the damage to the teeth is accomplished, the sugar is swallowed and eligible to accomplish its characteristic destruction of B vitamins and raise the blood sugar.

Did you know that there is even such a thing as chewing gum fever? It occurs when gum chewing produces a measurable rise in oral temperature from .4 degrees to 1.2 degrees Fahrenheit. Why this temperature rise should occur is not clear. However, elevated temperature is a sign of danger, a warning that chewing gum can lead to trouble. Chew on a piece of fruit or raw vegetable if you feel the urge to chew.

Childbirth

The Pain of Childbirth

From fire to atomic fission, there has always been reason to suspect that the "blessings" of advancing civilization may well be curses in disguise. Usually they turn out to be both. This is certainly true of childbirth anesthesia, which, in judicious and expert use, can be a saver of life and a sparer of excruciating pain, but which carries grave dangers along with it and is probably being used far more today than it should be.

It is natural to fear and avoid pain. This is an instinct that plays a vital role in the birth process. As described by Alan F. Guttmacher, M.D., Clinical Professor of Obstetrics and Gynecology of the Columbia Medical School, in his book *Pregnancy and Birth,* ". . . the baby's head pressing on the tissues of the lower vagina and bowel makes her (the mother) bear down involuntarily, with a reflex desire to expel the offending mass. With each labor pain, because of the powerful force generated by the contraction of the large, muscular uterus, aided by the mother's vigorous straining, the baby descends lower and lower, and soon its scalp appears at the entrance to the vagina. . . ."

This is the normal process of childbirth, in which the pain that is present hastens the delivery and minimizes possible damage to mother and child.

Today, however, while most leading obstetricians endorse the natural childbirth methods of Dr. Grantly Dick Read, or a very similar technique they refer to as "Educated Childbirth," there remain far too many that choose to ignore the dangers and difficulties of anesthetics and pain killers and use them far more than is necessary. This is an easy road to popularity, and also to birth complications, stillbirth and damage to the child.

Pain Killers Dangerous

Dr. Guttmacher, in *Pregnancy and Birth,* points out that "most drugs given the mother, no matter by what route of administration, rapidly gain access to her blood and forthwith pass through the placenta into the fetus' blood. This is the case when analgesic (pain-relieving) drugs are used. As a group, the analgesics are nerve depressants, depressing not only the sensation of pain, but other nervous mechanisms, including respiration. The mother's breathing center, located in the brain, is relatively resistant to their depressing effects, but not so the respiratory center of the new born, which is highly susceptible to such inhibitory influences."

In other words, even though Dr. Guttmacher uses discreet language calculated not to give alarm, what he is saying is that the pain relievers used so often during labor make it more difficult for the newborn child to start breathing. He also points out that they can slow up and prolong labor, and can endanger the safety of the mother as well as the child.

The Barbiturates

The most popular and commonly used of the analgesics in labor, according to this doctor, are the barbiturates (seconal, nembutal or amytal) in combination with demerol and scopolamine. This supposedly "modern" combination of drugs resembles the old "Twilight Sleep" introduced in 1907 by the German, Dr. Gauss. This was a combination of morphine and scopolamine. Like the modern group, which substitutes a barbiturate for the deadlier morphine, in expert hands, this was more a pretense of pain elimination than an actuality. Knowing the dangers, the conscientious doctor would use very little of the drug combination and would rely on the amnesic effect of the scopolamine to make the new mother *forget* the pain she felt. Using enough to eliminate the pain, however, was recognizedly hazardous, and still is.

As early as 1927 and again in 1933, Sir William Willcox was warning in the British medical journals that barbiturates are dangerous drugs, and pointing to such symptoms as mental depression, dizziness, hallucinations, slurring of speech, double vision and muscular paralysis. Dr. Guttmacher says of the patient under analgesia, "It is likely that the sides of her bed are equipped with movable metal guard rails, which are kept raised except during an examination. Analgesia makes one behave as if drunk, and the guard rails protect the patient, restrain her from jumping or falling out of bed if she is momentarily left alone."

Exercises to Minimize Pain

If this is the effect on the mother, imagine what is happening to the child about to be born. How infinitely more sensible, we say, for the prospective mother to take the trouble to learn the natural childbirth techniques and to prepare herself through learning and relaxation exercises to minimize in a natural way the pain of labor. To do so will not keep her from having anesthesia at the actual time of birth, if it should prove necessary. It *will* strongly reduce the terrifying possibility of having a "blue baby," by making absolutely unnecessary any preliminary analgesic drugs.

Even more to the point, we recommend the natural childbirth techniques because they minimize the need for anesthesia. It must be admitted that there is frequently a need for anesthetics in the delivery room. Often, surgical techniques are necessary in a birth, and these without anesthesia would be unthinkable. Still more often, the perineum is torn or must be cut. The conscientious obstetrician who is not obsessed with making things easy for himself can surely be trusted, and is the best judge, to determine the type of anesthetic to use and how much. Much of his decision will depend on the knowledge and expertness of the anesthetist he has available, for all anesthetics are dangerous and only the highly expert use of them will minimize the danger.

Thus, though it is our tendency to frown on general anesthesia in childbirth (nitrous oxide, ether, sodium pentothal, etc.), we'd still consider it preferable in the hands of an anesthetist, expert with it, to spinal anesthesia with which he is unfamiliar.

Anesthesia Can Kill

Why do we frown on general anesthesia? Because it can kill. Dr. David M. Little, Jr., of the Hartford (Connecticut) Hospital, called the anesthesia death-rate "alarming" before the West Virginia State Medical Association in 1958. Professor C. Lee Buxton, Chairman of the Department of Obstetrics and Gynecology of the Yale University School of Medicine told the Medical Society of the State of New York, in 1956, that anesthesia had reached fifth place as a cause of maternal deaths in New York City. The *New York Times* (May 11, 1956) quoted him as saying: "It is only reasonable to suggest that any obstetrical technique which can in any way reduce the amount and frequency of analgesia and anesthesia . . . is of profound practical value for this reason alone."

So dangerous is anesthesia, that it is frequently only by the patient's face turning blue (cyanosis) for lack of oxygen that the anesthetist is warned to take corrective measures. For this reason, Negro mothers, whose color makes cyanosis harder to recognize, suffer many more anesthesia-childbirth deaths—27,000 of them in 1956, which was considered a great improvement over previous years.

Oxygen Lack Produces Brain Damage

Dr. Lyon P. Strean, Ph.D., in *The Birth of Normal Babies,* states that "Lack of oxygen for even short periods could produce brain damage to the fetus. General anesthesia for childbirth should be reduced to a minimum for the prevention of brain damage to both mother and child."

These things being so, obstetricians have tended to prefer conduction anesthesia, of late years. This is the more localized (or regional) type of anesthetic that does not enter the mother's blood stream and therefore, does not affect the child. For this purpose, according to Dr. Guttmacher, it is usually one of the cocaine drugs that is used. Depending on the type of solution used, such a drug injected into the spinal canal will either anesthetize the entire body below the navel, or produce the so-called "saddle block" anesthesia in just that portion of the body that would come in contact with the saddle when riding a horse. Both types can be used only for birth pain as, used too soon, they halt labor. They can only be administered by highly expert anesthetists, and even then, frequently cause steep drops in blood pressure and severe and protracted headaches.

Caudal anesthesia is a variation of this technique with continuing injection into the area just below the spinal canal. Technically enormously difficult, it is not widely available and quite expensive, requiring constant vigilant attendance of a doctor or nurse over many hours. It has the same inherent dangers as the other spinal techniques.

For the woman who has succeeded in achieving the relaxed state at which natural childbirth aims, when anesthesia is required, it may be enough to give her local injections to numb the perineum and the vagina, Dr. Guttmacher states. This, of course, is all to the good from our point of view. The less anesthesia, the better.

For the same reason, we prefer conduction to general anesthesia, while cautioning that it requires great expertness of the anesthetist for proper administration. Improperly administered spinals have resulted in drawn-out nervous conditions, sensations of numbness and tingling, etc.

What We Recommend

While we dislike and fear anesthetics, we are compelled to recognize that they will continue to be widely used in childbirth. We recommend the natural childbirth method, yet must admit it is not for everyone, nor is instruction in it available everywhere. We do *not* advise anyone, without competent medical care and guidance, to try to have a child without any anesthesia. This would be as foolish and harrowing as undergoing major surgery without anesthesia. It is simply one of those cases where one must accept the lesser evil—in this case, anesthetics.

What we do advise, strongly, is that the pregnant woman build her general health by good nutrition, thus improving her child's ability and her own to withstand the toxic effects of whatever anesthetics may be necessary. (Vitamins C and the B complex are especially useful in aiding the body's processing of toxic substances.) We also consider that special emphasis on vitamin E, the vitamin that helps the body utilize oxygen better and oxygenates the entire system, will be of definite assistance in preventing anesthetic damage due to lack of sufficient oxygen.

Children

The Amazing Poor Health of Our Teen-Agers

Teen-agers have a famous talent for eating almost all the time. Their parents attribute this insatiable appetite to their children's growth period, or to the strenuous activities these youngsters engage in. While both of these are likely reasons, we think there is another one that is largely ignored: teen-agers are eating all the time, but they seldom eat any real food. Breakfast is usually skipped, and this results in the need for a snack at midmorning—usually a candy bar gulped between classes. For lunch, it's a coke, a hot dog, potato chips and more candy. After school, a chocolate malt or a sundae on the way home takes care of ruining dinner. By 7 or 8 o'clock, however, it's time for another snack, this time pretzels or cookies while watching TV, or doing homework. By 11 o'clock, they need a bedtime nightcap of cake and/or ice cream with coffee to top off the day. This is not a far-fetched summary of teen-age eating, as many mothers can tell you.

Knowing this to be the case, is it not surprising to see how little interest there is in improving the eating habits of our younger people? We are constantly told by our health agencies how well fed we are. Devitalized and downright bad foods are hawked by television announcers as desirable for our children, and no one seems to care. Youngsters are encouraged on all sides to eat what is worst for them —candy, soda, ice-cream, etc—and they do. The result can only be reports such as the one made public by nutrition authority, Dr. Pauline Berry Mack in *Newsweek* (May 4, 1953).

Teen-Agers "Gravely Undernourished"

Dr. Mack made a 10-year study of 2,536 boys and girls between the ages of 13 and 20. Her final judgment was that American teen-agers, even those of high income families, are "gravely undernourished." Only one-quarter of the youngsters she examined were eating sufficient energy-making foods to keep the body running efficiently. That means that three quarters of these children were somehow defective in their health, and were using up whatever reserves they had to keep their bodies going.

Protein, one of the most basic of bodily needs, usually suffers in the teen-age diet. By the time starches and carbohydrates, both dear to young people's hearts, have been taken in, there is no room for protein foods such as meat, eggs, fish and vegetables. Dr. Mack's findings bear this out, too. Nearly half of the girls and a few less of the boys lacked the proper amount of protein foods necessary to build and repair body tissues. This repair and rebuilding goes on every second, but from where is the material for this process to come, if not from the food we eat? If the raw materials for new tissues are not here, the body is bound to deteriorate.

Necessary Bone Materials Missing

Every one of the 2,536 teeners was lacking in calcium and phosphorous, so necessary for good health, teeth and bones. There is no surprise, then, in finding that only 7 girls and 12 boys, out of the entire group, had perfect teeth. One does not get calcium and phosphorus from cake, candy and soda. Fresh fruits and vegetables, eggs and bone meal are rich sources of these minerals, and growing children should be especially careful to get their quota of these foods. The fidgety actions of many children are due to what Dr. Mack calls "nutritional nerves." Forty-nine per cent of the boys and 48 per cent of the girls suffered from this. The blinking, twitching and nail biting that make adults wonder if youngsters are electrically wired is nothing more than the result of careless eating. The B vitamins perform the function of maintaining calm and healthy nerves. How many teen-agers manage to eat liver, whole or desiccated, at least once a week, or brewer's yeast or wheat germ? How many make an effort to avoid white sugar and products containing it, which deplete the vitamin B supply in the body? Serious shortages of the B vitamins were found in most of Dr. Mack's subjects, just as they would probably be found in most adults, if such a test were made. American customs in eating rule out, to a large extent, foods that are rich in B vitamins, and processing removes a good share in the few of the vitamin B-rich foods we do eat.

Eye Trouble and Poor Skin

Vitamins A and C were also found to be lacking in many of the children examined by Dr. Mack. The vitamin A deficiency showed up in the fact that there were three-fourths of the adolescents examined suffering with eye trouble that could be traced to poor diet.

Rough skin and acne were the rule, especially among the girls. Vitamins A and C are both credited with effective help in maintaining a clear and healthy skin. There is no mention of colds or infections in the report, but with a lack of these two nutrients, the incidence would have to be high. Fresh fruits and vegetables, and rose hips for vitamin C, are necessary for a steady supply of these two vitamins.

Investigation revealed that income was not a factor in the lack of good diet. A well-balanced, healthful diet need not include fancy food. Selection and proper cooking of good foods, which would have been cheaper than the barren foods being eaten in many cases, would have given these children the nourishment they needed.

Misguided Effort to Keep Figures

A clue to the problem of proper eating in the case of high school girls lies in the emphasis placed on a good figure, says *Food Field Reporter* (November 12, 1956). Girls are found to be the worst offenders of nutritional standards, and it is often because they limit their intake in order to stay slim. It is unfortunate that they are not educated to know that eating properly will result in a proper weight level. If a high school girl, or anyone else, will follow a well-balanced, healthful diet exclusively, she will soon see a trend toward the weight level she should carry, the weight at which she is most attractive, most efficient.

In this same article, it was noted that 4,458 average children had been examined, and *56 per cent of them failed to meet even minimum health requirements.* The opinion was offered, by Dr. J. Obert, that this poor record was due more to inadequate diet than lack of exercise. In any case, such figures should shake us out of the complacency we entertain about the health of our children.

A Concerted Plan for Good Nutrition

Appalled by findings, similar to those related above, in his own area, a Louisiana parish (county) Superintendent of Schools set about promoting a better-life campaign for the children, to be brought about in part by selecting proper foods and developing healthful eating habits. A 1944 survey had shown that less than 2 per cent of the children in white schools had what could be called good eating habits. In the Negro schools, the percentage was even lower. By 1950, the count for good-diet students had gone up to 31 per cent, while those eating a fair diet included 64.3 per cent, and only 4 per cent were eating what was classed as a poor diet.

The reform began with public meetings that were well-attended, due to the inducement of door prizes given to those who came, to build interest. A grant came from the State Education Board and a nutritional expert was hired. Everyone cooperated and health consciousness spread everywhere. In classrooms, arithmetic problems were reworded to use food examples; in spelling, food words were frequent, compositions were written about good food, and skits and playlets on nutrition hammered the message home. Children even kept score cards on the kind of meals they were eating at home.

Why Not a National Campaign?

The general interest generated in promoting this program is what made it successful. It was begun by a person with the leadership and authority to make it work. Government officials are the likely source of such a movement for the entire country. It is doubtful that the indifference to nutrition shown by our people would continue if they were better educated to its importance during their school days. It is not enough to devote one or two hours a week in high school to hygiene classes, in which the children are bored and skeptical. How can they take it seriously when the cafeteria run by the school features everything they have just been told is dangerous to health, and encourages them to buy it? No, the teachers must talk good food whenever they can; candy machines, cigarettes and sodas must have no place on school grounds; proper menus must be offered in the cafeteria, with fresh fruits and nuts for dessert. The students must become convinced that the rules of good nutrition apply to everyone, young and old alike. Then perhaps the levels of good health in our young people will begin to rise.

While you are waiting for such changes to come about in the schools your children attend, stress good nutrition with your own family. See that they get healthful foods and supplements such as brewer's yeast and vitamin A and rose hips to keep them healthy. There is no reason for anyone to be poorly nourished in such a land of plenty.

Children Need Guidance in Diet

We've been reading, on and off, about the enviable health of Americans, and even more about the enviable health of American children. The assumption is, of course, that because our country is so wealthy, our kiddies eat better and live better and their health is better than that of children of any other country. Few food economists seem willing to say in print that our children's diet leaves much to be desired. Our school children eat little that is worth eating, and those not old enough for school do as badly, or worse, on strawberry-flavored milk, cereals that spell words and all but speak in the bowl, cookies, ice cream and marshmallow-laden crackers. Well, Mrs.

American Mother, your child is not physically all right. He's sick and getting sicker each year! You can look for the answer in a hundred places, but before you do, ask yourself how much food with any real value your child eats. How much meat (not the deep-fried, breaded stuff), how many fresh vegetables, how much fresh fruit? Does he get any supplementary help with his nutrition? Any bone meal, rose hips, brewer's yeast, cod liver oil? If the answer is none, you are probably typical. If you are typical, your child is quite probably in physical trouble or on the verge of it.

Scope (April 4, 1959) reported that one-fourth of the operations performed in the United States are performed on children. The Metropolitan Life Insurance Company reports that, as of September, 1959, heart disease is responsible for about 10,000 deaths a year *in children under 15*.

Ulcers Not Rare

In the *American Medical Association Journal of Diseases of Children* (February, 1960), an article appeared which discussed the frequency of peptic ulcers in children. ". . . . peptic ulcer in children should not be considered rare," said the authors. Recorded cases ". . . undoubtedly represent only a small portion of the total number of children with the disease." Out of 1,000 adult patients with duodenal ulcer, 26 of them had symptoms traceable to when they were 4 years of age. Out of 1,000 with gastric ulcer, 16 of them had symptoms dating from childhood.

The classic treatment for ulcer is regulation of diet. Often, with careful diet management, an ulcer will disappear. Why not, with careful diet management, prevent its appearance in the first place? Fried foods, one of the most common of all forms of cooking in America, are high on the list of foods forbidden to the ulcer patient. Many American kids eat fried foods at least once a day. Aspirin is another suspected cause of ulcer. Do you know any child who is not well-acquainted with aspirin? They even come especially made for children—candy-coated!

Diabetes is showing up with increasing frequency among children. Cancer, especially leukemia, is also becoming common among children, to the extent that cancer-ridden children have a whole hospital to themselves in Boston, and we are sure others will follow. In *Scope* (March 9, 1960), we read of the findings of Dr. Daniel Stowens, presented to the annual meeting of the California Medical Association. Dr. Stowens reported that a post-mortem study of 285 children who died of leukemia showed: 10 per cent of the children had sugar in the urine; 25 per cent had a history of diabetes in the family (usually a grandparent), while this was so in only 4 per cent of non-leukemic children; significant changes in the Islets of Langerhans existed in all leukemic children autopsied.

Dr. Stowens said leukemia is not a blood disease, but a disease of the whole body, showing most dramatically in the blood. Can there be any reason for a disease of the whole body which is not closely allied with a nutritional deficiency? A proper supply of the necessary vitamins and minerals would be a strong deterrent to that very situation. The fact that diabetes appears to be linked with leukemia emphasizes even more the likelihood that leukemia is the unhappy result of careless diet.

Shot Full of Vaccines

The American child is shot so full of vaccines that his arm should resemble a Swiss cheese. Our preoccupation with vaccines of all kinds is a dangerous one. Through them, we force the body to experience many illnesses it might ordinarily avoid, and often the intensity of the vaccine is too much for the system.

In *Scope* (September 5, 1956), it was reported that 8,000,000 of our school-age children need some form of professional eye care. Hearing defects were estimated to be present in 3,000,000 children. A survey of 100,000 school children in Philadelphia showed that 15 per cent were suffering from actual malnutrition. The *Archives of Pediatrics* (June, 1958) carried an article which estimated that 25 to 40 per cent of school children are physically unfit.

How the Sweets Habit Begins

We are convinced that most of the physical problems of a school-age child, or anyone else, are due to poor diet. Sweets are one of the biggest offenders. Children who eat large amounts of sweets are bound to eat little else, and the lack of good, nourishing food soon shows itself in weakness and disease.

How do some children get the sweets habit? The *Indiana State Board of Health Bulletin* (December, 1958) fixed the blame quite properly. In an article by Joyce Meyers, we saw this statement: "Adults can, without realizing it, cause children to develop a desire for sweet foods. Sweet formulas are not uncommon in infancy; excessive sugar on fruits and cereals, heavy desserts, soft drinks and snacks frequently continue throughout childhood. The child who acquires these habits will find it difficult to change . . ."

What kind of food habits are you teaching your children? It is you who will teach them whether or not a bowl of sweet berries needs to be sprinkled with white sugar or whether a piece of fruit is dessert instead of a piece of pie or a dish of ice cream, or that a fig, a date or some nuts are a better snack than a candy bar.

In the formative years of their children, parents have a great influence which can be channeled toward giving the children good eating habits which will keep them healthy through life. You are the source of their food supply. You can give them only what they should have. Let your child learn how good an apple can be, and he will probably choose it over a piece of cake when he wants a snack. Let him drink fruit juice instead of soda, and the artificiality of soda will not appeal to him. Keep the good foods around, and don't have any refined sweets in the house. If the first few years of life are geared to this kind of eating, half of the battle is won. At least give your child this early chance at good health through selective eating.

Children Need Natural Foods and Supplements

Several years ago, a mass study was made of the "Nutritional Status of 9-, 10- and 11-Year-Old Public School Children in Iowa, Kansas and Ohio." The conclusions drawn from this survey presented a dismal picture concerning the state of health of American youth. In plain words, the diets of the children were simply inadequate—inadequate in the vital nutrients needed to keep their bodies running efficiently. Samples taken from the blood of school children in the age bracket mentioned above told the true story of just how good the diets of these children were. And the answers the researchers got should be enough to dispel any trust we Americans have in the statement that our kiddies eat better and live better than the children of any other country. How can this be true when the findings of this survey showed that ⅓ of the children tested had a vitamin C deficiency and ¼ of them had less than the minimum of 20 to 30 milligrams per 100 milliliters of vitamin A in the blood stream. Bear in mind that vitamin C functions everywhere in the body, rebuilding tissues, helping in the formation of teeth and bones, healing of wounds and resistance to infection. And vitamins A and C are both credited with effective help in maintaining a clear and healthy skin and warding off the dangers of the common cold.

Children Reported Anemic

And what about the robust good health characteristic of our children? Can we really accept this assertion when 63 per cent of the children of Kansas were below the minimum of 11.5 grams of hemoglobin per 100 milliliters of blood. Remember, hemoglobin is the red coloring matter in the blood. About 75 per cent of the body's iron is concentrated in the hemoglobin. Without the minimum of 11.5 grams, a child was considered anemic. Sixty-three per cent of the Kansas children in this age bracket were anemic! What about the rest of the United States? Do we have any reason to think this figure would not approximate the condition of our youth in the other states? Is this one of the results of our best-in-the-world diets?

Dr. Harold D. Lynch, in the *Lafayette* (Minnesota) *Journal and Courier* (December 6, 1958), said that "the chubby, half-starved glutton"—the American child—has become one of our nation's major health problems. He said that the children are growing flabby on foods they don't need while they starve for protein-rich foods that are vital to proper health and growth. Dr. Lynch goes on to say that a low-protein diet in young children can cause extreme susceptibility to infection, moderate degrees of *anemia,* irritability, constipation, flabby muscles, lethargy and tooth decay.

Nutritional Value of Modern Food

This is the direct outcome of that wonderful American diet that needs no supplementary nutrients, the same diet of the children of Kansas, Iowa and Ohio, which the Ohio researchers found so woefully deficient in vitamins C and A and which resulted in such a shortage of hemoglobin. What kind of faith can we put in the statements of nutritionists and scientists which assert that the necessary elements for healthy bodies can be gotten from the foods we usually eat? We have just seen above what such foods can do for our children's bodies. Can you call a body suffering from anemia, constipation, flabby muscles and tooth decay a healthy one?

We think it's high time that parents realize the value of the food they are feeding to their children isn't what it's cracked up to be. Alarming as the deficiencies in vitamins C and A were in the Ohio test, one can't help wondering how the children would have fared had they been tested for the vital but scarce B vitamins. The B vitamins are almost strained out of most foods fed to the American youth. His white bread and cereals are bled practically free of them, and few children can be found who eat eggs instead of cold processed cereal for breakfast. And, parents, how much meat does your child eat? Does he get the vitamin B-rich organ meats with any kind of regularity?

Whether due to a sense of misplaced generosity or ignorance on the part of many parents, children are guided largely by television shows and newspaper ads in their choice of foods, not by sound parental authority and knowledge of basic nutritional needs. But they don't know any more about it than the children do, nor do they ask any questions. The result: parents usually buy the processed and devitalized, popularly advertised foods. Little attention is given to foods which are natural and organically grown.

Dietary Supplements the Answer

Since the food-buying habits of the modern mother make her shun those foods which would give her family the needed vitamins and minerals, what can be done to provide those needed nutrients which are lacking in children's diets? We think the best way to provide these missing links is through a program of nutritional supplementation. Bring the vitamin and mineral intake up to full quota by adding to the diet rose hips and fresh fruit for vitamin C, desiccated liver, brewer's yeast and wheat germ for vitamin B and cod liver oil perles for vitamins A and D. Then this rounded diet will result in healthier, more robust American children.

In light of the previous studies discussed at the beginning of this article, the researchers at the Ohio Agricultural Experiment Station in Wooster decided to plug the nutritional gap existing in the youngsters' diets with vitamin A and vitamin C supplements. The results of their efforts again point out, in no uncertain terms, the fact that youngsters simply don't get the required amounts of vitamins and minerals through the meals they eat. In most cases, even after supplementation, the diets were still lacking in the required allowance of nutrients. Here are the details concerning this study.

Survey of the Children's Diets

Seventy pupils (37 girls and 33 boys ranging in age from 8 to 12 years) from an Ohio elementary school were selected for this study. Their diets were carefully observed over a period of 3 years, the first year, or period A, being an observation period without supplementation, while the second (B) and third (B') years were periods of supplementation. The dietary supplements included 50 milligrams of vitamin C (ascorbic acid) to be part of the regular school lunch, along with 2,500 International Units of vitamin A and 360 International Units of vitamin D. (Remember, in the pilot study, the Ohio researchers found the children's diets to be drastically lacking in these nutrients.)

To determine just how much of each vitamin the children were getting in comparison to the amounts recommended by the Food and Nutrition Board of the National Research Council, the children's diets were classified into the following groups:

Group I—diet consisted of all nutrients which were 100 per cent or more of the recommended allowances. Group II—diets consisted of some nutrients less than 100 per cent but none less than 67 per cent of the recommended allowances. Group III—diets consisted of at least one nutrient below the 67 per cent level of the recommended allowance.

At the end of the first year (period A), only 10 per cent of the children's diets fell in Group I (all nutrients satisfactorily meeting the recommendations of the National Research Council). Classified in Group II were 60 per cent of the children and 30 per cent were numbered in the Group III category. Isn't it a sad state of affairs when only 10 per cent of a representative group of American children can meet the minimum daily requirement of essential nutrients? What about those children classified in Group II? Their nutrients ran between 67 and 99 per cent of the recommended allotments. And in Group III, some nutrients were even less than 67 per cent of the total. The report says, "In general, those diets in Group II failed to meet recommended allowances for more than one nutrient whereas the majority of diets in Group III were below 67 per cent for one nutrient and at the 67 to 99 per cent level for most of the others. Diets were placed in Group III because of low calcium values more often than for any other nutrient."

What more need be said about the reason for the poor health of our American children? In most cases, they are getting only the recommended allowance of one nutrient. How can a body be kept running at full capacity if the necessary fuel isn't present?

Findings Not Uniform

Now, what would be the effect on these diets if we added extra amounts of nutrients in the form of vitamin A and vitamin C supplements? The logical assumption would be that these deficient diets would be brought up to full strength, nutritionally speaking. However, we think the findings of the survey prove that this was not the case in most instances. Consider the following statements taken from the Ohio Agricultural Experiment Station's *Research Bulletin 887,* as proof of this point:

"During supplementation, the percentage of participants getting recommended amounts (of protein) decreased, with a small percentage getting less than two-thirds of the allowances."

"Before supplementation, all of the children who ate the school lunch got at least 67 per cent of their recommended allowances for calories. Little change in this was noted during the first year of supplementation. During the second year of supplementation, however, fewer met the recommendations and more were in the less than 67 per cent category previously."

"More of the children met their allowances for vitamin A, ascorbic acid and for thiamin in B′ than in the previous periods, but fewer met their allowances for calories, protein, iron, riboflavin and niacin in both supplementation periods than in the unsupplemented period. As the study progressed, not only did a larger percentage fail to meet their allowances, but they did so by a greater margin." The reasons the researchers give for their apparent success in vitamin A and vitamin C supplementation is that they had better control over the amount and way in which they gave these supplements. Can these same strict controls be applied to every child throughout the country whose diet, like that of the experimental children, is also lacking in vitamins A and C? We think not.

Natural Foods Are Best

Perhaps the best answer to the why of this downward, instead of upward, trend in the amount of nutrients during the supplementation periods is found in this statement taken from the findings of the Ohio committee: "Many of the children, as they became older, did not increase their food intake sufficiently to keep pace with the higher recommended allowances." In other words, as the child grows older, naturally, his body will demand increased amounts of nutrients for its proper functioning. Does this mean greater amounts of food? Yes, to a certain extent, but far more important, we think, it means supplying the body with greater amounts of vitamins and minerals. To be sure, if the mother is going to feed her children foods robbed of almost all their nutrients, then it certainly will mean increasing the quantity of these foods to bring up the nutrient count. But this same purpose could be better achieved by serving her children natural foods—foods which have their complete store of vitamins and minerals intact. Children fed on such a diet would need little or no supplementation to acquire the recommended daily allowance of the vital nutrients.

Results of Blood Tests

The blood samples (also part of the Ohio test) which were taken from these children revealed the same results. Children, as they grew older, tended to have lower values of the nutrients in their blood streams. "Further, higher percentages of children 8 years of age at the start of the study had mean dietary levels at or above the recommended allowances and higher mean serum levels (amount in blood stream) of ascorbic acid throughout the study than did older children." Comparing this study to the earlier study conducted on the children in Kansas, Iowa and Ohio, we find that, during the 3-year study, in spite of the fact that the children were receiving supplements, 69 per cent at some time fell below the recommended level of vitamin C. The earlier study showed that 56 per cent of the Kansas children, 37 per cent of the Iowa children and 30 per cent of the Ohio children fell below the minimum vitamin C requirement.

Our Conclusions

We can conclude, then, from the findings of these two tests, that the diets of our American children are seriously lacking in essential nutrients—deficient to such a point that even supplementation will not bring many of the dietary essentials up to the minimum recommended allowances. This is, to be sure, a sorry state of affairs, especially since it pertains to the children inhabiting one of the wealthiest countries in the world.

The answer to this situation lies in the realm of foods which have what nature intended them to have in the way of vitamins and minerals. Since we have seen that processed and refined food can't do the job, even when extra dietary supplements (especially synthetic supplements) are added, then it's high time we switch to healthful foods and supplements. Children should have fresh fruits and vegetables plus fresh meats that have not been treated with objectionable chemicals. And they should be assured that their every nutritional need will be met by providing them with natural food supplements, like wheat germ and desiccated liver for vitamin B and rose hips for vitamin C. The natural food diet will result in healthy American children who are way above average in nutrition.

"One Great Big Milk Shake"

The troubles of America's youth were rolled into a neat package by Dr. Stanley M. Garn, anthropologist and nutrition expert at Antioch College (*Newsweek,* March 14, 1960). He says that, while our children gorge themselves on a diet that has been called "one great big milk shake," exercise opportunities are diminishing. "There is room at the curb for father to lather the car, but precious little space for the child to play tag."

Dr. Garn says that overweight is becoming a more serious problem in our children each day. Heart and artery diseases, particularly hardening of the arteries, "far from being exclusively adult predispositions actually begin with overweight in childhood." What kind of a diet is causing this? "Through the stimulation of advertising, tap water is being replaced by sugared juices, milk and carbonated drinks. Snacks have become a ritualized part of the movies, and candy and nuts are inseparable with television viewing."

Dr. Garn's answer to the whole dilemma is much too simple to earn any attention from mothers. "Keep the 6 year old from eating his way into a premature grave at 60, even if it means making life less joyous in the childhood period."

We agree—almost—with everything Dr. Garn says. We do not believe, however, that candy and other harmful foodstuffs will make or break the joyousness of being a 6 year old. If a child becomes used to eating fruit as his sweets from early childhood; candy will not mean much to him beyond its curiosity value. As for nuts, we think they are the one worthwhile snack our children eat of their own accord. They are high in nutrients, and certainly much better than candy, cookies or potato chips which have been fried to a "fare-thee-well" in deep fat.

Chiropractic

The Case for Chiropractic

Most chiropractors cheerfully admit that a large percentage of their patients come to them for the first time after they have exhausted all other medical possibilities and found no relief. Sometimes, chiropractors can do what medical doctors could not do. The spinal adjustment they make turns the trick and the patient is cured. From a humanitarian viewpoint, one would think that such results should make everyone happy; that the chiropractor should be pleased with his success, and the medical doctor should be glad to know that his patient has been helped after all. Perhaps that is the feeling in some cases, but, for the most part, organized medicine has fought a long and bitter battle to ridicule, defame and legislate chiropractic out of existence, in spite of the results it achieves. It would appear that all of this effort has been wasted.

The case for chiropractic received some much-needed clarification in an article, carried in *McCall's* magazine (Otober, 1959), by Samuel Grafton. It comes not so much from the fact that Mr. Grafton approves of chiropractic (he has some reservations), but that he gives an objective impression of what chiropractic is, and is meant to be. He describes the average examination and treatment by a chiropractor, and the kind of person who goes to be treated by one. One feels the mystery which seems to surround chiropractic begin to evaporate. Chiropractors sound much like any other doctor, but with a different approach to the treatment of disease, and this is essentially true. Among medical doctors, it is not unusual to find opposing views on the treatment of a simple disease. For example, one doctor will advise complete rest for a heart condition, another will order steady, if not strenuous, exercise. One doctor will order a bland diet for an ulcer patient, another will allow roughage. Medical doctors do not rise up in protest against either of these views; they do not promote the passage of civil laws intended to bar dissenting doctors from practice. Yet, they do exactly that where chiropractors are concerned.

The Basic Idea of Chiropractic

The chiropractor views disease as caused by pressure on the nerves, due to a misalignment or dislocation of a vertebra. His solution is, therefore, to restore the offending vertebra to its proper position by manipulating and adjusting. This relieves the pressure on the nerve and restores proper function and health to the distant part of the body by once more allowing the proper flow of nerve energy. In chiropractic, the perfect adjustment of the body's bone and nerve structure is considered to be the means of maintaining health.

180

Usually, chiropractic patients—especially new ones—are suffering from an indefinable ache, in the limbs or the back, which medical doctors haven't been able to help. The examining chiropractor has the patient get into a gown, open in the back, so that the spinal column is exposed. He uses either X-ray or a meter intended to measure temperature change caused by a congestion of blood at the point of dislocation. Sometimes, special lights which indicate these congested areas through changes in skin coloration are employed. The chiropractor might then touch the painful spot to make certain of the area of pain, and following this, he will work the neck to free its nerves. Then he makes what he calls an adjustment to a part of the spine with his hands. Depending upon the extent of the injury, the patient might get off the table free of pain in a matter of minutes. In some cases, a series of adjustments might be required. But the record of success either way is surprisingly good.

A Massage or Psychology

When opposing medical doctors are reminded of this undeniable fact, they attribute the patient's improvement to a rubdown, and contend that a masseur could achieve the same effect. But a chiropractor does not give a rubdown, he often uses only one or two swift movements. Other M.D.'s say that chiropractors use psychology, that they talk their patients into feeling better. If this be true, it would seem wise to have medical doctors learn the technique, for chiropractors are often successful where M.D.'s have failed.

"Low back pain" is an area in which chiropractors claim especial skill, and 500 dollar-conscious insurance companies in America back them up by paying the bills for policy holders who are treated by chiropractors for this condition. Whiplash is another type of injury with which chiropractors say their methods are particularly successful.

Individual chiropractors told Mr. Grafton some interesting stories of cures they had effected. One young doctor told of a young girl brought to him who had a history of epilepsy in its milder form, known as petit mal. The girl would have 20 or 25 short blackouts a day. The doctor had never before treated epilepsy, but he took a preliminary X-ray at the request of the girl's uncle. She was found to have a severe pressure point in the neck area, a pronounced distortion. He began with adjustments 3 times per week, and in the first month, the attacks went down to 5 or 6 a day, and there was a definite change for the better in her mental attitude and behavior. She did better work at school, was relaxed, and began to make friends for the first time. Her adjustment schedule was reduced to one every month. At the end of 8 months, her attacks were occurring at the rate of one every other month and she was planning to attend college, encouraged by her excellent school marks. Even the doctor was surprised with these results, and he said he would not presume to say that every case of epilepsy would respond similarly to chiropractic; however, it would be worth a try.

A Humble Beginning

The chiropractic approach to healing was originated quite by accident and in a most humble way. In 1895, Daniel David Palmer of Davenport, Iowa, was engaged in conversation with a hard-of-hearing janitor. Palmer was a rather inquisitive man, and in the course of the conversation, he asked the janitor how his deafness had come about. The man told Palmer of how he merely bent down one day, heard something pop in his back, and became almost completely deaf at once. Palmer had the man take off his shirt, and the janitor's back showed an obvious lump which turned out to be a misplaced vertebra. Palmer put him on a table and simply tried to push it back into place. The janitor's hearing is said to have improved at once, and it got better with each additional treatment until his hearing was completely restored.

That was the start of a profession which has grown to 30,000 members in the United States alone. Forty-six of the 50 states recognize chiropractic by license. Chiropractors practice, as well, in the 4 dissenting states, New York, Louisiana, Massachusetts and Mississippi, but they are forced to make use of subterfuge and technicalities to do so. Even in states which do give a license, the pressure is never off. Chiropractors are sometimes forbidden to use the title "Doctor," or to make diagnoses or use diagnostic instruments such as blood pressure gauges and stethoscopes.

Traps for Chiropractors

In New York, chiropractors are not allowed to name a patient's ailment. Some years ago, it was quite common for spies from the district attorney's office in that state to pose as patients and try to get the chiropractor to make a diagnosis, or use the blood pressure gauge or stethoscope. The authorities would then bring charges against him for illegally practicing medicine without a license. If the "patient" could show the district attorney a good case, an order for arrest would be issued. A state trooper would visit the doctor, seize the offending equipment as evidence, and might even take the chiropractor along as a prisoner. Usually, that is as far as it went. In all the history of New York State, only one chiropractor has been convicted for "practicing medicine," and he pleaded guilty to avoid the delay of a trial, since he had plans for a European trip.

The complaints that lead to these skirmishes usually come from M.D.'s aggravated at the chiropractor who has just set up shop down the block. Often, the chiropractor is not new, however, and has been practicing at the same place for perhaps 15 years, and in exactly the same way, with many satisfied and continuing patients. Such a man could be hustled off to jail just like a criminal.

"Harassment" Is the Word

Such harassment and discrimination takes other forms, too. For example, in many states, chiropractors may not use the facilities of hospitals supported by public funds, nor may they make examinations for insurance policies. In Massachusetts, the word "chiropractor" may not appear on a shingle. In Louisiana, an injunction can be procured to force a chiropractor to "cease and desist" his work. The same state bases its objections to chiropractors on the court ruling that they practice medicine. Across the river, in Mississippi, they are refused a license on the grounds that a chiropractor does *not* practice medicine. In Minnesota, a chiropractor is not allowed to do anything classed as physical therapy, and may not prescribe vitamins.

An item in the *New York Times* (May 25, 1961) announced that the New York State Health Department was putting into effect a regulation which prohibits chiropractors from using X-ray equipment. The regulation does not name chiropractors specifically, but limits the use of radiation equipment to doctors, dentists, osteopaths and podiatrists. A test case was decided against the chiropractors on the ground that they had failed to make a case against the regulation.

In commenting on the decision, the State Health Commissioner, Dr. Herman E. Hillebro hailed the regulation as being of "great significance in protecting the health of the people of the state and particularly of future generations because of the harmful effect of unnecessary X-ray exposure."

Aware as we are of the dangerous effects of X-ray exposure, and as much as we are opposed to the use of X-ray as a therapeutic measure, we fail to see what qualifications a medical doctor has over a chiropractor for the use of X-ray. We have heard and read of many instances in which radiation was unnecessarily and clumsily employed by medical doctors. We remember the suit in which a medical doctor was convicted of causing skin cancer by means of his injudicious use of X-ray. If medical doctors are truly concerned over the genetic effects of unnecessary X-ray as used by chiropractors, we hope they will concern themselves as well with this same danger in relation to their colleagues' use of X-ray. The danger is certainly there, but to imply that an osteopath or a podiatrist is more responsible than a chiropractor is the most blatant kind of politics and nothing more.

What it all means, actually, is that the patient is deprived of his choice of the type of doctor who is to treat him. If X-ray treatment is indicated, he must choose one of those practitioners who are legally permitted to use the apparatus. If he would prefer a chiropractor, or if he has faith only in chiropractors, the patient cannot be treated according to his preference.

Why chiropractors are subjected to such legal manhandling is not readily explained on the objective merits of the situation. The acceptance of chiropractic all over the world as a legitimate and effective form of treatment takes it out of the category of quackery. The long line of practitioners over the past 75 years would preclude the judgment that it is an upstart cult that will soon be forgotten. Nor can it be held that the chiropractor is ignorant, and ill-prepared by study to treat the human body.

School for Today's Chiropractor

Today's student of chiropractic attends school with about a thousand fellow students in one of 16 accredited chiropractic colleges in the United States. Among his classmates will be men from many foreign countries, including France, Australia, Canada and New Zealand. He will probably have had at least two years of college before beginning the 4-year course in chiropractic. During that time, he will take over 4,000 hours of instruction (equal in length to medical-school standards) in such subjects as embryology, histology, chemistry, obstetrics, gynecology, endocrinology, roentgenology, pediatrics, etc., plus the practice of chiropractic. In some states, he will take the same basic medical-sciences examination as an M.D., and will do very well.

It is obvious that chiropractic is doing its best to raise the standards of its practitioners and increase their prestige in medical circles, as well as among laymen. The advance from Daniel Palmer's days has been swift and impressive. The modern chiropractor is an educated practitioner of a form of therapy which is recognized throughout the world as legitimate and beneficial. The interference he experiences in the United States as he attempts to practice is difficult to reconcile with the obvious legality of what he is doing. Chiropractic is based upon a reasonable and physiologically sound premise. Those who believe that proper alignment of the spine is the best way to regain good health should certainly be free to pursue it. To pass laws denying chiropractors the right to use the term "doctor," when others, with even less education, in other fields, use it freely is degrading and insulting. To hold these men, who have studied as much medical science as many M.D.'s, liable to prosecution for using a blood pressure gauge or verbally identifying a disease is absurdly discriminatory.

Chiropractic Has a Right to Unbiased Evaluation

For many persons, chiropractic has been the only answer to years of pain and invalidism. Is the man who put them on their feet and relieved their misery to be outlawed because he did not do it with drugs or surgery? We believe, first of all, in avoiding disease through proper diet and exercise. Once disease has struck, the cure of it should be effected by means which will interfere as little as possible with other bodily functions. If a series of adjustments will do the job without the dangerous side effects of drugs or the risk of an operation, we can see no reason for not having them. Of course, there are some illnesses which chiropractic cannot cure, but then other medical treatments are not able to claim universal effectiveness either. A patient should have the right to choose the type of therapy he prefers. This choice should not be dictated by the results of political wrangles among legislators and doctors of opposing ideologies, who seek to maintain a strangle hold on the treatment of disease in the United States.

In West Germany, a group of 200 M.D.'s, including members of medical-school faculties, has formed an organization for research and work in chiropractic. A professor of surgery at the University of Hamburg, D. L. Zukschwerdt, has praised chiropractic in the German medical press. Why hasn't such unbiased investigation and comment been forthcoming in this country? Here a chiropractor is referred to disparagingly as a "spine pounder," with little effort made to find out whether or not his work is productive of results. As Dr. Zukschwerdt has recommended, it would be wiser that physicians "not neglect the application of so worthwhile a method."

Cholesterol

Miscellaneous Notes on Cholesterol

The debate still rages—is cholesterol in the diet responsible for hardening of the arteries—largely, partly or not at all? Does it do any good to avoid animal fats like butter and fat meats and concentrate on diets which contain very little animal fat and more vegetable fat like salad oils?

Here are some conflicting opinions that have appeared in medical literature during the past years. Reading through them, you may realize how difficult the problem is and how many angles must be considered. These brief notes represent a tiny fraction of all the writings on this subject.

* * *

Trappist monks, who are strict vegetarians, have less cholesterol in their blood than Benedictine monks, who do eat meat, according to *Science News Letter* for April 2, 1960. Although the two kinds of communities are similar, it is true that Trappists devote their lives to contemplation, prayer and physical labor. They neither smoke nor drink. Benedictines are teachers and preachers and are not prohibited from smoking or drinking. We also discovered, in another report of this same survey, that the Trappist monk's "strict vegetarianism" includes plenty of milk and eggs.

*   *   *

There is a relationship between high cholesterol blood levels and heart attacks, according to Ancel Keys, of the University of Minnesota, speaking at the Atlanta Graduate Medical Assembly. He reported that a recent Finnish study of 1600 men, 40 to 59 years old, supports the theory that high blood cholesterol is a major factor in developing coronary disease. Men of East Finland were found to have higher cholesterol levels and more heart attacks than those of West Finland. Dr. Keys added, "We have found no evidence to support the theory that Americans, busy setting the pace for the modern world, naturally have higher blood pressure and more heart attacks . . . the highest frequency of hypertensive disease (high blood pressure) was in Japan, but Japan has only ¼ to 1/20 the rate of heart attacks we have in the United States."

*   *   *

Emotional makeup influences changes in the way our bodies use fats, including cholesterol. Certain behavior traits were found to be positively correlated with high cholesterol levels—the need for dominance, social achievement and drive, aggression, hostility, inflexibility and rebelliousness. Those with low cholesterol levels turned out to be mostly people who had fewer open conflicts in life, were better satisfied with themselves and accepted their position in life. *Roche Report* gives this summary of a speech given by R. Bruce Sloane of Queens University, Ontario, before the American Psychosomatic Society.

*   *   *

Two physicians offered evidence that high levels of cholesterol do not necessarily mean hardening of the arteries or heart attacks, in a report to the American Public Health Association, reported in the *New York Herald Tribune,* October 23, 1959. In a study of 1,400 white and Negro children, the doctors found that cholesterol increases at the same rate in children of both races from 8 to 20. In spite of this, there were 4 times more fat deposits in the arteries of the Negro children than in white children of the same age. And, in direct contradiction, Negroes seem to suffer less from heart attacks.

*   *   *

A study made of farmers in the northern states shows that their incidence of heart attacks is roughly half that of city dwellers. Physical work seems to be the clue here, although, it is admitted, the modern farmer spends more time sitting in a tractor seat and less time in hoeing than his ancestors did. The study was reported in the *New*

York Times for December 28, 1959. Heavy, prolonged smoking also raises cholesterol levels, according to this report.

* * *

Large doses of niacin, one of the B vitamins, were shown by two Mayo Clinic scientists, to reduce levels of blood cholesterol, according to *Newsweek* for November 9, 1959. We recommend getting niacin in vitamin B-rich foods like liver and wheat germ and food supplements like desiccated liver and brewer's yeast.

* * *

Two Johns Hopkins professors carried out tests on the cholesterol level of students taking their final exams and compared these to the same students during the much less anxious activities of regular study. They found, according to the *Journal of Chronic Diseases* for December, 1958, that the cholesterol levels were significantly higher during the exam periods.

* * *

Two physicians of the University Hospital at Lund, Norway, experimented with giving rabbits a diet completely devoid of cholesterol. They ate sugar, starch, milk protein, vitamins, coconut fat and minerals, but no cholesterol. In spite of this, the rabbits developed high cholesterol levels within a few weeks, and thickening of the arteries followed.

* * *

One researcher, Robert E. Olson of the Falk Clinics, Atlantic City, believes that lowering the protein content of the diet will lower the cholesterol content of the blood. He claimed, in a statement which appeared in *Food Field Reporter,* that adding as much as almost a fourth of a pound of butter did not cause the cholesterol to rise, so long as the protein content of the diet was low. This is in striking contrast to most researchers which show that a high-protein diet is protective.

* * *

The *Journal of the American Medical Association* for January 18, 1958, gave some facts on cholesterol. They revealed that the "normal" level of cholesterol is not known. The *average* level in this country is 240 milligrams for males, 225 milligrams for females. Daily variations of the level of cholesterol may be as great as plus or minus 20 per cent. Tests for cholesterol must be done by a physician or in a laboratory. It is not possible to test oneself for cholesterol level in the blood.

* * *

Two Montreal researchers report, in *Union Médicale* for February, 1959, on 720 patients who were analyzed for cholesterol levels of the blood. Of these, 392 had hardening of the arteries with heart disease and high blood pressure, and 328 had rheumatic or congenital heart disease and other diseases not connected with heart and arteries. Of the first group, 37.2 per cent had high levels of cholesterol in the blood. Of the second, only 1.34 per cent had high levels. This seems to indicate that high cholesterol in the blood is indeed related to heart and vascular conditions, more than it is to other disorders.

*   *   *

Henry A. Schroeder of St. Louis, Missouri, as long ago as July, 1955, wrote, in the *Journal of Chronic Diseases,* that deficiency in pyridoxine, one of the B vitamins, produces hardening of the arteries in monkeys. He shows how the modern diet is almost completely lacking in this vitamin. He also stated that many "abnormal" metals are present in American tissues—aluminum, lead, tin and nickel were present in surprising quantities. Dr. Schroeder mentions that nickel is used in the hydrogenation of fats. These are the fats believed to contribute to cholesterol deposits and hardening of the arteries—the fats that are solid at room temperature—lard, margarine and the white shortenings used for baking. In countries where there is little "civilization," there is practically no hardening of the arteries and high blood pressure. Granted that the diet there is different, Dr. Schroeder says, there are other differences, as well. These people are not exposed to trace metals in canned and processed foods, to the products of petroleum combustion (furnaces and automobiles) and water piped through metal pipes. There is little or no experimental evidence *against* this theory, he adds.

Citrus

Why We Still Object to Citrus

If America is citrus-happy, it's because we've been educated to think a breakfast without orange juice is no breakfast at all. Several years ago, we startled many folks by announcing that we opposed the indiscriminate use of citrus fruits and their juices. The main reason was that the high acidity of these fruits has a corrosive effect on the teeth. The situation hasn't changed, and our view is reinforced by a continuous flow of research material proving that the person who uses large amounts of citrus juice can expect to have trouble with his teeth because of it. Notice that we say *large* amounts. A small glass of orange juice once or twice a week probably won't do any harm; and an orange in the lunch pail now and then is certainly preferable to candy or cake. But Americans aren't moderate about such things. They hear that orange juice is an easy way to good health, so they drink it by the quart each morning if they can. They are not likely to notice that the endorsement and encouragement to "drink it every day" has come from a citrus-growers association, whose main purpose is to find new ways to get people to drink citrus juice, and to use the whole fruit.

Position of the British Health Ministry

Britain is in a peculiar situation as regards citrus fruit and juice. The Ministry of Health has been supplying free orange juice to young children because of the nutrients it contains. Such a project is a commendable one—at least in purpose. However, the *British Dental Journal* (May 6, 1958) carried a report showing the serious dental problems being caused by drinking orange juice. The *Journal* noted that acid is accepted as a major cause of tooth erosion. It follows that an acid-containing food taken into the mouth will have a similar effect. The experiment included soft drinks as well as acidic fruit juices. The soft drinks showed up as worse offenders to the tooth enamel, but the sucrose they contain for added sweetening was blamed. The acid in soft drinks and citrus was responsible for general loss of tooth substance, extreme sensitivity of the teeth to heat, cold, sweets, etc., and reduction of surrounding natural materials, so that fillings actually stood above the biting surface of the teeth.

It was also found, in these experiments, that the length of time the acidic substance was in contact with the teeth played a part in determining the amount of damage done. Actually, the harm done by citric acid might outweigh the good of the vitamin C in citrus. It would seem logical then to encourage rinsing the mouth by drinking plain water after eating or drinking citrus. As for the effect of citric acid in the stomach of an ulcer patient, we have seen no research, but the situation seems worthy of investigation.

Infants and Orange Juice

New mothers are usually encouraged to give their babies orange juice as early as possible. It is the usual thing for mothers to divide their infants' liquid diet between orange juice, milk and water. The *Journal* report observed that sucking orange juice concentrates from a baby's bottle was associated with the erosion of teeth. The general view of the 3 authors was summed up in this sentence: "It is suggested that, in man, under special conditions, fruit juices may damage tooth enamel and this is most likely to occur in children."

In November, 1957, the *New York State Dental Journal* made similar observations in an article by Adeeb E. Thomas, D.M.D. He told of the destruction of tooth enamel in patients who ingested the juice of whole lemons. The people he included in this observation were routine clinic patients whose reasons for the ingestion of lemons or lemon juice ranged from pregnancy to merely a special desire for the fruit. They all showed a pitting of the enamel, or concave, trough-like areas with rounded margins.

Dr. Thomas concluded that, "slight modification in enamel to-
pography (surface) is possible in human teeth following daily ingestion of 12 or more ounces of grapefruit juice or a carbonated beverage such as Coca-Cola (or of 18 or more ounces of orange juice)
over a period of 4 weeks or more."

The modern diet is plenty hard on the teeth as it is. There are
many materials in it now which are especially damaging to our dentition—not the least of which are sugar and white flour. Coupled with
these, orange juice and the other citrus juices taken consistently, even
in small amounts, can cause tooth trouble. They are just more fuel
added to an already raging fire.

The Intestinal Problem

Aside from the effects on the teeth, the *Journal of Pediatrics*
(October, 1953) tells us that the protein in orange juice does not
appear to pass through the intestinal wall readily. This means a slow
down in digestion and can mean real internal distress. Some persons
have such a violent reaction to orange juice that drinking it can bring
them close to death. Of course, this is true of many foods, but the
Journal of the American Medical Association (May 21, 1960) carries
a story of a woman whose allergy suddenly appeared after she had
eaten oranges all her life. The attack (she'd had one other—a milder
one) had her in the hospital with chills and shock, among other things.
Her blood pressure was affected and she was severely, dangerously
ill. Had she been aware of the possible consequences, she might have
been more cautious about drinking orange juice after the first warning. Many people break out in a rash upon eating citrus. When one
is that sensitive, one should avoid all contact with citrus. The next
time might be the one that will cause a really serious reaction.

It is true that citrus fruits are rich in vitamin C, but this means
the pulp and white lining of the peel as well as the juice. If you are
depending upon orange juice alone as your major source of vitamin
C, you are probably short of this precious nutrient. Expand your diet
to include other fresh fruits and vegetables which are rich in it and
do not have this undesirable effect on the teeth.

Some natural vitamin C supplements are made of citrus rind;
are these harmful? The small amount of citrus one gets in these pills
would hardly cause problems with the teeth or retard the digestion.
However, even this small amount is likely to affect those who have
an allergy to citrus fruits. If this is your problem, we would suggest
that you get your vitamin C from rose hips instead. Most natural
supplement houses that offer one also have the other.

The important thing is to avoid an overemphasis upon citrus
juices. They are not healthful in large quantities, contrary to the publicity we see almost daily.

Pure Orange Juice in a Carton?

Housewives across the United States have fallen in love with a new product—fresh orange juice delivered by the milkman. The packagers seem to choose only the sweetest oranges. They squeeze them, remove seeds and large pieces of pulp and put the juice in handy wax cartons that sit outside the back door, beading with wet coolness. No defrosting, no mixing. The carton says "Nature Made It—Nothing Added." Health-conscious people were not so quick to snap up orange juice that was in a carton for hours. Some vitamin C was bound to be lost. But for most people who are not particularly health-conscious, the convenience of the product was appealing. Furthermore, it was better, they thought, than no juice at all for their children. Pure orange juice ready to pour? Of course they'd buy it!

Well, one corporation, at least, has been doing plenty to its "nature made it—nothing added" pure orange juice, a suspicious Food and Drug Administration discovered. Cal-Tex Citrus Juices, Incorporated, who sold Vita-Pakt and Meadowgold in 22 states as unadulterated orange juice, was found, on analysis of its product, to be selling orange juice that may have been pure when it came into their plant, but was half orange juice, half sweetened water when it went out for sale. (Drew Pearson told the story in his column of April 24, 1961.)

When Cal-Tex officials were confronted with this analysis, Pearson says, they claimed they'd been framed. Why would anyone do such a thing to that wonderful golden liquid? It was a monstrous thought!

Meanwhile, back at the plant, the sugar and water were dumped into the vats of juice, as usual. After all—business must go on, even if the bosses were testifying before the Food and Drug Administration.

Well-Camouflaged

The Food and Drug Administration sent a special investigator to the plant to check on operations. They were still skeptical in spite of the hurt looks and pious promises about the purity of their products, which Cal-Tex officials offered. However, on each visit, the inspector found the plant as clean as a whistle—no sugar to be seen, no water being added, pure orange juice going into the cartons. Apparently, they were making the product as it was supposed to be made. They were while the inspector was there.

In a vacant apartment across from the plant, 3 FDA investigators took up residence and began to keep a close watch on the Cal-Tex plant. They used high-powered field glasses and movie cameras to be sure that nothing escaped them.

They thought it interesting that, during a period of 11 days, only

4 truckloads of oranges were delivered to the plant. During the same time, on numerous occasions, an unmarked panel truck pulled up to deliver something, then was hosed down before leaving. The cargo was found to be sugar in loads of 2,000 pounds at a time. The washing down was to remove telltale sugar crystals from the truck.

The sugar, contained as it was in 100-pound sacks, could easily be hidden behind a flat wall of packing cases in an outbuilding beside the main plant. Men carried it, a bucket at a time, into the plant as it was needed. These men all became stars in the movies taken by the investigators. Then, with a search warrant, the agents raided the premises, and this time they knew where to look for the sugar. They also discovered that Cal-Tex had arranged to pay for the sugar by cashing small checks at the bank, made out to Cal-Tex petty cash, then exchanging the cash for the sugar to eliminate records and receipts.

The owners of the company were charged with and convicted of conspiring to violate the Pure Food and Drug Act.

We are, of course, gratified at this action of the FDA, but we can't help wondering how many such operations are missed. Certainly, not every carton of juice can be analyzed. Not every one is adulterated, but are you sure yours is pure orange juice? So were the Cal-Tex customers. We say you can be sure the orange juice, or any other juice you drink, is pure if you make it or see it made. Sure it's more work, but it's the kind of work that makes sense. Suppose a diabetic had been drinking that "pure" orange juice and was getting more sugar in a single glass than he was intended to have all day.

Natural Foods Best

Are you giving your children orange juice for its food value? Why bother, if it's been squeezed so long ago that the vitamin C is gone out of it, the bioflavonoid-rich pulp is eliminated, and sugar to destroy teeth, rob B vitamins and lower blood sugar is there in good measure? You would do as well to forget his nutrition if this juice is the only measure you plan to take.

If you don't want to bother squeezing oranges, give the child a whole orange, quartered, to eat on his own. It's infinitely better for him than the juice alone, even good pure juice. Furthermore, orange juice can have a corrosive effect on the enamel of the teeth, if taken too frequently. We say use any citrus food with moderation.

What happened with the orange juice in this story has probably happened, and is probably happening, with items we buy and eat every day. The label says they're pure, we believe it, and we end up with an adulterated food. The only way to be really safe is to eat as few processed foods as possible, so that you won't have to rely on labels. Remember, it is just about impossible to buy a packaged food that hasn't been treated in some way.

Cleft Palate

Cleft Palate Is Preventable

One of the most common of birth abnormalities is cleft palate. It is the condition which occurs when the roof of the mouth, growing in the fetus from both sides of the upper jaw, has not met at the center. The two sides have not grown far enough or fast enough, as they normally should, to form what is called the normal palatal arch.

One of the most persistent beliefs as to the cause of cleft palate has long been that the mother might have suffered some shock during her pregnancy—especially during the sixth to twelfth weeks of pregnancy, at which time this part of the fetus is forming. For some time, medical science sternly put down such theories as superstitious old wives' tales. However, in *Time* magazine (September 17, 1956), the idea that stress, both emotional and physical, may be a precipitating factor in causing cleft palate and harelip (imperfect meeting of two sides of the upper lip below the nose, often an adjunct to cleft palate) is recognized as a strong possibility. Of 228 cases of cleft palate at Newark's (New Jersey) Hospital of St. Barnabas, 40 per cent were among first-born children. Going back over the mothers' experiences during the critical weeks of pregnancy, the doctors found that 25 per cent had been ill and 68 per cent recalled emotional disturbances. The investigators reasoned that severe emotional disturbance, of whatever kind, stimulates the adrenal glands to pump out extra hydrocortisone; this checks the formation of connective tissue between the two sides of the palate, or may actually dissolve tissue already formed.

The Theory Is Tested

To test their thesis, the doctors pumped cortisone into female mice at the corresponding stage of pregnancy when the palates of the embryos were forming. They produced cleft palate in 87 per cent of the newborn mice.

Similar findings have been recorded elsewhere. In the *Lancet* (July 14, 1956), a letter to the editor from Dr. Michael Oldfield said, in part, "Cortisone prevents healing of wounds and causes cleft palate in animals; it might be assumed, also, that it may prevent fusion (of the palate) in the development of the human fetus."

Then Dr. Oldfield voiced a thought that has crossed our minds often in the area of cleft palate, and other physical defects as well. He wrote: "Surely it is time that a careful research program was started in this country to find out the cause and the way to reduce the number of babies born, or stillborn, with congenital deformities. . . . The preliminary animal experiments have been carried out."

The Question of Cortisone Is Discussed

The article which prompted Dr. Oldfield's letter appeared in the *Lancet* on October 6, 1956. Two doctors wrote describing a case history to show the possible relationship between cortisone in pregnancy and cleft palate. A 25-year-old woman became pregnant while taking 100 milligrams of cortisone and 400 milligrams of tolazoline hydrochloride daily after a clinical diagnosis of lupus erythematosus. "The baby was born prematurely, weighing 2 pounds, 11 ounces. He died 14 days after birth, from bronchopneumonia. There was a cleft palate which involved the soft tissues; no other developmental abnormality was found.

"This patient received a moderate dose of cortisone during the relevant period of development of the palate."

The article brought a letter corroborating the theory of the cortisone-cleft palate relationship all the way from Spain. The two Spanish doctors who signed the letter (October 19, 1957) noted that they had published similar information on "the dangers of the prescription of corticosteroids in early pregnancy."

Nutrition Is the Tool

There is much evidence that there is a tool to be used as a sort of insurance against cleft palate in the newborn child. That tool is careful attention to nutrition. There are several nutrients which have been shown effective in preventing cleft palate and harelip. In the *Chicago Daily Tribune* (September 11, 1957), a news story covering the 22nd annual meeting of the International College of Surgeons told of one of these. Dr. Lyndon A. Peer told the group of his experiments which have reduced the number of such abnormalities by 65 per cent in laboratory animals given daily injections of two B vitamins, folic acid and pyridoxine.

Pregnant mice were first injected with cortisone, described by the newswriter as a powerful body chemical which can cause interference with vital life chemistry, 4 times daily. Cleft palates developed in 85 per cent of their offspring. When pyridoxine was injected with the cortisone, such abnormalities were reduced to 45 per cent, and the folic acid in the combination reduced the cleft palate number to 20 per cent.

On the basis of these experiments, Dr. Peer said he had been giving the two vitamins routinely to human mothers who had previously borne cleft palate children. At that time, he said, all children born to these mothers had been normal.

In the *New York Times* (March 22, 1957), we read that "massive doses of vitamins A and B in early pregnancy appear to hold great hope for women likely to bear children with harelips and cleft palates." This was the opinion of Dr. Herbert Conway, Professor of

Clinical Surgery at New York Hospital, Cornell Medical Center. He reported that there is a tendency by mothers to repeat cleft palate births. At New York Hospital, however, a group of 59 women who have had an affected child received the vitamin treatment early in pregnancy. All bore normal offspring.

A Logical Conclusion

A study of 400 pregnancies which resulted in offspring with cleft palate was reported in *Plastic and Reconstructive Surgery* (22:442-449, November, 1958). The authors' conclusion was this:

"On the basis of the protective effect of vitamin B_6 (pyridoxine) and folic acid on mice, these vitamins are being given to all mothers with children with cleft lip or cleft palate, during a subsequent pregnancy, to determine the value of such medication in humans as a protective measure. The recommended oral administration is a daily dosage of 10 milligrams of vitamin B_6, 5 milligrams of folic acid and one tablet of the stress formula vitamins. (Editor's Note: We imagine this last to be vitamins B and C in a multiple vitamin capsule.) When possible, vitamin therapy should begin at least one month before a planned pregnancy and continue through the fourth month." Why shouldn't each and every pregnant woman be receiving these B vitamins from the beginning of her pregnancy? Who knows, her third or sixth baby, as well as her first baby, could be born with cleft palate? What's wrong with having a little insurance?

In spite of the work that has been done, many doctors still insist that cleft palate cannot be controlled or prevented. They *will* allow their pregnant patients anything they care to eat, with no restrictions on sweets, the very foods which interfere with the body's maintaining a proper level of vitamin B_6 and folic acid. They *will not* prescribe food supplements, and will laugh it off if the question arises. They *will* give steroid drugs to a pregnant woman if they want to. No food faddist is going to tell them what to do! And we are sure that a larger percentage than need be of their patients *will* give birth to babies who are afflicted with cleft palate.

Clothes

The Health Problem in Wash-and-Wear

The lure of wash-and-wear has captured the imagination of the American housewife as well as the American bachelor. Most customers find the fact that an item is wash-and-wear second in importance only to how much it costs. While there are some items that are deceiving with such a claim, the shirts and blouses, dresses and suits which do live up to the advertisements are indeed convenient and, in the long run, economical.

The National Cotton Council of America tells us that 3 billion yards of easy-care fabrics were marketed in 1959. The Council offers several reasons for this phenomenal product acceptance in the short space of 10 years. For one thing, Americans are once again having large families, and mothers welcome the opportunity to omit the chore of ironing; then, too, we wear more sports clothes, and impeccable smoothness is not vital to these. Almost everybody has an automatic washer these days, so the washing part is easy, but the ironing is still a job unless you use wash-and-wear. Also, in these days, married women work; they do not have the time to fuss at an ironing board.

Increased Exposure to Poisons

All of the reasons make sense, and there are more which would be easily acceptable. Unfortunately, wash-and-wear, or easy-care, fabrics have one unforgivable fault. They increase our exposure to deadly poisons, in addition to those we already inhale from the atmosphere and ingest with our food.

There are 4 principal methods for obtaining or improving the easy-care qualities of a fabric: chemical finishing, use of 100 per cent synthetic fabrics, blending and utilization of fabric construction and surface effects. A combination of fabric construction and chemical finishing may produce better results than either alone, or chemicals may improve the performance of blended fabrics. In the final analysis, almost all easy-care fabrics have chemicals as an integral part of their manufacture.

A Word of Warning

It is in that area that we must warn people about wash-and-wear fabrics. The primary chemicals used are these 4: urea formaldehyde, ethylene urea formaldehyde, triazines, triazones. Of these, the formaldehyde mixtures are by far the most common. The formaldehyde is a very volatile substance (turns into a gas or vapor with very little encouragement). Perspiration, with its heat and moisture would easily be enough to cause such a vaporization of formaldehyde. Just hanging a wash-and-wear garment in a warm and humid area would be enough to make the formaldehyde in it go up in a cloud.

Irritation of Nose and Throat

The *Dispensatory of the United States, 25th Edition,* tells us that, "The vapor from formaldehyde solution irritates the mucous membrane of the nose and throat . . . Because of its local irritant effect, formaldehyde is rarely used for disinfection of body tissues . . . In the past, formaldehyde vapor was extensively used for disinfection of rooms and other closed spaces . . . Inhalations of formaldehyde vapor have been employed in the treatment of pulmonary disorders . . . the treatment is so irritating to mucous membranes that it probably does more harm than good . . . Following absorption, formaldehyde depresses the central nervous system; vertigo (dizziness), depression and coma may be observed. . . . About one fluid ounce of the official solution may be fatal to an adult. . . ."

The danger of unforeseen exposure is not remote. In the fumigation of rooms, formaldehyde was once sprinkled about in regular solution, and the fumes that spontaneously occurred were considered a fumigant strong enough to kill insects and their eggs. As further evidence of this subtle danger, may we refer to a short note, printed in the *Journal of the American Medical Association* (November 1, 1958), which reported considerable difficulty with irritation from formaldehyde vapors in retail establishments selling wash-and-wear garments. The writer said that the warm weather releases these vapors from the garments and circulates the fumes by means of air conditioning. The skin, eyes and nasal mucosa seem to be most affected, and certain manifestations of formaldehyde allergy show up in serious dermatitis and asthma.

Three Choices

Can there be any doubt that body heat, even in winter, let alone summer, would cause these fumes to escape from wash-and-wear underwear, skirts and blouses as they are worn?

There are 3 choices open to us. We can write to the manufacturer of the easy-care materials or garments we usually buy, or plan to buy, asking if formaldehyde has been used in preparing the material. If so, we can urge him to use a substitute and, in the meantime, buy untreated fabrics. We can simply avoid all wash-and-wear materials, to be absolutely safe. Finally, we can (as most people who read this will) do just what we've been doing: Buy the convenient clothes whenever we can find them, and take our chances on poisoning.

If you should choose to do the latter, at least make sure you fortify your system against this poison with plenty of vitamin C and the B complex supplements (rose fruit and brewer's yeast). The formaldehyde we breathe, or that which comes in contact with our skin, in easy-care garments, is one of hundreds of poisons we're meeting these days. Try to counteract at least some of the ill effects of these, by extra dosages of natural vitamins and unprocessed foods.

Colds

Colds and How to Avoid Them

Are you one of those people who can expect at least one bad cold a year? Don't you envy those few who march confidently through the winter months knowing full well that no cold will take them out of circulation? How do they do it? How can they be so sure?

First of all, they eat properly. They take food supplements to fill any unknown gaps in their nutrition. Finally, they get the rest they need to rebuild tired bodies.

We believe that some colds are the aftermath of a busy work schedule or too many social engagements, where the individual hasn't allowed himself a chance to rest and regroup his forces. But this kind of fatigue is easily recognized. "We've been doing too much," is a phrase husbands and wives often exchange. When this is true, the sensible person slows down.

How often do you hear this: "My protein intake is off lately," or "I should be eating more vitamin C-rich foods, and getting some extra B vitamins with my dinner." Not often. People don't talk about such things very often. Most of them don't even think of it. But such concerns are the ones that might keep you from a week in bed or a few days out of work.

Many persons who suffer from colds and say they have tried everything, haven't done a thing about their diet. One of the most common causes of cold is an allergy to wheat products. Editor Rodale has written frequently of bread as a cause of colds. It is this reason, and others in connection with bread's adverse effects on many individuals, that has led Mr. Rodale to campaign against universal acceptance of bread as the staff of life.

The Way a Cold Attacks

In the *Journal of the Medical Society of New Jersey* (October, 1959), I. J. Sobel, M.D., called the common cold "the largest single cause of absenteeism in industry and commerce." Exactly what causes colds doesn't seem to matter very much to the man who gets one, although, since 1948, 70 viruses which are labeled as cold-causing have been discovered. But the general path of a cold is the same as that of other viral infections. The initial damage is to the small blood vessels and capillaries. Once these are penetrated, it is easy to see how quickly the virus is passed on to other parts of the body as the blood moves on.

To test this theory on a live subject, virus particles were injected into the blood stream of a chick embryo. After 45 minutes, the walls of the blood vessels were invaded, causing destruction of the cells and blood leakage. During the next two to four hours, still more blood vessels were attacked by the virus until several areas of hemorrhaging became visible. The capillaries were partly or completely destroyed with subsequent inflammation of the other local tissues. It has been shown that a virus can and does release enzymes which have the effect of weakening capillary walls.

The proper functioning of the capillaries—the many little cross-pipes which draw off blood from the main vessels to serve the body's tissues—has been shown, in *Biological Review of the Cambridge Philosophical Society* (19: 81, 1949) and elsewhere, to depend upon the mucous cement substance covering the pores of the capillary walls. Once the virus particle reaches the capillaries of the mucous membranes of the respiratory tract, this cement substance is destroyed and the blood vessels are penetrated, permitting a spread of the infection.

The Results of 176 Cases

It is obvious, with the above information in mind, that vitamin C and the bioflavonoids would act effectively to prevent infections, since they are both responsible for maintaining capillary strength and manufacturing and fortifying the cement that binds the cells. As proof of this, Dr. Sobel reports on his experience in treating 176 cases of common cold with a citrus, bioflavonoid and vitamin C compound. The patients received 400 milligrams of bioflavonoids and 400 milligrams of vitamin C every 4 hours. Of the 176 cases, "160 responded promptly. As a rule, a complete abatement of symptoms occurred in 24 to 72 hours in most of those cases apparently uncomplicated by bacterial involvement . . . the overall response obtained from the bioflavonoid therapy in this series of 176 cases gave us a definite impression of its salutary effect."

In a related experiment, 62 patients were given bioflavonoids as a protective or preventive medication at two capsules (we presume they contained 400 milligrams each) daily for a period ranging from one to two years. They were selected for this study because of a past history of extreme susceptibility to common colds and influenza. "Twenty-two of them did not have a single attack of common cold or influenza while on this 'preventive therapy.' The remaining 40 patients each had but one episode of 'cold,' which was very mild and subsided within two or three days." Where these colds had been frequent and of long duration, now the few colds that did develop were so mild that they did not interfere with daily activities.

Dr. Sobel quotes the book, *Current Therapy,* by Howard S. Conn (W. B. Saunders Company, 1958), as saying that "there is no evidence whatsoever that any of the presently used antibiotics or sulfonamides have any antiviral effects." The book goes on to say that the routine use of antibiotics or sulfa drugs, all of which produce some side effects, is an inadvisable practice. "In patients with

chronic disease (e. g., cardiac involvement, hypertension, diabetes),"
writes Dr. Sobel, "it may be even hazardous. On the other hand,
bioflavonoid therapy produces no side effects and, in fact, often
produces an improvement in well-being."

In *Archives of Otolaryngology* (34, 787, 1941), an effort was
made to evaluate the effect of vitamins A and D on the prevention of
colds. Irwin C. Spiesman, M.D., then of the University of Illinois
College of Medicine, wrote that his colleagues told of patients who,
on receiving large amounts of these vitamins, had claimed that both
the severity and frequency of their colds had diminished appreciably.
The doctors who told him this had done no tests, nor had they made
any controlled observations for a scientific evaluation of their claims.

Experiment with Vitamins A and D

Dr. Spiesman set out to study the effects of vitamins A and D,
both singly and combined, on a group of subjects. He wanted to
discover whether any reduction in the incidence of colds could be due
to intake of these vitamins, and whether one or the other of the
vitamins was alone responsible for the effects, or if both were
necessary.

Fifty-four patients figured in the study. They all belonged to the
group called "chronic or frequent cold sufferers," and usually had
5 to 7 colds a winter. The colds were accompanied by high fever
and lasted for a week or two weeks. Many of the patients required
rest in bed. The patients were separated into 3 groups: I—received
only vitamin A; II—received only vitamin D; III—received both
vitamin A and vitamin D. Children under 12 years of age were given
half the adult dosage.

The results were interesting. None of the patients who received
either vitamin A or vitamin D alone were benefited by the treatment.
In the group that received both vitamins, 80 per cent of the subjects
showed a significant reduction in both the number and severity of
common colds. The number of colds dropped from 7 to 3 a year, and
the average duration was 5 days with little temperature elevation.

We have seen much evidence on the value of vitamins A and D
—especially vitamin A—in avoiding colds. It is vitamin A's special
function to maintain the moisture of the mucous membranes in the
nose and mouth, etc. When these areas are dry, it is an indication of
cell breakdown. It should be said here that Dr. Spiesman's use of
enormous amounts of carotene vitamin A had some ill effects, as
would be expected with this vitamin. But the dosage (up to 900,000
International Units per day) was much higher than one would use on
one's own. Twenty-five thousand to 50 thousand International Units
of vitamin A per day is considered by most scientists to be perfectly
safe.

The "Adequate Diet" Confusion

After reading about Dr. Sobel's and Dr. Spiesman's work, it is hard to imagine why doctors don't use vitamins all the time for treating colds. Instead, we see statements like this, even in responsible publications: "Vitamin pills added to an adequate diet are a waste of money." Now, of course, the statement as it stands is true. But no one sees a statement of what an adequate diet really is. To most people, an adequate diet is one that keeps them from going hungry. Others think they're eating well if they eat 3 meals a day with some protein, a little starch and some carbohydrates. To younger people, milk shakes and hot dogs constitute an adequate diet. For all of these people, vitamin supplements are a must for cold prevention and for the prevention of any other sickness. "Adequate diet" should mean a daily intake of food that gives the body all of the nutrition it needs or can use in the course of a day. It must allow for sudden stress, exposure to disease, tense situations, intense heat or cold, etc.

Such pre-planning is impossible in our society, because there are so many complexities involved that one cannot take account of all of them. Few of our days are exactly alike. We meet new people on the job, ride with hundreds of strangers on public transportation; we are always under the pressure of world events, and we breathe auto exhaust, eat sprayed foods and drink polluted water. All of these things affect our needs for nutrients. In each of us, the need is different and unpredictable. The only way to be ready is by using a daily intake of food supplements which we hope will exceed our actual needs, so that some reserve is always present. We believe that no one actually eats an "adequate diet," because the demands made on the nutrients we get in food are usually more than any normally eaten foods can meet. Even the most careful of us needs a food supplement program.

For those who are hoping to have the whole problem settled by a vaccine, we refer them to the *Journal of the American Medical Association* (June 4, 1960) for a report on such a product. There was a controlled trial of bacterial vaccine among 293 fliers of the Royal Air Force in Britain. After 18 months of testing, "It was clear from the results that autogenous bacterial vaccines are unlikely to have any practical application in dealing with the problem of the common cold among the flying personnel of the Royal Air Force." We don't believe vaccines are safe or worth waiting for. We'll pin our hopes for avoiding colds on a good intake of the vitamins, especially vitamins A, C and D.

Constipation

Foods You Can Use against Constipation

When irregularity in elimination becomes a problem, most people turn to laxatives for relief. Doctors warn that laxatives used in this way can become a lifelong habit and cause much more misery than they ever correct. As might be expected we are in favor of a careful review of dietary procedures for a clue as to why constipation has set in. We believe that most people who are bothered by constipation are eating the wrong foods—or, perhaps, the right foods prepared the wrong way. After all, maraschino cherries are not digested with the same ease as fresh cherries, and deep-fat fried, breaded fish sticks present a problem to the intestines that doesn't occur with fresh flounder, simply baked or broiled.

Why Processed Foods Are a Problem

Why do processed foods present more of a problem to the digestive system than fresh, natural ones? Because they have been robbed of their nutrients in the processing, and vitamins play an important role in avoiding constipation. In the standard work *Dietetics Simplified* by L. Jean Bogert, Ph.D., and Mame T. Potter, M.A., we read: "We have known for many years how important is the vitamin and mineral content of the diet in preventing constipation. There is a great disturbance in the movements of the intestinal tract in vitamin B deficiency, for instance. . . . The emptying time of the intestine is twice as long in vitamin B-deficient animals. And such animals respond with a greatly improved activity of the intestines when vitamin B is added to their diet. . . . Vitamins A, C and B_1 and B_2 are all needed to keep the mucous lining of the digestive tract in a healthy condition. Constipation and many ill-defined digestive disorders frequently clear up when additional amounts of these vitamins are given."

This view is supported and amplified by many other authorities. To be sure, there are other causes of constipation, but a lack of specific nutrients is a major one which should be considered in treating every case. It should be noted, too, that some of the most unstable vitamins (those which are lost most easily by exposure to oxygen and to heat) are the very ones which figure most prominently in the control of constipation. Therefore, efforts to preserve these in the foods we eat, and efforts to eat foods rich in them, should be made.

However, there are many of America's millions of constipated citizens who rarely include a piece of fresh fruit or a raw vegetable salad in their daily diet. They make no deliberate effort to eat vitamin C-rich foods, and these same persons are addicted to fruits and vegetables that are so highly processed, that even the incidental vitamin C they might possess has been wrung out of them.

Imbalance with the B Vitamins

The B vitamins present a different type of problem, but basically their shortage can also be laid to the processing of food. Here we are faced with some synthetic B vitamins added to foods by manufacturers, causing an imbalance. The lone synthetics borrow other B vitamins from the body for proper processing. In the end, rather than enhance the body's store of B vitamins, the added synthetics often lead to, a shortage!

Another problem presented to proper elimination by modern living begins on the farms where our foods are raised. They are saturated with insecticides. These poisonous sprays have this result, among others: they kill bacteria indiscriminately. The same is true of the antibiotics we use. We tend to lump all bacteria into a category of undesirables. This is a serious error. Elsewhere in these pages you will see evidence of their value in preserving the intestinal atmosphere needed for good digestion and proper utilization of the nutrients in the foods we eat.

Fighting Bacteria Loss

In order to combat the loss of friendly intestinal bacteria—intestinal flora—we can endeavor to use only organically grown foods and avoid drugs, and we can reinforce our diets with foods which encourage the growth of intestinal flora. Prominent among the foods which do this work are yogurt, acidophilus milk and buttermilk. Each of these carries with it the hardy and prolific bacteria which will multiply quickly in the gut and supplement the action of hydrochloric acid there. This acid decreases in supply as people grow older. And this might well be the main reason for frequent constipation in the aged. Paradoxically, babies suffering from constipation respond to yogurt equally well. This indicates to us the value of yogurt's preservative action on intestinal flora, as well as its effect on the action of hydrochloric acid. Presumably, babies have the necessary supply of hydrochloric acid in their stomachs.

Our disapproving attitude toward milk products is suspended in the case of the cultured milks, since it is evident to us that the basic character of the milk is transformed by the addition of selected bacteria. Most of what is good in milk is retained in cultured milks, while most of what is undesirable is eliminated. No need to drink these milks everyday, but a cup now and then would certainly not be objectionable.

Value of Potassium and Calcium

Calcium and potassium, according to nutritionist Adelle Davis (*Let's Eat Right to Keep Fit*), are important dietary factors in preventing constipation. She writes that plenty of calcium in the system prevents cramps or spasms in the intestines. These spasms are called by physicians spastic colitis or spastic constipation. Added calcium brings relief. Miss Davis cautions that too much fat in the diet can result in a lowered calcium supply. The fat and calcium combine into a soapy substance which hardens in the excretory path and causes constipation. (This would appear to contradict several popular dietary manuals which encourage the liberal use of fat in losing weight and maintaining good health.)

Potassium should never be a problem. It is in plentiful supply in fruits and vegetables, but cooking brings about serious losses of this important mineral. Salt is another thief of potassium in the system. Eat plenty of fresh raw fruit and vegetables if you would keep up your potassium supply, and avoid salt.

The Value of Bulk

One of nature's most effective means of maintaining proper elimination is its handling of bulk in the intestines. Many foods yield the vitamins and minerals they have and leave a large residue of useless bulk which the body must then discard. This bulk is capable of absorbing large amounts of water and expanding as a sponge would. As this expansion occurs, the mass pushes at the walls of the intes-tines, thus stimulating the peristaltic action (a wave-like motion of the intestinal wall) which serves to push all waste through the intestines so that it can be eliminated.

Cellulose is the name given to this bulky constituent in foods, and it is obvious that constipated individuals should be certain to include liberal sources of it in their diet. The bulky juicy foods are the important ones—tomatoes, melons, figs, dates, grapes, plums, apricots, raisins, also dried peas, beans, nuts, seeds, etc. The rougher foods have a slightly abrasive effect on the intestinal wall, and prod the muscles into the desired reflex action which moves the waste.

How far should one go in concentrating on cellulose foods? Certainly, common sense must be our guide. Rich as many cellulose foods are in vitamins and minerals, they cannot take the place of the needed protein meat and eggs supply. Furthermore, too much cellu-lose can literally engulf the protein you ingest, thus limiting its avail-ability to the body. So, if you increase your intake of celluose foods to combat constipation (and you should do so), be reasonable about it. If you get a great deal of it at one meal, cut down on cellulose-rich foods at the next. Try to eat most of your protein at a meal that is not too rich in cellulose-containing foods. That way the protein will have a chance to do its job, unhampered.

How Much Water Should One Drink?

In mentioning cellulose, we called attention to the moisture which inflates the sponge-like cellulose. It is important to the process of elimination, then, that there be sufficient moisture available to be absorbed in this way. Water can come to the body only as water is drunk, or from foods with water content, or by the body's oxygen mixing with the hydrogen, liberated from the foods we digest, to form H_2O. This supply of water in our bodies is drained through urine, perspiration, feces, exhalation in breathing, sputum, menstrual flow, nasal secretions, tears, etc.

With these varied avenues of water loss, it is easy to see the need for making certain that the supply is continually replenished. This is especially true of those who are bothered by constipation. Illustrative of this need is a paper by James A. McKenny, M.D., which appeared in the *American Journal of Digestive Diseases* (March, 1946). He tells of a study carried out in California in which the observers looked to discover the relationship of water intake to constipation. A record was made of those taking water before, during or after meals; also, the use of laxatives was recorded. It was shown that those taking water with their meals did not require laxatives; conversely, those not doing so were users of laxatives.

Dr. McKenny concluded his paper with this statement:

"The use of large quantities of fruits and vegetables is frequently effective as a remedy for constipation, but in the final analysis, perhaps some of their effectiveness is due not only to their water content, but also to their ability to retain and carry water further along the digestive tract. The use of water before breakfast, also before and after meals was noted, but after extended observation, the conclusion was reached that it was the water which was taken along with meals, that was the most efficient in overcoming the symptom of constipation."

The patients who took part in the experiment of which Dr. McKenny speaks, took two or more glasses of water with each meal, apart from any juice, coffee, tea or other beverage served.

No Harm in Trying Water

Our attitude on water drinking has been that one should drink when thirsty, and that instinct will tell one when the body needs liquid. This is probably quite true where primitive peoples are concerned. However, modern living may have repealed that rule. We can't always stop what we're doing to get a drink, nor do we eat as many moisture-rich fruits as we should. Modern man may need to remind himself to give his body the water it needs. Mealtime is considered the best, by several physiologists McKenny quotes, for drinking water that will act with the foods you eat to prevent constipation.

We can see no real objection to trying this system as a means to controlling constipation. Water is certainly not harmful in these amounts, and if it is bottled spring water (recommended by Editor Rodale as the safest for drinking and cooking), one can rest assured of its purity.

Exercise Necessary for Proper Elimination

Exercise appears to be a necessary factor in proper elimination. Any kind will do, of course, but the moderate and regular motion of walking seems best suited to everyone's needs, and it is the one exercise we feel free to recommend for everyone.

We have offered here a few valuable aids to fighting constipation which are sound and which have no danger in them. They all revolve around eating a natural diet and taking some exercise. No researcher we have seen will recommend processed or fried foods to alleviate this condition, nor will he tell you to avoid some mild exertion. Some do suggest careful use of laxatives, but when they do, they admit that laxatives are no true solution. We say laxatives are *no* solution.

Before resorting to patent medicines or drugs for treating constipation, give these natural suggestions a try. A month on natural foods and an occasional intake of cultured milks should certainly be enough to demonstrate their value. Many people have been using laxatives for years with no improvement in the basic condition. We believe most of them would be grateful for a chance to escape from that trap.

Contact Lenses

Contact Lenses Endanger the Eyes

When the idea of contact lenses first originated, the reasons for using them were much clearer than they are today. Movie stars and athletes were the chief consumers, and the need was obvious. The styles of glasses, until 10 or 15 years ago, were far from flattering. They were either encased in a round, solid gold or silver metal rim, or they were rimless and angled. Glasses were anything but attractive, and for anyone whose livelihood depended upon pleasing appearance, contact lenses seemed to be an answer to a prayer. The glasses in those days were fragile, too. If they were dropped, they were gone, so athletes were faced with a real problem in trying to keep them from being broken at a game. Contact lenses would at least be a practical consideration here.

Now let's look at the situation today. The shapes of the new frames, and materials used in them, have made eyeglasses a fashion focus for the ladies. It is the style now to call attention to eyeglasses, by studding them with rhinestones, shaping them exotically and coloring them to match any ensemble. Some women with good vision are actually envious because they can't take advantage of the fashion values of cleverly designed spectacle frames.

Not only are the frames beautiful, but they are made so that the lenses can take a lot of punishment. The plastic frames have a valuable resilience, so that the shock when they drop is lessened, and because they can be set deep in a plastic frame, the lens surface is not likely to be scratched or cracked when they are dropped. Actually, the original reasons for the development of contact lenses have just about disappeared, yet they are more sought after than ever before. About 6 million Americans now wear contact lenses, and the number is increasing by 500,000 a year. It's a $200,000,000 business. If all these contact lenses are being used, why are we not willing to go along with the thousands of doctors who recommend and prescribe them? We do not believe contact lenses are safe.

Can Lead to Serious Impairment of Vision

One eye specialist after the other has expressed caution or true fear at the prospect of prescribing contact lenses. In the *New York Times* (June 2, 1960), the House of Delegates of the American Medical Association was quoted as saying, ". . . the use of such lenses (contact) is not entirely without hazard . . . this House views with grave concern the use of contact lenses." Said Dr. R. O. Rychner, ophthalmologist of the National Medical Foundation for Eye Care in New York, "The use of contact lenses can at times lead to serious permanent impairment of vision."

How true that statement is can be gathered from what an AMA meeting in Miami was told by Captain R. K. Lanshe, an eye specialist serving with the Marine Corps: corneal strangulation can result from wearing contact lenses with too sharp an inner curvature. This lens curve creates a suction cup effect that can prevent the metabolic exchanges of gases, hypertonic tears and heat.

The *U. S. Armed Forces Medical Journal* is quoted in *Newsweek* (August 8, 1960) as warning of "potential danger of eye infection and of injury" from wearing contact lenses. *Good Housekeeping* magazine (June, 1960) tells of 5 leading ophthalmologists who observed cases where corneal damage resulted. One specialist in lens fitting said, "Corneal abrasions are not uncommon. Though they heal quickly in most cases, you can get scarring and reduced vision. I tell all my patients that there is danger in wearing contact lenses." A routine sampling of 16 ophthalmologists across the United States brought out some startling facts: 15 of them had treated corneal injuries resulting from contact lenses, and 4 out of these had handled cases in which the eye was lost as a result of the damage.

Trouble and Expense

The whole contact lens procedure is so much trouble and expense, aside from the real danger always present to the eye, that one wonders why anyone has the patience to bother with them. The price is prohibitive: it averages about $200 for a pair. But perhaps the words of a contact lens purchaser who told of his experiences in a letter to *Consumer Bulletin* (January, 1960) would be of greater persuasion than ours. He says, "At a contact lens specialist, I bought a pair of contact lenses. The standard price is, or was, $180.00. This, in my case, included a pair of reading glasses to be worn with them and a bottle of liquid, which I was directed to use every time I used them. Because of the ever-present danger of losing the lenses by misplacement or having them fall out of the eye, I was advised to buy an insurance policy. Annual premium $15.00 . . . I could see quite well with the lenses. There the satisfaction ended. Putting them in the eye requires the use of a special fluid, considerable skill and practice, a mirror and, preferably, privacy . . . Taking them out is another trick . . . This I know: Any talk about 'throwing away' your glasses is pure deception. You will need them.

"Having thought contact lenses primarily suited to outdoor activities, on boats (or swimming), my experience of losing them is just another time I was played for a sucker and should have known better. Nothing could be what the ads say contact lenses are. Fortunately, the financial loss was not serious for me, but I do regret the evenings I spent with the cussed things in my eyes, crying copiously, looking down only, night after night."

That's one man's misery, but his feelings are not unusual. The discomfort and precautions involved in getting used to and wearing contact lenses are monumental, even for those who are said to have made the adjustment with relative ease. As a rule, the wearer suffers stinging, burning and the sensation of a foreign body in the eye at first, and these annoyances often last for several weeks. No wonder. The lens is a thin plastic disc a little smaller than a dime, and it rests directly on the cornea, separated only by a film of tears which holds the lens in place. The wearer always feels as though there were something in his eye, and indeed there is—something as big as a dime, when even a tiny speck of dust is enough to cause discomfort!

One person tells of a visit to his ophthalmologist, who had just finished with a patient using contact lenses. The doctor told him that the previous patient was unable to endure wearing contact lenses for more than one hour. When the man suggested sunflower seeds to help strengthen the eyes against the irritation of the contact lenses, the doctor was skeptical, but decided to give it a try. The patient, after using the sunflower seeds for a short time, reported that the contact lenses could be worn for 3 hours without removal, and attributed the improvement solely to the sunflower seeds. If you know someone who is suffering similarly, perhaps your suggesting that he do the same would save him much discomfort.

Endless Restrictions

And do you think anyone could possibly remember all the restrictions concerning contact lenses? Here are some from *Scope* (July 3, 1960): "Patients must be warned never to experiment with the lens, nor engage in competition for length of wearing time with other patients.

"They must not build up the wearing time too rapidly or irregularly, nor wear the lenses for irregular periods from day to day or while sleeping. The lenses should be removed when conjunctivitis (inflammation of the eye-covering membrane), blepharitis (inflammation of the eyelid itself) or upper respiratory infections are present. Strict personal habits of hygiene must be followed (using saliva for cleaning the lenses is unthinkable), and gentle insertion and removal of the lens is absolutely necessary."

The *Good Housekeeping* article mentioned above adds these dissuaders: Certain people should never even try to wear contact lenses—diabetics, those with chronic colds or sinusitis, extra dry or teary or abnormally protruding eyes. And those who do wear them must constantly be on the alert for lenses roughened in use; dust, dirt, nicotine on the lenses; rubbing the eyes; wearing lenses while eyes are irritated by colds, hay fever or styes. Any one of these can cause a scratch on the cornea, which can lead to serious eye infection. Any break in the surface of the cornea gives germs a chance to enter, multiply and cause infection. These can cause corneal scars that may reduce vision, or worse, an ulcer may develop which, in some extreme cases, requires the eye's removal.

That's the story on contact lenses. How anyone who is seriously interested in the health of his eyes could even consider using them is something we cannot understand.

Cooking

What About Cooking Temperatures?

Some time ago, we asked a knowledgeable biochemist what the cooking temperature is at which the fats in meat or other foods may become dangerous. Many researchers claim that too great a heat can produce harmful compounds in fats—indeed, these compounds have been shown to be cancer-causing.

He answered that there is no answer, for the way you are doing your cooking controls the results and there is an infinite variety of circumstances which may be involved. For instance, let's say you're broiling a steak. If you like it rare, you may broil it for a short time beneath a fairly moderate flame and the temperature may be so low as to leave the entire inner part of the steak completely raw. On the surface of the steak you may have achieved a temperature high enough to form chemical substances dangerous from the point of view of health. If you broil the steak at high enough heat to char it, then you have certainly created substances that are suspected of being quite dangerous. But, of course, the same is true of a burnt crust of bread, toasted to that temperature.

If you put a roast in the oven to cook, some of the same problems appear. Searing the roast at a high temperature before putting it in the oven may produce dangerous fatty substances on the surface of the roast. But, if you like to cook your roast at a moderate temperature, the inside of the meat may be just warmed by the time you are ready to serve it. If you enjoy eating the charred parts of the roast and avoiding the softer part of the meat, you will certainly be more likely to get a potentially dangerous substance.

Other Considerations

The length of time you cook the food also enters in. This is most easy to observe in cooking bacon or some equally fatty meat. Up to a certain point, the meat cooks slowly. But, suddenly, almost in a moment, it burns and chars. This is the point at which the dangerous temperature was reached. But you can cook bacon slowly for a much longer time and get little or no burning, seeming to indicate that no danger is involved. On the other hand, cooking at fairly high heat over a very long period of time may result in a final temperature high enough to do some damage.

If you cover something which is cooking on the stove, you increase the amount of heat to which the food is exposed. Leaving the cover off allows some of the heat to escape. Turning the slices of whatever you are cooking reduces the amount of heat to which they are exposed. So they are much less likely to burn or char.

The size and original temperature of the food you are cooking also influence the result. Foods chopped fine cook much more quickly than large pieces because more total surface is exposed to heat. So it would seem to be less likely that you would reach dangerous temperatures cooking something like ground meat or chopped vegetables which can be tossed quickly in a skillet. On the other hand, if you cook a meat loaf until the outside is burned in order to make certain that the interior is fully cooked, you have certainly created some dangerous fatty substances on the surface of the loaf.

Deep Fat Frying

Deep fat or French frying is dangerous from several points of view. You don't want the food fried to be fat-soaked and soggy. So you keep the fat at a very high temperature so that the food will be coated with a crisp layer of fat. Undoubtedly, this fat has been raised to a temperature high enough to be dangerous.

Then, too, since so much fat is used in French frying there is a tendency to use the same fat over and over, keeping it (often unrefrigerated) between fryings. Not only does the unchilled fat become rancid (a very dangerous kind of food to eat) but in the heating and re-heating, there is certainly a degeneration of the fatty substances into compounds that are bound to be harmful. Many people who fry in deep fat use hydrogenated fats (solid at room temperature like lard, butter or commercial shortening) which are deficient in unsaturated fatty acids.

What about the temperature of your food to start with? Was it room temperature, as most cookbooks recommend? Or did you take it right from the freezer or the refrigerator? In either case, the temperature of the food is bound to influence the length of time needed to complete the cooking and hence the possible influence of high or low temperature.

The kind of utensil you use will influence the results. A thin frying pan heats quickly and just as quickly burns the food within it. Cast iron, steel, enamelware, glass—each of these has its own rate of heating up and of holding heat, so that the utensil is of considerable importance, too. If you want to heat food slowly and steadily, use thick, heat-retaining and heat-distributing utensils.

Our Recommendations

If you are going to use fats in cooking—and we think it is permissible to a limited degree—use oils that are liquid at room temperature—olive oil, corn oil, cottonseed oil, peanut oil, sunflower seed oil, etc. Cook foods for as short a time as possible at as low a temperature as possible. The shorter the cooking time, the higher the temperature may be, within limits. And the longer the cooking time, the lower the temperature should be—again, within reason.

In general, what we are recommending is braising—that is, cooking the food first in a little oil to prevent it from sticking to the pan. By so doing, the food is coated with enough oil to prevent it from losing valuable vitamins and minerals throughout the rest of the cooking process. Then you can put a lid on the utensil and turn the fire quite low to complete the cooking economically and healthfully. This kind of fat-cookery should not produce dangerous by-products.

Our biochemist asked at this point if he had convinced us that there is no do-or-don't answer to the problem of what temperature is dangerous in cooking fatty foods. He told us that he and his wife, in order to clarify the subject in their own minds, had planned to do experiments themselves in their own laboratory. But when they began to list all the possible combinations of circumstances, to say nothing of different kinds of food and utensils—as we have outlined above—they decided that this was a mammoth job which they could not undertake. Undoubtedly complete experiments will be done some day and we will be glad to print the full results then.

Copper Pipes

On the Fence about Copper Pipes

The medical fraternity is often found on the fence in making a pronouncement on a health matter. No matter how convincing the evidence might be, the doctors hem and haw when it actually comes to saying that a thing is dangerous to health. Their motives for this are sometimes obscure to us, but we do feel that their attitude is a disservice to those who look to them for guidance.

To be specific, we offer the case of copper as used in cookware, piping, etc. We have, long ago, on the basis of good scientific evidence, made our position clear on the use of copper in connection with food or drinking water: it is dangerous and should be avoided. There is no doctor who has not had access to the same information we saw, yet in the *Journal of the American Medical Association* (October 1, 1960), there is a letter from a New York doctor, describing in great detail, his problems with copper and asking for advice. He tells of sinks and the bathtub stained green, a plastic "glass" in the bathroom that has a green deposit, a dog's dish and a synthetic sponge all stained with copper. He wants to know how dangerous copper is in such amounts.

Journal's Answer

The answer is not easy to figure out. It begins with the statement that "copper has a relatively low toxicity in man"—whatever that means. Relative to what—cyanide or applesauce? The reply goes on: "Ordinarily, some of the salts of copper are insoluble and when ingested, may not provide amounts of the mineral in quantities sufficient to cause trouble." This means very little, really. It means that some salts may provide amounts that can cause trouble. From it, one can gather only that it is rather unusual for people to be poisoned by copper. Of course, that is true. It is rather unusual for people to be poisoned at all.

The answer goes on to say that, "Absorption of small amounts of copper over a long period may result in the deposition of the metal in the tissues, primarily the liver, where a pigmentary cirrhosis may develop. Other results of toxicity may include some injury to the kidney, capillary damage and excitation of the central nervous system followed by depression. It is believed that copper cooking vessels or copper piping do not ordinarily impart any significant quantities of copper to water or the food which they hold."

The answer is certainly indefinite. One comes away with the impression that copper pipes and vessels aren't anything to worry about—in spite of the damage copper from them can cause to the liver, the kidneys, the capillaries and the mind. The statement that "it is believed" that copper pipes and cooking vessels do not "ordinarily" impart significant quantities does not convince us. The doctor who wrote in contradicts that statement. If his are not significant quantities, what are?

Any substance which can cause damage to the system, especially if it is cumulative, should certainly be avoided whenever possible. If we were in such a position that our utensils and sinks were being stained by copper in the water, we would quickly change the piping, move or certainly drink bottled spring water. If we were building a house we would avoid copper piping. If someone were to ask us if copper from pipes or pots is dangerous to health, we would say "yes" as definitely as we know how.

Cosmetics

Dangerous Chemicals in Your Make-Up

Perhaps the things we write here about the dangers in using today's cosmetics will not cripple the cosmetics industry, and perhaps most women who read this will go right on using every dye and cream they used before, but surely some few will recognize that the situation is serious. The source of our information may carry some weight among skeptics who think we are unduly alarmed. It is an article by A. J. Lehman, M.D., from the Division of Pharmacology of the Food and Drug Administration, in *Drug and Cosmetic Industry* (June, 1960), a major trade publication. Time after time, Dr. Lehman mentions specific poisons being used in cosmetics. These cosmetics are being bought and used by you, the consumer. These poisons are poisoning you!

Dr. Lehman deplores one of the modern wrinkles in the industry —that of employing pharmacologically active substances in the formulations. By this, he means the inclusion of antibiotics, hormones, antiseptics, etc., in skin creams, lipsticks and lotions. The incorporation of such drugs in cosmetics poses serious problems of safety for the user. These things are hazardous, even when the user is aware of their possible activity and takes them as a necessity on doctor's orders. To take them indiscriminately, merely because they occur in a cosmetic preparation, or to use them only because they might help to enhance the skin's texture at the risk of causing serious injury, is very immature reasoning.

No Provisions for Varying Skin Type

The majority of cosmetic injuries result from local toxicity reactions, due to surface irritations from so-called "surface-active" agents. These agents appear in most types of cosmetics, and no one has ever determined just what different effect they have on clear skin or blemished skin, skin that is porous as opposed to that which is firm, the skin of a healthy person compared with that of one who is ill, young skin or old skin. Yet everybody who uses cosmetics uses them every day, whether they feel fine or rundown, whether they are working or in bed at the hospital. They begin using cosmetics in their early teens and continue into old age. No provisions are made for the changes in skin by the manufacturers. Doesn't the constant reintroduction of these irritants on aging skin invite skin difficulties, or even health problems involving the rest of the system? Nobody really knows, but very little effort is being made to find out. Where is the federal government at such times?

Dr. Lehman discusses a few of the most commonly-used beauty aids and some of the hazards involved in using them. For example, it was found that, if the neutralizer of a certain hair waving product accidentally got into the eye of the user, serious, acute damage could occur. The surface-active agents were responsible.

Chemical Changes for Waving

Most of the surface-active ingredients ("surfactants") are classified as cationic, anionic and nonionic—in order of toxicity. Active ingredients in hair wave lotions must be able to produce chemical and physical changes in the hair to cause it to wave. If it is powerful enough to do that, the agent is likely to cause unforeseen effects on the skin itself, as well as the rest of the system if exposure is frequent and extensive. Of reported injuries from permanent waves, 80 per cent are similar to a regular chemical burn. There are occasional reports that permanent wave preparations cause the development of dangerous changes in the blood. Dr. Lehman says that such claims have not been substantiated, however they are so persistent that one wonders at the possibility.

Depilatories and Hair Dyes

The shaving of legs and underarms by women has been displaced, in many cases, by depilatories; that is chemical preparations which literally burn the unwanted hair from the skin. The convenience factor, of course, of these preparations is a big selling point, but their use on such delicate skin areas as the underarms is extremely hazardous. They include in their formulas the salts of thioglycolic acid, which causes frequent chemical burns of the skin, and sometimes kills the hair follicles so that the skin is completely denuded permanently. What systemic effects such powerful chemicals can have we do not know.

The thought that "only her hairdresser knows" has lured millions of American women into the hair dye habit. Their use has become so commonplace that a dye job to match a favorite dress or for a single special occasion is not unusual. Dr. Lehman reports that the darker hair dyes contain the dangerous ingredients, paradiaminobenzenes and aminophenols, and reports of sensitivity to these are fairly frequent. Interestingly enough, 24 per cent of all complaints about cosmetics are attributed to hair dyes. The FDA strongly advocates patch testing before using a hair dye. How many people bother with this important step?

Coal-Tar Dyes and Toxic Metals

Reports are received occasionally that tell of blood changes produced by dyes. Again, Dr. Lehman says that these changes are not substantiated by laboratory experiments. But no one denies that the coal-tar colors used in the dyes are dangerous. As a matter of fact, the law forbids their use around the eyes (how many of us knew that before now?), for they can be extremely dangerous to the mucosa of the eye. In California recently, several high school girls used such dyes in make-up for a play. Injuries were serious enough to cause hospitalization.

What about deodorants and antiperspirants? The deodorants mask the odor of perspiration, while the antiperspirants actually inhibit the flow of perspiration by blocking the normal function of the sweat glands. Aluminum compounds are usually used in these preparations, and reports on injuries from these products are characterized by Dr. Lehman as "fairly numerous," and he goes on to say in typical bureaucratic understatement that, "it must be concluded that these cosmetics are, in general, poorly tolerated by some individuals."

What about shampoos? Well, most contain the toxic metal salts, selenium and arsenic. But then these poisonous salts turn up everywhere. Lead comes with just about every hair dye, and mercury was used in a variety of cosmetics, and still turns up in bleach-cream preparations. Mercury is not only very toxic to the system, but is notorious for producing skin damage. Dr. Lehman says, helplessly, "It is our conviction that it would be in the best interest of the cosmetics industry if these toxic metal salts were eliminated from cosmetic formulations." Whose "best interest" should come before the consumer's where the Food and Drug Administration is concerned? It seems to us that the United States taxpayers are paying, not for the FDA's advice to the cosmetics industry on what would be good business practice, but for their guarding us against business practices that can harm our health. If these ingredients are dangerous, why not pass a law that will preserve us from them?

Are We Protected?

The lists of objectionable cosmetic ingredients go on and on. We know about the cancer-causing lipstick dyes, but we have yet to get any legal protection from them. There are preparations for anchoring false eyelashes to the eyelids which produce serious irritation. Now we have tanning preparations that can be taken orally, and preparations that are meant to be rubbed on the skin. They're being made by the carload and sold by the millions of packages, yet no one has any idea of their safety or lack of it.

Cosmetics are really one thing a health-conscious person can and should avoid. For the woman who doesn't "feel dressed" without a touch of lipstick, a completely natural lipstick is available now. For a beautiful complexion, clear eyes and healthy hair, a good diet is the best and safest insurance. Don't risk serious health problems by falling for the advertisements that promise miracles for your appearance. They don't work, and even if they did, is being falsely beautiful, but sick, better than being normally attractive and healthy?

We Need Protection from Cosmetics

For one brief moment in April, 1959, the Food and Drug Administration stood up to an industry and announced that the law protecting the health of Americans would be enforced, regardless of commercial considerations. It had been found in experiments, as defined by law, that certain dyes being used in lipsticks were hazardous to health. The law says that any such ingredient must be removed from the product or the product will be banned for sale.

The decision of the FDA followed after two years of tests that proved "definite injury" in animals was caused by the ingestion of 7 of the banned colors. (A group of rats had been fed relatively large amounts of the dyes for 90 days. They developed damage to the liver, kidneys, spleen and blood-forming system as a result.)

It was revealed that only these 7, of the 17 being used, had been tested, but that the other 10 were so similar in composition that they would also be ruled off the cosmetic market. The spokesman for the FDA said that, unless the present law were changed, it had no choice but to ban the use of these colors by lipstick manufacturers.

"Vital"—"Absolutely Essential"

At this news, the Toilet Goods Association exploded, saying that such a ruling could destroy the art of lipstick manufacture. In the *New York Times* (April 17, 1959), Stephen L. Mayham, a vice president of the Toilet Goods Association, estimated that one or more of these dyes are contained in 90 per cent of all lipsticks produced by such cosmetics houses as Coty, Elizabeth Arden, Revlon, Hazel Bishop, Helena Rubenstein, etc. He said, further, that 9 of the 17 colors are considered vital in lipstick manufacture, and 4 of these 9 are "absolutely essential."

This was the opening blast in the war the cosmetics industry waged to have this ban rescinded. The Toilet Goods Association wailed piteously that "It does not seem possible that any satisfactory substitute colors can be developed." This statement appeared in *American Druggist* magazine (May 4, 1959). For an industry that has come up with iridescent lipsticks, eyeshadows that won't smear, waterproof hair dyes, etc., this cry was hard to believe. Apparently, 10 per cent of the lipsticks produced by the above-named houses were utilizing something else, why not the rest, if need be?

If You Can't Obey a Law—Change It!

Of course, it was obvious to the cosmetics men that the FDA could not simply look the other way and allow these coal-tar dyes to be included in the lipstick formulas, else they would be breaking the law themselves. The answer lay elsewhere. It lay in a statement by Shelby T. Grey, director of the FDA's bureau of program planning, to a meeting of the Cosmetic Career Women, quoted in the same issue of *American Druggist*. He disclosed the fact that the agency already was "drafting proposed legislation to amend the Food, Drug and Cosmetic Act to allow continued use" by lipstick manufacturers of any coal-tar dyes for which "safe tolerances can be established." You see, the solution was easy. No one would dream of breaking the law, but if obeying or enforcing it becomes inconvenient, simply change the law!

The law for lipsticks is the same as for internal medicines, and it demands that laboratory tests prove that any dye used in such a product be completely harmless. The reason lipsticks, especially, are included in this category is that they get into the digestive system, and so must meet the same safety requirements as products actually intended for human consumption. The reasoning couldn't be more logical.

Larger Amount to Experimental Animals

The lipstick men resorted to the old device of pointing out that the rats were given a much larger amount of the dyes than a woman would get in 90 days from using lipstick. That is true, but do women wear lipstick only 90 days of their lives? Most women wear lipstick as their first cosmetic in their early teens, and they continue to do so into old age. The poisons from coal-tar dyes have been proven to be cumulative, so the lady who has worn lipstick daily for 50 or 60 years is sure to have matched the rats' ingested quota several times.

The argument for a safe tolerance is even more absurd. How could a safe tolerance be set for a thing like lipstick? Who knows how much is used by each woman? Some touch up their lips a dozen times a day, and others get by with a dab before work in the morning and another at night, before dinner. Could anyone be certain, in deciding on an amount of coal-tar dye to be put into a lipstick, that there would be no overdoses, even in women who use excessive amounts of the stuff—often in several layers.

No Fatalities? Who Knows?

The articles on this controversy are all careful to point out the fact that no fatalities have been known to result from the use of lipsticks employing these dyes. Who knows what deaths have been caused by this substance? Have you ever known of a doctor who considered lipstick in casting about for the cause of a patient's cancer, or damage to liver, kidneys or spleen? Is there any way of testing for its actual effect on a human being? No, just as there are no simple tests for the effects of industrial air pollution, or smoking, or fluorides. We must go by what we've seen in experimental animals or the statistics we can analyze. Experiments on rats tell us these dyes are injurious to live tissue. Why not avoid them? Use something else, and if there's no substitute, use nothing. If a woman were made to realize that she might have to pay for reddened lips with ill health, and possibly death, we wonder if she would still feel the necessity for lipstick.

If the law can be changed, in this case, to accommodate the lipstick industry, then why not change it to suit every other industry? If we are not affected by the reports of damage caused by lipstick dyes, why be bothered by the dyes used in oranges, in sodas, pink and blue popcorn, etc.? We must take a definite stand somewhere! A food additive should be proven absolutely harmless before its use is permitted, and the tests should be done by the manufacturer and the FDA. In that way, complete objectivity could be better served.

This whole altercation almost erupted 6 or 8 months earlier. In the *Consumer Bulletin* (September, 1958), there was a report of a request by two cosmetics firms for an amendment to existing legislation, which would permit so-called harmless coal-tar dyes to be used in eyebrow and eyelash preparations. The request was turned down because no evidence of harmlessness could be shown. The case was dropped there, perhaps because eyebrow and eyelash preparations are not as big money as lipstick, and because they've found other unobjectionable substances to use.

Coal-Tar Colors Found

Drug Trade News (May 1, 1961) told the story of Food and Drug Administration seizures of eye make-up products "on the ground that they contain non-permitted coal-tar colors," and other seizures, said an FDA spokesman, are "quite likely." A number of colors have been provisionally listed as safe for use in the area of the eye, but apparently manufacturers are not satisfied to use only these.

The FDA announced the seizure of "eye-liner violet" pencil leads from a southern manufacturer of eye pencils for the entire cosmetics industry. Many well-known cosmetics houses have been named as sellers of illegal eye cosmetics in this and other instances. Of course, all immediately promised to withdraw the offending pencils. But as S. L. Mayham, executive vice president of Toilet Goods Association, has said, no cosmetic maker should market an item unless he is certain that it conforms with all FDA regulations.

We were interested to see the comment of an FDA spokesman who "emphasized that none of the seizures involves possible danger to users, but all are grounded on failure to obtain safety clearance." How can a product fail to meet safety standards and still pose no possible danger to the consumer? Furthermore, the law that prohibits these coal-tar dyes has been on the books since 1938, what legitimate reason could there be for their being present in any cosmetics? In more than 20 years, manufacturers whose livelihood lies in cosmetics should have become accustomed to what is and is not allowed in their products. Also, coal-tar dyes are not accidental contamination. The product must be planned around them. For the FDA to pretend it believes the presence of these illegal dyes was unintentional is malarkey. These cosmetics manufacturers should be prosecuted, instead of hailed for their cooperation. Let them obey the law and cooperation is accomplished by that alone. How many coal-tar dyed eye pencils do you suppose have been sold and used since 1938?

The use of cosmetics is extremely common among women of the United States in spite of the dangers involved. If they will be used, then we need laws that will assure us of their safety and purity, and these laws must be enforced to the fullest.

The Perfumes That Surround Us

Did you ever stop to think about the substances that may be in the bottle of perfume you open and sniff at the perfume counter? Remembering that you slosh the stuff over yourself pretty generously, doesn't it seem wise to discover a little more about what perfumes, colognes and shaving lotions contain?

What's happened to perfumes since grandfather's time seems indicative of what has happened to many aspects of our life which used to be pleasant, natural and harmless, but which today are far more stimulating, brilliant, intense, and who knows, possibly harmful.

An article in *Drug and Cosmetic Industry* for December, 1960, discusses perfume for men, giving considerable information on how these scents used to be concocted, compared with the formulas used today.

Nothing could be more natural and pleasing and less likely to harm one than the ingredients used in perfumes in earlier days. Citrus oils, plus flowers and herbs of various kinds were blended to make the perfume. Here is the formula for an early one: bergamot, lemon, sweet orange, bitter orange, rosemary and lavender. This combination of oils was put into a still and distilled with alcohol and water to give a clear solution.

"As simple and ancient as this formula is, it is still attractive when converted to a finished product with alcohol and water in our modern manner," says J. R. Elliott, perfume consultant, who wrote the article in *Drug and Cosmetic Industry*.

Fifty years ago, everyone would have been familiar with the delightful fragrances mentioned in this old recipe—the bergamot, rosemary and lavender would be growing in practically every garden, for in days when aerosols were unknown, when houses were tightly closed and shuttered against the cold, when baths were infrequent and in some places almost unknown, the freshness and spiciness of these herbs was an absolute necessity for anyone who had a sensitive nose.

Since such a perfume is agreeable and easy to make, why do we not use such formulas in today's perfume factories? In the early part of the twentieth century, according to Mr. Elliott, there was a rapid advance in the use of "synthetic" perfume materials. There was a sharp division in, the ranks of manufacturers on the use of synthetics. According to Mr. Elliott, claims and counterclaims rang through the air, appeared in ads, editorials and even handbills. The use of synthetics was attacked as sacrilegious: "natural oils were made by God and should be kept pure and undefiled." One perfume maker went so far as to claim that inhaling the fumes of his competitor's hair tonic would rob an individual of his manly vigor.

As a result, says Mr. Elliott, "synthetic" became a nasty word whose bad reputation lasted well into the twenties.

The synthetics which were added to the old recipes contributed "brilliance and depth," according to this perfume consultant. We don't know what these words mean as applied to perfume, but we guess they mean just about what similar words mean applied to the food industry. We are told that maraschino cherries, jams, preserves, canned fruits and confections must have a "brilliant" color or the consumer will not buy them. Lipsticks must be dyed with "brilliant" dyes, so that they leap out from women's faces like neon signs. And the first impression one has of a lipstick in which only wholly natural colors are used is that it is "dull" compared to the "brilliant" ones which are commercially available. However, one quickly becomes fond of the "dullness" and then the other kind of lipstick looks garish and vulgar.

Why Do They Use Synthetics?

So we see that the synthetics added to perfumes contributed just what synthetics added to other aspects of life contribute— falseness, which is made to seem more real than the real thing. Cherries dyed with coal-tar dye are redder and lusher looking than any real cherry ever could be. Oranges dyed with coal-tar dyes are oranger than any citrus fruit ever could be. So, because of the fake, hopped up, artificial "brilliance" which surrounds us on all sides, we are gradually losing our appreciation for the less violent, less concentrated hues of nature. So it is with perfumes. Anyone who has raised lavender believing he would get something that smells like the lavender toilet soap for sale in the drug store is going to be disappointed, for nothing in nature could ever smell like that.

Here is the formula for a basic cologne as it was made from natural oils: rosemary, bitter orange, French verbena, lemon, oil of limes, rose otto, orange flower and peppermint. In modern times synthetic chemicals are added to create "brilliance and depth." Here is a formula using the synthetics:

H and R Jasmaketon 10% in DEP
H and R Mulgoflor (Verona)
H and R Decylaldehyde acetal (Verona)
Methyl naphthyl ketone
Geranyl acetate
Linalyl acetate
H and R Agrumen aldehyde N (Verona)
H and R Verdural F 10% in DEP (Verona)
H and R Jasmin 6066H Reconstitute (Verona)
H and R Hesperidol H/5 (Verona)
H and R Neroflor Extra (Verona)
Lavender, rosemary, oil of lemon, petitgrain, orange oil,
    bergamot

This formula shows, says Mr. Elliott, that the essential bergamot, orange, lemon, lavender and rosemary are still there. The reason for the addition of the synthetics is that they add "showiness," "sparkling quality," "brilliance."

Suppose then, that you had lived 100 years ago and had used perfume or cologne several times a day. Not a chance that anything harmful could result, any more than harm could result from carrying around a rosebud or a twig of lavender in your pocket. But today, if you apply perfume several times a day and, especially if you douse yourself with cologne as many people do after a bath or before going out in the evening, there are, apparently, a number of synthetic chemicals involved which may or may not do you harm.

So far as we can discover, no one has ever done any research on the possible harm of the synthetics in perfumes, just as no one has done research on the possible harm of using a chlorinated water supply over a lifetime. Until we can rouse enough concern about chlorinated water to bring about a change in this method of water purification, there is nothing one can do to avoid the chlorine but buy bottled spring water. How about avoiding perfume? It seems easy enough to avoid buying commercial perfumes and colognes and shaving lotions. Just don't buy them. Depend on fresh, clean skin and clothing to give you an acceptable fragrance in even the fussiest surroundings. Keep your bed linen and personal lingerie fresh-smelling with sachets of real lavender and real rosebuds.

But one realizes how impossible it is to avoid these perfume chemicals completely when one reads an article like the one that appeared in the *Kiwanis Magazine* for December, 1960-January, 1961. It tells us that perfumes conceal the natural smell of just about everything these days—the unpleasant odor of such things as synthetic fabrics, rubber, adhesives, insecticides, fertilizers and detergents. A certain plastic used in making the inner doors of re-frigerators was found to be causing off-odors and tastes in food. The doors were "smell-conditioned." Housewives, buying new dryers com-plained about not being able to smell the "clean laundry smell" of clothing dried in the open sunshine. So the perfume makers invented a smell that approximates the fresh-washed smell which is metered into the bottom of dryers to scent the clothes.

Everything Must Have a Synthetic Smell

Nor is the requirement always for a pleasant or concealing smell. Modern fishermen, we are told, miss the tarred-hemp smell of old rigging and sails when they use new equipment made of nylon. So the makers paid to have the nylon gear impregnated with a syn-thetic smell approximating the old tarred hemp smell.

Furs are scented with heavy, exotic perfumes to conceal the odor of the tannery. Leather-scent gives a genuine air to things made of plastic and imitation leather. The smell of a new car (solvents, glues and plastics) has been made into an aerosol which can be sprayed on old cars to give the buyer the feeling that he has bought something newer than it is. Floor waxes, furniture polishes, paints, lighter fluids, wax candles, charcoal briquettes, scouring powders, etc., are heavily scented.

If the housewife is not satisfied with the many aromas spread around by these household products, she can buy aerosols that smell like (well, a little like) lavender, spice, mint, cedar, pine, apple blossom, etc., to spray into the air if she burned the dinner or upset the garbage pail. We do not know, but it seems reasonable to assume that most of these new scents are made from synthetics. So, in addition to perfumes we apply to ourselves and the fumes which rise all day long around us, we are also exposed to many, many other sources of synthetic scents.

What to do? Avoid all of it that you can, we suggest. Undoubtedly, one must use a certain number of household products. Use as few as possible and use them in well-ventilated rooms. Keep the doors and windows open when you apply waxes or polishes. Never, of course, use a room deodorant or an aerosol. The effect on one's lungs of breathing in droplets of moisture spread about by such concoctions is undoubtedly not healthful, even if the substance being sprayed or wafted were not poisonous—and ten to one it is.

So far as personal perfumes and colognes are concerned, we believe that you would be lots better off without them unless you can find ones in which synthetic chemicals have not been used. In some parts of the country, you can buy the natural oils of woods and flowers—sandalwood oil, for instance, which is a popular base for perfumes. Rosewater is available from your local druggist. You can grow sweet-smelling herbs like lavender, rosemary, bergamot, mignonette and the various geraniums and simply make little sachets of the dried leaves or flowers. Mixed with spices like clove, nutmeg and coriander, flower petals and leaves of herbs make up the potpourri ladies of yesteryear used to mix for keeping in bowls on their living room tables, or carrying about in a purse or pocket. And delicious were their scents, too!

Dairy Products

Some Facts on Dairy Products

Cheese is one of the most popular dairy products in this country as well as abroad. How are cheeses made and what chemicals go into their manufacture?

In general, cheese is made by coagulating the casein, or protein, of milk, skimmed milk or milk enriched with cream. The coagulation is accomplished by means of rennet or some other suitable enzyme, souring or a combination of the two. Rennet is a digestive fluid from the stomach of a calf. It breaks up the milk protein and reconstitutes it into a different form. Sometimes sour milk is used for cheese.

The curd, or solid, coagulated mass, that results is then processed by heat, pressure, molds or other special treatment, depending on what kind and flavor of cheese is wanted.

Hard cheese is made by souring milk and adding rennet. This

is then heated, stirred, the solid part (curd) separated from the liquid part (whey). During the process, calcium chloride may be added, salt is added and the rind of the cheese may be coated with paraffin or vegetable oil.

Processed Cheese Most Objectionable

Processed cheese is, as its name implies, a product that has gone through several more processing steps. It involves mixing several kinds of cheese with an emulsifying agent to produce the consistency so much admired for the topping of casseroles or grilled cheese sandwiches. The emulsifying agent is, we are told, any of the following: monosodium phosphate, disodium phosphate, dipotassium phosphate, trisodium phosphate, sodium metaphosphate, sodium acid pyrophosphate, tetrasodium pyrophosphate, sodium citrate, potassium citrate, calcium citrate, sodium tartrate or sodium potassium tartrate. Are these chemicals added in minute quantity so that there is only a remote possibility of their doing you any harm? Quite the contrary. Regulations state that they may be added to make up 3 per cent of the final product. Artificial coloring is added, and an acidifying agent may be added, such as citric acid, acetic acid, phosphoric acid, etc.

The two dyes that are used to color cheese, margarine and other dairy products are two of those suspected by scientists of being cancer-causing. Alginic acid is also used in processed cheese as a stabilizer to give uniformity of color and flavor. Methyl cellulose is used as a thickening agent in processed cheeses. Sugar may be added if the flavor demands it. The smoked flavor some cheeses boast of is prepared by precipitating wood smoke. The hydrocarbons produced by this burning process have also been incriminated as possible cancer causers.

The wrappers of processed cheese have long been the source of trouble. These wrappers may be coated with preservatives—mold inhibitors and like chemicals. Of course, no company making dairy products wants to lose profits through spoilage. So the processed cheeses, especially, are treated to thorough dosages of preservatives before they reach grocery shelves.

In 1956, the cheese industry decided to use a chemical insecticide on the cheese itself to prevent attacks from the cheese mite. The insecticide is made of pyrethrins and piperonyl butoxide. It is applied to the rind cheeses like cheddar after it has been made into blocks. It is coated with paraffin, then the insecticide is applied. This insecticide is so strong that it guarantees that the cheese will not be attacked by insects during the entire time that it is aging or "ripening," which may be many months. How much of it seeps through the paraffin covering into the cheese? Is it harmful? We do not know.

Just as yellow dye is added to many cheeses because the milk from which they are made does not contain enough vitamin A to color the cheese, so other milk must be bleached in order to make Swiss cheese, which, the cheese institute says, must be pale-colored, or consumers will not buy it.

Cottage cheese is made from sweet skim milk, making it low in fat. Calcium chloride and salt may be added.

Cream cheese is made from cream or a mixture of cream and milk, skim milk or powdered milk. In preparing cream cheese, various gum products may be used to produce the right texture and body. These are natural products in that they have a vegetable source, but they are surely not "natural" to dairy products.

Other Dairy Products

Buttermilk is made from pasteurized, skimmed or partly skimmed milk to which a bacterial culture is added to sour the milk. Although buttermilk looks as if it contains lots of fat, because of the small specks of fat in it, in reality it is very low in fat.

Whey is the liquid left after the milk curds have been used to make cheese. It consists of water, lactose (milk sugar), milk protein and most of the minerals of the original milk. Whey has been used by doctors as a food for normalizing the intestinal tract in cases of constipation, dysentery and so forth. Apparently, it is effective in changing the intestinal flora, so that harmful bacteria are discouraged and helpful ones are encouraged.

Yogurt and acidophilus milk are two fermented milk products which also achieve this purpose.

Dried or powdered milk products are recommended by many nutritionists because they provide, in highly concentrated form, all the protein, vitamins and minerals found in liquid milk. However, this product is even more highly processed than other dairy products, so, of course, we do not recommend it.

Our Recommendations on Dairy Products

We do not recommend milk as a food for adults. We believe it has been greatly overrated as food and that the agricultural practices on dairy farms have made the modern cow a milk machine and nothing more. Then, too, milk these days is contaminated with antibiotics and other drugs used on sick cows. The antibiotics have been so plentiful in milk at various times and places that cheese could not be made from it, for the antibiotic killed the bacteria necessary for making the cheese. Someone trying to avoid antibiotics because of a sensitivity to them may find that he is getting considerable quantities of them in milk.

The processing through which modern dairy products go is another basis for our complaints against them. Pasteurization, homogenization, emulsifiers, stabilizers, preservatives, dyes, possibly toxic wrapping materials, insecticides—all these must be taken into account these days when the health-seeker considers milk as a food. From the evidence we have produced above, it seems that cheese is an even worse bet than plain milk, since it may contain so many objectionable things.

We recommend deleting milk and dairy products from your grocery list or taking them in extremely small quantities. You can make up the minerals by taking bone meal and the B vitamins with brewer's yeast.

Dancing

Over-Twisting

Kids will probably say that we're trying to spoil their fun, but we can't pass by the obligation to inform parents that the latest dance craze, the Twist, can have serious physiological repercussions. An orthopedic surgeon, Dr. Bernie P. Davis, was quoted in the *New York Times* (December 3, 1961) as saying that the Twist is almost as hazardous as playing football.

Dr. Davis said that he found knee injuries generally associated with football turning up among teen-agers who had performed the Twist. One boy suffered a torn cartilage and had to undergo surgery. A girl dislocated her kneecap and has her leg in a cast, and a third teen-ager suffered severe strain of the knee ligaments.

The surgeon explained that the injuries were caused by severe rotation of the knee required in the dance. This rotation results in strong side motion of the knee, thus straining the ligaments. Under normal conditions, when excessive strain is put on the ligaments, the resultant pain causes the person to stop whatever is causing the pain. In the Twist, teen-agers seem not to notice the strain on the knee.

Chiropractors have objected to the Twist on the grounds that the dance strains the lumbar and the sacroiliac regions. One chiropractor said that dancers "will be wise to practice moderation instead of excess, because casualties are occurring."

We are aware that trying to stop teen-agers from doing the latest dance is akin to halting an avalanche, but we do agree that one might try to instill some restraint into the youngsters by making them aware of the possibility of injury from overenthusiastic participation. We believe, too, that bone meal in the diet will provide the tensile strength that will keep twisting bones from being damaged.

Deodorants

Something New in Deodorants

The core of the perspiration problem in mature persons lies in the apocrine glands concentrated in the underarm area and the glands in the groin. The secretion, itself odorless, which is released by these glands mixes with bacteria ordinarily present on the skin surface, creating the characteristic unpleasant odor most of us find so offensive.

United States manufacturers have two basic methods of approaching the problem. They offer either antiperspirants, which are designed actually to stop the normal flow of perspiration, or they offer deodorants, which are intended to neutralize the unpleasant odors of perspiration.

Our objection to antiperspirants lies in the fact that these preparations interfere with nature's plan to rid the body of waste materials and to cool the skin. A chemical is applied to the skin, and it creates a slight irritation of the skin. Tiny blisters form with just enough swelling to close the sweat ducts and to confine the perspiration inside the body. This moisture, we believe, should come out. We also believe that any irritation of the skin, such as is promoted by this action, should be avoided whenever possible.

The deodorant preparations also have unsavory records, as can be seen in an article which appeared in the *Journal of the American Medical Association* (November 3, 1956). It told of an increase in unusual skin eruptions in the underarm area. In each of the 4 cases mentioned, the authors were convinced that the eruptions were due to the daily applications of deodorants two to five weeks prior to examination. The article recommended further tracing to find the offending mechanism. *Consumer Research Bulletin* offered a similar appraisal of the problem of deodorants 3 years earlier, in September, 1953. It recommended minimal use of such preparations.

A Better, Safer Way

Now there is a new theory which meets these objections nicely. The idea behind this preparation is neither to stop perspiration, nor to neutralize it by chemical action. Instead, the perspiration is absorbed as it flows, and before it can react with skin bacteria to form the components which produce strong body odor.

The basic ingredient is a natural absorptive, known generally as "fuller's earth." Its peculiar natural property is to attract and to hold moisture. It is the product of the weathering of igneous rocks and is found in a free state in many parts of the United States. The special type of fuller's earth being used in this preparation is known as attapulgite. It is an especially absorbent type of fuller's earth. The attapulgite deposits are mined as ore is. Then, at a processing plant, crushing, drying, grading and sterilizing operations are carried on, and that is all that is done to treat the attapulgite which is used in the anti-body-odor product of which we approve. To the attapulgite is added natural, non-alcoholic essences, whose pleasant smell, not their chemical reaction with the skin or with bacteria, is their only objective.

Are We Preoccupied with Inconsequentials?

We are frequently chided for our seeming preoccupation with inconsequentials. Why, for heaven's sake, should one worry about the little irritation that can come from a deodorant? Why be concerned with one part per million of sodium fluoride in drinking water? Why make a fuss over a little coal-tar dye on orange rinds?

We have two reasons which we consider to be quite sound. First of all, who knows how inconsequential any of these things actually are? We use the coal-tar dyes, the fluorides and the deodorant and antiperspirant chemicals, just *presuming* that they will do no more harm than we can observe on contact. What happens to them as they accumulate inside our bodies, as they mix with other natural and synthetic compounds we ingest, as they pile up in this or that organ? No one knows. Who can say, then, that they are inconsequential?

Reason number two for our preoccupation with these seeming inconsequentials is our awareness of the way they are taking over every aspect of our living. These minute amounts of chemicals appear in just about everything we eat and use. Can you buy anything in a super market today that has not met with an additive or an insecticide on its way to you? Certainly, no piece of meat, no fruit or vegetable is free of one or more of them. It is merely a question of degree. Has it only been sprayed? Or has it also been emulsified, preserved, disinfected, plasticized, colored and artifically flavored, as well? Then there's the polluted air we breathe and water we drink. The "inconsequentials" really add up!

That's why we carp about minute irritants such as deodorants. Why should we approve of still another avenue for chemicals to reach us? There are many we can't avoid. After all, we must eat, we must breathe and we must drink water, and sometimes we must take them as they come. But deodorants do not constitute such a necessity. If they present a physical problem, we can avoid their use. We can wait for a safe, non-irritating type to be perfected.

This may be interpreted as a narrow view, but we feel that it is the only sane one. One must take a stand, adopt a point of view on modern living and stick to it. If not, one drowns in useless gadgets and poison-filled, additive-infested foods. New gadgets may be novel and amusing, but they often prove impractical over the long haul; new "foods" may be easy to prepare, taste fine and they may be filling, but will they keep you healthy and help you live as long as you should? We think not. We say avoid them, and anything else you can that could interfere with your body's natural functions.

If you are going to use a deodorant, we say use a safe one, since it is available. Every purchase of such a natural product is a vote against the commercial ones to which we object. The more natural deodorants we buy, the less synthetic ones will be sold. It could be enough of a factor to make the major companies re-evaluate their product, and offer their own natural one for those who prefer that type. Economical arguments are often the most convincing ones.

Desiccated Liver

That Something Extra in Desiccated Liver

"For many years, investigators with experience in nutritional disorders, have stressed the necessity for complete therapy. This, of course, requires the inclusion in the therapeutic regime of an adequate amount of a satisfactory source of the as yet unidentified essential factors," says Dr. Morton S. Biskind writing in the March, 1953, issue of the *American Journal of Digestive Diseases*.

By this, Dr. Biskind means that, although we have investigated scientifically many of the vitamins, proteins, enzymes and minerals that exist in foods, there are perhaps just as many that we know little or nothing about. However, since our bodies have been using these elements, as well as the known and well-researched ones for many years, we must admit that the unknown ones are probably just as important for our good health as the known ones.

Liver seems to be a food rich in known nutriments, which also seems to contain many other as yet unknown factors also vitally important.

Dr. Biskind tells us that he has treated many deficient patients with supposedly complete vitamin and mineral formulas without any benefit at all, or possibly with the patient becoming worse. The addition of desiccated liver or some other form of liver has invariably resulted in a "dramatic and lasting improvement, often evident within a few days." Do we need any more evidence of the effectiveness of liver?

Dr. Biskind quotes about 15 references from medical literature describing the work of scientists who have found that liver achieved results which no synthetic vitamin preparation and no other food produced.

Unknown Substance in Liver

There is, for instance, some substance in liver which will heal certain kinds of mouth inflammation (glossitis). We know that many disorders of the mouth are linked with a deficiency in the B vitamins. But apparently we have not as yet found out what all of these vitamins are, for liver contains something extra, something special, which is not as yet known, and hence cannot be included in vitamin formulas.

There is, in liver, some substance which is essential to normal liver function. If this substance is not supplied in the diet, the functions of the liver will suffer. There is something in liver which helps in the production of certain blood elements. Animals given estrogen (a female sex hormone) and put on diets free of B vitamins develop a certain kind of dermatitis. Something in liver, apart from its B vitamins, prevents this skin trouble.

We think such a finding as this one is most important for us in these days when we are all receiving a certain amount of sex hormones in the food we eat, since they are regularly fed to animals to fatten them more rapidly. Since most Americans are at the same time eating diets in which the B vitamins are certainly not plentiful, perhaps the taking of liver could prevent much of the damage done by this combination of circumstances.

Liver for Animals

Certain parts of liver are essential for the health of certain animals—the fox and the mink—so that these parts of liver must be included in a healthful diet for such animals. There is a substance (we do not know what it is) that occurs in desiccated whole liver (but not in the liver extract commonly given by doctors for anemic patients) which protects animals given too much thyroid extract. There is a substance appearing in desiccated liver which is involved in producing a certain important enzyme in the intestines. There is a substance appearing in whole liver, but not in water-soluble extracts, which protects against certain kinds of anemia. There is a substance in whole liver, which is not present in either a water-soluble or a fat-soluble extract of liver, which seems to protect against cancer. There is a substance in whole liver which protects against fatigue.

Liver and Fatigue

B. H. Ershoff, M.D., writing in the *Proceedings of the Society of Experimental Biology and Medicine,* July, 1951, tells of testing for an anti-fatigue diet in his laboratory. He used 3 groups of rats on 3 different diets, which he fed for 12 weeks. The first group ate a usual laboratory diet to which were added 9 synthetic and two natural vitamins. By this we mean that the synthetic ones were made in a laboratory of the various chemical substances of which the vitamins are made. The natural ones were extracted from foods—brewer's yeast, wheat germ or something like that.

The second group of rats had this same diet, added vitamins and all, with, in addition, a batch of B vitamins—all the known B vitamins. The third group ate the original diet with 10 per cent desiccated liver added instead of vitamins. Desiccated liver is liver dried at low heat (to conserve vitamins) and powdered.

Now for the test. Each rat was placed in a drum of water from which he could not climb out. He had to keep swimming or drown. So, as you can see, this was a real test of endurance and anti-fatigue. The first group of rats swam for an average of 13.3 minutes before they gave up and indicated that they had no strength left. The second group swam for an average of 13.4 minutes and gave up. The third group—those which had the desiccated liver in their chow—broke all records. Three of them swam for 63, 83 and 87 minutes. The other rats in the group were all swimming vigorously at the end of two hours when the test was ended. Now, notice please, we did not say that Dr. Ershoff gave these super-rats a shot of something, nor did we say that they took liver for a day and then could perform this feat of endurance. We said that Dr. Ershoff fed them liver for a period of 12 weeks, which corresponds to a number of years in human beings, and *then* they were able to swim almost 10 times longer than the ordinary rats, or the ones which had been taking synthetic B vitamins.

Of course, since most of these factors in liver are at present unidentified, we may eventually find out that they are the same thing —it may be the same vitamin or enzyme or protein which protects from fatigue and also protects against the poisonous effects of certain drugs. But whether we eventually find that there are only two or three factors responsible for all these important results or whether there are many, it certainly seems evident that liver (whole liver) is a treasure house of valuable nutriments which simply are not available from any other source—and certainly not from synthetic vitamin preparations which contain, of course, only those B vitamins whose chemical composition is known.

Is Liver the Best Source of B Vitamins?

How about brewer's yeast in comparison to liver? Yeast is a fine source of B vitamins, undoubtedly, but, as Dr. Biskind says, there seems to be a number of elements in liver that yeast does not contain. For instance, he tells us of a case of hypertrophic gingivitis (inflammation of the gums), which improved rapidly when 6 teaspoonfuls of desiccated liver were given daily. When the liver was stopped and brewer's yeast substituted, the condition returned. When powdered liver was given again, the condition disappeared. This illustrates what all nutritionists have learned, he says, that liver supplies some fraction which yeast does not.

"Similar observations have repeatedly been made by the author and his associates," continues Dr. Biskind, "in treating a variety of nutritional defects and their resultant endocrine (gland) disturbances. Suitable liver preparations, and especially desiccated liver, were found to be incomparably superior to yeast and rice bran extract as a source of therapeutically effective nutrients. Yeast and rice bran are, nevertheless, very useful and do provide some of the necessary unidentified factors when given in sufficient dosage. For whole dried yeast, this would represent from 3 to 6 ounces a day. (How nearly insignificant then are the few grains of brewer's yeast per capsule or tablet included in numerous commercial vitamin preparations as a source of accessory factors!) Yeast extracts, however, considerably more concentrated, are effective in correspondingly smaller doses, two or three heaping teaspoonfuls a day. Yeast extract or rice bran extract, or both, may effectively be combined with liver preparations."

Take Desiccated Liver

It seems to us, from the above, that the person who is healthy and wants merely to prevent illness should seriously consider adding desiccated liver to his food supplements, whether or not he is taking brewer's yeast, rice bran or wheat germ (which contains much the same material in the way of B vitamins).

In the case of readers who are taking food supplements in a pitched battle against some chronic disease, we certainly recommend adding large amounts of desiccated liver to the supplements taken, at least until one has determined whether or not a lack of B vitamins and other things related to B vitamins is involved. It seems that taking desiccated liver powder would be preferable to taking pills of liver, since in this way one can get much more. Many people find the taste and smell of liver disagreeable and would have to conceal the powdered liver in a strongly flavored fruit drink or salad. Don't expect to get full benefit from the B vitamins in the desiccated liver if you use it in food which is then cooked, for heat destroys B vitamins.

In pointing out past misconceptions about liver, Dr. Biskind tells us that, since liver preparations for fighting anemia have been available, it has been assumed that such products as this contain all the elements in liver that are effective from the nutritional point of view. Nothing could be farther from the truth. Doctors who use the liver-anti-anemia preparations are then disappointed when they cannot achieve remarkable results with this in cases where anemia is not involved.

For instance, the liver extracts which are purified especially for treating anemia contain very small amounts of the B vitamins, which are so important for preventing other conditions. Dr. Biskind points out that there is terrible waste involved in processing liver for anti-anemia extracts, for much of the rest of the liver is discarded. "The whole liver from which the extracts are made, if used as food, would provide dramatically superior results for maintenance and treatment," says Dr. Biskind.

Unknown Factors in Liver Are Valuable

He tells of giving a patient anti-anemia liver extract for 30 days to combat a severe condition of mouth inflammation. There was no improvement. Giving by mouth whole cooked liver in much smaller quantities than were needed to prepare the liver extract brought about quick relief.

For years, he tells us, one manufacturer of vitamin products had the best vitamin B complex preparation on the market, because he used parts of the liver remaining *after the anti-anemia liver extracts were prepared.* So his supplement included many unknown factors which other products did not. Even so, says Dr. Biskind, including the whole liver with all of its nutritional riches intact is the best idea, for anything less than this is bound to lack some of the important factors.

In a final word about desiccated liver, Dr. Biskind covers other elements present in addition to B vitamins and things associated with them. Trace minerals, for instance. These are minerals which we need in extremely small amounts and which we are likely to be short on, because our present farming methods leave soils in deficient states. Says Dr. Biskind, "When whole desiccated liver is used as a source of the as yet unidentified but essential nutritional factors, both trace minerals as well as a certain amount of protein of highest quality are simultaneously provided. Although, in actual practice, it has rarely been necessary to supplement such therapy by addition of further trace minerals, the mineral content of liver products must of course vary from batch to batch and it is not certain that the entire need for all trace minerals can always be supplied by this source. Hence supplementation with these elements may often be advisable."

We advise getting trace minerals in bone meal and kelp. If you grow some or all of your own food organically, this will help in assuring you of your quota of trace minerals. But meanwhile, don't think of desiccated liver as a source only of B vitamins or the other as yet unknown nutrients. It is also a fine source of protein and the trace minerals.

Powerful Food Elements in Desiccated Liver

An article in the *International Record of Medicine,* July, 1959, brings us enlightening information on the effectiveness of desiccated liver in the treatment of cancer. The article says:

"Precancerous conditions of the oral cavity were treated with a special dietary supplement containing desiccated liver, vitamins and riboflavin, reported George S. Sharp (Pasadena Tumor Institute) to the annual meeting of the James Ewing Society in New York City. Patients lacking in hydrochloric acid were given acid supplementation. Oral erosions and ulcerations cleared in one or two months and mucosal atrophy and inflammation in a slightly longer period; areas of leukoplakia improved somewhat."

Leukoplakia is the most serious of the precancerous states described above. It consists of hard, smooth, whitish patches on the inside of the mouth, tongue or gums.

We have not been able to get further information from the Institute. But it seems perfectly clear that the combination of food elements included in liver, and complete vitamin supplements including lots of riboflavin, can do much to reverse the cancerous process and put one on the path to health once again.

Desiccated Liver Hailed

However, Dr. Sharp was not the first to conduct experiments using desiccated liver. As long ago as 1951, experiments at the Sloan-Kettering Institute for Cancer Research proved that desiccated liver is a powerful weapon against cancer. The *Journal of Nutrition* for July 10, 1951, carried a report of the work of Kanematsu Suguira, who conducted the experiments. He tried out various food substances for preventing cancer in animals which had been exposed to a substance known to produce cancer—butter yellow. This is a dye which was once used in food, but which is today prohibited. Mixed with rice, it will produce liver cancer when it is fed to laboratory animals in given quantity.

A group of rats was put on a diet of butter yellow and rice. Another group was given the same diet plus 10 per cent desiccated liver. All 50 of the animals in the group receiving no liver had cancers within 150 days. The rats to whose diets desiccated liver was added were completely protected from the cancer. But when the amount of liver was cut to 2 per cent rather than 10 per cent, the protection was less. It was also found that the liver supplement did not make for permanent protection. After it was discontinued, cancer developed in most of the animals.

Brewer's Yeast Helps in Tests

At the same institute, brewer's yeast was successful in tests for preventing cancer. For complete protection against liver cancer, a diet, which consisted of 15 per cent brewer's yeast was necessary. Believing that the protective substance in the yeast and the liver might be riboflavin, a B vitamin, Dr. Suguira then gave this vitamin to his rats. When the rats were fed daily with only riboflavin along with milk protein, there was almost no protection from the liver cancer. But when the daily consumption was increased, the protective effect was striking.

Now we have a California doctor, Dr. Sharp, who uses riboflavin along with desiccated liver plus all the other known vitamins and reports the above excellent results with human beings. Incidentally, the hydrochloric acid given to some of the patients was undoubtedly given to make sure that they would be able to absorb the vitamins.

Do you see any reason why orthodox medicine should continue to insist that they do not know what causes cancer and that the only treatments acceptable or known to have any effect on cancer are radium, X-ray and surgery? Would you call this California doctor a food faddist? Would you say that, as soon as he discovered the effectiveness of desiccated liver, riboflavin and other vitamins for the treatment of cancer, he should have concealed his findings rather than risk being called a faddist or a crank?

Dietary Facts Should Be Made Public

And, finally, in all the slick but meaningless words of the latest releases from the American Cancer Society and the National Cancer Institute, has the American public ever been told that B vitamins, plus desiccated liver or brewer's yeast are a powerful protection against cancer, even when you are exposed to a certain cancer-causing agent? So far as we know, these facts have never been made known to the general public. Why not? If the inclusion of these harmless substances in every day's diet will give one even a small bit of protection against the great killer, can you see any reason why everyone should not know it?

Detergents

Should We Be Using Detergents?

All of us have read about or know someone who has had a skin problem caused by the use of detergents. But annoying and dangerous as skin irritations can be, the problems involved with detergents only begin with them. Since washing dishes is one of the main uses of detergents, the question of residue left on the dishes is of concern to us. Chemicals so strong that they will cause serious skin irritations of the hands will certainly damage the more sensitive tissues which make up the body's inner organs and stomach lining. The adherent qualities of detergents, to dishes and glasses, as well as silverware, appear to be quite pronounced. Sometimes, even thorough rinsing is not enough to remove the almost invisible film that they leave.

The detergent left on the dish for the next meal is likely to find its way into your body. It might come from the plate with a piece of meat, a sauce or a cup of tea. You could get it from a spoon or fork, or drink it with a glass of water.

Nursery Bottles with Deadly Residue

Can such small amounts of detergent cause serious aftereffects? The tragic answer to that question was printed in the *Chicago Tribune* (October 11, 1951). The story told of a suit for 15,000 dollars, filed by Aloysius Braehler against the wholesale grocer whose detergent product was used at a hospital for washing babies' bottles. Braehler alleged that his infant son died from boron poisoning, as the result of this grocer's detergent leaving a poisonous residue in the bottles. Along with the Braehler infant, 3 other babies died, and 16 were made ill from the detergent. The lips of the dead babies all showed rather severe burning. None of the hospital's breast fed babies were affected. It was concluded that the tragedy was due either to detergent which clung to the bottles after washing or which was accidentally spilled into the milk. The latter guess seemed highly unlikely, since such an error, affecting 19 babies, could hardly have gone unnoticed.

Contaminated Syringes

A similar situation was reported in the *Journal of the American Medical Association* (September 19, 1953). In this case, it was a detergent residue remaining in syringes, due to faulty cleansing, which caused serious complications following spinal injections, as in myelography (a means of measuring the fatty tissue which covers nerve fibres) or spinal anesthesia. The detergent was the cause of severe demyelinizing (loss of the fatty tissues covering of the nerve fibres) and spinal arachnoiditis (inflammation of delicate membranes found in the brain and spinal cord).

Out of 25 cases with severe spinal arachnoiditis, 11 were thought caused by improper cleansing of detergents from the syringes used in anesthesia. In 10 of the remaining 14 cases, spinal arachnoiditis developed only after multiple spinal injections had been given. No cases developed among the patients of one physician who consistently washed his syringes in sterile water. It was concluded that the damaging syringes contained detergent which became pulverized during the sterilizing process, and dissolved subsequently in anesthetic solution.

This is how the infinitesimal amounts of detergent left on the sterilized glass walls of nursery bottles and syringes can react in the body. Could there be better reason for caution in the use of detergents for dishwashing?

Detergents As Chickenfeed?

As with other harmful synthetics, just not using detergents in your home dosen't mean you won't be getting any. *Farm Journal*

(February, 1952) announced that certain detergents give the same boost to chicken growth as antibiotics. The following month (March 23, 1952) saw an article in the *New York Times* telling farmers that, in an experiment with 3500 chickens, broilers needed 8.61 pounds of regular feed to achieve a weight of 3 pounds. With detergents in the feed, another group of 3500 chickens got to 3 pounds by eating only 7.44 pounds of feed. There was evidence that this detergent-feed could work as well with other animals. Do farmers use this feed on the poultry, beef and pork we buy? We don't know. It is possible though, since antibiotics with even greater dangerous potential are not outlawed, and are used to aid the speedy growth of most of the animals producing the meats we see in the stores.

Watch Your Plumbing

Once detergents go down the drain, they begin to plague the house and city plumbing systems, as well as the sanitation of our streams. *Consumer Research Bulletin* (September, 1954) says detergents cause corrosion of domestic equipment and plumbing, lessen efficiency of sewage plants and result in excessive foam on the rivers where sewage is discharged. The *Medical Journal of Australia* (November 24, 1956) adds this warning: ". . . detergents may, by removing curds and grease films, either encourage corrosion of metal appliances and pipes, or expose corrosion which was formerly hidden." A need for a change in the types of metals generally used in plumbing may result from the increased use of detergents.

An idea of the oceans of detergent which find their way into our waterways came in the *Houston* (Texas) *Post* (October 23, 1954) which showed a mountain of suds, looking like a huge snow bank, outside a sewage plant in Roanoke, Virginia. In Santa Rosa Creek, California (*Chemical Week,* September 5, 1953), a large amount of detergent from dishes and washers, which had somehow by-passed the city's sewage treatment plant, bubbled around while fish swam in it, and ate from the water. While the fish seemed all right at the time, these trout were probably destined to end up on a platter eventually. If someone were to become ill after eating the fish, would anyone remember, or be able to uncover, the fact that the fish were contaminated by detergent water? We doubt it. Of course, water from such streams as these is drunk by many people. Does the purifying system of cities whose water supply is a river or a stream remove the detergents from the water before it is sent through pipes into faucets? We rather doubt that all the detergent pollution can be removed.

Use of Chemicals Bound to Affect Health

The complications of modern life don't always allow for observable cause and effect. As with the chemicals in our food or the poisonous gases in the air, the effect of detergents on our dishes, on our skin, in our waterways, might not be dramatically sudden, but when we are so intimate with dangerous chemicals, the effect is bound to show up in our health somewhere. Why not stay away from detergents and use soap for clothes and dishes; it always worked well enough before and it was kinder to hands and to plumbing. Yet soap is hard on your hands, too, so use as little of it as possible, to get the cleaning job done.

Diagnosis

Be Persistent about Finding a Cure

Persistence is a major asset in tracking down the cause of a physical problem. This point was well illustrated by a letter to the *British Medical Journal* (December 12, 1960) from a Dr. M. Aston Key. Dr. Key wrote to comment upon a previous article on the subject of migraine. He said that eye conditions of patients should be considered in treating this problem. Dr. Key then related a short history of a friend who was subject to migraine headaches. He would occasionally fall down unconscious from them in the subway and have to be lifted out at the next station, lying on the platform until he regained consciousness.

It was suggested that his eyes might be responsible, so he consulted one oculist after the other until he had been to 5 of them, but he saw no change in his condition. When he consulted the sixth, his glasses cured him of migraine completely. He had suffered from mixed astigmatism that required a very accurate correction. Without this persistence, which, we admit, was far above the usual, the man would never have been cured.

Nutritional Therapy

We believe that one should not be easily satisfied by the words of a doctor who despairs of a cure. We are constantly hearing of bursitis victims who have had hot packs and injections, even surgery, to no avail. They have been told their problem is hopeless, that they must endure the pain for the rest of their lives. The doctors they have consulted may not have known of the treatment with injections of vitamin B_{12}, which has been amazingly effective in treating this condition, with results within two weeks. Many doctors ignore nutritional therapy, perhaps the next one consulted would not ignore it.

Suppose an inability to have children or to carry a conceived baby to full term, had led to consultation with 5 or 6 doctors, and no results. The seventh might know enough about nutrition to prescribe vitamin E, because it has shown itself effective in so many of these cases. He might insist that the prospective parents stop smoking (a proven source of some infertility) or he might prescribe more of the very necessary vitamin C.

One could go through countless other symptoms—the brittle bones that need calcium, the nerves that are short of B vitamins, the eyes that could be helped with vitamin A, the infections that would respond to vitamin C—that many doctors give up on. They are drug-oriented, and fail even to consider or learn about other approaches to a disease. You may have to search quite a while to find the doctor who is able to use nutrients as a tool for curing a disease, but until you do, you haven't done everything that can be done. This is not to say that nutrients are a sure cure, nor that they are the only treatment worth trying. But they are a treatment, and an effective, respectable, proven one at that. Insist that your doctor at least consider using them, and if he refuses, find a doctor who will!

Drugs

The Terrible Effects of Certain Modern Drugs

We saw in a magazine of the embalming profession one of the most startling and horrifying articles we have ever encountered in all our research. In the *De-Ce-Co* magazine (June-July, 1960), published by the Dodge Chemical Company, Professor Ray E. Slocum discusses body conditions in the dead person which are likely to give trouble to the embalmer. In every case, he relates these conditions to drugs that have been given to the person while he was alive.

For example, the so-called steroid drugs (cortisone, ACTH, etc.) which are used, he says, in treating arthritis, skin disorders, rheumatic fever, asthma, allergies, cancer, etc., may produce in the patient, ulcers of the digestive tract with possible perforations and bleeding. Ulcerative colitis may be a complication. The drugs also make the membranes of the cells less permeable—that is, more resistant to fluids—so that passage of fluids into cells and tissues is blocked.

The estrogenic hormones (progesterone, etc.), which are used in pregnancy, menstrual disorders, cancer therapy, etc., upset the salt balance in the body, causing accumulation of excess water, swelling, dropsy, etc.

Drugs which are given by mouth for diabetes (orinase, tolbutamide, chlorpropamide, etc.) cause liver enlargement, with cirrhosis of the liver a definite possibility. The tone of certain muscles is also affected.

Tranquilizers

The tranquilizers (happy pills) are used, as the author tells us, to treat mental depression and other conditions of mental ill health. These drugs cause disorganization or destruction of the red blood cells, enlargement of the spleen and liver, fatty deposits in the liver and other internal organs. They also cause kidney failure and accumulations of waste products from the kidney. There is also a degeneration of the sheaths in which nerves are contained and the muscles connected with these nerves.

Other tranquilizers used for treatment of mental patients and also for controlling high blood pressure cause, mainly, liver enlargement and "mild to severe jaundice." Another tranquilizer, used for asthma, high blood pressure and mental disorders, causes extreme liver damage and jaundice, general wasting of tissue and a group of changes in the body which resemble changes brought about by Parkinson's disease.

Thyroid medication, which is given for thyroid disorders, as well as diseases of the circulatory system, causes hardening of the arteries with "very brittle and degenerate blood vessels resulting."

The mustard drugs, which are used to treat leukemia, cancer, etc., produce intensive thinning of the intestinal walls so that they are likely to burst.

Effects of the Drugs

In commenting on these facts, Professor Slocum reminds his embalmer readers that one does not always know exactly the cause of death. But, to do a good professional job of making the body of the deceased look lifelike, there are certain well-known facts available which will help him. For instance, if the patient had diabetes, one does not know whether or not he was taking one of the new diabetic drugs that are taken by mouth rather than injected. However, if the ankles and feet are ulcerated, "one may assume that these were used." One may also anticipate that the blood will be clotted! If the patient was fed intravenously, the arteries may be filled with a jelly-like substance which apparently is quite difficult to remove during the process of embalming.

Nowadays, a majority of people use tranquilizers in one form or another, Professor Slocum goes on. Most of them do not use them in sufficient quantity to produce the conditions mentioned above *unless* they were mentally ill or had some circulatory disorder. (Such a category includes, we suppose, many millions of Americans.) Some patients from mental hospitals may *not* have been taking tranquilizers, he goes on, but it is well to assume that they have. In most mental cases, there is a fatty cheese-like substance found throughout the body tissues—due to a fault in the functions of the liver and kidneys.

Do you suppose there is a psychiatrist or a doctor in a mental hospital who knows that such conditions are typical of mental patients? If so, why do they not relate such conditions to the patients' diets and physical health, and realize once and for all that mental illness, like all other illnesses, gets its beginning in poor diet, resulting in disorder in many body processes!

Other tranquilizers which are used for asthma or high blood pressure produce jaundice, Professor Slocum says, which is difficult for the embalmer to conceal. He adds, "In heart diseases, it must also be remembered that the blood will be heavy and clotted." Patients who have died of leukemia or cancer may have intestines so thin that they cannot withstand the injection of embalming fluids into the veins or the arteries.

Although medical literature is full of references to the damage done by modern drugs, we have never come upon anything quite so horrifying or so graphic as this article. There is no reason for the embalmer to gloss things over, you see. He doesn't have to prove that, even in spite of all the bad side effects, the drug was an effective one. All he has to do is to find some way to work around the horrible and extensive damage that has apparently been produced by these drugs. There is no reason for him not to be frank about it.

And the casual comment that "a majority of people" now take tranquilizers, bringing always the possibility of the kind of damage he describes, leaves us little hope for the future of mankind.

We Cannot Tolerate Carelessness in Medication

Carelessness is about the most serious charge that one can apply to a doctor, outside of downright criminal intent. This includes not only carelessness in the examinations or operations he performs, but carelessness in the way he informs himself on the progress of his profession, and on the drawbacks of the medications he can use. Is he aware of the new uses for nutrients as therapeutic agents? Does he keep an open mind on what can be accomplished by remedying a vitamin deficiency? Does he exercise care in keeping up with the findings on new drugs? Is he conscientious about being aware of their limitations and their dangers? Does he weigh the harm they might do against the good he hopes to accomplish, or does he use new drugs because they're new?

We come across more warnings in the medical journals and newspapers on the dangers of medications than on almost anything else. Often they appear in the same organ which rushed into print to announce the development of the drug in the first place. One can't help but wonder how many patients used the drug, suffering the side effects for months without knowing the true cause. One cannot help but wonder how many patients died from the side effects of the drug without knowing what killed them. It is easy to see from this why great caution must be exercised by a doctor in prescribing medications. If there is an older drug that is known to do the job, and has shown its safety and its limitations through years of use, why not use it rather than experiment with a ballyhooed one-shot wonder whose ultimate effect on the body had no time to show? Even the best established drugs have shown some dangers, how can we assume the new ones are safe?

Antibiotics and Low Blood Pressure

The antibiotics seem to show a new stripe almost every day. In *Antibiotics and Chemotherapy* (August, 1960), the world was informed that intakes of relatively large amounts of chloromycetin, streptomycin, dehydrostreptomycin, oleandomycin or tetracycline would produce a marked fall in blood pressure. These same antibiotics also produce electrocardiographic changes and, occasionally, arrhythmias (variations from the normal heartbeat). In experiment, isolated rabbit hearts were depressed by each of the antibiotics mentioned, and heart rate and blood flow actually decreased with streptomycin. All of these drugs depressed the contractions of isolated rabbit ilium (part of small intestine) and in cats, all except chloromycetin inhibited the contraction of the nictating (blinking) membranes. These are the more recent discoveries to be added to an already bulging file on what dangerous things can happen when any of this group of antibiotics is used.

Impotency Induced by Ulcer Drug

Ulcers among men are more and more common every day. One of the newer and most used medications in this field is propantheline bromide. The *Medical Journal of Australia* (September 24, 1960) carried a letter from a physician announcing a side effect of this drug which no brochure ever mentioned—impotence. On treating 5 males, ranging in age from 35 to 45, with this drug, each experienced impotence, 4 of them for from 12 to 14 months, while the fifth had reasonable sexual relations, but this was adversely affected by minor illness and tiredness, when impotence would return.

A similar drug, methantheline bromide (Banthine), exhibits a like effect, according to a report in the *New York State Journal of Medicine* (1952). The authors, Schwartz and Robinson, wrote " . . . symptoms of impotence begin soon after therapy and disappear shortly after its discontinuance." The reason for this unpleasant consequence has to do with the fact that the penile erection depends physiologically on the functioning of the nervous impulses. These two drugs interfere with the transmission of these agents, and as a result, frustrate the natural course of events.

Here again, we wonder how many men were told of this hazard by their doctors, before starting a course of these drugs. How many of them suffered the mental anguish of supposed impotence, believing it was due to something that could not be remedied? Who knows how many other drugs interfere with the psychological processes which adversely affect potency while the victims resign themselves in ignorance to this unhappy state?

Drug for High Blood Pressure

Many high blood pressure patients complain of a feeling of intolerable weakness. Perhaps they are the unwitting victims of the side effects of bretylium tosylate, a drug being used to reduce high blood pressure. The *Lancet* (October 8, 1960) printed an evaluation which states frankly that this drug "may produce a derangement of muscle-cell function by direct action. . . ." By way of illustration, the authors include a case history of a 64-year-old man, who, within a few days of being treated with bretylium tosylate, complained of severe muscular weakness in the shoulder, so that he found it difficult even to comb his hair and shave. By the end of the day, his muscles were so weak that he had difficulty in performing the simple act of opening his eyes and swallowing. How many heart patients using this medication are warned by their doctors to expect this kind of exhaustion? How many doctors who prescribe it have been careful enough to check on such side effects?

Tranquilizers Unsafe

The unwanted effects of the drugs used to treat mental illness have not yet been fully explored. More evidence on this point appeared in the *British Medical Journal* (October 1, 1960), in a letter which describes the psychotic effects induced by antidepressive drugs. The writer tells of 4 cases in his own experience, in which the treatment seems to have led to worse psychoses than were originally observed.

Another correspondent, in the same issue of the *Journal,* recounted some of his experiences with the same drugs (phenelzine or "nardil" and impramine or "tophanil"). In 10 cases of recurrent depression treated with these drugs, 6 experienced marked reduction of blood pressure. The 6 felt giddy and had fallen, even upon getting up from a resting posture. One of the other 4 had a drop in his normal (130/80) blood pressure to 80/60 after 4 days on the drug. The rest had similar drops.

Not Always Obvious

Erwin Di Cyan, Ph.D., in *Drug and Cosmetic Industry* (September, 1960), wraps up the concept of side effects as well as anyone we've read. He writes: "True side effects are common and may occur with many drugs. However, the absence of clinical symptoms does not mean that no side effects have been caused by a drug. There may be biochemical changes such as a disturbance of enzyme metabolism, as, for example, increased transaminase activity, reduction in the blood of TPN or of glucose-6-phosphate dehydrogenase."

The deleterious effects of drugs, like the effects of poisons in foods, do not have to be obvious and dramatic to count. The changes that can occur in our systems due to these substances are often subtle and sometimes not understood even by experts in biochemistry. A doctor cannot be too careful about the way he uses drugs. If he is not absolutely sure of what a drug will do, he is doing his patient a true service if he refuses to use it.

Iatrogenic Diseases

The number of diseases which follow as the result of the use of new medications has increased to a staggering amount. In the *South African Medical Journal* (March, 1960), Dr. A. Landau, former president of the Cape Western Branch, Medical Association of South Africa, comes up with a whole series of afflictions, some new, some old, due entirely to the use of the newer medications. He begins by proposing a basic rule: "No one is entitled to prescribe a medicament who knows only the specific effect claimed for the remedy. It behooves him equally well to know the complications which may result from the therapy." If this rule were followed, the problem would be much simpler. At least, physicians would not be carried away by the professional drug salesmen who ballyhoo hundreds of new drugs each year as being miraculous and infallible. They are advertised to be effective in every type of illness and to have no appreciable side effects. The doctors who use them are easily persuaded that this is so, and there are very few of them who run precautionary tolerance tests on individual patients before administering the drug.

A New World of Side Effects

But, Dr. Landau remarks, a whole new world of side effects has opened, and the results are not always so readily apparent that a physician could spot them at once. Penicillin might be safe for 40 shots, and the 41st could be fatal.

In the case of broad spectrum antibiotics, the patient using them often develops severe diarrhea. This is presumed to be the result of upsetting the intestinal flora, but Dr. Landau goes on to say that this same alteration in flora may be the cause of staphylococcal colitis, a condition which can be rapidly fatal unless diagnosed and treated. And what other effects will follow the alteration of the intestinal flora? Will there be unfortunate changes in our digestion, in the absorption of our nutrients? These things are dependent on proper intestinal flora. Does the doctor make provision, after using such a medication, for extra vitamin supplementation until he is certain that the proper function of the disturbed intestinal flora has returned? It is staggering to contemplate the number of symptoms that show up in such a situation.

Is the physician who was merely trying "something new" ready to look for these changes and treat them properly? Is a shot of broad spectrum antibiotic given, as it so often is, for sniffles or something else just as inconsequential, worth the chance of incurring a serious, possibly fatal disease? All such injections given "just to make sure nothing develops" seems to be the height of foolishness, or worse, incompetence.

Getting Rid of Tissue Fluid

Many overweight conditions are due to the body's tissues retaining an undue amount of fluid. In most cases, a salt-free diet would remedy this situation. Instead, medications known as diuretics are given. These are intended to expel water from the tissues through the kidneys. Unfortunately, they also remove a great deal of needed sodium from the tissues, to the point at which the sodium must be replenished by excessive salting of food or taking salt tablets. If this is not done, the patient suffers from muscle cramps, nausea, shortage of breath and general weakness. How much safer and easier to have eliminated added salt in the first place, thus avoiding the use of the diuretic, by achieving a good sodium level and proper fluid level in the tissues naturally. This problem also frequently develops with the body's potassium supply when diuretics are used.

The Unsavory Sulfa Reputation

The sulfa drugs have a reputation that is most unsavory. Their unrestricted use has done a great deal of harm, especially by causing serious liver involvements. Dr. Landau notes another less publicized problem caused by the sulfonamides. It is an inflammatory disease of the coats of the small and medium sized arteries of the body with symptoms similar to blood poisoning and other systemic infections.

Then there is a drug, hydralazine, used extensively in the treatment of high blood pressure. In quite a few cases, patients treated with this medication have shown symptoms resembling rheumatoid arthritis with pain at the joints and muscles. If therapy is stopped at the early signs of these effects, they quickly clear up. If not, fever, skin rashes, inflammation of the lungs, enlargement of the spleen and disease of the lymph glands can result.

Steroid Treatment

Patients receiving cortisone, ACTH and other steroid therapy are in serious danger of death from "adrenal exhaustion" when exposed to new stresses, such as surgery, accidents, burns and even childbirth. The adrenal gland, which normally releases hormones to help the body to meet these emergencies, is lulled into relative inactivity by the injection of hormones which actually do the job of this gland. So when the emergency arises, the necessary response is lacking. Therefore, it has become necessary for physicians to administer steroids before surgery, and often afterwards as well, to anyone who has been receiving these hormones 3 to 6 months prior to the operation. Without them, the patient is in danger of death. We wonder how many surgeons investigate the patient's background sufficiently enough to determine the need for the support offered to a shriveled adrenal system by cortisone injections before surgery. Also, we wonder how many doctors are aware of the serious complications they invite by using steroid treatment when it is not *absolutely* indicated.

Aside from the above, the reactivation of latent tuberculosis conditions can follow the use of steroids; peptic ulcers are another frequent aftermath of the use of these hormone preparations, and when treatment is stopped, severely unpleasant withdrawal symptoms follow, including headaches, nausea, vomiting, joint and muscle pain and general restlessness—not unlike the withdrawal symptoms of heroin.

Rauwolfia and Seizures

When rauwolfia was first discovered, mental and heart patients were literally gulping it down on doctors' orders. It was, and is, a calming influence for many, but now there are numerous reports of the occurrence of an illness similar to Parkinson's disease (a shaking palsy) and of convulsive seizures in patients receiving this therapy.

Diseases interfering with proper function of bone marrow have resulted from drugs used for weight loss (dinitrophenol), the sulfas used for infections of all kinds, anti-thyroid drugs (thiouracil, methimazole, etc.), gout and arthritis treatment (phenylbutazone) and certain antihistamines (pyribenzamene and antegran).

Serious anemia can result from treatment with epanutin, an antiepileptic drug and from sulfanilamide and acetanilide. Both drugs were used extensively in medicine not too long ago.

Antibiotics have been on the carpet before, but the use of them is unabated, in spite of staphylococcus, fungal infections of the mouth and tongue, anal pruritus and pain, deafness, neuritis and interference with the body's proper use of vitamins B and K, among other disturbances, which they are known to cause.

Complete kidney shutdown can result from use of the sulfas and incompatible blood tranfusions and other kidney diseases can follow the use of tridione and intravenous infusions of glucose, sucrose, urea and acacia.

The lists could be extended and, if one were to speak in terms of individuals, variations on drug and treatment dangers would be infinite. Dr. Landau warns that the doctor must realize that he is responsible for foreseeing possibly dangerous reactions. He must ask himself the question: "Is the treatment which I am ordering potentially harmful, is the risk justified, is the treatment going to be worse in its effects than the disease treated?"

Don't be a guinea pig for some drug company's new product. If you must take a drug, be certain your doctor knows what its effect on you will be. Better yet, stay well by following a good health program, and you will not be exposed to such dangers of treatment.

Vitamins Versus Toxic Drug Effects

A monthly newsletter issued to the medical profession by Hoffman-La Roche, Limited, of Montreal, Quebec, Canada, the *Courier,* carried an interesting two-part series in its February and March, 1959, issues. The series dealt with the use of vitamins in the treatment of toxic side effects of drugs. It has been shown that many drugs deprive the body of its nutrients as they are used, often without a visible and pronounced side effect. However, sometimes the anti-vitamin effect of certain drugs is so strong that it must be classed as an iatrogenic (medicine-caused) disease. The *Courier* acknowledges this fact, but remarks that, "Often, they (side effects) must be accepted as the lesser evil when balanced by therapeutic value of the preparation." Of course, it is true that one would be foolish to hesitate in using a drug because of a rash it might cause, while one's life hung in the balance. But side effects are often more serious, and the drugs are used much less judiciously than in matters of life or death.

If a drug is the only answer, we say use it, of course. But to spare yourself possible side effects, always increase your vitamin intake and cut down on those habits and environmental situations, such as smoking, drinking, stress of temperature or emotional situations, etc., which cost the body nutrients. Drugs take more vitamins from the body than you can afford. If you put them back as quickly as possible, the body can continue to function with some efficiency; if you do not, the lack will quickly show itself as actual poisoning. It is for treating this poisoning that the *Courier's* article was written. Any disease that responds to nutritional therapy need never have occurred if a sufficient amount of that nutrient had been present in the first place. Never take the chance of permitting a vitamin shortage to exist in yourself.

Why Vitamins Are Helpful

The exact reason for the salutary effect of vitamins in cases of drug toxicity is not certain, but one explanation is offered by the *Courier:*

"As biocatalysts, the vitamins have a variety of regulatory functions in the metabolic processes. Sometimes they form part of enzymes, sometimes they act as redox (oxidizing) agents, protecting biologically important substances from inactivation. . . . Under these circumstances, it seems quite plausible that such substances should exert a favorable influence on iatrogenic disturbances, as they are able to compensate the dysmetabolism (upset in the body's nutrients) by their regulatory activity."

A common cause of toxicity is anesthesia. Certain of the anesthetics are almost sure to make the patient vomit, or headachey. Sometimes, an anesthetic is as likely to cause death as the disease or the operation employed to correct that disease.

Post-anesthetic symptoms are caused by an overloading of the blood with acid metabolites, principally pyruvic acid. The levels of this acid are always highest in the blood of those with the severest post-anesthetic illnesses. Markees, et al (*Schweizerische medizinische Wochenschrift,* 80, 1079-81, 1950), found that, if these patients are given vitamin B complex or cocarboxylase (thiamin pyrophosphoric ester), the pyruvic acid levels fall rapidly, accompanied by an improvement in the patient's comfort.

W. Hugin, in another German publication, *Anaesthesist* (2, 193-96, 1953), told of giving patients 3 intravenous injections of 100 milligrams of cocarboxylase during the first 24 hours after operation. Patients receiving this treatment felt much better than untreated controls and were less frequently sick. Another researcher, Stieve, is cited as describing cellular damage in a dog caused by anesthesia, which was sometimes incurable, and which could be prevented by administering vitamin B complex.

Some researchers experienced excellent results in postoperative situations by using vitamin B_6 (pyridoxine). One doctor, K. Wedel, reported in *Anaesthesist* (4, 122-23, 1955), that he used 100 milligrams of pyridoxine, injected subcutaneously (under the skin) after surgery. No vomiting was seen as a sequel of ether anesthesia in 79 per cent of this group, while only 49 per cent of those who were not treated with the vitamin escaped postoperative nausea.

Antibiotics Not without Dangers

Leaving the discussion of anesthetics, the *Courier* tells us that the use of antibiotics "is not without its dangers—toxic effects such as hearing impairment, neuritis and digestive disorders, to name only the most important. They occur despite careful supervision, because toxicity varies from patient to patient. In post-antibiotic enterocolitis (inflammation of the large and small, upper and lower intestinal tracts), neither onset nor severity of symptoms is dependent on dosage."

It is for this reason that we repeat again our strong warning against indiscriminate use of antibiotics. Here is a drug manufacturer who admits in his own bulletin that it is impossible to predict the reaction of an individual to an antibiotic drug. It is the height of foolishness for a patient to insist, for example, on a shot of penicillin to knock out a cold—and it is worse for the doctor to agree to such a request. Antibiotics can control life or death and should be used with that in mind.

Why antibiotics react so strongly upon the body has yet to be fully understood. It could be due to any of these: disturbance of the balance of the intestinal flora; prevention of vitamins combining properly; the development of resistant strains; moniliasis (an infectious disease of the skin, nails, bronchi, lungs, etc.); disturbance of progressive cell metabolism; and bacteriolytic endotoxins (destruction of bacteria working from within the cells).

Bacterial or fungus super-infection (staph, for example) leads to the suppression of certain organisms, giving rise to intestinal upset, or malfunction. To prevent or lessen such disorders, H. P. Kuemmerle (*Medizinische*, 1957, 715-19) recommends a combination of: pantothenol, ascorbic acid and acidophilus baccilli, plus the natural components of sour milk.

Treatment for Antibiotic-Induced Digestive Disorders

The *Courier* offers this set of principles for the treatment of digestive disorders induced by antibiotics: administration of the all-important vitamin B complex (oral administration if absorption and serum protein levels are normal; otherwise, injections of the B vitamins are suggested until a normal absorption of protein state is arrived at); oozing intestinal hemorrhage in the absence of other causes implies vitamin K deficiency and should be treated by vitamin K preparations, orally or by injections.

The usefulness of streptomycin sulfate has been restricted by its toxic effects on the acoustic nerve. Therapeutic amounts could not be given without running the risk of injury to the ear. However, when mixed with the B vitamin, pantothenic acid, the toxicity of streptomycin was reduced greatly. This applies, as well, to neomycin and viomycin. When either is mixed with pantothenic acid, the therapeutic result is as good and the drug is safer. Vitamin A is also used to reduce or prevent the acoustic nerve injury by streptomycin and neomycin. The dose of A used to accomplish this is high—300,000 International Units daily.

One of the most frequently used of the anti-tuberculosis drugs is isoniazid, an item which may cause toxic inflammation of the nerves in high dosage. The symptoms—paresthesia (tissue abnormality), feelings of deafness, burning and weakness are probably due to a disturbance in pyridoxine metabolism. Daily doses of this vitamin largely or entirely relieve the symptoms. If the pyridoxine is given in amounts of 50 to 450 milligrams per day from the beginning of isoniazid treatment, the neuritis never occurs at all!

Barbiturates are increasingly common on the American scene, in the form of sleeping pill preparations. Their danger does not seem to limit their popularity. Only those who have experienced the awful consequences of prolonged use of barbiturates seem to fear them. It is known that they may impair the oxidative processes in the tissues of the nervous system and elsewhere. The body's use of carbohydrates is chiefly affected. The electrical impulses of the brain also suffer interference when barbiturates are used in excess.

But here, too, it has been shown that the vitamins of the B complex are of great value in neutralizing the toxic effects. Interference with brain waves due to barbiturate therapy are relieved by use of the B complex. In acute stages of barbiturate poisoning, the prescription in the *Courier* is as follows: "Intravenous infusion or injection of 1.5 grams vitamin C, 1.0 gram vitamin B_1, 200 to 400 milligrams nicotinamide (nicotinic acid, a B vitamin), 20 milligrams vitamin B_2, 100 to 200 milligrams vitamin B_6 and 25 milligrams pantothenic acid, in addition to the usual measures, leads to a rapid regression of the symptoms and earlier recovery of consciousness. Such injections may be repeated every 4 to 8 hours if necessary."

There is much to be done in the field of vitamin therapy, but those who are wise are anticipating the findings by fortifying themselves before and after surgical and antibiotic therapy with vitamin-rich foods and natural food supplements. Especially valuable are brewer's yeast, desiccated liver, rose hips and flavonoid-C. We wonder that more doctors are not aware of this good news to pass on to their patients. Perhaps it would help to reverse the procedure. Maybe the patients should pass on the good news to the doctors.

The Risks of Digitalis

According to the *U.S. Dispensatory,* which is the official book for doctors and pharmacists on drugs and their uses, digitalis is used to bring about an increased force and decreased rate of heart contraction. It also has some action on the nervous system. "Practically nothing is known of the basic mechanism whereby digitalis affects cardiovascular function," says the *Dispensatory.* We know that it produces a decrease in blood pressure in the veins, apparently because it causes the heart muscle to empty the ventricle (one part of the heart) completely. It also results in giving the heart more time to rest between beats and more time for the ventricle to fill again with returning blood.

Experiments have shown, says the drug book, that, after digitalis has been given, the heart muscle is able to perform a given amount of work with less consumption of oxygen.

We are particularly interested in the subject of digitalis because
of a summary of its possible harmful effects, which came to us in
the November 12, 1960, issue of the *British Medical Journal*. Judging
from this article, written by Samuel Oram, Leon Resnekov and Paget
Davis of King's College Hospital, London, digitalis is responsible for
many different harmful effects. While the authors consider the drug
to be "the most useful single drug in the treatment of all forms of
heart failure," they tell us that the frequency and gravity of one form
of digitalis poisoning does not seem to be widely appreciated by
doctors.

Wrong Use Leads to Poisoning

There is no doubt, they say, that poisoning by the wrong use of
digitalis is increasing and is almost certainly due to a modern therapy
which affects the amount of potassium in the body. Potassium is one
of the minerals the body cannot do without; it is closely interrelated
to sodium in the body. In fact, it is a sort of enemy of sodium. The
more sodium (table salt) you take in, the more potassium you need,
or you will get out of balance.

It seems that there is a special heart difficulty, known as irregularity of heart action, which may be mistaken for another irregularity
called fibrillation. Fibrillation is an irregular contraction of the heart
in which each fibre of the muscle contracts individually and rapidly,
rather than all contracting together. The first kind of irregularity may
be caused by digitalis. But if the doctor does not recognize this and
thinks it is the second kind, he may give more digitalis. So, if the
patient is already taking digitalis, he may give him more, not realizing
that the trouble came from too much digitalis. "In certain circumstances," say our authors, "very little digitalis can prove fatal."

They go on to discuss a number of cases in which such misdiagnosis was made with serious results. It seems that digitalis reduces the amount of potassium in the cells. Patients who are taking
diuretics are already excreting large amounts of potassium, along
with sodium. Heart failure, in itself, causes a serious loss of potassium in cells. If nausea and vomiting or diarrhea add to the distress
of the patient, more and more potassium will be lost. Finally, says an
editorial in the same issue of the *British Medical Journal,* the patient's
condition will deteriorate and may even end fatally.

"Pure" Drug Is Even More Harmful

If the doctor recognizes what his doses of digitalis have done to
the patient, what should he do? Stop giving digitalis and give potassium, immediately, say the 3 London doctors.

Pursuing the matter further in our file, we found a number of
articles dealing with this same problem—some of them dating back
to 1951. From an editorial in the *South African Medical Journal*

(January 18, 1958), we learn that the modern digitalis drug has far greater potential for harm than the older ones—because the modern ones are "chemically pure," rather than being just preparations of the digitalis leaf. It seems that digitalis has a possibly harmful effect on the heart where another mineral is concerned, too. The body's calcium balance can be upset by this drug.

The March 1, 1952, issue of the *New York State Journal of Medicine* carried an article on digitalis poisoning in which two Brooklyn doctors commented on the "frequency of digitalis intoxication" and warned against it.

Relation between Digitalis and Potassium

In the *Proceedings of the Society of Experimental Biology and Medicine* for April, 1951, we read that the relationship between digitalis and potassium has been known for a long time. It seems that the drug becomes more dangerous as the patient's supply of potassium is depleted. Hence, any patient who has been losing potassium (because of any of a number of reasons) would be in greater danger from digitalis than another patient.

The *Journal of the American Medical Association* for July 14, 1951, states in an editorial that signs of digitalis toxicity can be introduced in a patient, then abolished by giving the patient potassium preparations by mouth. His doctor can then bring on toxic digitalis symptoms once again by giving the patient a diuretic made from mercury. This is a preparation to induce urination and hence to rid the body tissues of unwanted fluid. Mercury is, of course, a deadly poison which is used regularly for this purpose.

An article in *Circulation* for April, 1951, describes the extremely dangerous condition that digitalis can bring on when it is used wrongly, and cautions physicians to be ever watchful for such a condition. Even a suspicion of such a condition must be treated by immediately stopping the diuretic and the digitalis and giving potassium preparations.

We have related all the above facts to show the absurd and completely illogical lengths to which members of the medical profession will go in their determination to use harmful drugs. There is a wealth of material (all of it taken from medical journals) showing the great usefulness of vitamin E for treatment and prevention of heart disease, and disorders related to the blood vessels. Many doctors are using vitamin E themselves, for their own heart conditions, and some of these refuse to give it to their patients and refuse to be quoted on the excellent results they have gotten in treating themselves.

Why Not Take Vitamin E Instead?

Nowhere is there any evidence of toxicity in the use of vitamin E. It can be used with complete safety in small doses by anyone with any kind of condition. It can be used in massive doses by almost anyone, there being only a few conditions in which it could possibly cause discomfort and no record anywhere of serious or fatal complications.

Vitamin E does not produce any imbalances of minerals in the body—potassium, sodium, calcium or anything else. It does not result in damage to any part of the heart or peculiar flutterings or contractions of any part of the heart. It is a natural ingredient of food, a vitamin which is apparently essential to the proper working of all our muscles, including the heart muscle. Its serious deficiency in modern food is undoubtedly the cause of much of the heart and vascular disorder which is so common today.

And, finally, we know what vitamin E does that makes it valuable to the heart muscle—*it helps the muscle to perform a given amount of work with less consumption of oxygen.* If you will look back, you will find that this is exactly the way in which digitalis benefits the heart. Yet, involved with this beneficial action of digitalis on the heart, are all the risks and imbalances we have described above. None of these is involved with vitamin E.

Dosage of Vitamin E Important

According to Dr. Evan Shute of the Shute Clinic, London, Ontario, Canada, the world's foremost proponent of the use of vitamin E for heart trouble, the dosage of vitamin E is extremely important for getting good results in treating heart disease—but not because of any danger involved. The important thing is to take enough of the vitamin. This dosage must be tailored for every individual. If there is a history of high blood pressure, the dosage should be quite small to begin with, because there is a possibility of the blood pressure going up at the beginning of treatment.

Dr. Shute is working valiantly to persuade physicians to use vitamin E, whether or not they use other drugs for heart patients. Every time his ideas are attacked, he takes up his powerful and well-worn cudgels and strides into the controversy, quoting the many, many scientific articles published in this country and abroad to back up his statements. He is determined to get acceptance of vitamin E for treating heart trouble on the part of physicians. We are interested in this aspect, too, of course. But we are mainly interested in preventing heart trouble.

We believe that by following a healthful diet and taking vitamin E regularly, along with other natural food supplements, you can prevent heart disease, along with just about every other kind of ailment that bothers us in the twentieth century. Why take a chance on getting heart trouble later and being subjected to all the risks that attend the taking of digitalis? Now, while you are well, get plenty of vitamin E and assure the health of your heart and blood vessel system.

Danger in Using Nose Drops

The *German Medical Monthly* (April, 1959) told of the alarming experience of a mother who administered the well-known drug, Tysine (tetrahydrozoline), to her 8-month-old baby for the relief of nasal congestion. When one drop in each nostril did no good, she administered two drops into each nostril. The baby became sleepy after half an hour and lost consciousness soon afterwards. The breathing became shallow, the skin pale and cold. The child was in a comatose state and could not be revived. The child was rushed to the hospital and remained unconscious for 3 or 4 hours in spite of continuous administration of oxygen. He recovered, after a deep sleep, in about 24 hours.

Eventually, someone got around to reading the fine print on the container of the drops, and discovered a warning about possible "sedative side effects" in infants. Another well-known nose-drop product, Privine, may act in a similar manner in children. These two drugs are derivatives of adrenalin and ephedrine, both intended for constricting the veins. Overdosage of either of these causes excitement, tremors, sweating and cramps. Tysine and Privine also have a powerful depressant effect on the central nervous system in infancy.

The article goes on to say that many other drugs have a different effect upon children than they do on adults. Antihistamine drugs are offered as an example. They have a sedative, antispasmodic action in adults. In children, an overdose may actually cause violent and sometimes fatal spasms.

The unusual thing about the case history we quoted in the beginning is that the mother of the baby, the one who administered the drug, was, herself, a doctor. If such an experience can puzzle and alarm a trained doctor, what chance has a lay person who innocently makes use of such a drug with similar results?

The article says this: "The damage resulting from frequent and long continued use of nasal drops has been recognized for years." The continued interference with mucosal circulation by repeated local application of these drugs sets up a troublesome irritative condition of the nasal mucosa. There is a special warning against the use of nasal sprays, since absorption is more rapid and dosage is difficult to estimate.

". . . Tysine and Privine exert a powerful action on the circulation and the pharmacologic mechanism of their narcotic effect in infancy is not yet understood," says the last paragraph of the article. There is no word about prohibiting the common use of these drugs, just the statement that no one understands how they do what they do to the system.

We say stay away from nose drops and nasal sprays. They must contain harmful ingredients to have the desired effect. Why take a chance on a serious, possibly fatal, reaction for you or the members of your family?

Drugs and the New Born

In *Public Health Reports* (August, 1959), the results of experiments at the National Heart Institute, regarding the effects of drugs on the new born, are published. It was found that the enzymes required to inactivate drugs are absent in new born mammals during the first week of life. Further, the investigators found that the central nervous system of the new born is extraordinarily sensitive to barbiturates.

These findings were arrived at by comparing the ability of mice and guinea pigs of various ages to metabolize several commonly used drugs. The necessary drug-destroying enzymes were absent at birth, and did not develop fully for 8 weeks. The potential danger of giving drugs to new born infants was emphasized in the fact that one barbiturate drug given in very small doses put day-old mice to sleep for alarmingly long time periods—almost 100 times as long as it would if used on adult mice. The dangerous implications of these facts where human children are concerned is obvious. The use of drugs on infants or anyone else, unless it is absolutely essential to saving a life, is a perilous treatment that could result in immediate or long-range impairment of the body's vital organs.

How Drugs Are Tested

We trust our doctors and hospitals to give the best possible care to our premature infants, and usually we can feel safe. They do all they can, and use whatever facilities and medications they feel will be of help. However, the problem that seems to be increasing in all areas of medicine—drugs and their dangers—is making itself felt in the treatment of premature infants, too. We see an illustration of the problem in *Science News Letter* (April 29, 1961).

Dr. James Sutherland and William Keller, of the University of Cincinnati, reported on the bad effects of Novobiocin, an antibiotic drug, used to control a staphylococcal outbreak in an unnamed newborn nursery. The drug caused an epidemic of apparent jaundice among the infants. One infant who received Novobiocin died. Tests conducted later on newly born rats showed a yellow skin discoloration following a large dose of Novobiocin.

The sad fact is that the drug and others like it were given the prefunctory tests many drug manufacturers use, which could not possibly tell the whole story of a drug and predict how it will act in any given case. Novobiocin was tested on animals and on adult humans. The manufacturer did not see fit to mention that it had not been tested on infants, especially premature ones. No one at the hospital thought to wonder about its safety for these babies, either. They assumed, as many of us do, that each product we buy, whether drug or food, is perfectly safe, unless the label specifically warns that it is not. We should know by now how erroneous this impression is.

The dangers to babies from too much oxygen, sulfisoxazole, sulfadiazene, chloramphenicol and synthetic vitamin K were all discovered after the damage they did became obvious. Why do we not exercise more care about the use of drugs before they have proven unsafe so tragically? Testing them on normal adults and animals tells nothing about how they will react upon say a sickly staph victim, who has liver trouble. The combinations of possible harm are endless.

It is for this reason that we abhor the routine use of drugs by some doctors. These drugs are powerful mixtures that have a severe effect on the body. Using them indiscriminately is more dangerous, we believe, than simply ignoring the problem. Penicillin used for a simple cold is playing with fire. Penicillin is meant for dealing with such serious conditions as pneumonia. What is the body to do with the residual power of such a potent drug when it is given for a mere cold? Sometimes the body builds a resistance and an allergy to such a drug, so that another dose will be fatal. Why fool with drugs at all unless there is absolutely no choice to save a life? If you do use a drug, be sure it has been tested on your kind of person with your kind of disease.

Deadly Sales Across the Counter

You can buy potassium permanganate in almost any well-equipped drug store with no prescription necessary. In the *Journal of the American Medical Association* (June 11, 1960), a doctor's letter appeared deploring the ease with which it can be had and with good reason, too.

This preparation is sometimes used by women who wish to produce an abortion. The results, in many cases, are severe ulcerations of the upper vagina. Bleeding from these ulcers can threaten life. There is little use for this drug in today's medicine, if indeed there ever was. The author of the letter suggests measures prohibiting its sale across drug counters without some form of regulation.

We think that any preparation which can be shown to be lethal should be strictly controlled in sales. This would include aspirin, barbiturates, tranquilizers, etc. How much cooperation could such legislation expect from the drug companies?

Narcotic Cough Medicines

While much of the population suffers from winter colds, cough medicines disappear from the shelves speedily. Most people buy them because they taste good, not because of any proven benefit to be derived from taking cough medicines. In 1960, a *United Press International* dispatch, dated February 1, told of a Congressional move to give the commissioner of narcotics authority to curb a fast-growing abuse—the use of cough medicines by drug addicts.

It seems that drug users throughout the country are switching to certain brands of cough medicines as cheap, easy-to-obtain substitutes for narcotics. The syrups contain dihydrocodeinone, an opium derivative which can be purchased over the counter.

We do not see that the abuse is that of the addicts as much as that of the manufacturers. Why should they be permitted to use so dangerous an ingredient as an opium derivative in a product that will be given to children and others whose physical condition is already run down? Why should such a product, carrying an ingredient which is known to be harmful to human health, be permitted at all? No one can show a true need for it, and its curative powers are, scientifically speaking, unrecognized.

Any cough medicine is intended to soothe the irritated membranes of the throat. It does no more than that, unless it contains vitamin C (usually in minute amounts.) If you must use a liquid to soothe a sore throat, a hot herb tea or lemon juice with honey—two tried and true home remedies—will do the job as well as anything else. Plenty of vitamin C is both a preventive and a cure. It relieves irritation and promotes quick healing. It also reinforces against further infiltration of the infection. Even if the government won't act to protect you against useless medications, you can do your own safeguarding by simply refusing to buy any cough medicine.

AMA Opposition to Control of Drug Advertising

In the *Des Moines* (Iowa) *Register* (July 22, 1961), an *Associated Press* dispatch detailed a story, the implications of which were staggering. It described a Senate hearing in which testimony was given to the effect that 36 pregnant women had been delivered of sexually abnormal daughters after treatment with a synthetic hormone drug. It was charged by Dr. Martin Cherkasky, Director of New York City's Montefiore Hospital, that medical journal advertising of the drug carried no warning to doctors who might use it on future patients. The ads were printed in the *Journal of the American Medical Association* for 3 months after the appearance of an article on the drug, which described this chilling aftermath of its use. In none of the subsequent advertisements was there any mention of side effects of the drug, said Dr. Cherkasky. The *Associated Press* reporter noted that the *Journal of the American Medical Association* regularly carries assurances to its physician readers that they can rely on its ads.

Dr. Cherkasky was testifying on a bill which would tighten federal policing of the drug manufacturing industry. One provision of the bill would require drug firms to tell in their advertising and other literature about possibly dangerous side effects of their products, as well as the plus factors.

It was Dr. Cherkasky's view that there should be some assurance that doctors who administer drugs, such as the hormone discussed above, Norlutin, are aware of its possible side effects. In this case, the method of administration of the drug, as well as the drug itself, could have been the cause of the trouble. If proper information in the ads for Norlutin could have prevented the tragedy of babies being born with both male and female sex organs, it is incomprehensible to us that legislation forcing the inclusion of such information in the ads should meet even the slightest objection.

It is astounding to learn that one quarter from which opposition to the bill has arisen is the American Medical Association. This organization has opposed the bill's proposal to require proof of efficacy as well as safety before any new drug is allowed on the market. What would be more logical than to require such assurance? Why should doctors be willing to chance the use of drugs that might be unsafe or might not even work, when they could be instrumental in forcing legislation which would eliminate such chances?

Can it be that there would be difficulties in the advertising departments of their journals if such information were required to be included in the ads? Would it be possible for many big advertisers to list all of the side effects and warnings? Have many of the highly advertised products left unproven many of their claims to safety and effectiveness? Can it be in the best interest of the consumer, or the patient, for his doctors to be indifferent to the possibility of such protection?

Sweet Drugs—Sweet Poisons

Pharmaceutical houses have made quite a business out of manufacturing pleasant-tasting drugs of one kind or another to make them attractive to the kiddies. This effort is a two-edged sword. While it does make it easier to get children to take medicine when it is necessary, it also encourages them to repeat the pleasant experience when it is not necessary.

In the *Medical Press* (July 26, 1961), there appeared a letter from Dr. Robert Little. His letter begins: "This is a plea to make medicine unattractive. When medicaments taste like sweets, children may eat them with dangerous or fatal results."

Dr. Little goes on to tell of personal experiences in childhood and observations in professional life in which disastrous results followed children's taking swigs from bottles of "tonic," sugar-coated laxative pills, etc. He urges that pharmaceutical houses "make poisonous medicines unattractive. Medicine should taste like medicine, not sweets. This will prevent needless deaths."

It has been our observation that sweet-flavored medications, or so-called medications, are largely of the patent medicine variety, which rarely do any good and can do real harm. This includes aspirin, cough syrup, cough lozenges, laxatives, tonics, etc. Parents administer these as much for their own peace of mind (because they feel they must "do something") as for the benefit of the sick child. All of these can be damaging to the sick child, rather than be of help to him. First of all, they contain sugar, or some synthetic sweetener, which neutralizes what few B complex nutrients the child is getting in his diet, and upsets the blood sugar level. All types of laxatives can be dangerous, especially for a child. Aspirin has been shown to be deadly, even in small amounts. The cough medicines contain small amounts of barbiturates, tranquilizers, antihistamines, etc. Maybe not enough to cause serious illness with a single dose (and who really knows that?), but dangerous to the child who loves the taste and wants lots more of the same. When grownups aren't looking, the child might snitch enough candy-coated aspirin to kill himself.

When a medication is really necessary, parents will find a way to administer it, no matter how it tastes. Sometimes one wonders where this catering to the whims of children and adults will stop. We provide school buses to help children avoid what is often a relatively short walk to school. We insist that learning be fun, when it is actually hard work in many areas, and we find later that "Johnny can't read." (He didn't think it was fun, so he didn't learn.) Dad squirts weeds with chemicals, instead of pulling them, then wonders why his lawn is brown. Mom opens a can, or defrosts factory-cooked frozen dinners, and wonders why her family doesn't seem to thrive on the foods they eat.

We must learn to do some unpleasant things in this world if we are to build our bodies and our attitudes, so that we can withstand more severe illnesses and other crises. Maybe a good place to start is with medications that taste as one would expect them to taste, not the way candy or soda do.

We are against the use of aspirin, but many parents insist on using it for their children and themselves. If you must use aspirin, use it in its unpleasant tasting form. Don't give the children the idea that aspirin is a treat to eat whenever they can get hold of some.

A Dangerous New Patent Medicine

An American company which manufactures a fizzing seltzer tablet is mentioned, in a letter to the *Lancet* (December 9, 1961), a British medical periodical, as "launching a triple bromide preparation under the name of 'nervessa'." The product is also an effervescent tablet containing 617 milligrams of bromide, with one, two and not more than three tablets within a 24-hour period as the recommended dosage. We can expect to see plenty of advertising for this product, and people will probably be using it as freely as they do aspirins and alkalizers.

Dr. Lancer, the correspondent, urged that the medical profession condemn the unrestricted sale of bromide-containing products to the general public. His reasons seem sound to us. Why should a manufacturer be permitted to offer a product that can cause these chronic toxic effects: acne, gastrointestinal and neurological disturbances, plus mental effects "ranging from depression, lassitude and faulty memory to acute psychosis with dementia. The earliest symptom of bromism may be excitement and this may lead the user to the drastic mistake of increasing the dose of the drug . . . The drug should be stopped in any person who develops even slight symptoms of mental confusion . . ."

Once again we see the average drug store customer facing the possibility of poisoning from a patent medicine he will be led to assume is safe. No one will spell out the dangers involved in its use, and if the manufacturer should see fit to mention them at all, they will appear in minute print on a folder the user will probably toss away as he opens the package. Should he be unfortunate enough to experience any of the symptoms of bromism, the layman is hardly likely to pinpoint the source of them to a bottle of nerve pills he bought at the drug store. He might even buy more to relieve the very problem their use caused in the first place! The fact that bromides are excreted very slowly in the urine and can therefore accumulate in the system makes the possibility of continued use a very dangerous one.

If nervousness is a problem for you, check your diet for the B vitamin foods which are necessary for healthy nerves. Concentrate on their frequent appearance in the meals you plan—the organ meats are especially rich in B vitamins. If yours is a severe condition, see a doctor, but don't resort to a patent medicine as a cure for "nerves."

A Trail of Iatrogenic Cripples

How should one treat Bell's Palsy, a paralysis of a part of the face, due to an injury to the facial nerve, which results in a characteristic distortion of the face? For generations the prescription was a simple one: let it go and it will gradually heal itself. In the *Journal of the American Medical Association* (August 6, 1960), Dr. David Cohen offered a new treatment which calls for everything from ganglion blocks, through corticosteroids, to surgical removal of the vertical portion of the facial canal.

A rousing letter from Dr. Harold Stevens called the article full of "unfounded speculations" and said that it urged a "vigorous therapeutic attack which could leave a trail of iatrogenic cripples from here to old Olympus' towering tops." Dr. Stevens points out that Bell's Palsy is "a benign self-limiting affliction from which about 90 per cent of the patients recover completely. In the experience of most neurologists, the remainder have only minor sequelae (complications). Severe residuals are rare." To urge such radical therapy, sometimes only 3 or 4 weeks after the onset of the disease and before its true course can actually be determined, is certainly a procedure open to dispute. Are such emergency measures justified in this disease at all? Dr. Stevens says, "Bell's Palsy is an emergency in only one sense: if the physician does not hurry with the treatment, the patient is liable to recover spontaneously."

How many doctors, who read only Dr. Cohen's recommendations, do you think have been advocating his radical treatment with every case of Bell's Palsy they've seen since? Probably quite a few. It is doubtful that very many had the confidence or courage that allowed Dr. Stevens to criticize the treatment for the immoderate measure it is, or to favor their own judgment over Dr. Cohen's. The situation is not unique, and it puts us in mind of a treatment, seriously proposed several years ago, for doing away with the annoyance of sweating palms—it involved major surgery!

The strides made in surgical medicine and anatomical research are great, and their value is certainly not to be denied, but they should be used cautiously and with a certainty that their employment will aid the case, rather than worsen it. Too many doctors use new methods only because they are new, and in spite of the fact that there are older, more proven and more reliable measures that can be taken to bring about an equally beneficial or more beneficial effect.

Are Drugs the Answer to Insomnia?

The sleeping pill habit is encircling the globe and, apparently, it is as much of a problem overseas as it is in the United States. In the *Journal of the American Medical Association* (June 27, 1959), an article on the subject was abstracted from a German medical magazine. The piece estimated that, of those entering Swiss hospitals in 1956, 1,300 were suffering from poison due to sleep inducers. Thirty-one of these patients died.

One of the non-barbiturate drugs, Doriden, available in Switzerland without a prescription, has been claiming addicts with increased frequency. Patients who had ingested, regularly, 5 to 20 tablets per day over a comparatively short period of time, suffered from irritability, emotional instability, pronounced shortness of breath, emaciation, sunken eyes, twitching of the facial muscles, vertigo, headaches and fainting spells. Yes, it's available in this country and, though a prescription is required, no doubt any doctor would be glad to oblige.

The article goes on to say that barbital (Veronal) and its derivatives are the most dangerous drugs. They are not broken down by the body and must be excreted by the kidneys. Phenobarbital (Luminal) leaves the body so slowly that its presence can be detected in the urine 9 days after ingestion, and it is considered, by these authors, to be the second most dangerous drug. Doses as small as 3 grams of barbital may prove fatal. Doses of the barbital drugs which would not ordinarily cause death might prove fatal if there is sufficient alcohol in the body.

Don't take sleep-inducing drugs. No matter what kind of reassurance you receive as to their harmlessness, your case might be different. You could be the one in a dozen or a hundred whose kidneys can't handle the drug. You might become the one who can't stop using the drug, an addict. Why start? Be certain that your nutritional needs are being met and that you get sufficient exercise, before you look to other causes or cures for sleeplessness. If your body and mind are kept healthy, the sleep you need will come to you.

An Information Center for Drugs

With the speed of modern drug making, a recent development which occurred in the nation's capital was a natural result of a growing need. A service was inaugurated, "Mediphone," which hopes to relay the most up-to-date data on drugs now in use by the nation's doctors.

Nineteen doctors are employed by this service to handle calls from all over the country and give information on some 8,000 drugs currently in use. The doctor who would use "Mediphone" can do so for 3 dollars a call, over and above a yearly 20-dollar membership fee and the toll cost of the phone calls, says Earl Ubell, Science Editor of the *New York Herald Tribune* (January 9, 1962).

In a way, we must admit that such a service has its place in our modern method of practicing medicine. Many doctors are unaware of all there is to know about the drugs available to them. How can a busy physician be expected to keep abreast of 8,000 drugs? But we wonder who will be using the service. The fee, it is suggested, can be passed on to the patient. (After all, it is treating him that necessitated the call in the first place, isn't it?) What will the doctor do about a $5.00 phone call if the patient obviously can't afford to pay? Will he foot the bill himself or take a chance on using a drug with which he might be unfamiliar?

Great numbers of new medical drugs are created yearly. It is obvious that even the most conscientious doctor cannot keep pace with all them. He should be able to consult with experts for past experience with a potent drug.

Of course, it is our strong view that no drug should be used unless other safer measures have failed. Ask your doctor if his prescription of a drug for you is the only possible treatment. If it is not, ask him to prescribe something that is likely to be less dangerous. Otherwise, ask him if he has consulted with the new information service on the drug, especially if it should happen to be one with which he is unfamiliar.

Eating Habits

Snacking Preferred by Experts

Do you suppose the American Indians sat down for lunch at 12 noon, or that the cave man got the family together every evening at 6 for dinner? It is doubtful that there was any organization about mealtimes in primitive societies. Modern social structure dictates scheduling of meals. Factories with hundreds of workers interdependent upon each other's activities can't keep stopping production every few minutes because someone got hungry and left for lunch. Schools can't have students sauntering in and out of classrooms as their individual appetites dictate the need for a snack. Mothers can't cook several dinners each evening just to catch everybody when his appetite is high. Furthermore, with so many family members having individual outside activities in the evening, a set mealtime before such activities begin is the only practical way to see that everyone is fed.

Experiments on Rats

The *Journal of the American Dietetics Association* (May, 1961) suggests that this system could be the cause of serious metabolic diseases; that is, physiological problems, due to the way our bodies process the food we eat. Eating less food at a time, and eating more frequently would be the idea. In the *Journal's* article experiments with rats were discussed. One group ate full spaced meals, while the other was given frequent, small feedings.

The group on full meals, as contrasted with those on snacks, was found to have increased body fat, decreased body protein and water, altered thyroid and tissue enzymatic activities, increased hardening of the arteries and an increase in the severity of diabetes. Studies in man have shown that he reacts physiologically in the same way as do rats.

What is to be done? It would appear that, if one can arrange it, 5 or 6 meals, or snacks, should be eaten instead of the well-known "three squares." Need we point out that the snacks should be well-balanced among meats, fresh fruits, vegetables, nuts, etc. Snacks, to many Americans, mean ice cream, pretzels, potato chips, candy bars, etc. Obviously, such snacking isn't going to have a salutary effect upon one's metabolism. Also, if one can't be sure of getting all of one's nutrients by eating small meals throughout the day, better, then, to stay with the 3 full meals. The important thing in eating is to give the body the materials it needs to operate properly. Experiments seem to indicate that frequent small feedings help us to make the most of what we eat, but this does not mean that full meals are unhealthful. It means that full meals are somewhat less desirable than nibbling. So nibble healthfully if your schedule will permit you to do so. If not, eat high-protein, low-fat meals that will meet your nutritional needs.

Eggs

Eggs Belong in Your Diet

By J. I. RODALE

Regarding eggs let us take a walk up Park Avenue in New York City. On this wonderful street, from 45th to 96th Street, there are battlemented, luxurious apartment houses in which wealthy people live, and it has been discovered that their children rarely get rheumatic fever. But on Park Avenue above 96th Street, where there is nothing but squalid tenements and wretched poverty, rheumatic fever in children is quite common. The same condition was discovered in the slum-ridden stockyard area in Chicago. Investigators recently narrowed the cause down to eggs. The poor children rarely ate them because they were so expensive.

I got this information, strangely, from an article in a British medical journal called the *Lancet,* issue of April 16, 1960. This journal gave another example. In New York City, in the wealthy Brearley School for girls, there hadn't been one case of rheumatic fever in 10 years, but among poor children living near the school there were many cases.

To further incriminate lack of eggs as a cause of rheumatic fever, the *British Medical Journal,* issue of April 17, 1954, citing Wallis' theory about egg lack in rheumatic fever, stated that there is less of this disease in the period immediately following Easter when even the poor eat eggs.

Lecithin in Eggs

The medical investigators were not content merely to depend on trial-and-error observations regarding lack of eggs in the diet as a cause of rheumatic fever. They pinned down the exact factors in the egg that were responsible. They discovered that the blood of patients with rheumatic fever was low in the fats called lecithin and sphingomyelin and that eggs contained an abundance of these two fats.

Now, this piece of medical research does not stand by itself. I would like to refer to another that was described in the *Journal of Allergy,* issue of November, 1956, which proved that egg yolk had a protective effect on arthritis. This experiment was done with guinea pigs and showed that the guinea pigs raised on a diet containing whole egg powder showed about one-half as much joint swelling as guinea pigs with the same diet minus the egg powder.

What I think is very significant here is that, when lecithin was added to the diet of the no-egg guinea pigs, it protected them against the swelling of the joints. As you will recall, it was the lecithin in eggs that was one of the factors in preventing rheumatic fever. Incidentally, the taking of lecithin as a food supplement is one of the planks in the program I advocate for good health.

Protein and Vitamin Content

I think that eggs are one of the finest of all foods. Medical science calls the egg the number one protein, because it contains the best distribution of all the amino acids. Amino acids are what protein is made of. There are 32 amino acids. Eggs are also very rich in iron.

Another thing I like about the egg is that nature has provided it with a very fine closed package, and no spray poisons or chemical additives can get into it. Remember also that, in the egg, there is all the food needed to feed the chick that comes out of it. The poultryman never feeds the chick for the first few days. Nature has taken care of that and provided everything the chick needs for a full diet, until the chick is old enough to forage about.

Eggs are very rich in vitamin A, which is a factor in preventing colds. A deficiency of vitamins A and C is usually at the bottom of colds. I personally am extremely dependent on eggs, and if I cut them out for about two weeks, which I have done experimentally on several occasions, I invariably come down with a cold. If you are a "cold-catcher," eat eggs. They are the most wonderful of foods. Is it any wonder that an ancient rhymester said about eggs:

> Treasure houses wherein lie,
> Locked by nature's alchemy,
> Flesh and blood and brain and bones.

Eggs for Heart Cases

The question arises, what should a person with a heart condition do about eggs? The average doctor in the case of heart patients usually prescribes about two eggs a week, and some say, no eggs at all, on account of their cholesterol content. I think this is one of the greatest blunders. The heart patient needs the best nutrition he can get, especially in the way of protein. It is needed to prevent deficiencies in the blood, so that it can feed the heart tissues well and keep them in the best of condition.

First, the doctors overlook the fact that the egg contains large amounts of lecithin, which is an antidote to cholesterol. We saw in the Park Avenue research I referred to that it was a deficiency of lecithin in the blood that caused the rheumatic fever, and that it was the correction of this deficiency by the lecithin of the egg that cured this condition. Also, in the experiment with guinea pigs alluded to, the addition of lecithin to their diet protected them against the swelling of their joints. Lecithin is too valuable a substance in food to be disregarded.

Secondly, the latest researches indicate that the cholesterol on the artery walls and in the blood stream does not come directly from the cholesterol in the diet. The latest findings are that the body manufactures its cholesterol from basic substances in the body, and does this to excess when there is something wrong in the body, some disorder of body functioning or metabolism. For example, when there is lack of activity, or little exercise, then more cholesterol is made.

From my observation and in reading medical journals, I believe it is not the cholesterol *per se,* but the total fat in the diet that is the culprit. For example, in the average U. S. diet, there is about 44 per cent fat. In the average Italian diet, there is about 20 per cent fat, and the Italians have less than half the heart deaths that we do. But the Italians exercise more.

So, we must cut our total fat consumption down to 20 per cent. But please, let us not do it by cutting out eggs. Let's eliminate milk, butter, cheese, ice cream, the fatty meats and such foods. They don't hold a candle to eggs in their nutritional value. For one thing they don't contain much lecithin.

According to the opinion of a physician, Joseph G. Molnar, M.D., who conducts a syndicated newspaper column, eggs do not contribute to hardening of the arteries. He describes the case of a friend of his, another doctor, who eats eggs every day, and his cholesterol level is lower than when he began to keep a check on it. He states that a scientist he knows in Denver sometimes eats 5 eggs for breakfast, without any untoward results. I have a heart condition myself, although I have never had a heart attack, and have always eaten at least two eggs a day. At times, on experiments, I have eaten 7 or 8 eggs a day for weeks, without the slightest effect on my heart.

Eggs contain vitamin B, and the B vitamins are a protection against hardening of the arteries. The field of medical practice is full of fallacies.

Eating Eggs Raw

While on the subject of eggs, it might be a good thing to discuss the taking of the egg raw . . . the eggnog and such things. Cooking, of course, destroys a considerable part of the vitamins and all of the enzymes. Now . . . before we decide whether to eat eggs raw or cooked, we must be aware that the white of the egg contains a poisonous substance called avidin, but that cooking it renders it completely harmless. Years ago, before I knew anything about vitamins and such things, I decided to eat my eggs raw, and within a week or so, began to experience a funny dull feeling above the fore-

---

Ehrlich, Paul

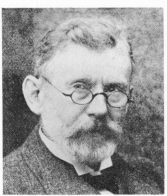

Paul Ehrlich's greatest contribution to medicine and science was his discovery of the chemical, salvarsan, or 606, as a potent weapon against the Spirochaeta pallida, the specific organism causing syphilis. Ehrlich, born at Strehlen, Silensia, Germany, March 14, 1854, received his medical education at the Universities of Breslau, Strasbourg, Freiberg and Leipzig. In 1878 Ehrlich began his studies on the effect of different chemicals upon living tissue. His first bit of research, and, in fact, all future research, dealt with the aniline dyes. Using their unique property of visibility upon being injected into animals, Ehrlich soon learned that certain chemical substances exhibit an affinity for disease organisms. With this knowledge, Ehrlich went on to make important discoveries in the histology of the blood, did research work in cancer and greatly improved the technique for the growth of serums used in modern immunology. However, Ehrlich is best remembered for his discovery of a specific treatment for syphilis. For this contribution to medicine, Ehrlich received the Nobel Prize for physiology and medicine—a joint award which he shared with Eli Metchnikoff.

head. Today, well-fortified with all my vitamins and following my healthful diet generally, I can get away with it without experiencing this feeling. But in my present diet, I do not consume any part of the egg raw.

For a while, I used to eat my egg yolks raw and cooked only the egg whites, but we found that to be too much trouble, and to me it smacked a little of hypochondria. A small amount of raw egg white can be taken, but in experiments with guinea pigs, larger amounts of raw egg white produced arthritis.

You might ask, why did nature put avidin in the egg white and thus spoil such a wonderful food? In answering, we might speculate. Nature provides ingenious ways to protect the species. Could it be that avidin has been placed in egg white so that animals which prey on eggs will discover that eventually eggs make them ill, because they consume the egg white raw, and then they will avoid them? Perhaps if there were no substance such as avidin in the egg, birds would have become extinct long ago.

In this case, it might be best to compromise . . . . that is, cook the egg and lose some of its value, but make it up by taking additional vitamins and minerals.

How to Prepare Eggs

What is the best way to eat your eggs? Shall they be soft-boiled, poached, scrambled, fried, hard-boiled? If you are trying to reduce weight, it would be best to eat them hard-boiled, because they remain longer in the stomach, thus not bringing back the hunger pangs too soon. I eat my eggs soft-boiled at present.

I am staying away from scrambled or fried eggs, because I don't think that people should eat fried foods. There is much evidence that raw oil is extremely healthful, but in experiments with animals, it has been shown that cooked oil can cause cancer. This might occur only in weakened individuals and only over a long period of time. It is possible, also, that our program for healthful living is such a strength to the body that it can resist the cancer-causing effect of consuming cooked oils. In such cases, a treat might be called for, occasionally in the form of scrambled or fried eggs, if one needs such a treat. What I am trying to say is that the follower of our program need not be a fanatic, although there are some items in the program regarding which exceptions should not be made, if at all possible.

For a treat I sometimes take my eggs as an onion omelette, using no salt in it. The onions give a superb flavor that takes care of the lack of salt. Another way to cover up the lack of salt is to combine raw chopped onion with chopped-up hard-boiled eggs. This makes a very tasty dish.

One lady advises a kind of omelette which contains no fat. She says, "Cut a large onion into small pieces and put this in the top of a double boiler with one tablespoonful of water and let cook until tender enough, then add two lightly beaten eggs. Cook until done. You will find the eggs light and fluffy. In cooking eggs in the top of a double boiler over boiling water, you keep them away from all fat. I put a lump of soybean butter in them when I serve them, but you do not have to do this."

Soybean butter can be purchased in health food stores.

While the egg contains unusually large amounts of vitamin A, it also contains many other vitamins and minerals, such as vitamin B, vitamin D and vitamin E. It does not contain vitamin C, which we get from vegetables and fruit, but it is one of the very few foods that contain vitamin D. Eggs also contain iron and the rare mineral copper.

If you live in the country, you should try to get your eggs from a farmer who lets his hens run with roosters in a barnyard. This insures their getting more minerals and other rare nutritional substances by natural means. The hen that eats earthworms and pecks about in manure piles is a much healthier hen than one that is kept in the artificial environment of a poultry house. She gives better eggs.

Then there is the question of storage. The fresher the egg, the better it is for you, quite apart from the fact that it tastes better. A little nutritional value is lost every day it is in storage. Frozen or dried eggs are not to be recommended. The whole egg does not freeze well and the yolk becomes leathery, which indicate a deterioration in its nutritional value.

Synthetic Eggs

I also wish to advise against food products that are supposed to contain eggs, but either don't or have them in a chemicalized form. Take the headline that appeared in a New York paper in 1957. It said, "Chemists are helping bakers to economize on eggs." But the question is, do those chemists know what they're doing? Do they know anything about nutrition? They suggest that, in making prepared dry cake mixes, whole eggs be replaced with methyl cellulose and a little extra milk, with, they say, very palatable results. They consider that up to half the normal amount of egg whites may be omitted from prepared dry cake mixes, if these chemicals are used.

Then there's the patent recently issued by the U.S. Patent Office for a process of preparing dried egg white where glucose oxidase and catalase are used. Then, an aliphatic polyhydric alcohol is used, constituting from 4 to 22 per cent by weight of the finished dried egg white products. One perhaps might not mind alcohol . . . but aliphatic alcohol is a horse of a different color. It is a chemicalized alcohol and has no place in egg whites. And who wants glucose oxidase and catalase in his egg white? Do you know who? The food manufacturer who saves money by practicing these shenanigans.

Infertile Eggs

One more thing about city-bought eggs. Did you know that a hen can lay an egg without a rooster? But it will be an infertile egg. No chick can hatch out of it. It's a sterile egg, and that's what people are eating these days. Today's chickens are raised by factory methods in crowded, unsanitary quarters, where a rooster would create a riot. But fertile eggs contain valuable nutritional substances that infertile eggs do not.

A French medical journal, *Compte Rendue Société de Biologie,* reports a research by a Dr. Riboullearo which showed that fertile eggs contain valuable hormones, whereas non-fertile eggs don't contain the slightest trace of such hormones.

Electricity

Water and Electricity

The danger that is inherent in the combination of water and electricity cannot be overstressed. In spite of many warnings, most people are not willing to pause to take the precaution of drying themselves before touching a plug or electrical appliance. Even worse, persons sitting in the bathtub will reach out to turn off a radio or answer the phone. Don't let yourself be fooled into thinking it can't happen to you. It happens to somebody (who probably thought that very thing) all the time!

In *San Diego's* (California) *Health* (May, 1960), a bulletin put out by the local Public Health Service, a few of the tragic incidents which could easily have been avoided are recorded. One evening in April, a 17-year-old boy was taking a bath. He reached from his water-filled tub and took hold of a metal floor lamp. He was pronounced dead an hour later. In other cases, two infants were being bathed in kitchen sinks. One died when water splashed on a nearby radio, the other was killed when he reached out and touched a radio. A housewife died when the socket of an electric heater attached to a wall outlet fell into the tub. Life ended for a girl of 15 when a lamp was pulled or fell into her tub.

Electric appliances of all kinds should be out of reach of the sink or tub. If you were tempted to touch them with wet hands, think just a second of what could happen—of what has happened—and we are certain you will be willing to sacrifice the few seconds it takes to dry your hands on a towel.

Enzymes

Enzymes Are Important to You

If the foods we eat may be compared to packages of nutrition, then we can consider enzymes the tools which open the packages and make the contents available to the rest of the body. From the moment a food is taken into the mouth, the enzymes begin to work on it, breaking it down into nutrients the body can absorb through the intestinal wall and use. Many of the foods we eat contain built-in enzymes which aid greatly in the body's most efficient use of that food. It is unfortunate, therefore, that in the processing and preparation of foods today many of these helpful enzymes are inactivated or destroyed. Without their active presence, the food which should contain them is less of a food than it could or should be.

The place of enzymes in the changes of our world from day to day cannot be overestimated. The Columbus, Ohio, *Health Bulletin,* in an article on the subject, called enzymes "life's chemists. . . . They control the green of the grass, the unfolding of a flower, the lethargy of a cow. . . . So, too, they control man as they control all life, from the instant of his conception to the moment he dies, his successes and failures, his characteristics and personality, his completed destiny."

They Come by the Billions

That is quite an area of control, especially for a substance of which one heard little until a few years ago. But enzymes are part of all living things, from the cells in a weed to the cells in the human brain. There are 650 known types of enzymes, and each type has its own specific purpose. The powerful influence of these tiny compounds becomes clearer when one reads that each cell of the body, of which there are many billions in each of us, is believed to contain at least 100,000 particles of enzymes.

The value of the enzymes becomes apparent when one imagines the effort it would take in the laboratory to break down a stick of celery or a piece of roast chicken into component parts of the human body. The enzymes do it with ease and dispatch.

The Columbus *Bulletin* article went on to say that the "amino acids originating in the muscle of the steer which becomes our steak are transported by the blood stream for the construction and repair of our bodies. Along the way, these acids are captured by enzymes and converted into human muscle, a radically different substance from the original. We chew a bite of bread and it becomes sweet. The starch in the bread, which is indigestible, has been changed into sugar by enzyme action. Invertase, an intestinal enzyme, can break down a million times its own weight in sugar and be ready for more."

271

This process occurs in one way or another, with just about every food we eat, because as we eat it, most food is not digestible (*i.e.,* ready to be absorbed into the blood stream to be transported through the body to where the nutrients are needed). So when one eats a piece of meat or a spear of asparagus, one is not eating fuel, nor energy, nor building material. One is eating the ore, as it were, from which these bodily needs will be fashioned by enzymes. Because of the enzymes, then, we have body heat and stored energy, to be used to blink an eye, run for a bus, figure a mathematical problem or a recipe—or keep the heart beating.

Disease Shows Up in Enzyme Increase

When disease strikes the body, it has been shown that the enzymes are prodded into unusual and frenzied activity. The Columbus *Bulletin,* to refer again to that brief, but informative article, says that "many medical and research authorities are of the opinion that most diseases originate from lost or deficient enzymes. Faulty enzyme behavior is at the root of leukemia and other cancers, some believe, with the possibility that synthetic enzymes of positive or negative action eventually may be utilized to hinder overactive enzymes or to assist those which have become ineffective to conquer many diseases with which man is saddled." Other diseases, such as mental disturbance, are linked to enzyme malfunction, say some researchers, and the answer to mental illness might some day reside in a pill which will straighten out the enzyme problem in the body.

Along these lines, we are fascinated by the findings of Dr. Felix Wroblewski, of the Sloan-Kettering Institute for Cancer Research in New York City. In the Toledo, Ohio, *Blade* (August 17, 1961), Science Editor, Ray Bruner, told of Dr. Wroblewski's work which indicated that certain diseases change the amount and composition of enzymes in the bodies of animals and man. The conclusion was that there may be an overproduction of one enzyme or an underproduction of another which somehow permits the disease to take hold.

Dr. Wroblewski found that an analysis of a blood sample for enzyme content, and comparison of the result with that of a normal sample, would indicate not only the presence of a disease, but specifically which disease. For example, the amount of a certain enzyme in the blood of a patient after a heart attack nearly tripled in the first 24 hours. After the onset of infectious hepatitis, which involves the liver, the enzyme, glutamic pyruvic transaminase, may increase in the blood as much as 10 times. Analysis of the blood at different intervals after the original diagnosis would tell the doctor the rate at which the disease is progressing, and indicate new steps to be taken in treating it.

Another enzyme, lactic dehydrogenase, has been found in tissue cultures of cancer cells, and in the blood of mice given experimental cancers. Of this phase of his work, Dr. Wroblewski is quoted as saying, ". . . all types of mice have been subjected to all types of experimentally induced malignant processes, including sarcoma and leukemia. In each case, the concentration of the enzyme in the (blood) plasma has risen before any other evidence of malignancy appears. When treatment makes the tumor or leukemia regress, the enzyme disappears from the blood in direct proportion to the improvement." Unfortunately, such biochemical analysis has not served to detect cancer in humans in advance of other symptoms. It is thought, however, to be a very promising field for further investigation. Scientists familiar with Dr. Wroblewski's work are, hopeful that urine, bile, gastric juices, cerebrospinal fluid and other body fluids might turn out to be useful in diagnosis through their enzyme content.

Trypsin for Blood Clots

Of a more practical nature to us at this time is the story of trypsin. Trypsin is an enzyme secreted by the pancreas, and it has been hailed as an aid in the solution of some circulatory problems. In *Drug Trade News* (November 19, 1956), we read: ". . . the value of trypsin in the treatment of thrombophlebitis (blood clots in the legs) was confirmed at a Conference held at the New York Academy of Sciences last fortnight." Investigators at Bellevue Hospital in New York City reported that trypsin was administered by injection to 82 cases of thrombophlebitis in a double blind test (that is, neither the physicians nor the patients know whether the substance under trial, or some inactive substance, or placebo, is being used until a coding system is translated by a third party at the end of the experiment). "An excellent response was seen in 72 per cent of the patients on' the drug, as opposed to 11 per cent response of those on the placebo. Poor results were observed in only 7 per cent of the patients on the active proteolytic agent, but 63 per cent of those on the placebo " Five of the patients who did poorly on the placebo were placed on trypsin, to which they responded well. It was emphasized that the enzyme had no apparent effect on the thrombus (clot) itself, but merely reduced the inflammation and edema accompanying the condition. It is presumed that the porousness of surrounding tissue is increased, "and the intercellular fluid is released. Biological continuity is restored and this in turn permits the multiple defensive forces of the blood to come into play. By this procedure, the edema, primarily, and secondarily, the inflammation are reduced." More simply, trypsin somehow dissolves protein, and clots are composed largely of protein.

A Personal Story

A more personal reaction to trypsin appeared in the *American Weekly* magazine (June 27, 1954). William Engle, science editor for that publication, wrote the story of John Allen, who "was suffering a while ago from chronic recurring thrombophlebitis . . . blood clots formed in the veins of his legs, over most of his body and in his lungs. . . . One doctor after another gave him up for lost. He himself, growing weaker, growing desperate, finally gave up. He conditioned himself for death."

About that time, Allen's doctor heard a lecture on trypsin by Dr. Innerfield of Mt. Sinai Hospital in New York. Dr. Innerfield was called to see John Allen. "I found him moribund (close to death)." He injected trypsin into a muscle, and within a day, the patient improved somewhat. Within a week, with continued injections, great areas of inflammation were clearing, widespread blood clots were dissolving. Within a month, John Allen left the hospital.

The William Engle article noted that earlier research had shown that trypsin injected into the veins of rabbits could be dangerous. It should be remembered, though, that the product used was not the enzyme that occurs in nature, but a synthetic one. Why not use enzymes as they occur in nature, for safety's sake? There could be no danger there, because the enzyme occurs as it does in any food and is presented to the body in a normal manner. All foods, as they are grown, contain large amounts of enzyme—it is, actually, the property which makes foods ripen and spoil. However, these enzymes are killed quickly by high heat, and it is this characteristic of the way most Americans prepare food that robs them of the enzymes they should acquire in their diets. Eating as much of your food as possible without cooking it is the best way to get enzymes safely, regularly and naturally. It is easy to see how a shortage of enzymes in the body could occur, when the way we cook seems almost calculated to destroy any enzymes we might have gotten.

A Possible Answer to Polio

Before we leave trypsin, we would like to mention a story carried in *Parade* magazine (no date), written by Robert P. Goldman. In it, Mr. Goldman told of some research work done with trypsin on polio. Two Wilmington, Delaware, hospitals studied 50 polio patients treated with trypsin and found this: " (1) Paralysis which usually continues for six or seven days after onset of the disease, appeared to be stopped after just two days among trypsin treated patients. (2) Muscle strength among the patients was increased over what would be considered normal during the period of recovery. (3) The patients were able to exercise and start rehabilitation work earlier. (4) Trypsin itself did not relax patients' muscles, but 'antistiffness' drugs given after trypsin worked better than usual. Of course, many more polio cases have to be studied before doctors can make any conclusions."

Could it be that trypsin might hold a surer polio preventive than the vaccines we are using? Isn't it worth more investigation?

The relatively new study of enzymes as a disease preventive and a cure has led to many interesting disclosures. In a *New York Times* article by William Laurence (no date), we read of a report on the annual meeting of the American Chemical Society in Atlantic City. At this meeting, the pancreatic enzyme, elastase, was named as a solvent for cholesterol deposits in the arteries of animals. Its human application in the treatment or prevention of hardening of the arteries was yet to be conclusively established.

Another enzyme, procollagenase, was reported by Dr. John C. Houck, of the Children's Hospital Research Foundation in Washington, D. C., to be capable of preventing or erasing ugly scars (*Science News Letter,* October 24, 1959). Disfiguring scars consist of collagen, a fibrous protein, and this enzyme can dissolve the form of collagen from which the scars develop. We have seen no more on Dr. Houck's work since 1959.

In *Drug Trade News,* December 23, 1956, there was a story on the pusliquefying enzyme, dornase. In tests of more than 100 patients, suffering from chronic bronchial and lung involvements, treated with the enzyme in aerosol form, there was usually a thinning of the sputum, greater ease of expectoration, a more productive cough and less constriction of the bronchial area.

In the London *Times* (May 15, 1960), an article told of treating boxing injuries with a combination of two enzymes, streptokinase and streptodornase, which were derived from streptococci. Once absorbed in the blood stream, they dissolved blood clots and broken down tissue. A spokesman for the Amateur Boxing Association, Dr. J. L. Blonstein, said, "We have been able to get a 50 per cent reduction of bruises and abrasions and a 15 per cent reduction of blood swellings, and cuts which would normally have taken 4 weeks to heal, have done so in one or two weeks."

An enzyme found in pineapple stems has been found to ease menstrual pain and, by relaxing the cervix, aid in childbirth. Dr. Ralph Heinicke of the University of Minnesota, told of the enzyme, bromelain, in a *United Press* interview printed in the *New York Times* (October 16, 1957). No further word on bromelain, so far as we know, except as an agent to keep beer from clouding.

Do You Need More Enzymes?

Normally, the body can take care of its own enzyme supply so as to keep up with proper digestion and assimilation of body-building protein. However, in these days, people whose diet is not what it should be, might go on for weeks or months without eating enzyme-containing foods, or they might be suffering from a disorder of the pancreas, the production center of most of the enzymes necessary for bodily function. In such a case, the body cannot acquire usable protein, and organs of the body begin to deteriorate, blood clots can form, bronchial congestion can occur.

Enzymes act to build prepared food into muscles, nerves, bones and glands; they assist in storing excess food in the liver and muscles for future use. Enzymes help in eliminating carbon dioxide from the lungs, help build phosphorus into bone and nerve, help metabolize iron and coagulate blood.

Can you add to your enzyme intake? Of course—if you're careful of the way your food is prepared. Wheat kernels contain enzymes, but the heat used in baking wheat flour into bread kills them. Raw wheat germ then, would be the only sure way to get enzymes from this source. Butter, milk and other dairy products lose their enzymes in the high heat of pasteurization. Only certified raw milk would offer enzymes. Canned fruit and vegetable juices also give up their enzymes in processing—as do other canned foods. You have to eat fresh or frozen fruits and vegetables to get their enzymes. Any sugar—even raw sugar—contains no enzymes due to the boiling process involved in its production, yet the original sugar cane is rich in enzymes. Cooking is the death of any enzyme. If you would get your enzymes, eat as much of your food raw as is possible.

Epilepsy

An Answer to Epilepsy?

"The evidence is still purely circumstantial, but . . . . it could open a whole new approach to the cause and treatment of epilepsy." So reads a part of a paragraph in the May 24, 1958, issue of the San Francisco *Examiner*. At any mention of epilepsy, our ears perk up, since persons who suffer from the disease are desperate for any news that offers them an escape from the constant use of drugs. Dr. Eugene Roberts, a biochemist from the City of Hope Medical Center, has concluded that a deficiency of vitamin B_6 might be a major cause of the disease. Another factor is the presence in the central nervous system of an amino acid, gamma-aminobutyric acid, or GABA. It is found in uniquely high quantities in the brain and spinal cord of mammals, and appears to be related in an extremely important way to the nervous system. A lowering of the GABA in the system results in seizures in animals, and these seizures bear a strong resemblance to the epileptic convulsions in human beings.

We do not know if more work has since been done on GABA,

though it does sound promising. However, vitamin B₆ is available as a natural food supplement, and can be acquired along with the other B complex vitamins in foods such as wheat germ, brewer's yeast, desiccated liver and all organ meats, to name a few.

Eskimos

Life among the Eskimos

"For the greater part of the long winter, no vegetables or berries are available to Eskimos, yet vitamin or other deficiencies are unknown so long as a large part of their diet consists of fresh meat and fish, mostly eaten raw and frozen." These words are those of Otto Schaefer, M.D., who lived for several years among the Eskimos in the Far North. "One would expect vitamin C deficiency to be prevalent in the North, since so many Arctic explorers died of scurvy, but it is actually never seen in people eating adequate amounts of fresh meat. Despite the long dark winters and inadequate ultraviolet radiation at all times, vitamin D deficiencies do not occur in Arctic peoples who live predominantly on native food and whose children are breast fed. Severe degrees of scurvy as well as rickets are to be seen in bottle-fed children who are not given vitamin supplements."

Dr. Schaefer's comments appeared in two issues of the *Canadian Medical Association Journal* for August 15 and September 1, 1959. The facts he reveals about the health of Eskimos are astonishing. Considering the great confusion that exists in the minds of most of us about life among the Eskimos, we feel that Dr. Schaefer has performed a real service in bringing these facts to light in an important contemporary medical journal.

He does not gloss over or excuse the changes for the worse in the health of Eskimos as soon as they are exposed to "civilized" food and ways. He tells us that no mineral deficiencies are known to exist among isolated Eskimos. He tells us that he regularly examined the iron level in the blood of the Eskimos expecting to find considerable anemia, especially among pregnant women and children. He found none, except in cases where accidents or disease had caused extensive hemorrhaging. On the other hand, Alaskan Indians he found to be slightly to moderately anemic. The reason? They lived chiefly on bannocks—a form of oatbread.

Until quite recently, he says, the Eskimos were regarded as being free of "degenerative and civilization diseases." He found that this is not completely true, but that so far as many diseases are concerned, the Eskimos are certainly far better off than we are. He says that most disorders of neuro-hormonal regulation (diabetes, arthritis, etc.), psychosomatic diseases, essential hypertension, presenile hardening of the arteries and some forms of neoplastic diseases (tumors) have never been observed in pure-blood Eskimos living in the old native fashion.

Absence of Circulatory Disorders

Diseases of the heart and blood vessels are now the leading causes of death in our civilization. Some reports have said that Eskimos never suffer from these conditions. Others say that they do. Dr. Schaefer tells us that some Eskimos do suffer from hardening of the arteries, high blood pressure and heart conditions *when they are old.* He says, however, that his impression, after examining more than 4,000 Eskimos is that these diseases are less common in old Eskimos than in old whites, and *that they do not exist at all among Eskimos below the age of 60.* Checking with another physician, Dr. S. Hanson of the Charles Camsell Indian Hospital, he found that Dr. Hanson agreed that he had never seen dangerous changes in artery walls of Eskimos below the age of 60. It is well to remember, in this connection, that large numbers of American soldiers killed in battle during the Korean war were found to have extensive damage to heart and blood vessels at an age certainly well under 60.

High blood pressure and resultant heart disease are practically absent in Eskimos, says Dr. Schaefer. He remembers only two patients whose blood pressure was above 100. What might some of the reasons be for this? Dr. Schaefer believes that the Eskimos' aversion to salted food is a large part of the reason. Even to be polite, they cannot and will not eat food salted as the average European or American salts his food. Their diet, consisting almost entirely of meat and fish, contains more sodium naturally than a purely vegetarian diet, and they do use a small amount of sea water in the water in which they boil their meat.

There is another and, it seems to us, a very significant comment Dr. Schaefer has to make on the total absence of high blood pressure among Eskimos. He says, "Important as diet may be as a contributing factor in the pathogenesis (cause) of arteriosclerosis and hypertension, it is probably overshadowed by factors of neuro-hormonal and neuro-vascular regulations, the balance of which seems often disturbed by the stress, frustration and constant pressures of our modern way of life. It is certainly wrong to assume that primitive people are not subjected to stress and pressure. I doubt if there is, or ever was, a carefree paradise for any people in this world. Certainly not for Eskimos, living under such hardships and constant threats to their very existence. Why and how, then, do stress and pressure exert pathological effects in our modern society? I have witnessed many examples of stress situations, including emotional pressures, in truly primitive peoples. These almost invariably led to an irresistible urge for increased and sometimes wild motor activity, which is the natural solution to stress, as stress evokes in animal physiology an increased readiness for motor action—to fight or flight. Our modern society has largely lost the habit or possibility for the motor 'work-out' of stress, while being constantly flogged by sensory overstimulation. Another important causative factor, providing much frustration and sustained mental stress, seems to me to be our loss of the genuine readiness of primitive peoples to modestly accept fate and our natural place in the world without ambitious revolting."

Another Good Reason for Exercising

We think this theory is an excellent one—and is a most convincing argument for exercise. The natural reaction to strain, fear, emotional upheaval or frustration should be "increased or even wild motor activity." Get out in the garden and dig or weed! Take a two-hour walk. If the weather is bad and you can't get outside, turn up the radio and do some exercises or dance for a while. With yourself? Why not? Make up your steps as you go along! The important thing is to work off steam; in other words, quite literally to use up the gland secretions your body has supplied for combating the stress or emotion you feel. The Eskimo is lucky. When he is afraid, he runs or he fights, for the hardships of his environment provide him with plenty of opportunity for blowing off steam.

Other Disorders Unknown

There are no cases of stomach ulcer or diabetes or asthma among Eskimos, according to Dr. Schaefer. Thyroid conditions are unknown. Birth control is unknown among Eskimos, he goes on, but their children are born evenly spaced, mostly 3 years apart. This pattern changes among Eskimos who go to work for white people and adopt some or all of their diet. Some researchers have believed that this may be because the large amount of carbohydrates supplied in the civilized diet furnish some fertility factor lacking in the Eskimo's meat and fat diet. Dr. Schaefer does not agree. He points out that, as powdered milk and pablum are more and more substituted for breast milk, there is a shortening or complete abolishing of lactation in the Eskimo mother, so she becomes pregnant more often. Eskimo mothers living on their primitive diet apparently have never heard of difficulty with breast feeding, so their children are given practically nothing but breast milk for the first two or possibly three years of life.

When a mother dies or a child is brought up in a foster home, milk is, of course, unavailable and so are nursing bottles. The baby is fed prechewed meat and fish, boiled or raw, from the mouth of the foster mother, much as a baby bird is fed. Dr. Schaefer believes this is an important factor in preventing deficiencies among children.

Gout is unknown among Eskimos, even though their diet consists mostly of foods rich in the purines which supposedly cause gout. Tumors do occur, but are less common and of a different kind from those of the white man. Cancer of the breast (commonest form of female cancer in white countries) is unknown. There is a conspicuous increase in breast cancer among Eskimo women who eat white man's food and take up his habits of life—chiefly a shortened period of breast feeding, or none at all.

Almost all Eskimos smoke, Dr. Schaefer tells us, but no lung cancer has ever been found among northern Eskimos. Stomach cancer is extremely rare. Cervical cancer, on the other hand, seems to be as prevalent among Eskimo women as among their "civilized" sisters.

Strangely enough, epilepsy is often seen in Eskimos. Congenital heart disease is seen occasionally, rheumatic heart disease does occur, though probably less frequently than in whites. Dental decay is unknown among Eskimos who eat their primitive diet and no refined carbohydrates. Eskimo teeth are often worn down by chewing raw meat, fish and whaleskin. Women also chew daily the skin clothing and sealskin boots to make them pliable again after drying. But their teeth, deprived of their protective enamel and worn down nearly to the gums, do not decay, but stay perfectly healthy so long as no "civilized" carbohydrates are eaten.

Skin parasites, such as lice and scabies, are frequently seen. But other skin diseases like psoriasis and eczema are unknown.

Dr. Schaefer concludes his articles with a plea for further study of these primitive people before they have been completely overwhelmed by the "blessings" of civilization. It is only thus, he says, that we can sort out those disorders which are hereditary and those which result from some factor in environment. Opportunities to study the Eskimo are fast disappearing.

Exercise

The Many Ways to Exercise

Athletes are getting all the exercise they need, and so are most active children. It is the average adults we are concerned with. How often do you have occasion to raise your arms high above the head during the day at the office? What about full range of motion for hips and knees. How often do you have to climb stairs if you live in a ranch-type house and work in a building equipped with an elevator? If you don't garden, how often is stooping or bending required, except in housecleaning or checking the tires for air? The middle-ager's stomach muscles don't do much but expand, as "potbellies" form and poor posture sets in. These are the ones who need exercise. These are the ones who are courting ill health, simply by neglecting the movements necessary to keep the body operating efficiently. Perfectly normal muscles lose their tone and "rust out" when left unused. The person who aspires to all-round good health will not neglect his daily exercise.

Disorders Can Be Prevented

In the *Medical Journal of Australia* (June 10, 1961), we saw an article on the subject of exercise by Dr. F. J. Gray. He emphasized that there are certain disorders of the joints and their supporting structures which can be prevented by proper exercise. Then he offers a set of exercises which, he says, ". . . will do much to improve general physical well-being, as well as cardiac, respiratory and vasomotor function. They are thereby calculated to lessen the severity of respiratory tract infections, to minimize vasovagal disturbances, and so on." The exercises Dr. Gray offers are especially for those who are engaged in non-active occupations, and are intended to supplement any infrequent forms of exercise. "One has only to picture the business executive filled with drive for his domestic as well as his financial advancement, moving 20 barrow loads of soil at the week end and wondering why he requires 3 or more weeks of daily physiotherapy for low back pain, or finding himself so short of breath at his very exemplary week end task that he imagines he is in the early stages of heart failure, to realize the importance of some form of planned exercise."

Dr. Gray admits that many of us are aware of the need for this exercise, and get some disorganized moments of it. But such exercise puts certain parts to strenuous use and leaves others in a state of disuse. With such non-thorough effort, one cannot depend upon freedom from all the troubles that exercise can prevent—only some of them. Complete exercise of the body, with studious regularity is necessary.

The paper then offers 8 exercises described by Dr. Gray. The exercises are not new, nor are they claimed to be new, and you will recognize them at once. But they do for the body what should be done, exercising those joints and muscles which are often neglected in daily activity. They should be done in order, as provision is made in the scheduling of each for the opportunity to catch one's breath, and they should be done at least each morning. The effort should be gradual—no exhaustion called for—and soon the average individual should be able to complete the entire cycle in 5 minutes.

Eight Basic Exercises

1. Beginning with arms at sides and feet together, on toes, jump to the position of both arms extended over the head and feet spread wide apart, then jump to bring yourself to the original position (50 times).

2. Beginning with feet 10 inches apart and arms fully extended overhead, touch the toes, exhaling and inhaling with each bend and stretch respectively (25 times).

3. Alternately flex and extend the neck by a slow, exaggerated nodding that stretches the neck as far back and as far front as it can go (25 times).

4. Plant feet firmly, hand on hips, then rotate torso and neck as far as possible, first to one side then to the other (25 times).

5. Extend the arms full length and cross wrists in front; then, without bending them, bring them to the back and cross them there, inhaling and exhaling deeply each time (25 times).

6. Start with feet apart, standing on toes, arms extended to the sides, then squat, bringing the arms to a forward horizontal position for the balance while squatting (25 times).

7. Hop from one leg to the other, stationary running, (25 times).

8. Start with feet wide apart and arms extended to the side in a horizontal position. Then touch the opposite toes with each arm alternately, inhaling and exhaling deeply with each movement (25 times).

In Dr. Gray's opinion, these exercises will do the job of keeping your muscles in shape. If it sounds like too much for you, do part of it. Do the exercises you can do; do them fewer than the recommended number of times if necessary, but do some of them, or something else to keep limber.

Running for Your Health

Maybe you'd like to try something more dramatic in the way of exercise. Maybe you'd like to try running. *Family Weekly* (September 17, 1961) told the story of a 65-year-old Syd Meadows, who celebrated his current birthday by running 10 miles on an indoor track. Mr. Meadows had been a heart attack victim some years before. He ran the 10-mile course easily, while skeptics who knew his history watched with fear for his life.

Of course, the approach to this feat was gradual. Under the direction of Bill Cumler, Physical Director of the Cleveland YMCA's Businessmen's Club, many such men have been led to good health through exercise. His approach starts very slowly (one client's first day workout consisted of walking the width of the pool once) and proceeds to the point of physical superiority.

The *Family Weekly* article ended with this warning to heart patients: "The lesson is clear. You must walk (or swim) before you can run. *But first consult your family doctor.* If he approves, walk one block vigorously each day for a week. Add an extra block each week. When you can walk a mile without tiring—and your doctor consents—you can begin jogging. Try 100 paces the first week, and build up gradually . . ."

The Walking Tour

Many people simply refuse to engage in any form of formal exercise. For these, we recommend such activities as dancing, cycling, gardening and, of course, walking. Editor Rodale is one of the most enthusiastic promoters of walking for exercise and enjoyment. One of the most attractive ideas we've seen for influencing individuals toward walking is the "Walking Tours" program advanced by the Museum of the City of New York. The idea behind this series is to get the people of New York interested in the history and character of the city. So, every Sunday during the pleasant-weather months, a group gathers to be conducted through the interesting streets of New York on foot by an experienced, knowledgeable guide. They do plenty of walking and love it!

We are certain that every American city has interesting things to see on a walking tour. Why couldn't such tours be arranged in Philadelphia, Cleveland, Pittsburgh or New Orleans? Why not in Bethlehem, Pennsylvania, Phoenix, Arizona, Peoria, Illinois or Dubuque, Iowa? This is something each of us can do for his own town. Why not write a letter to the local newspaper suggesting the idea, asking for the Chamber of Commerce or the YMCA to set up some sort of a trial walking tour program. It should be a huge success, since it won't cost anyone any money—except, perhaps, to pay a special guide—and it will be instructive as well as healthfully enjoyable.

A Curious Old Book on Exercise

In a book that is actually a curio today, *Book of Bodily Exercise* by Cristobal Mendez, a physician of the sixteenth-century Spain gave us the first full discussion of exercise ever printed. There had been other writings on the subject, but his is the first full book by a physician, translated by Elizabeth Light, and published by Waverly Press, Incorporated. Of course, the superstitions and misinformation of the age are evident, as ours will be to someone reading our medical literature in a few hundred years. Still, there is much in this old book that is true and worthwhile.

Let us present just a glimpse of the type of thing a "most skillful physician" of Seville in 1553 was telling his patients, and his methods of curing them. For him, as you will see, everything was quite simple. "Besides, the cure of any disease is so easy that many animals by natural inclination are able to obtain it . . . when a hawk feels weakness in his eye, it scratches fennel with its claws and some drops fall into its eyes and its sight becomes as good as ever. . . ."

This passage is typical of the keen observation, mixed with naiveté, which characterizes this book. Of exercise, Senor Mendez said, " . . . here are 3 important things the body accomplishes with exercise. The first places a greater power in the locations of the virtues, from which follow great ability to perform deeds and the impossibility of harming them. . . . The second is the increase in natural heat noticeable in the strong alteration of foodstuff, making digestion greater and more perfect and pouring throughout all the body that which is necessary to preserve health. It softens hard things and disintegrates obstructions by consuming the humor that causes them, because it makes the humidity more subtle, widens the passages and makes everything more perfect. In the third place, the movement of the spirits is increased, whence follows the opening of the pores in the body, and the superfluities pass out and are evacuated."

Book Is Amazingly Accurate

That's how important exercise was considered to be—"makes everything more perfect." It is praiseworthy that so much was known about the human body 400 years ago. Who could disagree with the theory that exercise endows the body with "great ability to perform deeds"? Is it not true that regular exercise is valuable in "making digestion greater and more perfect"? Of course, it is equally true that perspiration induced by exercise might be defined as the opening of the pores on the body, and "the superfluities pass out and are evacuated."

Senor Mendez was a strong advocate of exercise for poor eyes. He was "not apt to praise gentlemen who use spectacles continually because they are shortsighted, the eyes covered that way do not have any exercise. . . It is true what Don Garcia Ponce de Leon tells me, that after wearing spectacles he can see better. But if his Mercy could recall how much he can see now . . ."

The author suggested that one not wear spectacles continually, but only occasionally . . . "there is no better exercise than studying or reading without them . . ." Another bit of advice on the care of the eyes: ". . . it is considered good to wash your eyes in warm water in the morning for some time, and then to open them in the air, especially if there is a clean, soft wind." The warm water was supposed to soften any impurities, and the soft wind, dilute and expel what had been softened.

Was Unique in Thoroughness

Mendez is unique, we believe, in his thoroughness, as he advocates the exercise of the senses of smell, hearing and taste. To exercise your ability to smell, you should smell "very subtle things that are deeply penetrating like strong vinegar, aromatic wine, spiritous liquor, very fragrant odors of hot things like musk, amber, civet . . . Air is attracted and mixes with the vapor issuing from them and without doubt, consumes and dissipates a great deal of superfluities and thereby gives benefit." And as though he had foreseen smog and exhaust fumes, Senor Mendez warned ". . . not to smell things with bad odors that are capable without any doubt of killing a man." However, onions get a high recommendation, ". . . they produce great benefit by smelling them at very close range; it not only sharpens the smell, but also the sight and even does some good to the ears. . . . Sneezing is a very beneficial exercise for other organs as well."

"The organ of hearing is exercised by listening to loud sounds, strong voices, instruments which sound very high, or on one hand, by listening to many shots of artillery or thunder in the sky, or on the other by listening to triumphs or musical wind instruments of high pitch."

"The sense of taste rests in the tongue and has more ways of exercise. . . . It is cleaned in exercise by having subtle and warm things in the mouth that penetrate and dissipate what is bad in the morning with spiritous liquors, aged wine and chewing hot things like clove, cinnamon and ginger. . . To talk much and to shout is also great exercise for the tongue and this is why when you speak a great deal, you expel a very thick saliva. . . . because you have moved the tongue very much. Even the whole body exercises if you are standing as those who preach."

One really practical bit of advice comes in this statement: "Men without occupation, with ranches in the country very often might exercise and enjoy themselves doing what they order others to do to make a living." By this, Senor Mendez means gardening as practiced by a Spanish nobleman who "worked over two hours until he started to sweat and felt tired. Then he walked home, although it was a long distance. He changed into a clean shirt which had been warmed and exposed to the fumes of an aromatic lozenge, or even better, rosemary, which is a very healthful medicine; he washed his face and eyes with watery wine, he lay down for half an hour and then ate enough for 4 persons on the day he took his exercise." Did the peons on the ranch manage this elegant form of exercise?

Walking Best Type Exercise

Walking is endorsed by the author as the best type of exercise for the whole body—"the easiest and can bring the most benefit without harm." He complains of hearing the same excuses against regular times for walking that we hear today. " 'I do not have enough time . . .' Some want to spend plenty of time for things of much less importance and do not want to spend any time on their health. . . In walking, all the animal faculties are exercised . . . and the common sense is exercised in listening and seeing, the imagination and fantasy in everything you can imagine . . ."

Cristobal Mendez wrote more of exercise, who should exercise and when, the signs one should look for as reason to continue or stop, what exercise for ladies, what for young men and older ones, etc. The word for the appeal of this book is, we suppose, quaint. It has a great amount of charm and the picture of the era comes through quite vividly in the anecdotes and examples offered by Mendez to illustrate his points. One could hardly pull oneself from the grave by following the recommendations offered here, but some of the suggestions aren't bad, and the knowledge of physiology displayed by the author is remarkable.

We of the twentieth century seldom realize how far ahead of us were the ancients—even before Mendez—in their appreciation of the value of exercise. After all, our bodies were designed with a view to hunting our daily food and building our own shelters, fighting wild animals and other men for survival—not by pushing buttons or squeezing triggers, but with our hands alone. We need some form of this activity today to keep our bodies working at their best efficiency.

Five hundred years before Christ, the Greeks recognized this and perfected a system of exercise which is credited in part for the prominence of that nation in that time. As the Greeks came to drop the emphasis on exercise, coincidentally their influence on the world waned, too.

Build a House at a Desk

As man's environment changed, his activities became more limited. Cities rose and with them, specialization of jobs. Where a man, at one time, had to perform all of the operations involved in building a shelter for himself, the city man might do no more than write words on a paper to earn the money to pay a number of men, each to do some special part of building a shelter. He pays someone else to get his meat and someone else to carry him to his destination. No wonder modern man needs exercise—his body needs activity. Before this, vital activity was a part of everyday living, now it must be planned on, even manufactured in the form of games in order to be a part of modern life.

However you manage it, your body needs movement and health will be hard to hold onto without some regular form of exercise. Plan to do some form of manual labor, walking or calisthenics each day. And if it's labor you choose, it should be something other than what you do on the job or at home in the form of housework.

Exercise to Keep the Heart Healthy

Don't give up on the exercise if you want to keep your blood stream clear and functioning properly. Two British researchers (*British Medical Journal,* August 13, 1960) have discovered that exercise definitely influences the cholesterol level of the blood. After a fatty meal, the blood may show delayed clearing of cloudiness, which is thought by some researchers to indicate a high cholesterol level that may cause coronary heart disease. But tests have shown that a healthy person can speed the clearing of the blood by a little exercise.

Tests were made on 22 healthy medical students. It was found that when they walked or cycled after a standard meal containing 60 to 75 grams of fat, the plasma cloudiness was less than when they rested, in a statistically significant number of cases. And the standard meal was indeed that; no effort was made to arrange healthful foods or eliminate undesirable ones. For breakfast, the students were given cornflakes, medium-fat fried bacon, butter, a fried egg, two ounces of cream and 3 ounces of milk. No restriction was placed upon the amount of bread, coffee or tea or marmalade. Not ideal by any means, but fairly typical of what most people eat, who eat breakfast.

As can be imagined, the lunches and dinners we eat cloud the blood as much or more. This extra thickness might be just enough to couple with existing plaques and clog the blood's passages. So do a bit of exercising after each meal. No need to exhaust yourself, but a walk or some other simple exercise might help to preserve your life.

Eyesight

Your Eyesight Depends on Your Nutrition

By J. I. Rodale

Is there a connection between nutrition and eyesight? Medical research says there is. Can we eat our way into good eyesight? If you are a young child, yes. If you are older, proper nutrition can maintain the status quo, it can even improve the eyesight somewhat, but more important, it can prevent serious eye disturbances that so frequently attack older persons. Is overuse of the eyes a factor in harming vision? A physician has said, "It is almost impossible to damage the eyes by long hours of reading or sewing, even if great fatigue is experienced at those times." (J. H. Doggart, M.D., *British Medical Journal,* August 15, 1953.) General health is a factor in eye health. Thus, it is important to get adequate exercise, to be in the outdoors sufficiently, and to observe the recognized health rules. But nutrition is the most important of them all.

And what is the first rule of good nutrition? It is to be sure that there is plenty of good protein in your diet. The word *protein* is derived from the Greek and means "of first importance." Rarely has a word been so appropriately derived. That protein can improve the eyesight was proven in an experiment that was performed in Guy's Hospital, London (*Lancet,* May 19, 1958). The eyesight of two groups of myopic children was compared. One group had 10 per cent of their normal calorie intake altered to consist of animal protein, while the control group was given no dietary advice whatsoever. It should be known that it is generally regarded as a rule that progressive deterioration in eyesight takes place in near-sighted people until they reach the age of 20 or so. Yet, the children in this test over 12 years of age showed a definite arresting of such progress on the protein supplement. Some of the special diet children over 12 not only stopped getting worse, but actually had their sight improved. Those children under 12 continued to deteriorate, but at only ⅓ the rate of those not getting the prescribed protein. And those who took the most protein deteriorated least rapidly.

Another confirmation of the importance of protein to good eyesight is contained in a chapter of the book, *Modern Nutrition in Health and Disease,* by Wohl and Goodhart. This chapter is by Dr. J. J. Sterns of the Utica State Hospital, and states that a certain percentage of laboratory animals deficient in amino acids (which are the components of protein) always develop cataract. The cataract will disappear if the amino acids are fed before the cataract has progressed too far. Says Dr. Sterns, "The prescription of a diet high in protein and vitamins is, therefore, generally admitted to be possibly a valuable adjunct in treating early cases of cataract."

In 1942, when the Japanese took over Singapore and thousands of the unfortunate inhabitants were confined to prison camps on semi-starvation diets, a large number of them were affected by serious disturbances of vision and ocular diseases. In the medical reports, this was ascribed to the ingestion of an ill-balanced, excessive carbohydrate diet—too much rice especially. In children, one of the disadvantages of eating sugary carbohydrates between meals is that no room or desire is left for the more important meat and vegetables at the regular meals.

Vitamin A

As Dr. Sterns has mentioned, vitamins are a good adjunct to protein, in order to insure the preservation of vision. Let us check a few of them and see how they rate in connection with what they can do for the eyes. In this respect, the prima donna of them all is vitamin A, a deficiency of which is associated with night blindness. That is why so many people eat carrots. But it would require too many of this vegetable to give enough vitamin A to do any real good. I have come across health-conscious people who eat so many carrots and consume so much carrot juice that the palms of their hands turn yellow. Whether this is good or bad I am not prepared to say, but until it is proven to be of definite health value I would suggest eating a reasonable amount of carrots.

When England pioneered radar, they thought of a scheme to allay the Germans' anxiety as to why the British airmen were suddenly shooting down so many German planes. They circulated a rumor that their best ace, Cat's Eye Cunningham, accomplished his results by eating tremendous amounts of carrots. The Germans adopted the idea and vast amounts of carrots were consumed, but it did nothing for the acuity of the Luftwaffe's eyesight.

There can be no question that vitamin A is a specific for the eye. In 119 cases of conjunctivitis among school children, a vitamin A deficiency was discovered in all of them. Prompt improvement and recovery were the result of giving large amounts of this vitamin (*American Journal of Diseases of Children*, July, 1941). Conjunctivitis is an inflammation of the delicate membrane that lines the eyelids. In emergency cases, it is advisable to inject vitamin A, because in some persons, it may not be assimilated when taken by mouth.

Another condition caused by a lack of vitamin A in the diet is xerosis, a disorder in which the eyeball loses its luster and becomes dry. If not corrected, this will result in ulcers and finally, in perforation of the cornea of the eye. This condition is seen only in countries where food rich in vitamin A is unavailable.

Foods high in vitamin A are butter, milk, eggs, liver and carrots. It is also found to a lesser extent in fruits and vegetables. To get enough vitamin A, it is suggested that halibut liver oil capsules be taken daily as a permanent part of everyone's diet. Vitamin A has been called the longevity item. Animals, in experiments, always live longer when this vitamin is added to their rations. As far as dosage is concerned, the usual capsule contains 5,000 units. To do any good, 3 or 4 of them should be taken per day. The toxic point would be over 40 of them per day.

Vitamin B

It might come as a surprise that there are vitamins other than vitamin A that are necessary for the healthy functioning of the eye. The B vitamin complex, for example, is an absolute necessity, and even a partial deficiency in one or more of this complex results in serious eye symptoms. A lack of thiamin (vitamin B_1), for example, may cause pains behind the eyeball. Where there is a considerable lack of it, there can occur a true paralysis of the eye muscles. Vitamin B_1 will cure neuritis of the eye.

Other B vitamins are concerned in eye health. These include riboflavin, niacin, pyridoxine, pantothenic and folic acids. In certain forms of pellagra, for instance, giving just niacin will not cure the disease. These other members of the B family of vitamins are necessary as well. In pellagra, there is inflammation of the eyelids and loss of eyelashes, erosion of the eye tissues and clouding of the cornea. When riboflavin is lacking in the diet, the eyelids may smart and itch, the eyes grow tired, vision may be poor and cannot be improved by glasses, it may be difficult for the individual to see in dim light and there may be extreme sensitivity to light. This does not mean that the patient cannot stand any light at all, but rather that he suffers actual physical discomfort in the presence of bright light.

Dr. Sydenstricker, of the University of Georgia, studied 47 patients, all of whom lacked riboflavin. They suffered from a variety of visual disturbances. They were sensitive to light, suffered from eyestrain that was not relieved by wearing glasses, had burning sensations in their eyes and visual fatigue, and their eyes watered easily. Six of them had cataract. Within 24 hours after the administration of riboflavin, symptoms began to improve. After two days, the burning sensations and the other symptoms began to disappear. Gradually, all disorders were cured. When the riboflavin was taken away from them, the symptoms gradually appeared again and once again were cured by riboflavin.

A condition known as tobacco amblyopia is a dimness or loss of vision due to poisoning by tobacco. Patients complain of blackouts, headache and inability to read. Nearly all of them experience cold finger tips in the morning after the first cigarette. There is also a loss of the ability to see red and green colors. In every case, the patient who stops smoking soon regains full vision. In all of these cases, a vitamin B_{12} deficiency is found and injection of this vitamin brings about a cure. People who smoke strong pipe tobaccos are more likely to have the disease than are those who smoke cigarettes. Vitamin B_{12} is found in liver, also in egg yolk, and to a lesser extent in other animal products.

The safest way for the individual to insure that he is getting every part of the vitamin B complex is to take it in the form of food supplements such as brewer's yeast, desiccated liver, wheat germ and sunflower seeds, preferably all of them. They are of great benefit to the body's general health. It is dangerous for the individual to attempt to take individual parts of the B complex, as they occur in synthetic vitamin preparations, because serious unbalances can occur, due to the fact that they exert various effects upon each other, and excesses and insufficiencies may be harmful.

Vitamin C

The public is aware of the ability of vitamin C to prevent scurvy, but it does not know that this vitamin is of incalculable importance to the eye. Vitamin C is necessary for the oxygen uptake of the lens. In scurvy, there are hemorrhages of the eyelids and eye tissues.

Vitamin C performs an antihemorrhage function. Glaucoma and cataract are usually accompanied by very low levels of vitamin C in the lens. Extensive medical findings show that vitamin C is closely related to the health of the lens.

We prefer natural rose hip tablets to the synthetic ascorbic acid form of vitamin C. Rose hips are made from the berry which is the fruit of the rose plant and is 40 times richer in vitamin C than oranges or grapefruit. It also contains other vitamins and minerals, whereas ascorbic acid is a pure chemical formula, a fragmentation which is counter to the theory of what a food should be.

Foods rich in vitamin C are green peppers, broccoli, cauliflower, water cress, kohlrabi, raw cabbage, strawberries, collards, cantaloupe, tomatoes and fresh peas. We recommend only a moderate consumption of the citrus fruits because of their citric acid content. Overconsumption of the juices especially, sometimes causes *pruritus ani* (itching rectum) as well as serious digestive troubles. The pulp of the fruit contains vitamin P, which is not present in the juice. Vitamin P aids the body to absorb vitamin C.

Vitamin D

Vitamin D, the sun vitamin, is involved in cataracts. In experiments with chickens, a deficiency of it produced cloudy lenses. Vitamin D is found mainly in fish livers which are also rich in vitamin A. Vitamin D is also found in eggs and milk. The daily taking of halibut liver oil capsules will insure the necessary supply of A and D vitamins. There is no objectionable taste because the capsule does not open up until it reaches the stomach.

Vitamin E

Vitamin E is of value to every organ or part of the body because it causes an increased oxygenation of the veins and arteries. It forces oxygen to the most inaccessible parts of the body. In Italian experiments, 3 patients experienced improved vision when given vitamin E over a period of 3 months. (*Policlinico-Sezione Pratica,* 58: 1381, 1951).

In another Italian study, 3 doctors used vitamin E for ocular disturbances in 400 cases, and obtained uniformly good results in every one. In some cases, there was improvement in visual acuity and in several there were surprising results (*Annales d'Oculistique,* 186: 987-994, November, 1953). Dr. Shute of the famous heart clinic of London, Ontario, Canada, has shown that the use of vitamin E enables new blood vessels to form.

Sugar

There are some other factors in nutrition that should be considered insofar as the vision is concerned. There is hardly any other organ of the body that is so dependent on good blood chemistry as is the eye. The blood which feeds this organ should be as close to physiological perfection as possible. We should, therefore, avoid anything that distorts it. The overuse of sugar is the greatest offender in this respect. It causes a distortion of the calcium-phosphorus relationship of the blood. It also produces a condition of low blood sugar, strange as this might seem. Our teen-agers are more frequently fitted with glasses than their counterparts of previous eras, and in connection with this, we cannot overlook their jitterbug diet with its accent on candy, ice cream, cakes, pastries, soft drinks, etc. If sugar can cause cavities in the teeth, what is its effect on other more delicate organs? A note of caution is called for in the use of this category of food.

Rutin

A food product that is of proven value to the eye is rutin, a yellow powder extracted from buckwheat leaves. It is commonly used to strengthen artery walls to prevent strokes and hemorrhages. Dr. L. B. Somerville-Large, a famous English oculist, by means of rutin, was able to cure capillary fragility in the eye. In the interior of the eye, by means of a certain instrument, the oculist can see artery endings, and can observe the effect of giving rutin to strengthen them.

In Bicknell and Prescott's book *Vitamins in Medicine* (Grune and Stratton, 1953), an experiment was described in which rutin was administered to a group of patients with glaucoma, the tragic eye disease in which the pressure inside the eyeball rises. Among 26 patients who received rutin every day, 17 noticed a fall in the pressure inside the eye. Rutin may be safely taken by everyone as a preventive of capillary weakness all over the body.

Calcium

Dr. A. Huber, in a long article (*Ophthalmologia,* October, 1948), describes how he found the taking of calcium to be an effective means of clearing stubborn cases of inflammation of the pigmented layer of the eye, stating that a great amount of corroborative material has been accumulating in the medical literature. He quotes the work of 6 physicians who obtained the same results. He quotes, also, the work of other physicians who obtained results with calcium in a certain kind of conjunctivitis and in photophobia, which is an intolerance of the eye to light. He found it valuable also in excessive winking and in watering of the eye. Then he states, "The numerous reports of the efficacy of calcium therapy for the eye are now opposed, not only by the skepticism of strict scientific thought, but also by the hesitant attitude of many a practitioner."

In my reading of medical literature, and I subscribe to 30 medical journals, I find such skepticism quite general in connection with the medical profession's attitude towards the use of nutritional measures to combat and prevent disease. It is probably due to the training the medical student is given. He spends 99 per cent of the curricular time in studying the use of drugs and surgery. Nutrition still is the step-child of the medical sciences.

Milk is not the best food for obtaining calcium. There is evidence that pasteurization does something to the calcium in it that makes much of it unavailable to the human body. I don't say *not* to pasteur-ize milk, but if you are going to drink it with a feeling that you are getting calcium, you may wake up some fine day and find yourself calcium-deficient. Bone meal tablets are a sure way of getting needed calcium. Their effect in preventing cavities of the teeth is nothing short of sensational.

So much for specific elements of nutrition and their effect on the eye. But one word of caution. Many physicians are against the use of vitamins except in emergency situations. They say, "Get your vitamins with your knife and fork," but this is impossible, as can be seen by the extent of vitamin deficiencies prevailing in the public. There is an alarming decline in soil fertility that is reducing the nutritional quality of our food. There is much destruction of vitamins in the processing of food in the factories. Kitchen practices such as cooking, storing, soaking, paring, etc., take much out of food. Natural vitamins and minerals must be taken daily to restore that part of the food of which we are being robbed in so many ways, in the system of food production that our civilization forces upon us.

Soft Drinks

I have discussed briefly the possible effect of sugar on the eyes. May I speak for a moment or two about the effect of soft drinks on our vision? According to Hunter H. Turner, M.D., writing in the *Pennsylvania Medical Journal* (May, 1944), one of the predisposing causes of myopia, or near-sightedness, is the drinking of carbonated beverages. He states his belief that the carbonic acid they contain is the eye's worst enemy, and attributes the alarming increase in cases of myopia to "the pernicious guzzling of carbonated beverages by young children today."

In the stomach, he says, carbonated drinks break down into their basic ingredients of water and carbon dioxide, which goes to every part of the body. In the eye, it produces a chronic water-logging of certain important structures. An abnormal amount of fluid in the tissues of the white of the eye will cause a constriction of the vessels that traverse it and result in their congestion.

Yet, medical journals will regularly accept the advertisements of soft drink manufacturers. Here is a typical statement appearing in a recent ad: "The 'catalyst' of everybody's love of the carbonated soft drink is CO_2!" CO_2 is carbon dioxide, the very thing that should make the medical journal violently refuse such an advertisement.

Sunflower Seeds

Once I experimented with chickens on my farm, dividing them into two groups which were fed a uniform diet, except that one group received added sunflower seeds. The feathers of this group became more shiny and colorful, which is a sign of better health. I decided to eat sunflower seeds, too, to see what they would do for me. In about a week, I noticed a very startling thing. A slight intermittent quiver in my left eye went away. I usually suffered from this only in the winter when there is little opportunity for exercise or to be in the sun. This condition has never returned.

My eyes are not my strongest point. In the winter I would have trouble in walking on snow-blanketed roads. Before I became aware of the value of eating sunflower seeds, I left the house on the farm one day for a walk, but had to return after being out only a moment, as the excessive brightness of the snow interfered with my vision. In fact, it made the snow seem a pink color. After being on the sunflower diet for about a month, I noticed I could walk in the snow without distress. A little while later my car broke down and I had to walk over a mile on a snowed-up highway in bright sunshine. I had no trouble at all for the first three-quarters of the way. On the last stretch, the eyes smarted a little.

Because of this ability to stand snow glare, I imagined that sunflower seeds must be rich in vitamin A, but when I checked, I discovered that they contained only small amounts of this vitamin, but were unusually rich in vitamin B. And it is for this reason that they give the eyes a "resistance to light." Quoting from a French medical journal, "It seems that riboflavin (which is vitamin B_2) protects the cones in the eye from excess light, and that is the reason why it is found in the pigmented cells of the retina. It is probable that the pigment plays a very important role here. A deficiency in riboflavin brings about a lessening of visual acuity."

In pellagra, there is an injury to the cones of the eye, which makes them hypersensitive to light. During World War II, there was a condition of "camp eyes" and sun blindness which afflicted prisoners in concentration camps, and it was always traced to a pellagra condition caused by vitamin B deficiencies in the diet.

In the April, 1944, issue of *Organic Gardening* magazine, I published the details of my experience with sunflower seeds, and the reaction of my readers was dramatic and electric. In a few months, letters began to pour in by the hundreds. One reader wrote, "My eyes, which were causing considerable discomfort, seem much better." Another said, "After eating a handful of sunflower seeds each day for a month, I am able to fold bulletins without using my glasses, which I was unable to do a month before." Another one who needed glasses for sewing or other close work was able to dispense with them. Another wrote, "I have tried your suggestion and can see results almost instantly on the eyes." And so it went by the hundred.

It is a simple matter to try this experiment. Hulled sunflower seeds are now available from very many sources, so there need be no bother of shelling the seeds. If you are engaged in work where you are out in the sunshine, such as being a policeman, playing tennis, yachting, frequenting beaches, etc., start eating these seeds—a small handful or two a day and see if you won't be able to discard your sunglasses. You will be convinced that there is something in sunflower seeds that will enable you to withstand the glare of a tropical sun without using sunglasses.

As my own personal opinion, and not to be taken scientifically, I will hazard a guess that it is something in addition to vitamin B that exerts this mysterious power over the eyes. There is a phenomenon called heliotropism that can be observed in the sunflower. As soon as the head of the sunflower is formed, it always faces the sun, and as the sun swings its orbit across the heavens, the sunflower head turns with it, until, late in the day, it is facing due west to absorb the last few rays of the dying sun. The seed, therefore, is just drenched with sun vitality. It is a known fact, for example, the fruit growing on the outside of a tree, where it gets a lot of sunlight, contains more vitamins than that growing in the shady interior of the tree.

I cannot leave the subject of sunflower seeds without talking about Russia. You cannot talk to any Russian about these seeds without having him go into ecstatic raptures on the subject. Ivan does not know about their nutritional advantages, but he has always eaten them with zest. Russian table oil is obtained practically exclusively from sunflower seeds. In the old Czarist days in Russia, every soldier in the field received what was known as iron rations. These consisted of a bag of sunflower seeds weighing one kilogram (about 2.2 pounds). The soldier sometimes lived exclusively on these seeds. The army evidently was aware that they contained important nutritional values. Children in Russia prefer sunflower seeds to candy.

I have often wondered what the effect of this is on the Russian eyesight, and I obtained my answer when I recently saw a moving picture called *Inside Russia*. Rarely was a person to be seen who wore glasses. From what I observed, I would say that less than 10 per cent of the Russians wear glasses. In our country, 60 per cent of all adults are doomed to wear them, and the tendency is increasing. In the event of war between the United States and Russia, does this fact have some significance?

Conclusion

I have presented a great deal of data showing a direct connection between vitamins and minerals and the eyes, and that where nutrition went down, so did the ability to see. Does this hold any hope to adults; that is, to enable them to rid themselves of their glasses? I do not claim that. It can, however, prevent the onset of the terrible scourges of cataracts, glaucoma and senile blindness. It might also prevent the eyesight from further deterioration and assure full use of the eyes way into a healthy old age. It is part of the battle against general senility.

It is with children that the greatest hope lies. There the possibilities are far-reaching. There can be no question that, with a strong program to encourage proper nutrition, their eyesight can be preserved in all the strength conferred upon it at birth. In this regard, the Bausch and Lomb Optical Company has said, "As enzymes control all our metabolic processes and enzymes are composed of vitamins (or hormones or both), together with minerals and specific proteins, there is opportunity during the constructive stages of life to improve the condition of the eye through enhancing the nutritive values of the diet." (*Optical Developments,* February, 1957.)

Such enhancement of the nutritive values of the diet can begin in the home, but the schools can be a powerful influence, also, in teaching children about these nutritional practices that are harmful to the eyes. I would like to see developed an "eyesight" tablet made up of halibut liver oil for vitamin A, brewer's yeast for vitamin B, rose hips for vitamin C, vitamin E, bone meal and rutin, to be given daily to children in the schools. As part of the campaign, there could be large, blown-up photographs in the corridors of schools, of a goose wearing horn-rimmed glasses, with the caption, "Do you too want to be a four-eyed goose?"

Such a nutritional program will not only be conducive to an improvement in the general level of the country's vision, but it will build the health of the body generally. We must get the schools to make a thorough investigation of the facts enumerated in this discussion and take a strong hand towards adopting them into the school health program.

Faddists, Food

Answering Attacks on Food Faddists

Several of the women's magazines, many newspaper columnists who write on medical and health problems and some columnists who usually write about general subjects took up the current call to "beware of food faddists." "You are being gypped out of millions of dollars," they go on. They quote such authorities as the American Medical Association, the Food and Drug Administration and the Department of Agriculture. Without exception, every one of these warnings contains the statement that dietary deficiencies are rare in this country and most of our people get plenty of nourishment and their food supplies everything they need.

Why are such columns written and printed?

Other Articles

With this article in mind, we collected clippings of another sort at the same time the "beware" articles were appearing and in a few days, we got the following:

"In Perfect Health? Odds Say You're Not." A Tulane University study showed that 92 of every 100 persons studied in a 10-year survey had something wrong with them, even though they thought they were perfectly healthy. The majority of these folk were between 30 and 49 years old. Ninety-five per cent of the women who had trouble with their reproductive organs did not know they had it. Seventy per cent of those with hypertension (high blood pressure) did not know they had it.

Another headline: "U.S. Teen-Agers Are Starving Amid Plenty." Agriculture Secretary (at the time) Ezra Benson, whose department is so often quoted for attacking us faddists, said, in this article, "Never have the young people been more in need of wise advice and guidance on food. . . . Replacing their present faulty food habits with good ones will take the full cooperation of parents, teachers and teen-agers themselves." The figures which follow are discouraging, but not surprising, to any "food faddist." A Pennsylvania study showed that only 19 out of 2,500 teen-agers had perfect teeth. Of every 10 girls in a Montana survey, only 2 were rated adequately fed. A survey done at the University of California on 11 years of research on 4,000 students from 39 states revealed that the average intake of the girls was seriously low for calcium, iron, thiamin and ascorbic acid (vitamin C) or borderline low for calories and proteins. Another clipping tells us that a government survey shows that persons over 60 tend to eat too few foods containing protein, iron and the B vitamins, also vitamin A and vitamin C. "Diet of Aged Deficient" says the headline.

The 1960 White House Conference on Children and Youth, recognizing the seriousness of the situation, appointed two outstanding nutritionists to do further studies and make recommendations.

Finally, in the pages of the *Journal of the American Medical Association* for April 2, 1960, we found the following information in an article on "Farms and the Family Doctor." The total production of American farms can be tabulated in tons of grain and meat, etc. How much will this tell us about the eating habits of individuals? Very little, according to Dena C. Cedarquist, Head of the Department of Foods and Nutrition at Michigan State University. She said that people vary so much in their diets, that averages are practically meaningless. Records kept of what students eat may have little value because the students want to please by reporting a much better diet than they actually eat. "Much of the food faddism comes from dieticians like myself," she said.

So, according to this authority—and she is certainly just as competent an authority as any quoted in the "beware" articles—the situation is really much worse than the surveys indicate, and we actually do not have any way of checking on individuals, so, although an average may show a reasonably good diet, the individual diets of persons included may be much worse than the average.

Why the Attack?

Now, with facts like these on hand, why do articles appear attacking "food faddists"?

Most of the women's magazines are either owned outright by one or several of the big food companies or are controlled by them through editors or publishers who are on the board of directors or big stockholders in the company. These magazines are supported by their advertising and their advertising consists almost entirely of products which we food faddists warn against. Why should they not attack us editorially? We are taking money away from their advertisers with practically every article we write. Is any magazine which devotes 15 pages to cake recipes, so that its advertisers can sell cake mix, going to permit another magazine to say that cake eating is not healthful?

If you were editor of a magazine whose pages are filled with ads for dyed, chemicalized, refined, processed foods, wouldn't you do everything you could to discredit anyone who attacks such foods as being harmful? Once you realize that magazines of general circulation are completely controlled by their advertisers and that their editorial pages must say what their advertisers want them to say or the ads and the money they bring in will be withdrawn, then the whole picture becomes clear and easy to understand.

Hasn't it ever struck you as peculiar, with all the furor over chemicals in foods and the tremendous amount of evidence available showing that they may cause cancer, that no mention of that is ever made in any of the big women's magazines, even though they profess to be greatly concerned about their reader's health?

One of the silliest of all the "beware of faddists" columns that came in was on the subject of a "bird seed diet." This columnist, quoting a medical journal, ridiculed people who eat raw seeds like sunflower seeds, pumpkin seeds and so forth. He quoted the medical article as saying that eating such foods might cause one to avoid a "well-balanced diet" and thus be harmful.

We feel quite certain that such a columnist would believe a considerable part of a "well-balanced" diet to consist of cereals from which practically all nutrient has been removed by refining. Cereals are, of course, seeds. But anyone who likes to eat unrefined, unspoiled

---

Fleming, Sir Alexander

    One of today's most useful and at the same time most abused drugs due to indiscriminate prescription is the antibiotic, penicillin. Its discoverer was the British physician and bacteri-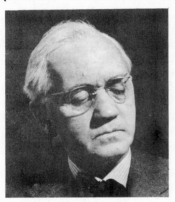*ologist, Sir Alexander Fleming. Fleming was born at Lochfield, Darvel, London Parish, Ayrshire, in 1881, and was educated at Kilmarnock Academy and St. Mary's Hospital School of the University of London. During his medical education, Fleming won practically every scholarship, award or prize given in the field of physiology, pharmacology, medicine, pathology, forensic medicine and hygiene. Due to this outstanding scholastic ability, Fleming was sure to make his mark on the world as a principal contributor to the science of medicine. And this he did, making two valuable contributions—the development in 1922 of the antiseptic Lysozyme and the discovery of penicillin. The latter find earned for Fleming together with Ernst Bris Chain, the Nobel Prize for physiology and medicine in 1945. Ten years later, on March 11, Fleming died in London, having given to medicine a weapon which, if used properly, is capable of destroying much suffering and disease.*

raw seeds in which all the rich nutriments are whole and unchanged is, *ipso facto,* a faddist who must be discredited. Now, just how silly can you get?

Dr. Stare's Position

Dr. Frederick Stare is head of the Department of Nutrition at the Harvard University School of Public Health. He is quoted almost everywhere as the outstanding authority on things having to do with nutrition. The February 14, 1960, issue of the *New York Times* announced that General Foods Corporation has made a grant of one million dollars to his department. A new 4-story nutrition laboratory will be built with the money.

Do you think Dr. Stare is going to find any fault with the products made and sold by this company? Or do you think instead that he will do everything he can to promote them and everything he can to attack and defame those who point out the deficiencies of many of these foods and the ill health they are certainly bringing to Americans? What would you do if you were Dr. Stare and wanted to keep your position in the world of science, your good job at Harvard and your good income?

Public Gets Misinformation

Incidentally, the Nutrition Foundation which is quoted as an authority on the dangers of food faddism is nothing more or less than an organization set up by the big food manufacturers partly to make statements of this kind. The Sugar Research Foundation makes statements "proving" that sugar is good for you, too. Why not?

They and the Nutrition Foundation have millions of dollars to spend in publicity campaigns to spread misinformation. They are just as blatant and just as blameworthy as the cigarette manufacturers who spend millions to tell you that cigarettes are good for you, except that the food people advertise in journals supposedly dedicated to the health and welfare of their readers. Directly or indirectly, they own the magazines.

The best program for meeting attacks like this is a two-point one. First, when friends and neighbors bring up the "beware of food faddist" articles, tell them some of the facts above, so that they will be better able to judge the truth of what they have read. Two, write to the magazines, newspapers or columnists and explain what the real situation is in regard to the inadequacy of our food supply.

Fallacies

How Nutritional Fallacies Get Started

Today's Health is the magazine published by the American Medical Association for the general public, the layman. While, it seems to us, very little that vitally pertains to health, as such, ever appears here, the questions of readers which are answered by the editors of *Today's Health* always interest us very much, for they represent the urgent questions that bother most families and the answers given represent, we suppose, the official position of the American Medical Association.

In the March, 1961, issue, we found a question from a reader asking whether a 6-month-old baby requires more in the way of vitamin supplements than 30 milligrams of vitamin C, 400 units of vitamin D and .5 milligrams of fluorine daily (as recommended by the reader's pediatrician).

The answer states that the Committee of Nutrition is studying whether or not fluorine or "fluoride iron" should be recommended as a dietary supplement. It goes on to say that "fluoride iron" has been shown in many studies to make the enamel of the teeth harder and more resistant to the formation of cavities. "Many experts interested in dental health have suggested the supplemental intake of sodium fluoride in amounts of .5 to 1 milligram per day—in areas where the water supply does not contain fluoride."

We have never heard of such a substance as fluoride "iron." However, the general impression given is that there certainly is such a substance as fluoride iron and that the AMA is seriously considering whether they should recommend that all children get some of this fluoride "iron" as a daily supplement.

Error Not Corrected

If indeed this was an error, it seems incumbent upon *Today's Health* to apologize for it and correct it in a later issue. We never saw such an apology or correction. If it was not an error, how could it happen that the highest authority in the land, especially on the subject of fluoride, could have been so misinformed as to believe that fluoride iron is something that has been tested in relation to tooth decay? Then, too, it is usual to speak of iron compounds as ferric or ferrous compounds. Thus, one would speak of ferric fluoride or ferrous fluoride—not fluoride iron.

We object to this kind of error for two reasons. First, because it is made by the very people who claim that *we* don't have the professional background to speak intelligently about nutrition and health. Secondly, because such misinformation, if uncorrected, starts nutritional fallacies. How many readers of *Today's Health* will read this page and go away with a confused idea that somehow fluorine is related to iron and hence necessary to prevent anemia and build strong bodies! Considering the welter of misinformation about fluoride already abroad in the land, one more erroneous idea will help to make the situation even more difficult.

In a town meeting or a city council meeting where the pro-fluoridationists have done everything they can to confuse the issue and bludgeon the unknowing into agreement, some reader of *Today's Health* is bound to arise and announce that fluorine is good not just because it's fluorine but because it contains iron as well—he read it in a publication of the American Medical Association and it's a well known fact that they don't make any mistakes!

Letters Not Answered

We have found that it is useless to write to *Today's Health* pointing out errors like this and asking for corrections, even though we are paid-up subscribers. We once challenged their statement that spinach is not a good food because it contains very little iron. We wrote to the author of the article every month for 5 months without receiving a reply. Then we wrote to the editor of *Today's Health*. No answer. Finally, we wrote to the President of the American Medical Association. No answer.

In every letter we pointed out that this was a serious misstatement of fact which would lead to entirely wrong ideas of eating among many people. We asked for a scientific source of such information, and we noted that many textbooks and scientific references indicate that spinach is a very rich source of iron, regardless of what other disadvantages it may have as a food. We were especially distressed because several other general publications had taken up this comment from *Today's Health* and reprinted it as fact.

Now, *Today's Health* has done it again, this time telling readers that fluoride "iron" is the substance which "in many studies" made teeth harder and more resistant to decay. This is how nutritional fallacies get started.

Fats

Fats in Food

Fats have not received the long-time study in nutritional laboratories that have been devoted to carbohydrates and proteins, so our knowledge of them is much more limited. And controversial. For, until we have quite a large body of knowledge on any nutritional subject, new discoveries are likely to set off a battle royal among those who do and those who do not accept any new idea. Especially is this true when large commercial interests are at stake and one side or the other is egged on by financial grants which, in a gentleman's agreement, are meant to guarantee that certain results will be found and certain conclusions drawn.

Several years ago, we began to investigate the importance of the unsaturated fatty acids—a certain kind of fat existing in food, which carries this awkward name because there are certain molecules of the fat which are, you might say, at loose ends. They are "unsaturated" and hence likely to be "filled" or "saturated" by any convenient substance which happens to be around, capable of taking over the unoccupied place in the chain of molecules.

Unsaturated fatty acids exist in largest quantity in foods of vegetable origin. Animal fats are richer in the saturated kind.

When oxygen is added to the unsaturated fatty acids, an atom of oxygen moves into the empty link, joins itself chemically to the other atoms and what happens? The fat becomes rancid. When hydrogen is added, it moves into the empty link, joins itself to the other atoms and we have what is called "hydrogenated" fat—a thick fat which is solid at room temperature. Unsaturated fats are liquid at room temperature. This suggests immediately that the unsaturated fats exist in far greater quantity in vegetable foods—and saturated fats in foods of animal origin—salad oils are liquid at room temperature; butter, lard and suet are solid at room temperature.

Most of the controversy in nutritional circles has raged around these two kinds of fats and much of the argument has appeared in newspapers and magazines of general circulation because of a very important relationship to the formation of cholesterol deposits. Many researchers believe that lecithin (a vegetable fat rich in the unsaturated fatty acids) should be taken in preference to animal fats, because lecithin apparently acts like an emulsifier, keeping the cholesterol moving along in little globules and doing no harm, just as it is supposed to.

In 1956, it was pointed out that unsaturated fatty acids have been successfully used for treating asthma and a number of skin disorders—eczema, psoriasis, etc. Arthritis, too, may be improved by including these fats in the diet, according to researchers. Later, it was reported that seborrhea and prostate gland disorders responded to diets in which unsaturated fatty acids played a big part.

Dr. H. M. Sinclair of Oxford University, England, believes that lack of the unsaturated fatty acids and an overabundance of the saturated kind may have a lot to do with many disorders we "civilized" nations suffer from. Dr. Sinclair found in experiments that rats who ate diets *in which there was no fat at all* suffered from cholesterol deposits. He believes this is because such a diet does not contain the important unsaturated fats which keep cholesterol in check. He says further, that the more *saturated* fats your diet contains, the more *unsaturated* fats you need to balance them. The kind of diet which produces hardening of the arteries and cholesterol deposits is one high in cholesterol and/or unnatural fats, and (equally important) low in the unsaturated fats.

"Unnatural" Fats Are Hydrogenated

By "unnatural fats," Dr. Sinclair means the hydrogenated ones —that is, vegetable fats processed with hydrogen so that their healthful, unsaturated fats become saturated with hydrogen. These are such fats as margarine, the white, thick shortenings sold so widely for baking, lard, which is usually hydrogenated and, of course, all the foods which contain such unnatural fats—and this means just about everything that has been processed—bread, crackers, bakery products, frozen prepared foods like TV dinners, restaurant foods, all commercially fried foods like potato chips, salted nuts, etc. When you stop to think of it, many Americans consume large quantities of this kind of food and practically never eat foods which contain the healthful unsaturated fats—salad oils and unrefined seed foods chiefly— nuts, cereal germs, beans, etc.

Is animal fat really destructive of human health in the quantities in which Americans eat it? Our conclusion is that most of us eat far too much animal fat, especially in relation to the amount of vegetable fat we eat and the amount of "hidden fat" which may consist almost entirely of hydrogenated, processed fat which can do serious harm. Nations whose fat consumption is extremely low appear to have a far smaller incidence of and mortality from heart and blood vessel disorders. Countries where animal fats were sharply rationed during the war experienced a sharp decline in such disorders. But, of course, other things were rationed, too (sugar, for instance) and this may have had considerable influence on what happened.

Natural Vegetable Fats Best

However, by 1957-58, researchers were tackling the problem of cholesterol deposits and hardening of the arteries by feeding likely candidates for these disorders with vegetable fats to the exclusion of animal fats, and were apparently getting good results. Dr. Sinclair at Oxford used safflower oil, other researchers used corn oil as the basic fat of diets which appeared to reduce the cholesterol content of the blood decidedly. Much evidence began to appear showing that milk may not be the "perfect food" it has long been called. A food of animal origin, it is high in saturated fats. Butter, cheese, cream and other dairy products are, too, of course.

After doing a considerable amount of research on fats good and bad, we came to this conclusion: All natural vegetable sources of fat are recommended. There is considerable fat in nuts, avocados, sunflower seeds and other seeds. Peanuts and soybeans are rich in good fats. Wheat and rice germ, pumpkin seeds, sesame seeds, peanuts—these contain lots of the natural, unprocessed fats of the valuable, unsaturated variety. Eating them raw assures us that the fats as well as vitamins present have not suffered any harmful chemical change. We believe that you should avoid fats of animal origin, in general, except, of course, for the fat that naturally occurs in meats, poultry, fish and eggs. Choose lean meats and fish and avoid dairy products, for the fats of cream, butter and milk are chiefly of the saturated variety. Most important of all, however, avoid the processed, hydrogenated fats and foods made from them.

Freud, Sigmund

Sigmund Freud, the Austrian physician noted as the Father of Psychoanalysis, was born in Freiberg Moravia, May 6, 1856. Under the patronage of a Jewish philanthropic society, Freud 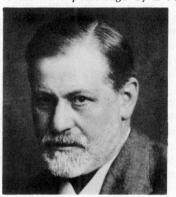 *entered the University of Vienna to begin studies toward his medical degree which he received in 1881. The next year found him at the Vienna General Hospital as a resident assistant physician. Here, under the influence of Theodor H. Meynert, Freud began to show a great interest in psychiatry. Pursuing this interest, Freud traveled to Paris to study under the famous neurologist, Jean Martin Charcot. There studies made their imprint on Freud, for it was their influence which started Freud on his life study of the psychological aspects of the mind. He first dabbled in the hypnotic treatment of mental ills which he dropped in favor of a method of free association —the "talking out" of a patient's innermost thoughts. This in turn led to Freud's doctrine of repression. Releasing these repressions from the unconscious through a process of talking out causes the patient to understand his true nature and thus readjust his life to include acceptable behavior patterns to replace them. This is the basic principle of psychoanalysis, Freud's important contribution to the conquest of mental illness.*

Vitamin B Essential to Fat Metabolism

As research continues in the field of fats, undoubtedly new ideas and theories will emerge. We will discover more about the relationship of certain of the B vitamins to the way our bodies use fats—a very important aspect of the whole affair, because without enough B vitamins in the diet, fats are not metabolized properly. Undoubtedly, even the simplest method of processing is important in our thinking about fats. Heating and re-heating fats is destructive of the nutriments and forms substances that are cancer-causing. This is why we caution against fried foods, especially those prepared by heating the same fats again and again.

Feet

Women with Sore Feet—Unite!

It is the women you see leaning against a wall downtown, taking off a shoe for a few seconds of blessed relief. It is the women who kick off their shoes in the movies or in a restaurant booth. It is the women who wear nothing but flats or bedroom slippers at home for comfort. These are the women who pinch themselves into dagger-pointed shoes and skyscraper heels when they leave the house, and who demand the same from the shoe clerk when they're out for a new pair of shoes. These are the ladies who protest to their foot doctors that they should put pressure on the shoe manufacturers to build sensible shoes for fashion.

At the American Podiatry Association convention, says Arthur Snider of the *Chicago Daily News* (August 29, 1960), the proceedings were interrupted so that a member might read a letter from a "prominent Chicago club woman." She wrote, "The long narrow and very pointed toes are crippling us. We have no room for our toes, especially for the large and small ones. Never have we suffered as we do now. I have talked with hundreds of women and all cry for relief." The writer went on to plead for a return of rounded-toed shoes.

At the same convention, a female podiatrist, Dr. Riesgraf, predicted that ultimately women's forefeet will become "just one big toe." She went on to say that, "No woman would tolerate gloves that deform her hands or eyeglasses which blind her, no matter how fashionable they are considered. But she will wear foot gear that is crippling her feet just because it is in fashion."

Sympathy for women who complain of uncomfortable styles comes hard when one is clearly aware that these women are happy in their misery. They adopted the style of the pointed toe and stiletto heel as though they had been waiting centuries for just such a gift.

There has never been a product yet that was a success if the consumers refused to accept it. Manufacturers react to the demands of those who buy their wares. If women were to go into shoe stores demanding to be shown shoes that are more practical and more comfortable, the word would soon get back to the manufacturer. If women would write letters, like the Chicago club woman's, not to podiatry conventions, but to shoe manufacturers conventions, a style change would come. But if women keep buying pointed shoes and heels that go higher and higher, they can expect the stores to get new supplies as soon as the old ones are depleted.

Consequences of Pointed Shoes

We were surprised and puzzled at this headline in the Allentown, Pennsylvania, *Morning Call* (January 17, 1961): "Winkle Pickers Set Just Lost Toehold." The article explained that "winkle pickers" is the name, in Scotland, for pointed-toed shoes—"They're so pointy you can dig a little mussel called a winkle out of its shell with them."

What brought "winkle pickers" into the news was a story of a young man, Mark O'Kane, who was faced with the concrete proposition: give up your shoes or your toes. Mark, a salesman in charge of the shoe department at a Glasgow store, had such painful feet—after wearing out 6 pairs of "winkle pickers"—that he went to a hospital. There doctors broke and reset 8 toes, and advised amputating two from each foot. "I'll give up my shoes, but not my toes," said Mark. He heaved his last pair of "winkle pickers" into the corner of his hospital ward.

Probably Mark's mistake was that he had not put any effort into gradually deforming his feet. In America, women wear what must be close to "winkle pickers" all the time. But they begin training when they are 9 years old, with cuban heels and narrower points to their shoes. By mid-teen age, they wear shoes narrow enough in the toe to be used for picking locks, and with heels so high and thin they could be knocked over by a stiff breeze. They grow so used to wearing such shoes that they don't even know that the painful legs and backs that are common to them, as well as the corns and bunions, are due to nothing but the kind of shoes they wear. Of course women's feet become deformed, only they don't feel the pain and recognize the need for correction, as Mark did, because the women have become used to this torture.

Relax with Your Feet Up

When you put your feet up to relax, you're really doing yourself a big favor. Aside from the fact that it feels good, having your feet higher than your head does wonders for your circulation. The *Lancet* (December 19, 1960) tells of actual observations, when the chest cavity was exposed, of the influx of blood from the limbs which was enough to start a heart beating after it had stopped. With this in mind, the author, W. W. Woodward, believes that, before one takes the drastic step of entering the chest cavity to massage the heart in dire emergency, one should first see if an elevation of the lower limbs will induce heartbeat.

Dr. Woodward gives 3 brief case histories in which the heart, though it was not actually involved in the surgery, stopped beating while the operation was in progress. In each case the quick-thinking attendants were able to elevate both arms and legs almost immediately. Within 15 seconds, the heartbeat began again, with sufficient strength to complete the operation in two of the cases, while the third was successfully completed after a few days.

This easy supply of blood to the heart and brain can come to you whenever you elevate your feet. The extra supply of oxygen to the brain via the blood, will make you think better and relax easier. Many people use a specially made "slant board" which gives the legs high support as one lies on it feet up. The contour chair also accomplishes this with the greatest degree of comfort. If you don't wish to buy special equipment, a couple of pillows under your legs as you lie in bed or on the sofa will do the trick.

If you nap frequently, don't waste the opportunity to elevate your legs, perhaps with a hassock, at least to the level of the seat you are using. You can give your circulation a boost without even trying.

Fingernails

Gelatin and the Fingernails

What are the true powers of commercial gelatin (unflavored) in treating brittle and fragile fingernails? Perhaps the answer lies in an article by Terence Lloyd Tyson, M.D., which was marked "Received for publication, November 19, 1949," and appeared sometime thereafter in the *Journal of Investigative Dermatology*. He tells of giving a patient gelatin by mouth in an effort to relieve muscular weakness. After 3 months, he noticed that her nails, always fragile and unsightly, had become practically normal in appearance and texture.

Encouraged by this chance response, Dr. Tyson observed 12 patients who had complained of soft, peeling, easily breaking fingernails for from 1 to 15 years. No detectable dietary deficiency was present. He gave each of them 7 grams of gelatin dissolved in water or juice once a day. In 10 of the patients, the nails took on a completely normal appearance in 13 weeks. In several of the patients, the toenails improved in the same way as the fingernails did. Several even reported improvement in the growth of hair and eyebrows. Two cases failed to respond, but it was not certain that they had maintained the daily dose of gelatin.

It is worth remembering that none of these patients had any *observable* deficiencies, yet 10 of them received some needed element from the gelatin which must have been missing before. Perfect nutrition in our modern world is almost impossible, and food supplementation is the only way to be certain of adequate nourishment. For those who wonder about the effectiveness of treating brittle fingernails with gelatin, we think Dr. Tyson's work is very convincing.

Fluoridation

Does Water Fluoridation Really Reduce Tooth Decay?

The old saying that "figures don't lie" is a fallacy. Today, we know that figures, or, as we call them, statistics, do lie very often. We know that they can be made to lie by ignoring certain parts of the collected figures, misinterpreting certain parts, leaving out certain parts or simply collecting an incomplete and hence unreliable set of figures from which to draw your conclusions.

The facts and figures on water fluoridation, accepted widely as proven and final, have now been shown to be faulty to the point of being almost completely meaningless. A full study and analysis of the figures appears in the book *Fluoridation, Errors and Omissions in Experimental Trials* by Philip R. N. Sutton. Dr. Sutton is no crackpot. He is Senior Research Fellow of the Department of Oral Medicine and Surgery of the Dental School of the University of Melbourne, Australia.

Dr. Sutton's Conclusions

Here are Dr. Sutton's conclusions on the statistical facts concerning the tests on water fluoridation, which form the *only* basis for promotion of this method of controlling dental decay! He says that the reliability of the results of the tests is affected by: (1) odd experimental and statistical methods used; (2) failure to consider several important aspects of such a test, for instance, the possibility of bias on the part of a dental examiner; (3) omission of relevant data; (4) arithmetical errors; (5) misleading comments.

In setting up scientific experiments, it is essential that controls be used. That is, if you are testing fluoridation in one city, you must compare the results you get with another city where water is not fluoridated. Furthermore, conditions in the control city must be as nearly similar as possible to the test city. Dr. Sutton tells us that, in the American fluoridation tests, controls were either doubtful or inadequate and no control at all was employed in one trial, which is regularly held up by fluoridation promoters as proof of the effectiveness of fluoridation.

Dr. Sutton says that the published data—that is, the scientific papers that have appeared in scientific publications—do not justify the statement that tooth decay rates remained the same in the control (unfluoridated) cities. That is, while decay decreased in the fluoridated cities, it also decreased in the non-fluoridated cities.

He concludes, "The sound basis on which the efficacy of a public health measure must be assessed is not provided by these 5 crucial trials"— that is, the 5 "test cities" pointed to as proof by the fluoridationists.

Control Cities

"It has been shown," he says, "that the reports of the controls used in these fluoridation trials contain arithmetical and statistical errors, and that results and relevant data were omitted. Also, misleading statements were made which denied, ignored or underrated the unexplained changes in caries attack rates which took place in the control cities and which suggested that the pre-fluoridation data from the test cities, and those obtained during the basic examinations in control ones, were more closely comparable than was the case."

For instance, in the fluoridation test which was set up in Newburgh, New York, a neighboring city, Kingston, was used as a control. While the fluoridators were publishing the startling facts that tooth decay had decreased among the children in fluoridated Newburgh, it soon became apparent from figures published in 1945-46 and 1949, that tooth decay was decreasing also among the children in non-fluoridated Kingston. Instead of investigating this significant fact, the Public Health officials in charge of the test simply stopped publishing any more figures on the decay among Kingston children. That's certainly one way to tailor figures to fit the case you mean to prove.

It is also true that the water supplies of Newburgh and Kingston are entirely different, as Dr. Sutton shows on page 49 of this book. The Newburgh water supply contains almost 6 times as much calcium and 4 times as much magnesium as the water supply of Kingston. Yet, the Public Health officials who set up the experiment announced that the waters of the two cities were "comparable" at the beginning of the experiment and remained so. Now when a scientist says "comparable" he does not mean that the test group is getting 4 or 6 times as much as the control group of important minerals like calcium and magnesium! This is the very question the experiment was designed to prove—the effectiveness of certain mineral substances in the water supply for preventing tooth decay. Why then should the experimenters have completely ignored this gross difference in mineral content of the two waters? Especially since calcium is extremely important for tooth health, as every dental researcher knows.

Proof against Fluoridation

We have given only a paragraph or two of the vitally important material this book contains. We urge that you read it in full. Dr. Sutton's arguments are unanswerable. They completely invalidate the claims made by the pro-fluoridators. The "proof" presented up to now of the decrease in tooth decay in fluoridated test cities is not proof at all. The published reports on the experiments show important omissions, deletions, misinterpretations.

And this critique of the scientific reports on fluoridation was made by an Australian researcher who started out with no prejudice in his views on fluoridation. He had no test cities to study first-hand, no pressure on him from groups who wanted this or that to be proved. He had only the published material on which the case for water fluoridation has been promoted.

Surely, there can be no doubt in the mind of anyone who reads this book that there is no convincing proof that fluoridation decreases tooth decay as we have been told it does. What more evidence do we need to decide that we want no part of this plan?

The name of the book is *Fluoridation, Errors and Omissions in Experimental Trials* by Philip R. N. Sutton, published by the Melbourne University Press, Melbourne, Australia.

The Safety Factor with Fluoridated Water

An opinion on the toxicity of fluorides in drinking water was expressed forcibly by two experts in the field, Herbert E. Stokinger, Jr., Chief Toxicologist, Occupational Health Program, United States Public Health Service, Cincinnati, and Richard L. Woodward, Chief of Water Supply, Robert A. Taft Sanitary Engineering Center, Public Health Service, Cincinnati.

The article appears in the *Journal of the American Water Works* for April, 1958. It deals with "Toxicological Methods for Establishing Drinking Water Standards." In a chart showing the estimated safety factor of minerals for drinking water, we find that arsenic has a safety factor of 10. Lead has a safety factor of 3 to 10. Cyanide has a safety factor of 40 to 125.

Fluorine has a safety factor of zero.

How should you interpret such a recommendation? "Safety factor" is a word used often in these days when poisons are all around us and some methods must be used to control them and to provide a minimum of safety for people who are exposed to them. Let's compare it to the expected load of traffic on a bridge. If the official limit of weight on a bridge is 2000 pounds, this does not mean that a truck weighing 2001 pounds is bound to crash through the flooring. A "safety factor" has been allowed for by the engineer. He has made the bridge strong enough to hold more than 2000 pounds. But, just to be on the safe side, he sets the official limit of weight at 2000 pounds. The difference between 2000 pounds and the actual weight at which a truck will crack through the flooring is the "safety factor."

No Allowance Made for Safety Factor

Water department engineers apparently think that arsenic (a deadly poison, of course) may be safely present in water up to .6 parts per million. The safety factor of 10 indicates that 10 times this amount of arsenic in water would still be safe "for a healthy adult," according to water toxicology standards. Nineteen parts per million of cyanide may be allowed in a drinking water supply, because you must have as much as 40 to 125 times this much of cyanide to endanger the health of adults drinking the water. Lead, we know, is a highly toxic, cumulative metal. Yet one part per million of lead is permissible in a water supply, say our engineers because there is a "safety factor" of 3 to 10. That is, 3 to 10 times that much would still be safe, so the engineers feel that they can allow one part per million.

Fluoride is the only water contaminant for which the safety factor is zero. The limit for water is 1.25 parts per million according to the chart. The safety factor is zero. In other words, this limit has not been set with the assurance that it takes 3 or 4 or 10 times this much to be poisonous. Anything over 1.25 parts per million of fluoride is likely to be toxic. That is what a zero "safety factor" means. And that is the safety factor set by toxicologists of the United States Public Health Service—the same outfit which is promoting water fluoridation the length and breadth of the country.

If they were trying to persuade us to add arsenic to our drinking water, we would still have a margin of safety. Cyanide, as lethal as it is, could be added in considerably larger quantities than it is usually found in water supplies, because there is such a big safety factor.

But fluoride is so dangerous that the amount *actually recommended by the Public Health Service is the largest amount* we dare to take in a water supply, without possible harm to "a healthy adult." There is no allowance made for a safety factor.

The table is based on the assumption that everyone who drinks the water is a "healthy adult." No allowance is made for children, for babies, for old people or for the millions of chronically ill.

Here is one of the most devastating arguments against water

fluoridation that we have ever come across, from an article by two Public Health toxicologists published in the official magazine of the American Water Works Association.

Who Is Against Fluoridation—and When?

We reprint here some excerpts from an editorial in the *Journal of the American Dental Association* for October 1, 1944. (We put in the italics for emphasis.)

"Comparison made by Arnold (in the *Journal of the American Dental Association,* April, 1943) of the dental caries (decay) picture in children living in communities where the water contains not more than 1.0 parts per million (of fluoride) and that of children living in communities using fluoride-free waters shows that (1) about 6 times as many children show no dental caries experience; (2) about a 60 per cent lower dental caries experience rate exists; and (3) there is almost a 75 per cent decrease in first permanent molar loss.

"While these data are certainly speculatively attractive as leading to possible mass treatment of caries, our knowledge of the subject certainly does not warrant the introduction of fluorine in community water supplies generally.

"Sodium fluoride is a highly toxic substance, and while its application in safe concentrations and under strict control by competent personnel, may prove to be useful therapeutically, under other circumstances it may be definitely harmful.

"To be effective, fluorine must be ingested into the system during the years of tooth development, and we do not yet know enough about the chemistry involved to anticipate what other conditions may be produced in the structure of the bone and other tissues of the body generally.

"We do know that the use of drinking water containing as little as 1.2 to 3.0 parts per million of fluorine will cause such developmental disturbance in bones as osteosclerosis, spondylosis and osteopetrosis, as well as goiter, and we cannot afford to run the risk of producing such serious systemic disturbances in applying what is at present a doubtful procedure intended to prevent development of dental disfigurements among children . . .

"With regard to the safety margin in the fluorine content of drinking water, the reported amount of fluorine in the water cannot be taken as the criterion for the amount taken in the system, as in an intensely hot climate much larger quantities of water would be imbibed and hence a much larger quantity of fluorine would be taken into the body. Another feature of the complex problem that demands consideration, in attempting to take advantage of the therapeutic value of fluorine, is the quantity absorbed by the system at various age periods of life.

"M. C. Smith and H. V. Smith, in their studies at St. David, Arizona, found that, of the people using drinking water containing 1.6 to 4.0 parts per million of fluorine at the ages of 12 to 14, 33 per cent had caries; at ages 21 to 41, nearly 100 per cent had caries; from 24 to 41, 50 per cent had all teeth extracted and replaced by dentures. The authors concluded from these data that the teeth of the individuals of a community in which comparatively large amounts of fluorine are found, in this case say 1.6 to 4.0 parts per million, are structurally weak; in some cases, the tooth structure being so impaired as to crumble on attempts to place fillings. (*American Journal of Public Health,* September, 1940.)

"Because of our anxiety to find some therapeutic procedure that will promote mass prevention of caries, the seeming potentialities of fluorine appear speculatively attractive; but, in the light of our present knowledge or lack of knowledge of the chemistry of the subject, the potentialities for harm far outweigh those for good."

The American Dental Association, in the pages of whose official magazine the above editorial appeared, is at present the most devout official champion of water fluoridation, with the exception of the United States Public Health Service.

What Has Changed?

What has changed in these passing years, gentlemen? Not the fluoride ion, which remains just the same as it has been for more centuries than man has been on this earth. Not human physiology, human tissue, human reaction to toxic substances. How does it happen that drinking water containing as little as 1.2 parts per million caused osteosclerösis, spondylosis and osteopetrosis, as well as goiter, in 1944, and does not cause them today?

Is it possible that there is some magic ingredient present when poisonous fluoride is poured into the hopper of a municipal water works which causes everybody in town to drink exactly the right amount of water? But no, back in 1944, the official spokesman of the American Dental Association warned us that there is a wide variation in the amount of water drunk by various people at different times of the year and in different climates. What has happened in the interval to change these facts?

Drs. H. V. and M. C. Smith of the University of Arizona, for many years the world's greatest experts on fluorides and their action in the body, were regarded in 1944 by a spokesman of the American Dental Association as authorities whose findings of tooth extractions and crumbling teeth should be taken with utmost seriousness. Why are these findings dismissed today as the work of crackpots and fanatics? Are not these facts just as true now as they were then?

What are we to make of a statement in the *Journal* in 1944 which says that sodium fluoride is a highly toxic substance which can be administered safely *only under strict control by competent personnel,* and the present-day attitude of the *Journal,* that anybody who works at the city water works is perfectly capable of throwing a bag of sodium fluoride into the drinking water and, by this gesture, assuring everybody in town of getting "strict control" of the proper amount of this "highly toxic" substance?

Opinion Changed

If you write to the *Journal of the American Dental Association* (222 East Superior Street, Chicago, Illinois) and ask for a copy of this issue of the *Journal,* then show it to the fluoridation promoters in your locality, they will probably assure you that everything has changed since then. Now we know, they will tell you, that fluoridated water is harmless.

Ask them how it happens that fluorides caused diseases in 1944 and do not cause them today. If they say the *Journal* made a mistake in the facts in the 1944 editorial, ask them how we can be sure the *Journal* (and everybody else concerned) is not making a mistake today. Poisoning everybody in a community is a pretty serious error to be making, especially since the only excuse for doing it is dental decay in children, which can perfectly and easily be controlled by a few simple changes in diet—and no one knows this fact better than a dentist!

Some Fluoridation Gobbledegook

The January, 1961, issue of the *Research Reporter,* put out by the Oklahoma Medical Research Foundation, contains a guest editorial by Paul W. Goaz, D.D.S., that is really a "lulu." Dr. Goaz is Head of the Dental Section. His editorial is on a "New Type Fluoride Now Under Study."

From his first paragraph, we learn that "a project being undertaken by the Dental Section . . . might go a long way toward taking some of the wind out of the anti-fluoridationists' sails."

Since it is *our* sails he is talking about, we naturally became interested. His second paragraph contains statements that make you stop and wonder about the peculiar brand of science we are dealing with in fluoridation, or whether it is science at all.

Some of His Statements

Let us consider some of these statements. His new fluoride compound, Dr. Goaz writes, "has been shown to be 7 to 8 times less toxic than the fluoride compounds that have been employed to date for the purpose of reducing decay." From this, anyone would conclude that Dr. Goaz recognized that presently employed fluorides are toxic, and therefore pose some health hazard.

But his next sentence says, "There is absolutely no danger involved in the use of the fluoride compounds now being employed, in the manner recommended."

If the fluorides now in use have "absolutely no danger," that can only be because they are absolutely non-toxic. Therefore, how can Dr. Goaz' new fluoride compound be "7 to 8 times less toxic" than preparations having no toxicity at all? If you have nothing to begin with, how can you possibly get one-seventh or one-eighth of it?

When you really dig into this fluoridation gobbledegook, this is what you always end up with—nothing.

Of course, you may also wonder about the Oklahoma Medical Research Foundation. Why does this research center spend money for Dr. Goaz to test a new fluoride compound that is supposed to be safer than fluorides which are now in use and which, according to Dr. Goaz himself, have "absolutely no danger"? You would think that the Oklahoma Medical Research Foundation would be aware of more important medical problems in which it would invest its limited funds.

But this is fluoridation, not science, that we are dealing with. And the two are worlds apart. Keep that in mind and you will be able to understand a lot of things that are being done and said on behalf of fluoridation.

Scientific Support for Fluoridation

Now let's look at something else that Dr. Goaz wrote: "At this point, lest the continued mention of toxicity becomes alarming, it can be stated that the use of fluorides, for the control of decay, has, without a doubt, as much, if not more, scientific support for its safety and effectiveness than any other public health procedure now in use or contemplated."

Let us assume, as Dr. Goaz wrote, that there is "absolutely no danger involved in the use of fluoride compounds now being employed, in the manner recommended." If Dr. Goaz really believes that, why did he write his editorial with "continued mention of toxicity" that he felt might become "alarming"?

We who are opposed to fluoridation repeatedly sound an alarm because we know it is dangerous. Dr. Goaz, on the other hand, keeps talking, in his article, about the toxicity of fluorides which, he claims, have "absolutely no danger."

Perhaps you can make some sense out of his contradictory position. Frankly, we cannot. But perhaps it is necessary to read his article while standing on your head because fluoridation is such a mixed-up, crazy, upside-down sort of thing. Perhaps then, fluoridation would be understandable, and such contradictions as Dr. Goaz' might seem perfectly all right. We are, therefore, now practicing headstands.

But let's return to that last statement by Dr. Goaz, which we've quoted above. According to Dr. Goaz, fluoridation "has, without a doubt, as much, if not more, scientific support for its safety and effectiveness than any other public procedure now in use or contemplated."

Hard to Substantiate 3 Big Assumptions

This is really a big order, for what Dr. Goaz implies is that: (1) He has evaluated the relative scientific support for *all* possible public health measures. You name it—cancer, heart disease, mental illness, nutrition, etc.—and Dr. Goaz has already evaluated the thing! (2) He has considered *all* public health procedures that are not only now in use, but are contemplated. This covers *all* public health work from now until the end of time; it includes everything in the future from here on in forever! (3) Finally, Dr. Goaz declares no public health procedure that may ever be instituted at any time and at any place can possibly have more scientific support than fluoridation now has.

After regaining consciousness and picking ourselves up from the floor, we would be forced to agree with Dr. Goaz . . . if we considered only such cases as the Salk vaccine and the antibiotic mess which Dr. Welch created in the Food and Drug Administration, for these things are as phoney as fluoridation.

If what Dr. Goaz wrote were true, it would mean the end of American science, and ultimately the end of our great nation. We seriously doubt this.

From another point of view, however, it may be in order to congratulate the Oklahoma Medical Research Foundation which is fortunate in having Dr. Goaz on its staff. No other institute, to the best of our knowledge, has anyone who can evaluate the relative scientific merit of *all* public health measures that are now in use or may come up anywhere in the future between now and the end of time.

Scientists admit they cannot make such predictions and don't try to do so. Fluoridationists, on the other hand, apparently feel they can and do so. That is why we say that, when you are dealing with fluoridation, you are not dealing with science.

Conclusion

In conclusion, let us again point this out. Dr. Goaz stated his editorial "might go a long way toward taking some of the wind out of the antifluoridationists' sails." We have examined his article, and analyzed it from a scientific point of view. It seems that, if Dr. Goaz succeeded, he would only have replaced the wind in our sails with a lot of hot air.

Actually, Dr. Goaz has done us a big favor. By again revealing the kind of muddled, contradictory pseudo-scientific thinking that is behind the whole fluoridation program, he has provided us with additional ammunition and motivation to fight this form of medical insanity. Far from "taking some of the wind out of our sails," Dr. Goaz has made it possible for us to sail on more rapidly and more directly toward our goal. When we realize that we are fighting not only against fluoridation, but also against the kind of unscientific thinking revealed in Dr. Goaz' editorial, we are that much more confident that we must win and that we will win.

Is Fluoridation Corrupting American Science?

Throughout the world, there has been extensive criticism of conflicting, incomplete and unscientific reports by American promoters of fluoridation. Some of this criticism has been based on re-evaluation of facts and figures or on inaccuracy of data.

Given a set of conditions on which to base an experiment or test, different researchers might conceivably arrive at different conclusions, depending on how they worked out the problem or interpreted the results. But a researcher, blindly dedicated to a proposition like fluoridation, would have difficulty, we believe, in accepting results that were contrary to what he wanted to prove. In spite of efforts to be honest, he might be inclined to interpret data according to the way he *wanted* the experiment to come out. This is certainly not scientific, but, human nature being what it is, perhaps this happens more often than we know.

Some people who studied this subject reported: "Recent studies in experimenter bias . . . have shown that experimenters are able to obtain from their human or animal subjects the data that the experimenters want, need or expect to get." This was published by R. Rosenthal and his associates in 1960 in *Perceptual and Motor Skills*.

Fluoride-Strontium Studies with Bone

Be that as it may, what are we to think when a scientist interprets his research on fluoride one way when he first reports his results, but then draws the very opposite conclusion in his later report of the very same research?

We are referring here to a report to the Atomic Energy Commission, Division of Biology and Medicine. This report is entitled *The Metabolism of Alkaline Earth Metals by Bone*. It was submitted to the Commission on March 23, 1959, by F. W. Lengemann, Assistant Professor of Chemistry at the University of Tennessee. The report was countersigned by Dr. O. W. Hyman, Vice-President in Charge of Medical Units. We may, therefore, assume that the contents of this report were carefully gone over, verified and accepted, not by one scientist, but by two.

This report, despite its title, is very pertinent to the problem of water fluoridation, even though Dr. Lengemann may not have realized it at the time he was doing his research. In his report, Dr. Lengemann tells how he studied, among other things, the effects of various poisons on the ratio of calcium to strontium in growing bone. To put it simply, he wanted to find out whether these poisons cause bone to take up more, or less strontium, in relation to the amount of calcium taken up by the same bone. Some of the poisons he studied were fluoride, arsenite, cyanide, lead and mercury.

Fluoride a Poison

The Atomic Energy Commission is greatly interested in strontium, because radioactive strontium is one of the most potentially dangerous elements in the radioactive fall-out which pollutes our atmosphere, due to atomic bomb tests. The poisons studied by Dr. Lengemann were enzyme inhibitors. This means that the poisonous effects they have on the body are due to interference with the normal activity of enzymes, which have important and necessary functions to perform. Fluoride is such a poison, along with cyanide, arsenite, lead and so forth.

In his tests, Dr. Lengemann studied the effect of different concentrations of fluoride. Some bone was not exposed to any fluoride at all. This constituted what scientists call a "control." It shows what happens under normal conditions. In this case, the normal condition is the bone alone without fluoride or any other poison present. Then Dr. Lengemann also tested 3 different concentrations of sodium fluoride, to which he exposed the growing bone. In plain simple everyday language, Dr. Lengemann studied, in this part of his research, the effect of fluoridation on cultures of growing bone.

Fluoride Increases Strontium in Bone

How did Dr. Lengemann interpret his results? In his report, he very clearly concluded, *"Fluoride . . . increased the strontium to calcium ratio."* These are his very own words. He drew this conclusion because that was what the data in his report showed. In view of the findings, which he submitted to the Atomic Energy Commission, that was the conclusion to which his experimental results led him. This, therefore, is a clear warning that fluoridation may well be increasing the amount of radioactive strontium that the growing bones of our children are absorbing. Bear in mind that Dr. Lengemann worked with growing bone which corresponds to the bone of our *growing children*. Also, both strontium and fluoride are boneseekers; that is, they accumulate in bone tissue.

Fluoridation and Strontium Retention

How relevant are Dr. Lengemann's findings to the horrors of fluoridation? An examination of his data quite conclusively proved that the strontium to calcium ratio was increased by the addition of fluoride. That is why he drew the conclusion that he reported to the Atomic Energy Commission.

Now, many people are concerned at present with finding something, anything, that will protect us against radioactive strontium. It appears, from Dr. Lengemann's report to the AEC, that fluoride *makes the threat of harm greater.* Hence, fluoridation is one of the things that we should avoid at all costs. The key words to remember, in the report submitted by Dr. Lengemann on March 3, 1959, are these: *"Fluoride . . . increased the strontium to calcium ratio."* In other words, increased the possibility of harm from radioactive strontium.

The Case of the Missing Data

Dr. Lengemann's report to the Atomic Energy Commission was a typewritten report, which relatively few people might ever see. Many scientists might not even know it existed. So, Dr. Lengemann published his work in the July, 1960, issue of the *Journal of Biological Chemistry,* which goes all over the world. Dr. Lengemann submitted his article to that journal on January 21, 1960, 10 months after he sent his report to the Atomic Energy Commission.

In his published article, Dr. Lengemann reported the very same experiment which we have just described, and gave *some* of his very same data. But he did not give *all* the results which he had reported to the Atomic Energy Commission. He completely omitted his findings from that part of his experiment where he tested the highest concentration of fluoride!

Hocus-Pocus! No Effect!

Then, to top it off, he clearly concluded in his published report that, *"Fluoride had no effect on the strontium to calcium ratio."* Note how different this is from what he reported to the Atomic Energy Commission.

Now, we are not scientists and we do not understand this switch-about. Will anyone, therefore, please explain to us how something that was proved to be a scientific fact on March 23, 1959, could turn into a diametrically opposite fact on January 21, 1960? How can fluoride increase the strontium to calcium ratio, and yet have no effect on this ratio? The fascinating thing about this situation is that we are dealing here, in both cases, with one and the same experiment. And the same individual, Dr. Lengemann himself, who did the experiment, is the one who drew these opposite conclusions. Moreover, no explanation was given!!! This is not a case where two researchers interpret the same experimental results, or where one investigator interprets the results of two separate experiments. In such situations, we could understand how different conclusions might be drawn. But Dr. Lengemann alone reported a different interpretation from the very same experiment, which he himself had carried out!

On March 23, 1959, Dr. Lengemann declared his experiment showed that fluoride increased the strontium to calcium ratio. Then, only 10 months later, the same Dr. Lengemann tells us that the same experiment shows that the same fluoride does not affect the same strontium to calcium ratio.

What kind of science is this? Is this what fluoridation is doing to American science? Why did Dr. Lengemann omit from his published article which the whole world sees, certain critical data which he felt were of sufficient importance to include in his report to the Atomic Energy Commission? Also, why didn't Dr. Lengemann's article in the scientific journal refer to his unpublished report?

Lengemann Supports Kerwin's Theory

The possibility that fluoridation might increase the amount of deadly strontium 90 in our bodies was also discussed in an article by James G. Kerwin, D.D.S., which appeared in *Dental Digest* for February, 1958. Dr. Kerwin's theory is that the simultaneous presence of strontium 90 and fluoride in the body may result in a greater accumulation of each of these two elements than if one were present without the other. This might be due, for example, to the formation of strontium fluoride or some other compound in which these elements occur together. Because of the low solubility of such compounds, the body could have infinitely more trouble excreting them. As a result, the deadly radiation of our cells by strontium 90 would continue for a longer period of time. There would thus be more likelihood of leukemia and other kinds of cancer developing.

The same conclusion about a possible interaction between strontium and fluoride inside the body was independently arrived at by J. F. Montague, M.D. He published his concern over this additional hazard from fluoridation in the October, 1958, issue of the *Journal of the International College of Surgeons*. It is interesting that both a dentist and a physician independently pointed out the same danger —that fluoridation may be causing an increased amount of cancer!

Dr. Lengemann's unpublished report to the AEC supports this possibility. He found that relatively more strontium is taken up by bone when fluoride is present. But scientists, reading his later report in the scientific journal, might know nothing of his earlier conclusion, or of the data which he omitted from his publication. Hence, they would assume that the relationship between these two elements is not physiologically significant. They would, therefore, not necessarily be concerned about the possibility that fluoridation might increase the incidence of cancer due to strontium 90.

Dr. Lengemann's unpublished report to the Atomic Energy Commission stated: "Fluoride . . . increased the strontium to calcium ratio." But his publication in the *Journal of Biological Chemistry* said: "Fluoride had no effect on the strontium to calcium ratio."

Why? Why? Why?

What happened between the time that Dr. Lengemann submitted his report to the Atomic Energy Commission and the time he sent his article to the biochemical journal 10 months later? Why did Dr. Lengemann omit from his published report, available to all the world, certain critical data and then reverse his own conclusions as to the fluoride effect?

We don't know the answers to these questions, but it seems to us to indicate a very serious change in the character of scientific research in this country. Are the promoters of fluoridation so determined to force this medication into an unwilling public, that they will distort scientific findings? If so, what will they not do next?

We don't, of course, know if that is what really happened. But if this is not the explanation, what is? Why did Dr. Lengemann present no explanation in his publication as to why he omitted certain key findings and then reversed the conclusion he drew? Was this because the explanation would have been more damning than the distortion itself?

What *You* Can Do

In his book, *Biochemical Individuality,* Roger J. Williams of the University of Texas discusses how we vary from one another in the biochemistry and physiology of our bodies. People differ considerably in the amount of fluoridated water they consume, and in the amount of fluoride their bodies excrete.

Dr. Joseph Samachson reported in the August, 1960, issue of *Radiation Research* that a wide range of retention (of strontium 90) can occur in adults, even on a single dietary strontium 90 intake, as a result of differences in the way each individual uses strontium and calcium. Variations of dietary intake further increase the range of body retention, he says. Dr. Samachson found that "the strontium 90 concentration in bone may vary by a factor of 1,000 or more from one individual to the next."

In the June 27, 1958, issue of *Science,* R. F. Palmer and his associates pointed out that the strontium to calcium ratio is "a measure of the potential hazard," and that a variation in this ratio in bone could "have an important effect on the evaluation of the strontium 90 fall-out hazard." It is precisely this kind of variation in the strontium to calcium ratio which Dr. Lengemann found in his fluoride research with bone.

Furthermore, Dr. Lengemann's published paper points out that the ability of bone to preferentially select calcium instead of strontium depends on the biologic functioning of the bone tissue and that living cells seem to be involved. But we know that fluoride is a deadly poison precisely because it interferes with cell enzymes and thereby affects normal functioning.

What can you do about this situation? You should write to your Congressmen and to the Secretary of Health, Education and Welfare. Ask them to institute a Congressional investigation to ascertain whether the United States Public Health Service and the American Dental Association, the two major agencies advocating fluoridation, may actually be increasing the incidence of cancer. Such an investigation should also reveal why *all* findings from Dr. Lengemann's research, *which was supported by public funds,* were not published, especially when the data appear to be so vitally relevant to the public health aspects of fluoridation and the strontium 90 fall-out danger.

The Second Battle of Concord

The first was fought in Concord, Massachusetts in 1775. The second was fought in Concord, New Hampshire in the twentieth century, and it continued for about 8 years. Both were fought for freedom: the 1775 battle was one of the opening struggles of the American Revolution; the twentieth century one was a classical battle in the fight to preserve individual liberty against mass medication—the battle against water fluoridation.

According to a New York *World-Telegram* writer who journeyed to New Hampshire to report on the battle of Concord, the state capital city of 28,000 still carries the scars of the 8-year battle which began when the city water was fluoridated "at the whim of the city manager."

Says Henry Walter in the *World-Telegram* for March 22, 1960, "Concord's water fluoridation ended January 1, 1960, after residents voted against it last November by a 2 to 1 vote. . . . Although even pro-fluoridationists agree the issue is dead now in Concord, the bitterness between pros and cons remains. Some old acquaintances do not talk to each other. And while most people freely expressed their feelings and opinions, several persons on both sides asked not to be quoted by name to avoid trouble with their neighbors.

"Each side accused the other of being 'hysterical' and 'emotional.' Each side claimed it had 'the facts', proffering yards of reports, books, magazines and clippings. Each side charged the other with making phone threats and sending 'poison pen' letters."

Name-calling was the order of the day. The pro-fluoridationists claimed that local doctors and dentists dragged their feet and did not go "all-out" for fluoridation as they were supposed to. The anti-fluoridationists claimed that the local newspaper devoted plenty of space to stories praising fluoridation, but relegated the information against it to the Letters to the Editor column.

Dentist Speaks Out

A courageous dentist who runs a free school clinic had this to say, "I serve children from the Penacook school and children from a school in Boscawen. . . . Both groups were similar in age range, both came from low-income families, both had similar oral hygiene habits.

"The Penacook children drank fluoridated water 7 years. The Boscawen children drank unfluoridated water. The Penacook children had as much, if not more, tooth decay than the Boscawen children.

"Moreover, I found 6 Penacook children between 8 and 14 with decalcified enamel (mottling) on the . . . teeth. I have found no such decalcification so far among Boscawen children. I do not know whether fluoridation caused this decalcification."

The State Dental Director answered this statement with a wild claim that the tooth mottling the local dentist had found was caused by a mysterious something in the soil which he could not reveal because it was the "subject of a top-secret report to President Roosevelt during World War II!"

Now, everybody concerned with fluoridation knows perfectly well that tooth mottling is caused by fluorides in the water. The nation's topmost promoters of fluoridation have admitted that a certain amount of mottling will be found, even under the most ideal conditions, when the water contains one part per million of fluoride and no more. No one knows which children will develop mottling and which will not, nor why. Is it just that some children drink more water than others (which, of course, they do), or is it something in the physiological make-up of some children which causes them to be more susceptible to mottling? No one knows. But to try to represent the well-known phenomenon of fluoride-caused tooth mottling as the product of some mysterious, top-secret element in the soil is villainy and demagoguery of the worst sort!

A Concord physician denied a report that he had lost patients because he privately told his patients that he opposed fluoridation, but he refused to let himself be quoted in the newspaper, because he feared that he might lose referrals from other physicians.

For more than 7 years, several hundred Concord residents carried water from a nearby artesian well, rather than drink the city water. You don't have to look far for the reason. A piece of pipe from the city water system was examined in a laboratory on November 18, 1958. A surface scraping of the corrosion on the inside of the water pipe was found to contain 8,000 parts per million of fluoride. It is interesting to note that this example of high fluoride build-up is from the section of Concord from which came the greatest number of complaints of dirty water, bad taste and odor, rust and corrosion of water tanks and household plumbing. Seven years circulation of water containing one part per million of fluoride built up *products of corrosion containing 8,000 parts per million of fluoride.*

In addition, it was found that water taken from a main in a side street contained 2.9 parts per million of fluoride. The Public Health Service and all other promoters of water fluoridation have stated emphatically that, to be effective, the water fluoridation program should maintain the fluoride level within in the optimum one part per million plus or minus .1 per cent. The variation of 180 per cent plus is all the more remarkable because, for one full month just before this sample was taken, no fluoride whatever was being added to the Concord water supply. This came about when fluoride supplies ran out and there was a delay in delivery.

Where were the 2.9 parts per million coming from when no fluoride had gone into the water for over two weeks? It came from the fluoride deposits inside the pipes that had been building up since May, 1952. Pipe cleaning or a change in velocity of water can dislodge these deposits at any time. These discoveries were made during a $200,000 water cleaning program which was necessary after 7 years of fluoridation.

Concord's Fluoridation History

A Brief History of Fluoridation in Concord, written by the mayor in 1959, states:

"The first official action taken by the City of Concord was at a meeting of the City Council held on March 12, 1951. At this meeting, the Director of the New Hampshire State Dental Services explained to the Council the objects of fluoridation and what it had accomplished. The Council then voted that the City of Concord should apply fluoride to its water supply, provided that this project should first receive approval from the Concord Dental and Medical Societies. Approval from each society was immediately forthcoming. The public affected had no knowledge of the proposal at the time and no voice in the decision.

"Personally, I feel that fluoride in our water supply is a violation of individual rights by enforced medication, as this was originally put in by the Manager and Council without any public hearing or referendum.

"Immediate criticism began to arise from our people in regard to the cost and a great many were definitely afraid of the effect of this chemical on the human body after continued use and it also began to be immediately apparent that more corrosion of the pipes was being caused. Previous to the installation of fluoride, our hydrants were flushed only once a year and all parts of the City received a natural good water supply. Now, the system has to be flushed every 6 weeks, at least. Since the installation of fluoride, however, we have been troubled with corrosion of copper tanks and copper pipes, together with brass and iron.

"This criticism from the public grew in volume and to the point where a bill was put in last winter's Legislature to provide that the use of fluoride by the City of Concord from and after January 1, 1960, shall be discontinued unless approved by a majority of its voters present and voting at the 1959 municipal election. There were some 6,000 voters present and they went against the use of fluoride at the rate of over two to one.

"Because of the great amount of corrosion to our water mains and private pipes, our Engineers, Camp, Dresser and McKee, suggested that we could partially remedy the effects of fluoride, at an expense of about 15,000 dollars, by the installation of a machine to add sodium hydroxide to our water, which would increase the pH and cancel the effects of the fluoride in regard to corrosion. This machine was installed in 1958, and of course, has not yet had a chance to prove its value.

"The use of fluoride is a matter that a great many people feel very strongly about, and in my opinion, its use should only be made by a referendum which will give each individual the right to speak for himself and avoid anyone's charge of an infringement of personal rights."

Calcium Fluoride Versus Sodium Fluoride

We reprint below a letter to the *Canadian Medical Association Journal* (December 1, 1959), showing the comparative toxicity of calcium fluoride and sodium fluoride. The former compound is the form in which fluorides appear in nature—in natural drinking water, in bone meal and in other food products. Sodium fluoride is the much more soluble form in which fluorides are being added artificially to drinking water. You can readily see that fluorine may be quite harmless or even healthful in one form (calcium fluoride), but becomes dangerous when it is taken in another chemical combination—sodium fluoride.

"TO THE EDITOR:

"There have been so few reports of the action of the fluorides by practicing physicians, that a bona fide survey of patients who have taken fluorides on prescription during the last 3 years is the subject of this presentation. It should bear more weight than much of the propaganda in favor of fluoridation, which is made up mainly of hearsay evidence, references, theories and unqualified affirmations.

"In 1959, a reliable pharmaceutical firm brought out two vitamin-mineral preparations containing fluorides. One was a syrup in which sodium fluoride was present in the amount of 3 milligrams per dose. The other was a tablet in which calcium fluoride was present in the amount of 25 milligrams, or more than 8 times the strength of the sodium fluoride.

"I gathered 9 cases from my files in which I had tested these fluorides by prescribing the above preparations. Five patients who had taken calcium fluoride in tablet form had no side effects whatsoever and are well today. Four patients who had taken the soluble sodium fluoride in the syrup form presented side effects. One patient was told by her employer to see her doctor as she looked so ill. She had not been examined for over 6 months in 1956, and had had her prescription refilled repeatedly. She had lost 6 pounds, her skin was a bad color, and she was wrinkled and shrunken to such an extent, that I was shocked by her appearance; her hair was falling out to an alarming degree and she felt as ill as she looked. I stopped the syrup after deciding that her symptoms were due to the sodium fluoride's robbing her body of calcium. In a little over a month, she had regained her weight and the other symptoms had subsided. The second patient returned after 6 weeks, in the middle of 1956, with bladder irritation, mental disturbances which made her think she was 'going mental,' lack of calcium as evidenced by softness of nails, deterioration of skin and falling out of hair. She was also advised to stop the syrup. The third patient could not take the syrup at all, as each dose made her nauseated. The last patient did not return for examination. That was the last time I have prescribed preparations containing sodium fluoride. In my practice I have little place for the fluorides and that is why so few were treated. Several bad results and the wise practitioner is through with the drug.

"A few words here about fluorine would be appropriate. There is clinical proof to show that the unstable forms of fluorine deprive the blood and tissues of calcium. In that way, they exert their poisonous effect, which is mild or lethal according to the quantity of fluorine present. Of course, calcium fluoride does not act in that way as it already has its full quota of calcium and is a stable product. To sum up then, these few chosen cases show that sodium fluoride is not to be taken internally while, on the other hand, calcium fluoride can be taken without apparent ill effects. That is the important result of this survey.

WILLIAM A. COSTAIN, M.D.
1567 Bathurst St.
Toronto, Ontario, Canada"

An Open Letter on Fluoridation

In December, 1958, Dr. Frederick Stare of Harvard University made a speech on fluoridation in Needham, Massachusetts. Below is a letter sent to Dr. Stare by Frederick B. Exner, M.D., F.A.C.R., of Seattle, Washington, a radiologist who has been in the forefront of the fight against fluoridation. Dr. Exner is coauthor of a book, The American Fluoridation Experiment. *Dr. Stare is the "authority" who writes voluminously for general magazines on subjects dealing chiefly with nutrition.*

Dr. Frederick J. Stare
Department of Nutrition, School of Public Health
Harvard University, One Shattuck Street
Boston 15, Massachusetts

DEAR DOCTOR STARE:

I have listened with great care to a recording of the fluoridation meeting at Needham, Massachusetts, on December 5, 1958. As you know, most of the meeting was devoted to answers by you to written questions from the audience. I am appalled at the casual disregard for truth exhibited in those answers, and at the abandon with which you fabricated "facts" to suit your convenience.

I am further disturbed at the manner in which you exploited your position at Harvard and at Peter Bent Brigham Hospital to impose on the credulity of the citizens of Needham. And the whole thing becomes somewhat funny when you, of all people, call " 'natural' food faddists" "purveyors of spurious information" and "pseudoscientists who insert quackery and misinformation in their publicity." (*Seattle Times,* January 20, 1959, page 40.)

To get down to cases: on December 5, you were asked why the Association of American Physicians and Surgeons, with over 15,000 members, had adopted a resolution condemning the addition of any substance to public water supplies for the purpose of affecting the bodies or the bodily (or mental) functions of the consumers.

Instead of answering, or saying you didn't know, you undertook to discredit the organization. You said it is not a scientific organization; that it was formed in the early forties for two purposes: to combat fluoridation and to combat socialized medicine; and that, far from having 15,000 members, it has only 5 to 6 hundred.

The Association of American Physicians and Surgeons, Incorporated (185 North Wabash, Chicago 1, Illinois) does not publish its membership. I am a member of its Board of Directors, and even I don't know the exact number. I can assure you, however, that 15,000 is a far closer estimate than 600.

As to your statement that it was formed to combat fluoridation

—it is not only utterly false, it is ridiculous on its face. Except for the original experiments, there was no fluoridation to combat when it was formed. Even today, you can find no mention of fluoridation in an official act of the Association.

However, the Association *has* condemned compulsory mass medication; and it has condemned the use of water supply as vehicle for drugs. In both instances, it was thoroughly understood that fluoridation was covered. Both, however, were actions on principle without reference to specific violations.

Your statement that the Association is not a scientific organization, happens to be true, but is wholly irrelevant. Neither, for that matter, is the American Medical Association. Both are professional organizations, with membership restricted to physicians. In neither case are members required to check their scientific training at the door; and it is safe to assume that the members of AAPS are as competent to understand the medical aspects of fluoridation as you are.

And even if AAPS were a scientific organization—it is not a function of *any* organization to pass on scientific truth. Authority of any kind has no place in science; and truth is not established by counting noses. AAPS is opposed, on principle, to "science by edict"; and so, by the way, is the British Royal Society, one of the world's truly great scientific organizations.

On December 5, you denied, at length, that fluoridation is mass medication. Your grounds were that it treats no disease—that it will reduce neither the number nor size of existing cavities. If you know anything at all about the practice of medicine, you know that medication may be either for the treatment or prevention of disease and that, actually, you treat people. You don't treat diseases.

You should also know that whether a substance is "a drug" depends solely on the purpose for which it is used. Any substance or mixture of substances *used for the purpose* of curing, mitigating or preventing disease or its symptoms is, by definition, a drug. Thiamin, when a constituent of the diet, is a nutrient. When it is administered *for the purpose* of preventing thiamin deficiency, it is a drug.

Yet you said it is "absolutely ridiculous to think that you are drugging anybody" by fluoridation. You even denied that fluoridation changes the physiological and biochemical processes of the consumer. Certainly you are aware that the very purpose of fluoridation is to modify the process of enamel formation so as to alter the ability of the enamel to resist decay.

To bolster your contention that fluoridation is not medication, you stated that fluorine is an essential "trace element in the diet" that, largely as a result of work by Dr. Harry Day at the University of Indiana, most nutritionists now classify fluorine as a "nutrient"; and that when, in two to four years, people understand that fluorine is just as much a nutrient as thiamin, the Christian Science religion will have no further opposition to fluoridation.

I don't know by what warrant you speak for the Christian Science Church, but I do know that no nutritionist worthy of the name regards fluorine as an essential nutrient. I also know that you misrepresented the work of Harry Day.

No human diet is so lacking in fluorine as to cause deficiency symptoms. Drs. Maurer and Day fed a highly purified, fluorine-poor diet to animals and could produce no symptoms of fluorine deficiency. The animals didn't even get tooth decay. The title of their article is "The Nonessentiality of Fluorine in Nutrition." (*Journal of Nutrition,* 62: 561-573, August, 1957.)

But all the talk about whether fluorine is or is not "medication," is or is not a "drug," is or is not a "nutrient," is just word games designed to fool the public. The right to decide what foods one will eat is just as fundamental as the right to decide what drugs one will take. And all the word games will not change the fact that "one man's meat is another man's poison."

One of your questioners stated: "One Dr. H. C. Hodge, states in the *Annals of the Rheumatic Diseases,* that crippling fluorosis occurs at 2 to 16 parts per million of fluoridated water." You replied that you knew Harold Hodge very well, and that you "would categorically deny that he makes that statement."

You went on to say that you would look up the article and prove it to anyone who was interested. If you looked up the article, you found, on page 379 (Steinberg, Gardner, Smith and Hodge, "Comparison of rheumatoid (ankylosing) spondylitis and crippling fluorosis," *Annals of the Rheumatic Diseases,* 14: 378-384, 1955): "Crippling fluorosis of industrial origin was fully described by Roholm (1937) in his investigation of the disease in Danish cryelite workers. The condition is also endemic in various parts of the world, India, China, Argentina and South Africa, where water supplies contain 2 to *16 parts per million* of fluoride." Actually it has been reported in India from 0.6 parts per million. But, be that as it may, have you told the people of Needham that you misinformed them?

When you were asked: "Doesn't fluoridation have a bad effect on bone structure, and isn't it bad for arthritis?" you said that "there was a very interesting paper published in the *New England Journal of Medicine* . . . approximately 8 to 10 months ago, where fluoride analysis was carried out on bones from . . . some 20 individuals who had died from severe arthritis and had come from communities that had fluoridated water, compared with the fluoride content of bones of individuals who had died of arthritis in non-fluoridated communities. And there was absolutely no difference in the fluoride content."

The article in question was also by Steinberg, Gardner, Smith and Hodge, (*New England Journal of Medicine,* 258: 322-325.) The people didn't die of arthritis. People *don't* die of arthritis. And there was a very considerable difference in the fluoride content in the bones of the two groups.

The study compared people in the fluoridated and non-fluoridated portions of Rochester, New York. Fluoridation had been in effect less than 5 years. The vertebrae of 10 persons from the non-fluoridated portion averaged 1,118 parts per million of fluorine, and their average age was 77. The average fluoride content for 13 people in the fluoridated area was 1,426 parts per million. (28 per cent higher) in spite of the fact that the average age was 11 years less (66 years).

What is more, the article started out by saying: "Deposition of fluoride in the skeleton is a known effect of fluoride ingestion. The recent trend in fluoridation of municipal water supplies . . . will naturally result in increased fluoride content of bone."

Moreover, it goes on to say: "Still unknown are the beneficial and ill effects that fluoridation of water may have on mankind."

When asked whether 10 years is long enough time for study of fluoridation as regards effect on adult population, you said that: "Actually, fluoridation for 7 million people in the United States has been carried on for generation after generation." And again you said, "There are about 7½ million people who have access to public waters where there is the proper amount of fluorine in the water and there is no necessity to add; these people have been receiving fluoridated water all of their lives, and there is no difference in the incidence of disease—of any type of disease at any age level—for people in these communities, as compared with other communities that do not have fluoridated water."

In 1949, Hill, Jelinek and Blayney reported (*Journal of Dental Research,* 28: 398-414, 1949) that 1,293,915 people in the United States *were then being served* water with between 1.0 and 1.5 parts per million of fluoride, and that an additional 1,714,242 were being served water with upward of 1.5 parts per million. Their figures may have been incomplete, but hardly by 6,000,000. Moreover, nothing was said about how long the waters had been in use, or how long the people had lived in the communities. Actually, very few people in the United States have used an unchanged water supply all their lives, and, again, it would seem that you made up the facts to suit your convenience.

Moreover, there is no support, and no conceivable possibility of support for your statement that there is no difference in the incidence of any type of disease at any age level in these communities as compared with others. You made that one up out of whole cloth. If there are two communities anywhere with the same incidence of all types of disease, no one knows it and no one could prove it.

You were asked: "How does the absence or lack of evidence via statistical studies prove that no harm is done when the syndromes of fluorosis are so complicated that only exhaustive study would enable a physician to even recognize these symptoms?"

You said: "There is nothing complicated about fluorosis. The patient complains of pain in the long bones . . . You can find out. Even a fourth-grade (sic) student, after he's had his course in X-ray analysis, ought to be able to give you a reasonably good idea if a person is really ill from fluorosis."

The symptoms of fluorosis, either in man or animals, are numerous and varied. Pain in the long bones is not one of the more usual symptoms. The flat bones and spine and the ligaments are far more commonly involved than the long bones. The X-ray changes are a *late* manifestation of fluorosis, and no physician can rule out fluorosis by X-ray examination.

In the questions and answers department of the *Journal of the American Medical Association* for March 15, 1958, a physician asked what methods were available to physicians by which they could make a diagnosis in cases where they suspected fluoride poisoning. The answer was that there are none—that the methods were too difficult to be readily available to physicians.

When it was asked how the dose of fluoride can be controlled when different children consume different amounts of water, you replied that, actually, there is very little difference in the amounts of *fluid* consumed by different people over a period of several days. That answer was not only false, but deceitful.

In the first place, there are enormous differences in the habitual fluid consumption by different people. In the second place, we aren't concerned with fluid consumption. We are concerned solely with the consumption of water from the public supply.

You were asked why the medical profession doesn't allow debate on fluoridation and you said it does. As proof, you cited the hearing before the Council on Drugs and the Council on Foods and Nutrition of the American Medical Association. You said the debate lasted about two days, that the two principal opponents of fluoridation (and you named Dr. George Waldbott of Detroit and me) had an opportunity to present their data—an "opportunity to present all their stuff," and that "there were one or two other people against fluoridation."

You failed to mention that the resulting report of the Councils knocks the "case for fluoridation" into a cocked hat. However, the hearing lasted less than one day. It was not a debate. It was not before the medical profession, and many of the members of the Councils are doctors of philosophy, not of medicine. In addition, Dr. Waldbott and I were the only ones speaking against fluoridation. There were no "one or two other people against fluoridation."

There has been no discussion of the case against fluoridation before the American Medical Association, or in its *Journal;* and there has been very little before other meetings of physicians. And in the last 40 years, there has been only one original article on chronic fluorine poisoning in the *Journal of the American Medical Association.*

These are just samples of the "spurious information" you have been giving the people of the Boston area on the subject of fluoridation. There are many more, both on the tape and in your letters to the papers. Even if there were a legitimate case for fluoridation, it would not be advanced by such tactics. However, there isn't.

I believe the people of Needham, and of the Boston area generally, have a right to know these things when their health and that of their children are at stake. This is particularly needed because you have employed the good name of Harvard. That is why I have made this an open letter.

Sincerely Yours,

F. B. EXNER, *M.D., F.A.C.R.*
Dental and Medical Building
Seattle 1, Washington

The Anti-Fluoridationist

By J. I. Rodale

There is an interesting story as to what started the whole fluoridation rumpus. The fluorides originated from a by-product of the aluminum industry and consisted of a slag that the companies used to dump into rivers way back in the old days, when health controls were practically nonexistent. Finally, it was discovered that these wastes were killing fish and were generally harmful to wildlife and farm stock. So legislation was passed banning this practice, and as a result, mountains of these waste slag piles began to accumulate.

Then it was that some smart cookie figured out the fluoridation wrinkle. It seems that there are certain communities in the United States, notably in the West, where the drinking water naturally contains fluorides, and it was found that there was less dental decay in those areas, so those who had fluorides to sell, figured that, by putting fluorides into the water, they could accomplish the same purpose. But they either overlooked or ignored the fact that there was a different kind of fluoride in the rivers than the kind of fluoride that could be made out of the aluminum wastes.

In the river water, the form of fluoride was the relatively innocuous, inert calcium fluoride, but the aluminum waste fluoride was the highly toxic, highly soluble sodium fluoride which is used as rat and cockroach poisons. It is like comparing milk of magnesia with carbolic acid.

Teeth Become Hard and Brittle

Another thing that is overlooked is the fact that in these naturally fluoridated areas, there is less dental decay in the youth, but the teeth become so hard and brittle that it becomes difficult to do dental repair work, and in these communities, therefore, more dentures per capita are worn than in the no-fluoride sections of our country. A survey by Smith and Smith of the University of Arizona, reported in *Fluorine and Dental Health,* published by the American Association for the Advancement of Science, showed that in St. David, Arizona, where the water is naturally fluoridated, 50 per cent of all individuals over the age of 24 had lost all their teeth and are now wearing dental plates.

Dr. Paul H. Belding, a dentist who edited a technical dental publication called *Dental Items of Interest* had an article in his January, 1952, issue entitled "Fluorine Has Its Limitations," and in it, he describes the case histories of two families who were his patients and who lived in a naturally fluoridated area. The Perry family's well contained more than two parts per million of fluorine, whereas in regular fluoridation procedures only one part per million is added. Of their 7 children, several began to show the characteristic fluorine mottling of the teeth soon after starting to drink this water. In addition, it soon became obvious, says Dr. Belding, that the structure of their teeth was such that they could not hold fillings satisfactorily.

But the pro-fluoridators never mention this difficulty with teeth in the naturally fluoridated areas, and they continue to cite these areas as an example of the benefits of fluoridation.

High Price for Waste

Well, here were the huge mountains of waste of the aluminum factories, which could be turned to gold if the proper sales pitch could be worked out. We must admit that we Americans are great ones when it comes to salesmanship and to selling something, and the aluminum boys ran true to form.

Here is a quotation from the trade publication called *Chemical Week,* a periodical that is read mainly by the top executives of the chemical industry. In its issue of July 7, 1951, appeared this note:

"Only one per cent of the nation's water is now treated (with fluorine); thus, the market potential has fluoride makers goggle-eyed. Any apathy or opposition on the part of the public is made up for by the United States Public Health Service's zeal in drumming up the program. It is asking for federal money to develop interest and there is talk of seeking federal subsidization of water treatment. . . . Standing to benefit from the boom are chemical companies and equipment firms. It adds up to a nice piece of business on all sides."

Well, they hit the jack pot. What used to sell for 1½ cents a pound now costs 15 cents and more, and all the wastes are gone. There is so much demand for the stuff that they have to make a lot of it from the ground up. Their theory is: if we can't give it to the fish, we will give it to the people. Nobody ever really worries about people too much when a dollar is at stake.

Delaney Hearings

In the Hearings of the Delaney Committee, there appears a statement made by Miss Florence Birmingham, President, Massachusetts Women's Political Club, that is unbelievable. Here is what she says on page 51 of this government report:

"In 1944, Oscar Ewing was put on the payroll of the Aluminum Company of America, as attorney, at an annual salary of $750,000. The fact was established at a Senate hearing and became a part of the *Congressional Record*. Since the Aluminum Company had no big litigation pending at the time, the question might logically be asked, why such a large fee? A few months thereafter, Mr. Ewing was made Federal Security Administrator with the announcement that he was taking a big salary cut in order to serve his country.

"As head of the Federal Security Agency (now the Department of Health, Education and Welfare), he immediately started the ball rolling to sell 'rat poison' by the ton instead of in dime packages. How?

"By using the pressure of the federal government he induced the city fathers of Newburgh, New York, Grand Rapids, Michigan, and Evanston, Illinois, to try a 10-year experiment with fluoridation to actually determine the effects of this 'rat poison' upon the dental caries of growing children."

Again, Oscar Ewing is mentioned on page 61 of this same government hearing by Mrs. E. Adams, President, National Committee Against Fluoridation, Incorporated. She says:

"It was Oscar Ewing who inaugurated the present intensive campaign to fluoridate the water, not only of this country, but apparently of the world, if possible, as a supposed health measure. His yearly budgets are said to have been considerably over a billion dollars and during the years of his administration, in addition to huge sums spent for high-priced propagandists, for other personnel assigned to this project and for advertising and propaganda material, some hundreds of millions of federal tax money, as subsidies, were poured out to State and local health boards on condition that under detailed instructions they would push this health program," meaning fluoridation.

Again, on page 195 of this federal hearing report, Dr. Ginns, Senior Dental Consultant of the Worcester City Hospital of Worcester, Massachusetts, said: "I would like to say this: It has been said here this morning that highly eminent authorities have been quoted in favor of fluoridation. Maybe it will answer your question, to some extent, if I quote some authorities."

MR. WILLIAMS (Congressman from Mississippi): Is the profit motive involved in any way?

DR. GINNS: Yes, begorry, it started with FSA (Federal Security Administration). They are objecting to federal interference. It all started with the FSA. I do not want to mention names. Perhaps I will stay away from that. But Oscar Ewing was Chief of FSA at the time he was chief counsel of the Aluminum Company of America. It seems to stem from there.

If you will read the Congressional Record, Congressman Miller has referred to it. You will find much of that in the *Congressional Record* of Congressman Miller a year ago.

(Then, after some discussion)

MR. WILLIAMS: My question is this: Does this argument stem primarily from that (legitimate differences of medical opinion), or does it go deeper and have its roots in some mercenary consideration of some selfish interest group of some kind?

DR. GINNS: I think it is both, perhaps. It has a mercenary background and it seems to be a blunder on the part of certain men who will not admit that they are wrong, although eventually they will. That is my bone of contention.

(Dr. Ginns is a violent opponent of fluoridation.)

So you pays your money and you takes your choice. "Was Oscar Ewing sent by the aluminum interests to sell their fluoride wastes?"

It is something you have to decide for yourself.

Why Children?

I have often wondered why the dentists have chosen such an unbalanced program in regard to the prevention of tooth decay— embracing a method which reduces tooth decay only in children less than 12 years old—especially since it has been shown that, as they grow older, the cavities catch up with them.

In the *Proceedings of the Royal Society of Medicine* (England) of May, 1948, the result of an investigation was published in reference to two towns in England—North and South Shields, one of which had fluorine in the water, the other had none. True, the 12-

year-old group in the fluoridated town had half as many cavities as in the town that was not fluoridated, but when they made a survey in both towns of 15-year-old children, the number of cavities was the same for both places. In other words, as the children keep eating ice cream, pastries, candies and soda pop, after 'the age of 12, they begin to get cavities. So the effect in this case was to postpone the progress of dental decay for 3 years.

There was a hearing on fluoridation before a committee of the House of Representatives in Washington from May 25 to 27, 1954, and on page 236 of the report of this hearing, George L. Waldbott, M.D., of Detroit, testified regarding a research on children's teeth by Smith and Smith, reported in Arizona Experiment Station Technical Bulletin Number 43. Dr. Waldbott said, "They found that individuals in fluoridated areas, who as children showed an apparent reduction in dental caries, after they had passed the age of 21, manifested much more extensive deterioration and weakening of tooth structures than those in non-fluoridated areas. A similar observation is related by Dr. Newman in the *New York State Journal of Medicine* for July, 1951, regarding two suburbs of Sheffield, England."

In the same report, Mr. H. L. Prestholdt says, on page 229, "Scientists, upon careful investigation, admit that the teeth are less prone to decay at an early age, but subsequent to childhood these facts are reversed. The fluoride content is then proven to be a masking operation. The teeth become infinitely more susceptible to decay and are so brittle, it is difficult for any dentist to accomplish needed repair."

Children as Patients

Regarding the question of children, here is something that bowled me over. In the United States government hearing report on fluoridation, p. 227, Mr. Thomas H. Allen, President of the Light, Gas and Water Division of the City of Memphis, Tennessee, testified against fluoridation from the *Journal of the American Water Works Association,* Vol. 41, p. 575:

"The dental society has investigated numerous statements on fluorine, but has failed to tell the public what a local dentist told a group in Memphis, which was that, in general, dentists do not like to serve children and that by putting in the same time on adults, they can gather in more money. Since, certainly, most dentists have received their education and training largely at public expense, they should feel obligated to serve all elements of the public, including children."

How do you like this? Children do not make good patients. They squirm and cry and yell and even bite the dentists, so the dentists want to bite us oldsters in return, forcing us to drink this treated water that could shorten our lives, instead of educating children to forego candy bars and soda pop. When the day of reckoning comes, as come it must, the dentists will be hard put to explain this.

The Wasteful Economics of Fluoridation

It is an admitted fact that fluoridation will only help the teeth of children of about 12 and under, and only partly. Then why should so much money be spent to fluoridate all the water of a city? In the average city, more than 99 per cent of the water goes for flushing toilets, laundering, bathing, sprinkling lawns, cleaning streets, swimming pools, factory uses of various kinds, fire-fighting, public fountains and such things. Yet, all these waters will carry the wasted fluoride chemical that has to be paid for by the taxpayer.

There are available in drug stores fluoride tablets that can be taken by children, if their parents are of the opinion that it will help them. But why should older persons be forced to drink fluoridated water when it is definitely known that it can't help them one iota? Why should people with dentures be forced to drink this chemicalized water?

But let us look into the economics of fluoridation as it affects the city of Allentown, Pennsylvania. The dentists have figured that it will cost Allentown 15,000 dollars a year for the fluoride chemical. Now, according to the *Bulletin of the 4th Annual Proceedings of Public Health Officers,* for every 700 quarts of water that leave the water works, only 1½ quarts are used for drinking purposes, which amounts to about .2 of one per cent. But since children in the benefited age bracket are but 10 per cent of the population, then only about .02 of one per cent of the total water consumed is used by children.

So, if we take .02 of one per cent of the annual cost of 15,000 dollars, it would mean an actual value of 3 dollars for the fluoride consumed by children out of a 15,000 dollar total expenditure. It is like sending a 15-ton Mack truck to deliver a packet of aspirin. It would mean that in 10 years' time, Allentown would be throwing almost 150,000 dollars down the drain for no reason whatever.

It would be different if fluoridation were practical from every other point of view, but there are so many holes in the idea, that when we add this serious economic flaw, we begin to wonder if those who are for fluoridation have not made other, even more serious blunders. A study of the whole subject will reveal that this is so.

Only One Part per Million

On one of the radio stations in Allentown, a commentator tried to quiet a lady's fear about the harmful effect of fluoridated water on her young son who is allergic to "practically everything." "Why it is only one little drop of fluoride to about ¾ of a bathtub of water," he said. "How can that hurt?"

It can hurt, Mr. Commentator. There are even smaller concentrations of substances than this that can hurt. In *Water and Sewage Works* magazine for March, 1951, p. 98, there is the story of fluoridation of water in Charlotte, North Carolina, in 1949. A week after its introduction, the entire ice manufacturing industry of the city reported a severe increase in the cracking and shattering of manufactured ice. This was accomplished by only one part per million of fluorine in the water.

You have heard of little drops of water wearing away the hardest stone. It is the continuous action every day of that little drop to every ¾ of a bathtubful that becomes a power to reckon with. Fluorine is a potent poison used in rat and roach killers. It can easily get out of hand if something goes wrong with the machinery, so that just a tiny bit more fluorine is released into the water.

Just as the one part per million had the power to shatter cakes of ice, so does it have the power to enter into the hard structure of the tooth in children and make it harder. Now, if only one part per million can do this, what other effects can it produce in the human body? When the fluoride chemical gets into the blood stream, it is drawn into every one of the billions of cells in the human body. That's because the fluoride is a soluble chemical and has strong power of flow.

When, by force, we cause to intrude into each cell even a fantastically tiny amount of a poison, we must be sure we know exactly what it will do there. Many scientists have said it doesn't belong there, and can do harm, but those who recommend fluoridation ignore this warning.

Effectiveness of Small Amounts

To give you an idea of how effective a small amount can be, a cancer research project at the University of Wisconsin took a substance called *Kinetin,* and using it in an amount of only one part in a hundred million, which is one hundred times smaller than the amount of fluoride used, made cells of plant tissue multiply by division. In other words, such a tiny amount caused cancer of this tissue.

In the branch of medicine called homeopathy, they use drugs in amounts that are millions of times smaller than the quantities of fluorine used in water fluoridation. The homeopathic physicians achieve effects with such smallness.

Viruses are so much smaller than bacteria, that many of them cannot be seen with the strongest microscopes, yet they can lead to virulent diseases.

In a book called *Selective Toxicity* by Dr. Adrian Albert, an experiment is described where a certain solution was applied to a culture of staphylococcus bacteria and the bacteria were able to live with it. But when the amount of this solution was *reduced* beyond a certain point, it acted as a poison and killed all the bacteria. In this case, smallness was the killer.

At the Biologic Institute at Stuttgart, Germany, in 1920, they experimented with the fertilizing effect of calcium on wheat seeds, on a reducing scale; that is, using 8 different quantities of reduction of calcium. With gradually lessening quantities of calcium, the wheat seedlings increased, the smallest quantity producing the largest size of wheat. The smallest amount of calcium fertilizer was one part of calcium to a hundred million parts of water, or a hundred times smaller amount than that of the fluorides used in fluoridation.

In the growth of plants, there are certain mineral elements, such as zinc, manganese, copper, boron, molybdenum, etc., which, for best plant growth, should be present in only "trace" amounts. For example, in the case of zinc, only up to 1/20 of one part per million in the soil is required for healthy plant growth. Larger quantities act as a poison.

Salt Water Experiment

At a European aquarium many years ago, a consignment of salt water fish had been brought in, but there was not enough sea water for them. It was decided, therefore, to make some sea water based on its known formula. The curators assembled the minerals and other compounds and made the water, but when they placed a fish in it, it soon died. The process was repeated several times, but in each case, the fish could not live in the artifically made sea water.

Then one curator at the aquarium had a bright idea. He said, "In the next batch of sea water we make, let us put in a tiny pinch of the real stuff. Perhaps it might contain a gleam of something which science has been unable to measure as yet, but which is essential to the life of a fish." And they did just that! In the next batch of sea water made, there was added the merest trace of real sea water—the slightest pinch of it—and lo and behold—miracle of miracles—the fish could live in it. It seems there is a living substance in sea water which is only a gleam, which probably must be measured by the millionth part of a millionth part, but which means life or death to a fish.

It has been discovered that detergents from household faucets can produce foam if the detergent is only one part per million of water. So you must be watchful that the people who want fluoridation don't mislead you with statements that the fluoride chemical is only one little drop in ¾ of a tubful of water. Let's find out what's in that little drop of fluoride.

100 *Cities Have Abandoned Fluoridation*

By J. I. Rodale

More than 100 cities in the United States have already banished fluoridation. Is this not enough evidence to show that this dangerous experiment is impractical? Yet, the dentists in their discussion of the subject never mention that a single city has ever abandoned it. Is this honest? Is this not pulling the wool over the people's eyes? We have written to these cities and would like to quote from some of the letters received:

From the mayor of Woonsocket, Rhode Island, December 28, 1960: "In reply to your inquiry dated December 20, 1960, concerning the reasons for Woonsocket's discontinuing fluoridation of its water supply, be advised as follows:

"The fluorides were being injected in our water distribution system in the main pumping station on the suction side of the pumps. After several months, it was discovered that the combination of fluoride and chlorine caused a high degree of corrosion to our pumps and other equipment at the pumping station.

"Further, it was ascertained that the dilution was improper and, for these reasons, the service was discontinued."

That the dilution was improper means that the people were getting more than one part per million of fluorides in their drinking water. This is highly dangerous.

Schenectady, New York

Here is part of a letter received from the City Manager, Arthur Blessing, of Schenectady, dated December 27, 1960:

"Fluoridation was originally started in Schenectady in 1954, at a cost of about 30,000 dollars. The City obtains its water supply from 11 wells and is pumped directly from the gravel strata into the distribution system. Hence, it is necessary for us to inject fluoride compounds in concentrated form directly into our mains at approximately 150 pounds per square inch pressure. This concentrated solution, under relatively high pressure, caused considerable damage to the mains and we were forced to discontinue the process about 4 years ago. Nevertheless, we replaced this equipment at a cost of approximately $20,000 (somewhat less than the original estimate) and resumed fluoridation about two and one-half years ago.

"During the last year, we experienced additional trouble with our fluoride pumps and feed lines and had to again discontinue the process."

Please note that the water supply of Schenectady is obtained from 11 wells. This is what all cities should aim for, rather than getting drinking water out of a river which receives the poisonous detergents and sewage effluents from homes and factories. In medical researches recently conducted in Holland, it was found that, in regions where the water comes from wells, there is less cancer than where the water comes from rivers. There are many cities in the United States where the source of water is from wells. Why don't doctors and dentists devote their time to crusading for such a pure source of water?

Mount Dora, Florida

Here is a letter received from the city clerk, M. R. Wagner, of Mount Dora, Florida, December 27, 1960:

"Concerning fluoridation in Mount Dora, a short time after adding it to the city water supply, various and sundry citizens began to complain of different ailments. Most, I feel certain, were imaginative. However, the city government decided to bring the issue to a vote of the people and it was decided to remove the fluorine from the water."

In this case, the city clerk takes it upon himself to say that the various ailments were imaginative, but there is much scientific evidence to prove that there *is* danger to various organs of the human body, through the drinking of water with only one part per million of fluorides.

Reading, Massachusetts

Here is another case where the fluoridation machinery broke down—the city of Reading, Massachusetts. We have a letter from Rudolf Sussman, the secretary of the Board of Selectmen, January 10, 1961:

"It would seem that fluoridation was rushed through a Town Meeting in Reading, Massachusetts, without a full study of all the aspects involved.

"The fluoridation machinery was installed and operation commenced; after a few months, the machinery broke down. By then, a group of citizens asked to have the case for and against fluoridation reviewed and the matter referred to a referendum.

"The Selectmen then set a date for the referendum, allowing several months for various individuals and groups to present the pros and cons through the medium of the newspapers, public meetings, etc. The referendum was held, and fluoridation lost by quite a margin.

"Chief arguments against: (1) no conclusive proof that cavities in children's teeth would become fewer by use of this method; (2) pipes in town were apparently affected by use of fluorides; (3) some people felt that, since only a small portion of the population might possibly benefit by fluorine in water, the larger portion of the people in town might suffer from an accumulation of fluorine in their systems.

"In other words, after all new and old evidence was examined by the people of Reading on the basis of circulated literature, group meetings and information available from other sources, the people voted to take out fluoridation."

Cuba City, Wisconsin

Here is a letter from the City Coordinator of Cuba City, Wisconsin, December 20, 1960:

"We have not discontinued fluoridation, it would only seem so, because after about 8 years of spasmodic operation, our equipment had been sent in for repairs.

"We now have it back and are getting it adjusted to deliver the desired amounts of fluoride. As far as results there is no concrete evidence for or against the use of fluoride."

The important thing here is that there has been no reduction in dental decay.

Tyler, Texas

R. H. Hays, Water Superintendent of Tyler, Texas, writes us under date of December 27, 1960:

"Your letter of December 20, 1960, has been referred to this office for reply.

"The City of Tyler had fluoridation a little over two years and were adding 0.8 part per million to our natural content of 0.2 part per million making a total of 1.0 part per million.

"A great number of citizens were opposed to fluoridation, some claiming it as forced medication, others claiming it was injurious to their kidneys and other parts of their bodies, others claiming it broke them out in a rash, and many other similar cases; therefore, it was put to a vote of the people.

"The referendum carried approximately 4 to 1 to discontinue its use, which was done immediately."

St. Helena, California

Here is a case where a city has stopped fluoridating its water because it was too costly. Marie Volper, City Clerk of St. Helena, California, under date of December 27, 1960, writes:

"At the present time, our equipment, which has been constantly breaking down, is not in operation. Due to lack of funds for repairing this equipment this project has been temporarily discontinued."

St. Petersburg, Florida

In the case of St. Petersburg, Florida, fluoridation was voted out on Setpember 1, 1959, Nadine Blesser, Secretary to the Mayor, writes us on December 28, 1960:

"The citizens seemed to feel that fluoridation violated their personal rights of freedom of choice, and that, since medical men themselves do not agree as to its merits or demerits, public officials should not decide as to its use."

Lake Geneva, Wisconsin

Lake Geneva voted some time ago to discontinue fluoridation, after 3 years, because of the "dirty" condition of the water as a result of the fluoride program. It seems that, according to the superintendent of water supplies, the fluoride was releasing and loosening mineral deposits formed on the pipes. He asked the city commission to discontinue fluoridation, which they did.

Akron, Ohio

A letter from the Superintendent and Chief Engineer of the Akron Bureau of Water and Sewage Department indicates that their fluoridation machinery broke down some time ago. Akron has since discontinued fluoridation.

Fulton, New York

" 'Action by Fulton's Common Council to halt the use of fluoridation of its water supply after 4 years was caused to a large extent by the fact that something in the water has been corroding the gears of water meters,' Mayor John S. Johnson, Jr. said today." (Syracuse, New York, *Herald,* March 8, 1956.)

Random Notes on Fluoridation

Progress in 1961

The year 1961 was a significant one in the continuing fluoridation battle. Despite an accelerated, high-pressure campaign by the United States Public Health Service (paid for out of *your* tax dollars, incidentally) to push artificially fluoridated water down the throats of citizens across the width and breadth of the country, *43 out of 56 cities* given the opportunity to vote on the question in 1961 *turned it down.* In this one year alone, voters representing some 2,500,000 water users rejected the mass-medicating proposal, while those of about 50,000 approved. (One of the more resounding blows was struck in Salt Lake City, where the vote was 35,864 to 10,389—a ratio of nearly 3½ to 1 in favor of pure water. In all, 5 Utah cities said an emphatic "no" to fluoridation in November elections—even after the vigorous, high-financed propaganda program of proponents. Other large cities defeating the water-tampering bill: Cincinnati (for a second time), Sacramento, California, and Saginaw, Michigan.

The House Listens

On the legislative scene, Congressman Walter S. Baring (Democrat, Nevada) attacked the role of the federal government in the promotion of fluoridation. A man who has earned a reputation as a crusading legislator in vital matters affecting the national security and health, Congressman Baring addressed the House of Representatives on September 17, 1961, calling attention to the increasing public rejection of the fluoridation program. He cited attempts by the United States Public Health Service to counter public reaction by "a new, accelerated, high-pressure program of the United States Dental Public Health Division that will be conducted through funds requested under pending House bill 4742 and Senate bill 917." This legislation he condemned as fostering continued harassment of the public.

Congressman Baring cited examples of "past errors that should have taught official agencies that they should not assume an air of infallibility and indifference to public wishes."

"Our citizens have certain fundamental and constitutional rights," continued the Congressman. "The sooner they are recognized, the sooner we shall resolve the fluoridation controversy."

"Certainly," concluded Congressman Baring, "when citizens have demonstrated unmistakably their rejection of fluoridation, and when there exists substantial disagreement within the scientific and medical professions as to the safety and efficacy in fluoridation, it should not, it must not be supported at a federal level."

What's Fair in Richmond?

At Richmond, Virginia, the fluoridation controversy has been raging for some time. The city is one where a decision of the city council has compelled the populace to try to continue living with fluoride-drugged water. The *Richmond News Leader,* a highly regarded and fearless newspaper, which reversed its early support of fluoridation, has been fighting for a public vote on the question. One of the *News Leader's* most forceful editorials and a very important letter which it quoted, appeared in its November 3, 1961, issue. The text of that editorial follows:

NOTES ON MILK AND WATER

A couple of wholly unrelated statements came across the desk this week from two respected physicians talking about two different matters. Their comments set a familiar train of thought in motion.

The first statement, from Dr. Walter W. Sackett, Jr., of Miami, was widely publicized. Dr. Sackett is chairman of the public policy commission of the American Academy of General Practice. He sounded off on the subject of milk. In his view, persons who drink substantial quantities of milk, once they have grown out of childhood, are courting trouble. Milk is high in cholesterol content. Too much cholesterol, he though, could mean "national suicide."

The second statement, from Dr. Edward A. McLaughlin, of

Providence, was not publicized at all. Dr. McLaughlin, now 68, served as State Director of Health in Rhode Island from 1935 until his retirement in 1959. He has been engaged in the practice of medicine for more than 40 years. He sounded off on the subject of putting fluoride in public water supplies. His statement, in the form of a letter dated August 11, 1961, was distributed by the Greater New York Committee Opposed to Fluoridation. The text of that letter appears below.

It occurs to us that the two incidents provide eloquent commentary on the difference between a voluntary society and a compulsory society.

The drinking of milk is a voluntary act. Families who may be impressed by Dr. Sackett's warning can cut down on their milk consumption or halt it altogether. Those folks who like milk, and doubt that the dangers are all that serious, can keep on having a cold glass whenever they want it. Maybe this will lead to an early grave. Maybe it won't. They can do as they please.

But in cities such as Richmond, where sodium fluoride is added to the public water supply, the consumption of fluoride is not a voluntary act at all. Only at immense inconvenience and substantial expense can the ordinary citizen avoid fluoridation. Dr. McLaughlin believes strongly that there are "inherent dangers" in this practice; and he is not alone: thousands of other American physicians, of unquestioned reputation and competence hold the same apprehensions.

For the time being, Richmond seems to be stuck with fluoridation. City Council will not even let the people vote on it. There will be other Councils, other years. Meanwhile, in the capital city of a state that prides itself on individual liberties, the very water we drink continues to be used as a vehicle for the compulsory treatment, indiscriminately, of all men alike.

FLUORIDE'S EFFECTS: 'TIME ALONE WILL TELL'

Dr. Edward A. McLaughlin, Director of Health for Rhode Island from 1935 to 1959, at one time endorsed the addition of sodium fluoride to public water supplies. On further reflection, he swung around to a completely opposite point of view. Several months ago, a resident of West Warwick, Rhode Island, wrote to ask him for a statement of his position. Dr. McLaughlin's reply follows:

DEAR MR. LEFOLEY:

The following are the reasons for my opposition to putting fluoride in our drinking water.

I believe that fluoride in the drinking water will produce a chronic fluoride poisoning similar to lead poisoning which painters suffered from in former days. There are small amounts of arsenic in the fluoride that is placed in drinking water supplies. In the past several years, I have seen so many cases of gastroenteritis and other physicians must have seen similar disorders. I am convinced that this disorder is not due to a virus as we previously thought, but due to some toxicity in our water supply. Regardless of how the fluoride is put in the water, there is always the possibility of human error or mechanical error where too much fluoride may be placed at different times in our drinking water supply.

In the past year, I have become very much interested in checking the teeth of my younger patients and find that they have just as many cavities as other children have had in the years prior to fluoridation. If the dental profession would concentrate on making application of fluoride to the teeth of youngsters twice a year or if parents would use the tablet which is available to put in milk, we would be more certain of obtaining the results that the United States Public Health Service, the American Medical Association and the American Dental Association expect to get by putting fluoride in our drinking water. By this method, the children's teeth would be taken care of—if it has been proven that fluoride would prevent decay (and I am very doubtful about this).

My opinion is that adults should not be exposed to the danger of fluoride in their drinking water when other methods can be used in treating children. It is my firm conviction that acute fluoride poisoning does result at times due to human or mechanical failure in operating the system by which fluoride is put into our drinking water. I firmly believe that there is a danger of chronic fluoride poisoning resulting in osteomalacia (softening of the bones) and osteoporosis (abnormally porous and spaced bone structure), not only in adults, but in children. Time alone will tell. When other means are available such as topical application to children's teeth and the tablets which mothers can use at home, I do not believe that the whole population of our state should be subject to the inherent dangers which putting fluoride in the water entails. I regret very much that in 1952, I approved of having fluoride in our drinking water system.

Very truly yours,

EDWARD A. MCLAUGHLIN, *M.D.*
August 11, 1961

"No Evidence of Harm," Say the Experts

The June 24, 1961, issue of the *Journal of the American Medical Association* published a letter from an M.D. in Corvallis, Oregon, stating that "certain citizens" there have maintained that they have noted a dermatitis both from contact with and from ingestion of fluoridated water. He says he has been unable to find reports of this in medical literature. Is it possible that fluoridated water can cause dermatitis?

The two experts assigned by the *Journal* to answer this question are both dentists. We don't quite understand how dentists have suddenly become experts on dermatitis, and we think it is strange that this question should not have been referred to some member of the medical profession—an allergist, for instance. There are two prominent allergists who have been campaigning against fluoridation for many years, precisely because they fear many people may be allergic to fluorides. But the warnings of these two, Dr. Jonathan Forman and Dr. G. L. Waldbott, have gone completely unheeded by the medical and public health authorities.

One of the dentists who answers this question in the *Journal* admits that "most substances known to man are potential allergens," but not fluoride. "There is no reliable evidence" he says, that fluoride could cause any ill effects. Such a statement means simply that this gentleman, for some reason, has chosen to ignore all the wealth of medical and scientific literature showing that fluorides may be dangerously harmful to many people and that, unless careful, unbiased scientific work is done immediately, we will continue to ignore many symptoms which may point directly or indirectly to serious or perhaps fatal harm from fluorides.

The second dentist confides to the worried Oregon doctor that there is no evidence that fluorine could harm anyone, giving as his chief proof the fact that 5 healthy young men who took fluorine doses for about 6 months did not suffer any harm. If one wants to follow such reasoning to its logical conclusion, one must assume that, if none of these young men was allergic to milk, then there is no such thing as allergy to milk. If none was allergic to shellfish, then there is no such allergy and so forth. A peculiar form of scientific deduction, we believe.

Dangers of Fluoride Toothpaste

The *British Medical Journal* for July 1, 1961, carried a letter from a physician, A. Kraus, on fluoride toothpaste. He states that fluorides destroy the activity of certain bacteria in the mouth. The complex relationship of these bacteria and the products they produce might be destroyed by fluorides. Yet, it is believed that this activity forms the basis for protection against certain harmful bacteria, which cause diphtheria, Vincent's disease and so forth. He concludes, "all these facts strongly indicate that regular and continued suppression of lactic fermentation in the mouth by fluoride-containing preparations may have far-reaching side effects, the extent of which is as yet unforeseeable. Their use should, therefore, be discouraged unless and until they can be proved to be entirely innocuous."

Now We May Fluoridate School Food

The Reading (Pennsylvania) *Times* for June 9, 1961, carried the news that, at a meeting of the school district's advisory health council, the president of the county dental society advocated fluoridating food in the school cafeterias. The director of medical supervision for the school district pointed out that "the primary purpose of the district is to teach, not to practice dentistry or medicine."

Then, strangely enough, the chief school dentist cautioned that such a procedure would necessitate permission from the parents of every child. No permission necessary for drinking fluoridated water, of course, but as soon as you put the fluoride into food, then a parent's consent is essential. You figure it out, we can't.

A Welsh Researcher Protests

Dr. R. A. Holman of the Royal Infirmary, Cardiff, Wales, writing in the pages of the *British Medical Journal* for April 15, 1961, makes the following comments on fluoridation: .

"Your leading article states that there is little doubt that caries (tooth decay) can be prevented to a large extent by the elimination of our so-called civilized diet. I agree whole-heartedly with this, but would also couple with it the elimination of the large number of chemical agents (many of which are enzymic poisons) which civilized man has allowed to pollute his food and drink. I do not agree that a reversal of the position is impracticable. Many eminent workers, including the Nobel Prize winners, Alexis Carrel and Szent-Gyorgi and more recently, Rene Dubos, have said that until we intelligently reform some of our habits of civilization, there will be no measurable reduction in the prevalence of the diseases peculiar to our time. In view of the widespread concern both in medical and non-medical circles about the mounting chemical adulteration of air, food and drink, it is my opinion that the time is ripe for the control of these hazards which have largely replaced the bacterial hazards so prevalent towards the end of the last century."

He goes on, "It is pertinent to consider the advisability of using sodium fluoride. Apart from the ethical side of regularly dosing thousands of people without their consent, and the debatable advantages to be gained by adults, the question of the long-term effects needs much more investigation."

Dr. Holman then proceeds to discuss a subject in which he is a recognized authority—the relation of enzyme deficiency to health and especially to cancer susceptibility. He says, "Fluoride is a well-known inhibitor (destroyer) of several enzyme systems. In some respects, sodium fluoride acts in the body as a whole like potassium cyanide. This is to be expected, since both fluoride and cyanide can form . . . compounds with the enzyme catalase, resulting in its inhibition (that is, preventing this enzyme from doing its job). Catalase poisoning has been linked with the development of viruses and the causation of a number of diseases, including cancer. One of the well-established facts about cancer is that, as the tumor grows, the cells become progressively deficient in catalase and the total body catalase is lowered. Many observers have suggested that agents which decrease the catalase in cells may predispose to tumor formation. Voisin has said, 'the method most likely to solve the problem of cancer is to ask why the cancer cell is lacking in catalase and try to prevent this impoverishment from taking place.' Since fluoride can inhibit catalase and since it is a cumulative poison, the danger of increasing the cancer-inducing potential in humans must be considered. Although there is not, to my knowledge, any good positive evidence as yet linking fluoride with known cancer cases, the whole question of fluoride intake from food, water, insecticides and industrial processes should be much more thoroughly investigated."

Another Englishman Protests

Another Englishman wrote a fine letter to the *Lancet* (another English medical publication) which appeared in the April 1, 1961, issue. C. G. Dobbs, also of Wales, wrote that he had inquired about the medical inspection given inhabitants of areas where fluoridation was being tested in England. He was told that a "medical check-up" was being given. This supposedly thorough and decisive check-up consisted of asking the local doctors to report any abnormal physical condition which they thought "might be attributed to fluorine."

Mr. Dobbs goes on, "Since skeletal fluorosis is the only recognizable effect upon adults of a high fluoride level intake and this is quite irrelevant at a fluoridation level of one part per million (or so I am assured by the advocates of fluoridation), the result must, of course, be negative and the whole procedure quite pointless and without bearing on the questions of the safety or desirability of increasing the intake of this substance, permanently, by every member of the population."

He continues, "This sort of argument can be applied to any type of pollution which it may be convenient to impose for some special purpose: a moderate increase in smoke, provided there is no obvious or statistically significant increase in bronchitis; a further increase in radiation, throwing the onus on 'objectors' among the public to prove that any single case of leukemia was specifically caused by it, and so on. What alarms me is that our public health authorities, from the Minister downwards, do not seem to realize that the effects of every such generalized increase in one toxic factor are hopelessly confused with those of every other operative factor, and that the impossibility of distinguishing them is not evidence for the 'safety' of such an increase.

"In the face of the appalling increase in chronic diseases far more deadly than dental caries, such a deliberate increase in pollution of the water supply can only create alarm, increase nervous stress and destroy confidence in the public health service. As for the approval of 'an impressive array of scientific bodies,' referred to by Dr. Alcock (in an earlier issue of the *Lancet*), this, I am afraid, is just what the layman is by now driven, cynically, to expect. It reflects, primarily, the successful activities of their more politician-like members. When I want a well-balanced and considered opinion of health matters, I consult an individual doctor, not the British Medical Association, or any other collectivity."

Old Age and Fluoridation

It looks as if the Public Health Service fluoridators are busy everywhere. The *Journal of the American Dental Association* for February, 1961, reports triumphantly that a recommendation for fluoridation of public water supplies was one of the results of a White House Conference on Aging. If anyone can tell us what "aging" has to do with water fluoridation, we want to know what it is.

Even the most earnest fluoridator knows that fluoridated water cannot possibly be of any benefit beyond the age of childhood, but we are asked to believe that hustling fluorides into the drinking water should properly be a vital concern of old people!

We are told that a report submitted at this conference states that "since fluoridation is a lifelong phenomenon, it is recommended that behavioral scientists focus attention upon the causes of resistance found in some communities toward institution of this public health measure."

So now, probably, tax money will be appropriated to provide psychologists who will devote themselves to studying the amazing (to them) spectacle of American citizens who disapprove of being asked to drink a potentially harmful chemical with every mouthful of water, simply because someone in Washington has decided that it might benefit some members of the community!

New Fluoride Toothbrush Appears

A toothbrush boasting of 2 per cent stannous (tin) fluoride in its bristles has appeared in drug stores. We could see no reason for putting fluoride into toothbrushes unless it would affect teeth in some way, so we wrote to the Food and Drug Administration and to the maker of the toothbrush, inquiring what purpose was served by such an addition and what guarantees of safety the buyer might have, should he use the toothbrush.

The letters we received in reply would be completely unbelievable, except that, apparently, nothing is impossible where fluoridation is concerned. Every new development is more fantastic than the last.

The Food and Drug Administration which has only one function—to protect the health of the American people—wrote telling us that their "medical advisers" concluded that the toothbrush was safe because the amount of fluoride that leaches out of the bristles during use is so small that it could not hurt anyone. They said they did not know of any usefulness resulting from inclusion of the fluoride in the bristles. If it is there to prevent tooth decay, the FDA apparently does not know it.

Obviously, a fluoride toothbrush appearing on a counter in a city embattled around the fluoridation issue immediately announces itself as part of the battle. The manufacturer doesn't need to say a word on the label except "fluoride." At once, those citizens who have listened to the alluring promises of tooth decay prevention by the fluoridators assume that the fluoride toothbrush is another part of the plan. They buy it eagerly! Who wouldn't? All the necessary advertising for the wonder drug, fluoride, has already been done by the Public Health Service and the Food and Drug Administration, although, of course, they never mentioned toothbrushes!

Our answer from the toothbrush manufacturer was even more astonishing. *He* knew why the fluoride was there—even if the FDA didn't—to prevent tooth decay, even though he could not say it. "While it is our firm belief that the stannous fluoride in the bristles will have a very good effect in use, our clinical data at this point is not sufficient, until the FDA rules for us, to make any claims regarding inhibitions of caries," he wrote. But you don't need to claim anything, sir—just put your toothbrush out on the counter and the American public will buy it, believing it will prevent tooth decay! In the welter of claims and counterclaims over fluoridation, how can an uninformed consumer know any different?

Fluoride Candy Next

We have a press release from a drug firm concerning an orange-flavored "lozenge containing sodium fluoride, vitamin C and vitamin D" for sale only in certain communities. The preparation could not be sold where water is fluoridated, say its manufacturers, because it obviously might result in serious overdosage of fluorine. So the company has planned, they say, an elaborate distribution scheme whereby the tablets will be available in towns and cities which are not fluoridated, and not obtainable in towns only two or three miles away that are fluoridated. The naiveté of such a proposition stuns us.

This company is apparently planning to sell so much of this candy-type preparation that they can put large sums of money into an organization to keep track of all fluoridation projects and switch their sales force accordingly.

What is to prevent someone from City A (fluoridated) from shopping in City B (3 miles away and unfluoridated) and purchasing a month's supply of the fluoride product for his family? It seems the only way to prevent this is to station guards at all roads entering City A to search anyone entering.

The makers of the fluoride lozenge state on the label just how the preparation is to be taken—and specify that it should be kept out of the way of children. Since its taste is a pleasant orange flavor, we can look forward to a rash of poisonings like those involving flavored aspirin.

Add up all the information above and you will see that we are faced with a veritable deluge of fluoride products. Willing to believe that if a little fluoride is good, a lot is better, many people will eagerly buy all the products available—toothpaste, toothbrushes, lozenges, pills and any new product that comes along in the way of creams, shampoos, chewing gum, dental floss or hair lotions.

Fluorine is one of the most dangerous poisons known. Even the tiniest fraction of fluoride over the specified one part per million is known to cause physical harm. With many different sources now available, in addition to all the fluoride we get in food and in air pollution, it seems certain that irreparable harm will be done by this chemical which has been so widely promoted by the United States Public Health Service.

How Can You Detect Harm?

How will we know when we have been harmed by fluoride? This question was asked by a Brooklyn physician in the March 15, 1961, issue of the *Journal of the American Medical Association*. He said, "Exactly what tests and office procedures can be used to determine individual idiosyncrasy or intolerance to fluorides? Are there practical tests available to the family doctor which he can use to determine whether various subjective complaints are actually caused by fluoride ingestion or just a fear reaction to artificially fluoridated water in a community—that is, concrete tests that can be used to identify early signs of fluoride poisoning, so that a family physician may be guided in his treatment and thereby prevent intractable, neglected cases of chronic fluoride poisoning?"

The answer given by the *Journal's* expert is, "What is here asked for does not exist. There are no simple tests for blood or urinary fluorides, such as may be carried out by the physician in his office or by the usual clinical laboratory. Precise tests require a high degree of chemical skill and equipment of uncommon nature . . . There is no evidence that the quantity of fluorides thus entering the body leads to any demonstrable indications of harm. This statement does not apply to water consumption when the natural fluoride content is excessive or to high industrial intake of fluorides. There are no confirmed reports of chronic fluoride poisoning from properly artificially fluoridated waters."

What does this official answer from the AMA say, in essence? There is no way to tell whether you have been irreparably damaged by fluoride—no tests your doctor can perform. The AMA thinks you probably won't be harmed by fluorides unless you happen to drink a lot of water or are exposed to fluorides in your work. But if you are harmed, there's no way of telling that the fluoride is responsible. And, we might add, no remedy for such harm, no way to repair the damaged tooth enamel, kidney, bone or thyroid gland involved. This is the situation we are asked, by people who call themselves scientists, to accept for ourselves and our families, including sick and old people.

It is interesting to look back on some older theories in regard to possible harmfulness of certain dangerous substances.

Did you know that radium was once thought of as not only safe, but positively beneficial? The virtues of radium therapy were extolled by C. Everett Field, M.D., in a speech given before the Washington Heights Medical Society in New York on November 23, 1915 and reported in the *Medical Record,* for January 22, 1916. Field, who at that time was apparently president of the society, submitted evidence which allegedly proved that radium was therapeutically effective in cases of high blood pressure and hardening of the arteries. And there were additional benefits as well. He felt certain that Bright's disease, for example, "may be wiped out."

As to safety, he claimed that radium was completely eliminated from the body and therefore does not accumulate. He declared, "radium has absolutely no toxic effects, it being accepted as harmoniously by the human system as is sunlight by plant." Deriding one authority who cautioned against radium, Dr. Field said, "If you assume that I have erred in conservative expression, let the excuse be that the worker in radium therapy grows enthusiastic as he manipulates that agent of greatest known energy, the product of the Almighty's laboratory, 'Mother Earth.' "

These are the words of a doctor whose first-hand experience included over 800 intravenous injections of radium chloride. Two other physicians, he reports, had previously given over 2,000 similar treatments. Others, too, had administered radium to human beings.

The deadly danger of radium is known to us today, yet 45 years ago, eminent physicians declared it "safe as sunshine," just as eminent authorities are today claiming that getting fluoride, from all the different sources being made available in water and various products, cannot possibly be harmful. And the experts today know the potential harmfulness of fluorides! But the profits to be made outweigh any sane scientific appraisal of the subject.

No Ill Effects from Fluoridation?

How often have you heard it—"There are absolutely no ill effects on any member of the community as a result of drinking fluoridated water." Here is one explanation of how such a statement is arrived at—in a letter to the editor of the *Canadian Medical Journal* for September 10, 1960. Says C. P. Harrison, M.D., of British Columbia, "In general, it works like this: A cursory examination of the vital statistics of the fluoridated area is undertaken. None of the diseases statistically listed is credited to the consumption of fluorides. It is not surprising then that there is no increase in these diseases in the fluoridated area, but this allows the statement to be made, 'No deleterious effects of fluoride have been found.' This is really a statement of ignorance as to whether or not there are any deleterious effects of fluoride, but, unfortunately, being ignorant is no bar to being positive and quite illogically, the statement is changed to read, 'It has been found that there are no deleterious effects from the ingestion of fluoride ion.'

"What little we know of the physiological effects of the fluoride ion does not redound to its credit. We know that it affects enzyme systems and that it is cumulative in the soft tissues as well as bone, but no clear-cut symptom has been established. We cannot detect early toxic effects of fluoride unless we know precisely what to look for. Possibly, in the dosage suggested, fluoride is not harmful, but surely it is incumbent upon us to prove its harmlessness from our knowledge of the action of the fluoride ion before we recommend it to the public."

One Victory on the Legal Front

In July, 1960, a St. Louis county judge decreed that fluoridation was illegal—that an ordinance authorizing fluoridation was invalid and unconstitutional. He called fluoridation "an unwarranted and unjustified invasion of the liberty guaranteed the plaintiffs and others under the United States Constitution." He also decided that fluoridation is contrary to the Missouri state constitution and the St. Louis county charter. "The plaintiffs," he said, "are deprived of the liberty of deciding whether they want to apply fluorine to their teeth for the purpose of preventing tooth decay." He went on to say that "while tooth decay may be termed a disease, it is not contagious in any way and in no way endangers the public health, in the sense that its existence in the teeth of one individual might adversely affect personal health in another individual. If fluorine is the key to dental health, and, as the evidence shows, fluorides are readily available to all who desire them, it appears that through proper education and persuasion, the people would accept application of fluoride and would not have to be compelled to be subjected en masse to fluoride."

Why Do People Object to Fluoridation?

An article in the *Journal of the Florida Dental Association* for summer, 1959, reviews the findings of a survey done in Northampton, Massachusetts, to discover who was opposed to fluoridation and why. Says the author, Delmar R. Miller, D.D.S., "Of great interest concerning the anti-fluoridation voters, was the fact that more than 90 per cent refused to accept as reliable the statements of qualified scientists and scientific groups who favored fluoridation. This is significant since nearly all scientists and scientific groups in the health field supported the measure . . . It might be pointed out, however, that this same group seemed to give great credence to the statements of a few scientists and professional people who opposed the measure."

Dr. Miller goes on, "The attitude of a large per cent of anti-fluoridation voters, on interrogation, seemed to be based on a deep-rooted suspicion of the scientific groups and individual scientists who favored fluoridation. They expressed fear that the United States Public Health Service and the American Dental Association were engaged in a conspiracy with large monopoly interests in this country. The impression that professional proponents of fluoridation were to profit from the program in some devious, underhanded way was rampant. To these people, the idea that dentists were to profit handsomely from fluoridation and that fluoride manufacturers were to reap a fortune from it, seemed perfectly reasonable."

If such an attitude is impossible for Dr. Miller to comprehend, let us help him out a bit. One of the foremost promoters of fluoridation (he tours the country with unlimited funds, apparently, at his disposal) is Dr. A. P. Black, Professor of Chemistry of the University of Florida. Dr. Black's son owns a business which sells fluoridation equipment. Now certainly there is nothing "devious or underhanded" about the benefits Dr. Black hopes to reap from widespread fluoridation. They are quite obvious and out in the open for all to see.

Dr. James Cox, outstanding fluoridation promoter from Pittsburgh, is Professor of Dental Research at the University of Pittsburgh. Financing of academic life at the University of Pittsburgh is inevitably involved with the Mellon interests, which are certainly closely tied in with the aluminum business. And fluoride is a by-product of the aluminum industry. Nothing "devious or underhanded" about the arrangement. It is all in the open.

The Department of Dr. Frederick Stare at Harvard School of Public Health was the recipient of more than a million dollars as a financial grant from a food company, many of whose products are under sharp attack by independent researchers as being contributory causes of tooth decay. It is not very hard to figure out why

Dr. Stare of Harvard would be on the side of the fluoridationists, now is it? Nothing underhanded or devious—the announcement of the million dollars in "payola" appeared in the *New York Times*.

The principal promoters of fluoridation (your servants in the Public Health Service in Washington) have staked their careers on the success of the fluoridation push. They dare not turn back. Incidentally, they are working in the Department of Health, Education and Welfare, some of whose activities were investigated by the Kefauver Committee. The head of the Antibiotics Division, you will remember, was found to be accepting quite a large salary from the industry he was supposed to be policing. This kind of disclosure might have something to do with the suspicions of the experts which Dr. Miller cannot understand.

We think it is the most encouraging development we have yet encountered—that Americans are at last waking up to the fact that the "experts" should be listened to only so long as there is no incentive (financial or career) involved in the scientific decision they are required to make. A man who foresees his livelihood or his career being destroyed if he makes a statement for or against a new concept in health, is not very likely to be objective in making the decision, scientist or no scientist. Our researchers today are so involved in financial obligations that they have almost ceased being scientists.

Finally, what is so surprising about intelligent people who are suspicious when scientific "experts" tell them that, in order to give medicine to a certain small segment of the population, *the entire population must take it?*

Possible Symptoms of Fluorine Poisoning

An excellent resumé of the possible symptoms of early chronic fluorine poisoning is outlined in a letter to the editor of the *Canadian Medical Journal* for July 9, 1960. William A. Costain, M.D. of Toronto writes as follows: "Now that fluoridation is receiving more attention, it would be desirable if doctors in fluoridated areas were to look for side effects from the taking of fluorine. In the past, there have been no leads. No one knew what to look for and consequently, no reports were forthcoming, but now, when the door has been opened, it is to be hoped that there will be many individual observations on this topic. The searching of medical history sheets for clues and recordings of early side effects of sodium fluoride are the necessary and important ones. Of these, the effects from lowering of calcium blood levels come first—a tendency to bleed evidenced by unfavorable results from surgical operations, both major and minor; undiagnosed skin lesions (disorders); all those conditions arising from edema (swelling) in the tissues as a consequence of slow clotting time; deterioration of skin and appendages; the ever increasing nervous and mental diseases aggravated by lack of calcium; and many others which will develop with time. . . .

"We do not know the proper fluoride doses nor do we know what manifestations may come from the smallest doses. There are no recognized normal fluorine blood levels and there are no known daily requirements for fluorine.

"Personally, I am convinced that dosage of fluorides is definitely in the microgram level, and that fluoridation dosage, based erroneously as it is on water levels instead of blood levels, is anywhere up to a thousand times too strong. Even at the microgram level, I have found and reported in the *Canadian Medical Association Journal* (Vol. 81, p. 954, 1959) cases showing side effects. Since that report, still further cases have come to my attention where skin and its appendages have been affected, and they all point to fluorine."

In the *Detroit News* for September 18, 1960, appeared an article by George L. Waldbott, M.D., a leading allergist. Among many provocative and stimulating statements, Dr. Waldbott says, "In a 14-year-old Detroit boy, the lens of an eye with a cataract, removed surgically, contained an unusually large amount of fluoride. In other lenses with cataract, not even a trace was found. Whence did the fluoride come? Who can assure Detroit citizens that this boy's ailment was not caused by fluoride? Why did it accumulate in his eyes and not elsewhere in the body?"

Dr. Waldbott reminds us, "Neither does it make any difference how many cities now have fluoridated water. Millions of people have been smoking cigarettes for generations. Does this prove smoking safe?"

Fluorides Contaminate Processed Foods

Contamination of processed foods by fluorides in the water supply of the city where the processing plants are located has been a major concern of the food industry. Many firms are using their own wells to avoid contamination.

The following concentration of fluoride was found in cereals by Northwest Testing Laboratory, Portland, Oregon, July 28, 1960: Post's Grape Nuts (Battle Creek, Michigan), 6.4 parts per million; Kellogg's Shredded Wheat (Battle Creek, Michigan), 9.4 parts per million; General Mills' Wheaties (Minneapolis, Minnesota), 10.1 parts per million. Public water supplies in these cities are fluoridated.

The average amount of fluoride naturally found in the cereals from which these products are made is ⅓ to 1 part per million. So it seems reasonable to assume that the rest of that high fluoride content migrates into the cereal from the water while it is being processed.

Suppression of Scientific Evidence

Back in 1959, we first read of the work of Dr. Ionel Rapaport of the University of Wisconsin Psychiatric Institute in, of all places, the *Bulletin of the National Academy of Medicine* (Vol. 140, pp. 529-531, 1956) in France. Dr. Rapaport, while studying the problem of Mongolism, noticed that such children have little tooth decay. He also learned, through study of the medical literature on Mongolism, that oxygen consumption in the brains of Mongoloid children is less than that of normal children. It is well-known that fluorine is an enzyme inhibitor (that is, it hinders the activity of enzymes).

With these discoveries in mind, Dr. Rapaport undertook a study of the incidence of Mongoloid births in 4 midwestern states, finding that there exists a relationship between the concentration of fluorine in the drinking water and the frequency of Mongolism.

Now, a letter from the Director of Dental Health of the state of Wisconsin tells us that the state Board of Health does not consider Dr. Rapaport's article on fluoridation and Mongolism to be scientifically accurate.

He enclosed information showing that a committee at the University of Wisconsin, consisting of the Dean of the Medical School and 5 members of the scientific faculty, have met on 3 occasions to discuss the affair. The committee decided that the statistical evidence does not prove that fluoridation is related to Mongolism and that further studies should be made. Such a conclusion is very interesting, because all that Dr. Rapaport did was to present figures for how many Mongoloid births there were in different communities and how much fluoride was in the water there. If such figures are of no importance, as the University committee implies, why should they recommend further study? And, if they recommend further study, shouldn't they also recommend that fluoridation of any and all communities be stopped or postponed until they have the results of further study?

The committee carefully points out, too, that Dr. Rapaport was called in and asked to explain. He stated that he made no effort to give publicity to his report and no claim that his studies revealed a cause of Mongolism. "Because of his desire not to be involved in a controversy, he published his results in France where this is less of a public issue," says the committee.

The above sentences, we believe, are among the most astounding we have ever seen in relation to a matter of scientific investigation. An expert university researcher turns up a fascinating and provocative piece of evidence which seems to show that a widespread public health measure may result in harm to future generations. But because of the controversial nature of the information, he felt that he had to publish his findings in a foreign country.

The very life's blood of scientific inquiry is controversy. Over the centuries, everything we have discovered, scientifically speaking, has been discovered because free, creative, inquiring minds have raised questions challenging old concepts. Invariably, the new concept is the subject of controversy—it has to be! Why should a scientist try to avoid controversy? It leads to further inquiry and, if he is convinced of the rightness of his idea, he is sure that further inquiry will result only in acceptance of it.

But the people who promote fluoridation want no controversy. They want no one to raise any question about the possible harmful effects of their drive to fluoridate. Surely nothing could be less scientific than this! Dr. Rapaport has worked for many years on his study of Mongolism. The University of Wisconsin calls in 5 scientists, none of whom seems to have done any work on Mongolism, so far as we know, and *they* decide what *we* should think about Dr. Rapaport's work. Surely nothing could be less scientific than this!

But saddest of all is the statement from Dr. Rapaport, that he published his article in France so that he could avoid controversy and that he has made no effort to give publicity to his findings. Statements like these reveal better than anything we could say the pitiful state of scientific inquiry in this country. Why shouldn't such a finding as this be blazoned on the front page of every publication in the land? The answer is that American scientists are living in an academic police state. The results of their experiments and observations must agree with the accepted, conservative view being promoted at the present time. If not, they are apparently submitted to intimidation.

Why should Dr. Rapaport, a respected scientific researcher at a university, have to explain to anybody why or where he published an article dealing with a subject of vital interest to every American? Why, instead, should he not have been honored for his work, why should not the University itself have taken up the cudgels in his behalf and declared their willingness to provide time and money for further inquiry along these lines, since the subject is so important?

We are afraid that the largest part of the answer lies in a small word that has been used to castigate another professional group—Payola. Universities receive financial grants from the United States Public Health Service. It follows that the findings reported from their laboratories will probably agree with the current programs of the Public Health Service. Won't they? Will the Public Health Service donate millions of taxpayers' dollars to universities which challenge the programs like fluoridation on which Public Health officials have staked their professional reputations? It seems unlikely to us.

Such payola is, of course, far more devastating to America than the TV quiz scandals. For true scientific inquiry cannot exist in such an atmosphere. Our universities and their students suffer, the American public suffers and devoted scientists like Dr. Rapaport suffer most of all.

Fluorine from Fish

Congratulations to Dr. Frederick Stare of Harvard for the first sensible word about nutrition he has said for a long time! Speaking at dedication ceremonies of a laboratory of the United States Bureau of Commercial Fisheries in Gloucester, Massachusetts, Dr. Stare declared that the battle over fluoridating drinking water to retard tooth decay can be solved by forgetting the water and leaving the job to fish. Fish from the ocean, he said, provide sufficient fluorine to protect dental enamel and prevent decay. According to the *New York Times* for June 19, 1960, he also recommended eating small fish, bones and all, for calcium, phosphorus and other elements essential to good health.

Better be careful, Dr. Stare—next they'll be calling you a faddist!

A Handy Jug of Fluorides

We wonder how the experiment announced by the Public Health Service in the Pittsburgh (Pennsylvania) *Post-Gazette* (August 10, 1961) is coming along. Three hundred families were to be asked to test a home gadget to fluoridate drinking water. The device looks like a metal jug, about half-gallon size, and is attached to the incoming water pipe of the home. It feeds one part of fluoride per million parts of water under any condition of water temperature, pressure or flow.

The cost is about 23 dollars to install and about 2 dollars per month maintenance. A safety feature provides for a shut-off of the device if, for some reason, it should fail to operate properly. So, for 24 dollars per year, after the initial cost of installation, claims the Public Health Service, a family can cut its children's dental problems by 60 per cent. (The *Post-Gazette* article says 33 per cent, but that's much more conservative than the figure one usually sees.)

We hope the jug does what its manufacturer claims it will do in properly controlling the addition of fluoride to the household water supply. Then those who believe fluoridation will lick the tooth decay problem can have fluoridated water just by turning on the tap. And we who doubt the validity of fluoridation's promises to reduce tooth decay and we who do not feel it is safe to drink fluoridated water, can have the pure water our taxes pay for, with nothing added but those chemicals deemed necessary to make it safe to drink.

Suppression of Freedom

Does the dental profession suppress the freedom of its own members to oppose fluoridation? Max Ginns, D.M.D., was "dropped" from the Massachusetts Dental Society "on 7 charges stemming from opposition to fluoridation" (*Boston Daily Record,* September 28, 1961). Dr. Ginns, senior dental consultant at the Worcester, Massachusetts, General Hospital and past chairman of numerous committees of his State and local dental societies, had obtained signatures of 119 dentists and 59 physicians from the Worcester area who opposed fluoridation. The petition sought repeal of the society's support of fluoridation. Referring to the injustice to which Dr. Ginns has been subjected, the *Springfield Union* (October 7, 1961) editorialized: "The Massachusetts and Worcester Dental Societies are penalizing Dr. Ginns for expressing his valid conviction that fluoridation is a hoax. Dr. Ginns has proven himself to be a noble asset to the humanity he serves by living up to his convictions."

Sodium Fluoride Is a Poison

The Merck Index, the standard reference book of the pharmaceutical profession, has some interesting notations under its heading on "Sodium Fluoride." Among *Uses:* "As insecticide, particularly for roaches and ants; in other pesticide formulations; constituent in vitreous enamel and glass mixes; as a steel degassing agent; in electroplating; in fluxes . . . for disinfecting fermentation apparatus in breweries . . ." Under *Human Toxicity:* "Severe symptoms from ingestion of 0.25 to 0.45 grams. Death from 4 grams. Sublethal: Nausea and vomiting, abdominal distress, diarrhea, stupor and weakness. Lethal: Muscular weakness, tremors, convulsions, collapse, dyspnea, respiratory and cardiac failure and death. Chronic: Mottling of tooth enamel, osteosclerosis."

Frankly, there's already a tremendously difficult struggle to remove increasing quantities of poisons from public water supplies. *Let's not foolishly put this one in!*

Food and Drug Administration

Government Scientists Recognize Health Hazards

We are often accused of fighting progress. This is not true. Who could sensibly be against a better, safer, easier, more enjoyable world? What we are against is progress at any price. If we must breathe and eat death-dealing strontium 90 in order to have atomic energy, we are against this form of progress. If we must pay with the very nutrients we need to keep alive and free from disease, in order to have "heat-and-serve" dinners and meats and vegetables that don't need refrigeration, we are against this form of progress, too. If progress means accepting poisonous additives to color our foods, keep them soft or hard, smooth or grainy, we deplore it. We deplore the progress that releases exhausts and gaseous wastes into the air so as to make it unfit to breathe, and we resist a progress that puts a definite poison in the water on the illogical theory that it will prevent tooth decay. In short, progress that is largely the synthetic product of the advertisers' art, is progress we are against wholeheartedly.

Government Often Adds to Confusion

The "progress" label on these things does not fool everyone. But it does confuse many of us. The government, to whom we look for guidance in many of these matters, only adds to the confusion. Government scientists say nuclear testing is suicidal because of fall-out, then the government tests nuclear bombs. The government says a coal-tar dye used to color oranges is cancer-causing, then proceeds to allow use of the color as before, for several more years. The government says air pollution is dangerous, but declines to make federal laws to control it.

When we say that government scientists feel the way we do, many people find it hard to believe, in view of the support the government gives the very industries which present these problems.

To show that the problems we recognize are also recognized by the government (in spite of its lack of action in combating them), we would like to quote from *Federation Proceedings* (Vol. 19, No. 3, Part II), a publication of the Food and Drug Administration. The article by E. M. K. Geiling and William D'Aguanno, Division of Pharmacology, Food and Drug Administration, is entitled, "Our Man-Made Noxious Environment."

For example, here is how our government scientists see the problem of radiation hazards:

"The potentialities (of atomic energy) for good are almost boundless; the consequences of the misuse of this enormous source of energy are terrifying. Even the peaceful uses of atomic energy are fraught with danger, and present serious problems. There is enough radioactive waste material in huge steel tanks at 5 different locations in the United States to cause severe pollution of all the land and water areas of the country. Fall-out, pollution of streams, soils and crops, and disposal of waste products are serious hazards which must be guarded against. Solutions for these problems are being sought by many thousands of scientists."

Chemicals Aplenty

Are they aware of the chemicals we face in every activity of daily life? Indeed they are. One finds it difficult to understand how the government can express such definite concern and yet take such spiritless action to protect us.

"The phenomenal growth of the chemical industry has made available thousands of new compounds, many of which are toxic, and

new ones are constantly being prepared. Production of new chemicals
has increased at an annual rate of 7 per cent since 1947. This rate
surpasses, by far, the impressive average annual increment of 3 per
cent for all United States production. By mid-1959, the chemical
industry ranked fourth in size among all industries in the United
States. At present, more than 10,000 chemical entities contribute to
some 500,000 products that are used industrially to produce innumerable durable and nondurable goods, which are integral components
of our environment. Predictions that the growth of this industry will
continue at an accelerated rate are supported by information from
the Manufacturing Chemists' Association. Expenditures on chemical
production and construction of research facilities will be nearly 2
billion dollars during the next 2 years. By 1975, the production
index will be 100 per cent higher than it is now. It is not at all
unreasonable to expect a proportionate increase in the already impressive 10,000 chemical entities—placing man in an environment
of a truly chemical age.

"The intrinsic injurious properties of many of these chemical
agents constitute potentially serious environmental hazards. The
readily accessible source of toxic or potentially toxic consumer products is evidenced by the thousands of pharmaceutical preparations,
chemical pesticides and household products. Toxicological investigations of many of these have been extensive. However, instances
have been reported in which chronic or synergistic effects are apparent only after a product has been marketed for some years.

"Within recent years, we have become acutely aware of the
importance of accidental chemical poisoning as a cause of death and
disability, chiefly, but by no means exclusively, in the home. In 1958,
accidental poisoning through ingestion of solid or liquid substances
caused 1,429 deaths in the United States. Of this number, 422
(approximately 33 per cent) occurred in children under 5 years of
age. Aspirin (mostly the candied variety) tops the list. Gases and
vapors were responsible for 1,187 deaths. An additional 3,958 deaths
occurred following the ingestion of either solids, liquids or gases
with suicidal intent. At present, it is estimated that there are approximately 700 nonfatal poisonings for every fatal case in children.
Among this number, many children and adults were either crippled
or made seriously ill, or required some treatment, either in the
home or in a hospital.

"The Public Health Service estimates that there are about 600,-
000 children who accidentally swallow toxic substances each year. In
the United States there are very few, if any, households which do
not have on hand several potentially poisonous preparations. These
may be either pesticides (vermicides, rodenticides, herbicides, etc.),
cleaning fluids, solvents, paints, deodorants and the like. These ma-

terials may be either solids or liquids or gases. Some are toxic when ingested, others when inhaled or absorbed through the skin.

"According to the testimony presented at a recent Senate hearing, there are over 300,000 toxic or potentially toxic trade-named products on the consumer market. In the case of drugs, pesticides and caustic-containing products, federal law requires that the ingredients be clearly stated on the label. However, cleaning fluids, bleaches, certain soaps, detergents, furniture polishes and a host of other hazardous substances and devices used in the home in ever-increasing numbers are, at present, not subject to the existing federal statutes. (There are a few states which do require informative labeling of such products which are not now subject to federal law.)"

The Farmer Does His Bit

When we come to the foods we eat, the problems are monumental. From the farm to the table, every form of treatment possible is dumped into food. Let the Food and Drug Administration's scientists speak on what the farmer and the factory do to the foods you eventually buy and eat.

"The increase in agricultural productivity in this country has had a proportionate impact on our environment. The result is that the role of the farmer has broadened considerably in our society. In 1940, the average farmer produced enough for himself and 10 others; in 1958, he produced enough for himself and 22 others. From 1950 to 1958, farm output rose 20 per cent, while the population increased 15 per cent.

"This increased productivity is the result of a number of contributory factors. Among them are: (a) the striking increase in the use of chemicals such as fertilizers, insectides, fungicides, herbicides, nematocides, coccidiostats, animal health protectants and medicated feeds; (b) more efficient use of machinery in practically all farming operations; (c) better seeds and improved strains of practically all breeds of farm animals; (d) more efficient training of larger numbers of students in our agricultural and veterinary colleges, as well as an increase in the many types of short courses offered to farmers in these institutions; (e) contributions for research from federal and state departments of health and agriculture, who also contribute in an advisory and regulatory capacity.

"The use of a wide variety of chemicals on the farm has undoubtedly been the most important single factor accountable for the marked increase in raw agricultural products. The toxicological significance of many of these agents is generally recognized. The concern expressed by regulatory officials and their continued emphasis regarding adherence to label warnings and directions is certainly justifiable. The farmer, by disregarding these warnings and direc-

Table 2: DRUGS CURRENTLY USED IN ANIMAL FEEDS

DRUGS	WITH-DRAWAL TIMES*	CERTIFIABLE ANTIBIOTICS
New Drugs:		
Arsenobenzene	5 days	Bacitracin
Bithionol and methiotriazamine	3 days	Chlortetracycline
Dienestrol diacetate	48 hours	Dihydrostreptomycin
Diethylcarbamazine (dog food)		Penicillin
Diethylstilbestrol	48 hours	Streptomycin
Diethylstilbestrol (poultry water)	4 days	Streptomycin
Hygromycin B		
Nicarbazin	4 days	Enzymes (except pepsin)
2-acetyl-amino-5-nitrothiazole	7 days	
2,4-diamino-5(p-chloro-phenyl)6-ethylpyrimidine		
3,5-dinitrobenzamide	48 hours	
Glycarbylamide	4 days	
Hydroxyzine hydrochloride		
Nithiazide	24 hours	
Nystatin		
Oleandomycin chloroform adduct		
Para-Ureidobenzene arsonic acid	5 days	
Reserpine		
Other Drugs:		
Acetyl(p-nitrophenyl) sulf-anilamide	5 days	4-Nitrophenylarsonic acid
Aminonitrothiazole	7 days	Iodinated casein
Arsanilic acid	5 days	Menadione sodium bisulfite
Aterrimin		Oxytetracycline
Cadmium anthranilate	30 days	Para amino benzoic acid, sodium or potassium salt of
Di-N-butyltin dilaurate		para amino benzoic acid
Dinitrophenylsulfonylethyl-enediamine		Pepsin
Dried rumen bacteria		Phenothiazine
Dynafac		Piperazine
Erythromycin thiocyanate	5 days	Piperazine hexahydrate
Furazolidone		Piperazine monohydrochloride and dihydrochloride
2,2'-dihydroxy-5, 5'-dichloro-diphenylmethane		Piperazine phosphate mono-hydrate
3-nitro-4-hydroxyphenyl arsonic acid	5 days	Piperazine sulfate
Nicotine	5 days	Sodium arsanilate
Nitrofurazone		Sodium fluoride
Nitrophenide	4 days	Sodium propionate
		Sulfaquinoxaline

*Required to free tissues of drugs under specific conditions of use and representation.

tions, can directly expose a large mass of our population to the toxic effects of the chemicals which he uses currently without benefit of special training and without any real appreciation of the problems and dangers of residual contaminants.

"The practice of adding drugs to the feed of domestic animals for both prophylactic and therapeutic purposes dates back many years. It is a simple as well as a convenient method of administering medicaments to large numbers of animals. Two of the main objectives of adding such drugs are to shorten the time required for animals to reach market weight and to increase the efficiency of feed utilization by the animals.

"Among the drugs incorporated in the animals' diet for these purposes are: diethylstilbestrol, dienestrol diacetate, iodinated casein, organic arsenicals, antibiotics, nitrofurans, sulfonamides, coccidiostats, organic tin compounds, parasiticides and many others. The widespread use of potent chemical agents introduces additional problems into the protection of the food supply of both man and animals. We are indebted to Dr. Charles G. Durbin, Veterinary Medical Director, Food and Drug Administration, for allowing us to reproduce in table 2 his list of drugs currently added to animal feeds. Drug residues which might occur in the edible tissues of animals are increasing in importance and causing a proportionate amount of concern. An example is the use of chicken feeds containing the coccidiostat nicarbazin, which results in the appearance of this drug in the eggs.

Table 3: ANTIBIOTICS PRODUCED FOR ANIMAL FEED SUPPLEMENTS, 1956*

Antibiotic	Pounds Manufactured	% of Total Output
Penicillin procaine	173,455	20.5
Streptomycin	8,250	0.9
Bacitracin	21,104	2.5
Chlortetracycline	465,197	54.9
Oxytetracycline	179,190	21.2
Neomycin	29	
Total	847,225	100.0

*By 1956, animal feed supplements represented over 27 per cent of total antibiotics output.

Table 4: OUTPUT OF LEADING ANTIBIOTICS

Antibiotic	1948 lb.	1956 lb.
Penicillin	155,873	1,059,704
Streptomycin	80,737	148,999
Dihydrostreptomycin	2,989	492,173
Chlortetracycline	661	560,663
Oxytetracycline		324,614
Tetracycline		220,074
All others	72	275,146
Total	240,332	3,081,373

"The term 'medicated feed' as commonly used is intended to designate a feed to which a drug or drugs have been added. The extent to which this adding of drugs has grown and the complexity of the scientific and technical problems involved, indicate that the feed manufacturer is in reality also a drug manufacturer. The addition of a drug to feeds makes the resulting product, in essence, a drug. Such a feed may now be subject to the New Drug as well as to the Food Additive sections of the Federal Food, Drug and Cosmetic Act.

"The large amount of drugs being used in medicated feeds makes the industry 'big business.' The antibiotics used in the medicated feeds industry represents roughly over 27 per cent of the total antibiotic output. The use of these potent drugs in medicated feeds is attended with potential hazards and requires careful observance of the directions for their use. To insure the proper use of a medicated feed, there must be competent personnel to perform each of the following steps in the process of manufacture: (a) the drug must be checked for purity and weight before use in the premix; (b) the premix must be properly prepared and assayed; (c) the final dilution of the premix with the feed must also be checked; and (d) full directions for use of feed must be clearly stated on the label on the feed container. The farmer in turn must not use the feed for the stated time prior to slaughter.

"It should be noted that animal feeds may incorporate an additional hazard, i.e., the accidental presence of pesticide chemical residues and other potential toxicants applied to the plants or added to the soil to improve the crop or to protect it against pests.

Therapeutic Use of Drugs in Farm Animals

"In recent years, many new drugs have been introduced into veterinary medicine. It has been estimated that 75 tons of antibiotics are used yearly in intramammary infusion for the prevention and treatment of bovine mastitis, probably the most important economic disease in dairy cattle.

"Milk from cows treated with the recommended amounts of penicillin may contain some antibiotic residue up to 72 hours after the last infusion into the udder. For this reason, the label is required to include a statement that milk from treated cows must not be used for human consumption for at least 72 hours after the latest administration. Withdrawal time for antibiotics administered parenterally have not yet been established. Studies to furnish the necessary data are still in progress.

"The very serious effect of small amounts of penicillin to individuals sensitive to this product cannot be overemphasized.

"It is not only on the farm that chemicals are being used in the production of our food. Large amounts of chemicals are employed in the food processing industry. *Increasingly, the consumer demands more processing of foods before purchase.* The trend in modern civilization is toward food prepared for immediate cooking or consumption. *A substantial number of chemicals, perhaps 2,500, have*

been introduced into our food supply to function as preservatives,
color improvers, extenders, flavor intensifiers, texture modifiers and
nutritional factors. Even the new types of packaging offer a potential
source of food additives, in that diffusion of toxic chemicals may
occur from the packaging to the food during storage. Many of the
chemicals may be of unknown toxicity or even of known high toxicity.
Data must be provided that either the chemical does not become a
component of food or that it is safe toxicologically in the amounts
present." (Italics ours.)

The Problem of Air Pollution

Is it silly to concern oneself over the dangers of air and water
pollution? We don't see how any thinking person can afford to be
indifferent to what appears to be a virtual choking off of our safe
supply of life's most vital elements. Geiling and D'Aguanno have this
to say in emphasizing the gravity of the situation:

"Air pollution has become an exceedingly serious public health
hazard in a number of localities in the United States and in most
industrial areas throughout the world. The air pollution problem was
already prominent in many industrialized cities more than a century
ago. The chief pollutant, then, was smoke from coal and wood. However, in the past 50 years, industrial production has increased over
900 per cent, and the number of automotive vehicles has increased
from 1,000 to 70 million. In the United States, the population has
more than doubled and has concentrated to the extent that more
than half the population lives in metropolitan areas which cover less
than 5 per cent of our total land space. This intense concentration
of population, coupled with the tremendous rise in industrialization
and increase in the use of automobiles in these areas, has led to an
intensification of toxicants emitted into our atmosphere. The chief
air pollutants today are oxides of nitrogen and sulfur, the aldehydes,
carbon monoxide, smoke, condensed fumes and organic vapors, often
referred to as hydrocarbons, of which there are said to be 200 in
automobile exhaust fumes alone. Statistical analysis and tabulation
of pollutants on a nation-wide scale have not yet been undertaken;
however, their magnitude can be envisioned by considering the fact
that data shown in table 5 are for New York and Chicago only.

"Health hazards from air pollution may be of an acute or chronic
nature. Acute air pollution episodes of a spectacular nature, such as
the Donora catastrophe of 1948, are not the most difficult part of the
problem. There are more subtle effects which may result in chronic
illness, disabilities and/or premature death. Toxicants emitted may
act as irritants on mucous membranes, by specific toxic reactions,
which may be cumulative by allergenic and possibly by carcinogenic
activity. Evidence is accumulating which suggests that air pollution

may be involved in the development of chronic bronchitis,
asthma, emphysema and lung
cancer. Dr. David F. Eastcott,
formerly Assistant Director, National Institute of Health of New
Zealand, recently stated that
'immigrants to New Zealand,
from highly industrialized Britain, run a risk of lung cancer
30 per cent greater than persons
born in New Zealand of the same
stock and way of life. If they are
more than 30 years of age on
coming to New Zealand, their
risk is 75 per cent greater.'
Similar evidence is available
from the Union of South Africa.
The serious effects may be discovered only after years of exposure—11 years in the case of

Table 5: ESTIMATED AMOUNT OF
TOXICANTS LIBERATED INTO THE
ATMOSPHERE IN TONS PER DAY*

Pollutant	New York	Chicago
Sulfur dioxide	2,170	3,197
Sulfur trioxide	133	182
Hydrogen sulfide	133	196
Nitrogen oxides (as dioxide)	1,355	1,103
Hydrogen cyanide	96	196
Ammonia	115	141
Hydrochloric acid	118	141
Formaldehyde	131	147
Organics, miscellaneous	4,330	3,836
Organic acids (as acetic)	1,542	1,732
Fluorides (as fluorine)	8	16
Solids (smoke, dusts, etc.)	12,693	26,236

*Data from *Literature Review of Metropolitan Air Pollutant Concentrations,* Stanford Research Institute, 1956.

the Donora episode. Preliminary data from the Donora incident indicate that the group made ill by exposure to the fog show a higher
disease and death rate than do the residents not affected by the fog.

"The yearly economic losses due to air pollution have been
estimated at 7.5 billion dollars. They include: damage to crops,
livestock and vegetation; corrosion; soiling; fuel losses; interference
with visibility; and interference with production or services.

Water Pollution

"The pollution of our water supply is due, in large measure, to
the fact that many of our major industries and population centers
are located along rivers or inland lakes. The most urgent problem is
the adequate handling of the many tons of nonliving contaminants,
which are discharged as waste, or otherwise, and find their way into
our water supplies. A number of these substances are as yet unidentified chemicals. There are often so many of these products present
in a single sample of water, that analysis takes many days of work
just to name the broad categories of chemical constituents. A great
deal of research needs to be done to identify these contaminants, to
determine their pharmacological and toxicological effects, and to
develop control methods. It is necessary to formulate the solution of
these problems on a broad base, and it requires the collaborative
efforts of well-trained scientists, including engineers, biologists, chemists, pharmacologists, toxicologists, physicians and statisticians. Such

individuals must have well-equipped laboratories in which to carry out their researches.

"The presence of radiological waste in some of our rivers, notably the Columbia River, adds a new hazard which, if not checked, may in time become a serious menace."

We are in trouble and it's getting more serious every day. We have only one recourse: protest. Write to anyone you can think of who is concerned in the situation—government officials, chemical companies, legislators, city fathers, farm associations, etc. Protest food additives by letting manufacturers know you won't buy products that have been treated, *and don't buy them!*

Food Processing

Food Research

By Robert Rodale

There is no better way to understand what the research scientists are doing to our food than to read the trade publications of the food processing industry. The December 11, 1961, issue of *Food Field Reporter* contains an article which is most illuminating, because it tells what the food technologists themselves are planning to make available for us to eat in the next decade. I will quote it in its entirety:

SIMULATED MEAT, "SPUN" PROTEIN, PLANNED FOR 1970's SUPERS

DETROIT—Despite no appreciable increase in the number of basic foodstuffs, there are some 6,000 food items in today's super markets, 4 times the number sold 20 years ago. Moreover, in the development stage today are half of the food products which will be in the super markets of 1970.

In fact, Dr. Harold W. Schultz, president of the Institute of Food Technologists, told scientists at the American Public Health Association, cupboards would be pretty bare were it not for thousands of new and improved food items developed by technologists.

There will still be the "convenience foods," but the technologists will, through scientific studies of structural, chemical and bacteriological aspects of food and through application of engineering skills and food processing techniques, build into them even greater nutritive value and desirability, it was stated.

There will be fabricated peas and simulated meat, poultry and fish resulting from a "spinning" of vegetable proteins, such as derived from soybeans, into fibers and incorporating them with binders, fats, colors, flavors and nutrients into ready-to-eat products, he stated.

According to Dr. Schultz, who is also head of the Department of Food and Dairy Technology at Oregon State University, the fabricated "peas" will probably result from a tasteful blending of starch, flavoring, color and a binder or "skin" to hold the materials together. Simulated meat will come in many new forms and at a lower cost than the original.

Dessert toppings will be marketed in pressurized cans or squeeze tubes and the constantly improving "instant" coffees will grow in flavor and favor. Dehydrated cottage cheese is a possible newcomer and there will probably be some un-aged cheese with all the characteristics of the well-aged cheeses.

Seafood lovers can look for more ready-to-warm-and-serve frozen seafood items and freeze-dried vegetables will be widely used. Canned breads, now made for military use, will be a "new" item in up-to-the-minute markets and beef and pork, tenderized by injections of enzymes at slaughter, will be preferred by the particular shopper, Dr. Schultz said.

Butter will spread more easily and there will be a greater variety of precooked poultry in the convenience packs. Freeze-dried fruits will probably be on all shopping lists and there will be a long list of special purpose foods prepared or modified to fit the special needs of infants, infirm people or those with special dietary requirements. These special purpose foods will eliminate extra work of preparing prescribed diets at home for individuals suffering from ulcers, heart ailments or obesity.

And because the food technologists have been so responsible for developing both the foods of today—as well as of tomorrow—they plan to have complete convenience meals available for every need, ranging from new forms of baby foods to tailored meals for ailing senior citizens, the speaker stated.

That article was not meant for reading by the people who are going to eat the foods of the future, but by the people who are going to sell them. Even so, why should *anyone* feel that there is an advantage to fabricated peas and simulated meats? Surely the peas and meat that nature produces are far and away superior to any product that man could concoct in a factory. It is in trying to find an answer to a question like that, that we get an idea of the spirit of modern food research and how it differs from traditional concepts of food preservation and preparation.

Meaning of Food Research

Until recently, food research was primarily concerned with finding the best ways to preserve foods between harvests or other periods of surplus. Back in the dim reaches of antiquity, men figured out how to smoke fish, dry meats, make sausage, bread and cheese, so that they could keep a stock of food on hand at all times. Then, as progress was made in solving the storage problem, men concentrated more on developing foods that would please their palate—like vinegar, pickles, sauces and desserts.

Today, food research has emerged as a science with vast power to influence what we buy and eat. Nothing that you buy in a food store today has escaped the scrutiny and attentions of the food processing scientists. Even the purpose of food research has changed. No longer is it simply the art of developing new recipes and ways of preparing food. Now it is oriented around products instead of appetites. The large food processing firms have hundreds of men and women at work in experimental laboratories and, even though they may not admit it, here are some of their goals: (1) to increase the percentage of the nation's food dollar that is spent on processing; (2) to create foods that make money for grocers, by combining long shelf life with high profit mark-ups; (3) and, as a result of the above two goals, to make more money for the food processing industry.

Of course, the food companies say that the primary purpose of their research departments is to make improved products that better serve the needs of the public. It is probably true that some of their work fits that description, although I am hard put to think of an example. The convenience foods that have been introduced in a great flood over the past decade merely cater to our natural tendency to avoid work if possible. They are inferior nutritionally to fresh foods. In fact, nutritional value is an after-thought in most food research projects. More commercial values, such as taste, shelf life and cost are considered first.

Statistics Tell the Story

The influence of expanded food research on the cost of food and on the profits of food companies can be gauged quite accurately through government statistics. Let's consider first the spread between the price the farmer received for his products and the price the consumer pays for food. Back in the 1947-49 period, the farmer's share of the consumer dollar was 50 per cent. By 1950, it had dropped to 47 per cent, by 1957, to 40 per cent and by 1960, to 39 per cent. What is causing the drop in the farmer's share? The answer is that food companies are constantly finding new ways to process food, thereby adding to its retail cost. The article in *Food Field Reporter* that I quoted points out that there are 4 times the number of food items sold today than were sold 20 years ago. What are those new items? They are such things as TV dinners, luncheon meats packed in plastic envelopes, instant hashed brown potatoes and powdered imitation orange juice. The farmer's contribution to such foods (in terms of dollar value) is considerably less than his contribution to fresh and natural foods.

According to the 1961 yearbook of *Canner-Packer* magazine, the production of processed foods hit a record total of 86 *billion* pounds that year, roughly 480 pounds for every man, woman and child in the country.

Government statistics also record the direct expenditures for food research and the number of people engaged in that work. In 1958, the food companies spent 67 million dollars for research. In 1959, they spent 79 million dollars and in 1960, 92 million. The figures for 1961 are not yet available, but the amount no doubt went over 100 million dollars. It is logical to expect that these greater and greater research expenditures are going to result in more and more new food items and a continually growing share of the consumers' food dollar being diverted into the treasuries of the food processing companies.

In 1959, 10,200 people were employed in food research, broken down as follows: 4,100 engineers, 3,900 chemists, 100 mathematicians, 1,600 life scientists (biologists, nutritionists, etc.) and 300 "other." Note that only a little over 10 per cent of these research workers are workers in the life sciences, and it is likely that only a fraction of those are trained in nutrition. The great majority of food researchers are engineers and chemists. Perhaps it is not fair to draw too firm conclusions from this breakdown of the training of food researchers, but it indicates that more of them are at home with the artificial aspects of food products than with what should be the basic goal of food research—nutritional value.

The primary tools of the food research trade today are chemical additives. Finding ways to use them to create new food products or "improve" old products are the tasks that keep food technicians busy. The following article from the Detroit *Free Press* of December 14, 1961, provides one example of how chemicals are being applied by food technicians:

Vegetables Kept "Youthful"

By John Millhone
Free Press Staff Writer

Celery that stays fresh for 3 weeks, even when left outside the refrigerator. Carnations that haven't faded long after other flowers turn dry and brown.

These are some of the wonders attributed to a recently discovered chemical.

A team of researchers at Michigan State University revealed fantastic applications for the substance. They are Dr. Richard R. Dedolph and Dr. Sylvan N. Wittwer, MSU horticulturists.

The chemical, N-6-benzylaminopurine, a white powder, has been available for 6 years.

The MSU scientists learned it slows down a vegetable's "breathing." It creates a suspended animation that retains the plant's youth.

"When you harvest a plant in the field, it has had its last meal," explained Dedolph. "The trick is to keep it alive as long as possible."

You can do it by refrigeration, controlled atmospheres, (such as a near vacuum) and now, a third way, chemical treatments.

The chemical works with plants that store some of their own food as carbohydrates, such as celery, broccoli, asparagus and probably lettuce, plus carnations and some other flowers.

Vegetables high in carbohydrates, such as sweet corn, aren't helped.

Dr. Dedolph said the chemical is harmless—nontoxic, tasteless and odorless.

It is being tested by the federal Food and Drug Administration and it may be cleared for use by the 1962 harvest season, Wittwer and Dedolph said.

"We are playing with some fundamental life systems here," Dedolph said. "When you start to slow down breathing, you are affecting some of life's basic metabolic pathways.

"Now we are trying to learn how the chemical slows down the breathing."

Nutritional Values Secondary Consideration

Aside from the fact that embalmed celery is completely undesirable and a fraud upon the consumer, it is interesting to note that no mention is made of what effect this chemical might have on the food value of the celery. As I said before, nutritional value is a factor that is given only secondary consideration in today's food research programs.

If nutrition is given little attention in food processing, the safety factor in the additives used to make foods more attractive, longer lasting, easier to handle, etc., is even more likely to be ignored by the manufacturers. Time and again, the effects of dyes and chemicals used by food processors have been questioned for the danger they present to the human body. The *New York Times* (August 21, 1956) carried a report on a symposium on cancer in which 42 cancer experts from 21 countries gathered in Rome and in which, says the *Times,* "A number of food additives used in the United States and Europe as dyes, thickeners, sweeteners, preservatives and the like were labeled cancer-producing. . . ."

Still Using Condemned Additives

The statement has had little effect, if any, on the methods of processing adopted by the food industry. We are still using the additives which were condemned. The laws which are intended to govern such things as additives are so wide open to varied interpretations that a processor can stay within the letter of the law while he openly flaunts the spirit, by using additives which present a grave danger to the consumer.

It is unfortunate that we have to give thoughts to protecting ourselves against the discoveries of food researchers, but it is necessary to do that. The way to do it is to strive to buy as much natural and unprocessed food as possible.

The Scientists Are Making Plans for You

Magazine stories sparkle optimistically with titles like "What the Scienists Plan for Your Food" or "Food You Can Store for a Year." In each, you will see a writer licking his chops over a new way to process the freshness out of your food, annihilate its vitamin content and grind its flavor into nothing. After each unspeakable new process comes into being, one is convinced that nothing could be worse, but the manufacturers are resourceful and it would appear that, so long as there is food to mangle, they will find a new way to do it.

For a good many years now, we've been doing quite well with eggs as they come from the chicken, with no interference from man in preparing them. Now, the processes with eggs are many and they grow in number each year. In *Farm Journal* (October, 1960), a few of the latest wrinkles are discussed. As an inducement for oiling eggs, we are told that "besides holding a high grade longer, they just look fresher longer." As you can see, an egg which holds a high grade and "looks fresher longer" is of no particular advantage to the consumer. The consumer has always bought only fresh eggs and, when less than fresh eggs were offered, she simply didn't buy them. With this innovation, it is presumed that she won't be able to tell the difference between grades.

The *Journal* also describes "an eggshell germicide" that reduces the number of "rots" and "exploders" in hatching eggs. The consumer is the fall guy here, too. She buys eggs treated not for her good, but the good of the producer.

Finally, her eggs are likely to be washed in a "one per cent solution of zinc sulfate at 110 degrees for 3 minutes." This solution, along with the oil and germicide, is bound to leave some part of its components inside the egg. Eggshells are porous and these poisons can easily seep through them. Why not check with your egg supplier on what happens to the eggs you've been buying between the time the chicken lays them and you buy them. It's probably true that the more being done to them, the less fresh they are when you get them. Find a farmer who sells fresh eggs, untampered with.

Who Sues Whom?

The food processors emphasize the point that no food is as germ-free as processed food. You can be sure a can or a jar has had its ingredients soundly fumigated, boiled and chemicalized before you eat them. A feature writer, Howard L. Oleck, writing in the Cleveland (Ohio) *Plain Dealer* (July 31, 1960), has a different story. He is discussing whom to sue if impurities in processed food cause injury to the consumer. If the food itself is not fit to eat, the retailer is responsible. Or the consumer may sue the manufacturer for negligence in preparing the food, if the negligence can be proven.

Such suits are not rare and accounts of them can be seen in newspapers from time to time. Mr. Oleck cites a few. A can of chicken chop suey was found to contain contaminating chicken bones; in New York, a purchaser of a jar of prune butter broke her tooth on a piece of prune pit in the spread. In the latter case, the question of who is liable was really scrambled. The lady sued the retailer and won. The retailer then sued the manufacturer for negligence in making prune butter with pits in it. The manufacturer proved that he took great care in sieving the butter and couldn't be held liable. Also, the retailer hadn't bought the prune butter directly from the manufacturer, but from a wholesaler. He then sued the wholesaler, but the outcome is not recorded in Mr. Oleck's column.

Bottled soft drinks have often been found to contain bugs, mice, cigar butts, pieces of wood and even coins. The bottler is responsible, legally, and if the consumer is made ill by such contaminants, he can collect.

Unfortunately, the consumer can't feel so well protected by the law where dangerous additives are concerned. Illness is hardly likely to occur after consuming one bottle of soda. Red dye that can cause cancer might appear in a soda, but the consumer won't be nearly as alarmed by its presence as by the appearance of a piece of wood or a coin. The customer can take care of himself in suing for clean containers, but he must depend upon expert guidance from government watchdogs when it comes to protection from subtle chemicals that can wreck his entire system.

Frozen Foods Quick to Spoil

It has always been our opinion that fresh-frozen foods probably offer the least denatured form of commercially preserved foods. Since it is possible for the manufacturer to freeze vegetables and meats without adding anything to them or treating them in any way beyond cleansing, such a product offers less chance of pollution with additives than canned foods. We did not include in our recommendation pre-cooked frozen foods, such as meat pies, TV dinners, frozen soufflés, etc. The additives in these are compounded beyond the wildest dreams of the canners, in many cases.

Of course, our views were properly scorned in many newspaper articles which urged one and all to take advantage of the convenience foods available, regardless of what "those quack food faddists say." But in its October 12, 1960 issue, the *Journal of the American Medical Association* reported that frozen pre-cooked foods "offer ideal conditions" for contamination. The report goes on: "The inherent protective mechanisms found in frozen raw meats, fruits and vegetables are not present in frozen, pre-cooked foods of a moist, bland nature, such as poultry pies and prepared dinners . . . They are often contaminated with bacteria in the food plants after they are cooked and offer ideal conditions for bacterial growth."

The report warns that frozen foods are "remarkably sensitive" to temperature changes. "Whereas most chemical reactions are 20 to 30 per cent more rapid when the temperature rises 5 degrees F., certain deteriorative reactions in frozen foods may double, triple or quadruple their rates with such a temperature rise." If you are using such foods, at least be certain to heat them thoroughly before serving, for in that way, at least one hazard is overcome, since high heat destroys most bacteria. Please understand: this makes the food less dangerous, but by no means safe for good health. Don't let frozen foods manufacturers do your cooking for you! They are in business to sell food at a profit. They do their best to insure that profit in any way possible, including the substitution of chemicals for natural flavoring and coloring and texture.

The "Freeze-Dry" Method

Business Week (October 15, 1960) spent a lot of space on a relatively new processing system called "freeze-dry." The food item, say steak, is frozen, then heat dried in a vacuum that sucks the moisture away as vapor. The steak gives up 75 per cent of its weight in the process and emerges hardened, almost brittle. No further refrigeration is needed. If the food has been pre-cooked before processing, as any meat probably would be, the housewife merely takes it from the shelf and pops it into a pot of hot water long enough to restore the water—reconstitute it—and serve.

Does it taste like steak? Well, sort of—that's one of the problems to be licked. These foods seem to lose some flavor in the process. For that reason, Minute Maid Corporation abandoned a freeze-dried orange juice it had on the market in 1946. "It just wasn't as good as our frozen orange juice." A Minute Maid vice-president said the juice "fell off" in flavor during long storage periods. Some experts question the nutritive value left in these foods. We certainly do.

Aside from the nutritive and taste problems, freeze-drying creates trouble with the appearance of the finished product, especially if it is meat. Professor Robert Dimarco of Rutgers University says,

"Equipment manufacturers still haven't licked the problem of meat browning." During the freeze-drying, "browning" is a reaction that takes place between the sugar and amino acids in raw meat, causing it to fade slightly in color and lose some of its flavor. That is why freeze-dried meat is usually pre-cooked. The "browning" then isn't so evident. No one knows, or tries to explain, how the changes in the make-up of the meat affect the finished product, nutritionally, or how the product affects the consumer's health.

The processors who realize the limitations of freeze-drying are experimenting with refinements on the process. One firm quick freezes perishables with liquid nitrogen, a cold gas. The freezing temperature is then maintained in an insulated carton and can be stored several weeks without refrigeration. Another firm removes only part of the moisture from the food item, thus, requiring refrigeration, but reducing weight and space. The processors appear determined to save money in terms of spoilage, shipping and storage by selling these products to you. Unless you make it known that you want no part of foods further processed than they already are, you will soon be able to buy little else.

Food Supplements

Food Supplements Are No Joke

The use of food supplements is usually good for a laugh when doctors meet at a cocktail party. Comedians find vitamins and kelp a fertile field for jokes. Wheat germ and yogurt are also words that seem to carry built-in humor for people who are ignorant of their nutritive value. The interesting thing about this is that the researchers who write in medical journals and other scientific publications take a much more respectful attitude toward food supplements. These nutrients have proven themselves in the laboratory, time and again, to be valuable and necessary in preventing and curing disease. We would like to bring our readers up to date on some of these findings.

In *Dental Abstracts* (April, 1959), we read of a Polish dentist who reported on excellent results from the use of garlic oil in treating dental root canals. The oil is known to have bactericidal activity (about the equivalent of 15 penicillin units per milligram), though the exact source of this activity is not fully understood. The patients upon whom the garlic was used to prevent infection were called back 3 to 18 months after completion of the root treatment. No changes, either in the X-rays or in an occurrence of new symptoms, could be found. The garlic oil was given credit as unquestionably possessing antiseptic qualities that remain active for long periods of time. Also, garlic oil is safe for the body and will not endanger the tender areas of the gums and mouth.

The *San Francisco Examiner* (May 24, 1958) carried a boost for the value of protein and vitamin B_6. Dr. Eugene Roberts, a research biochemist from the City of Hope Medical Center, found evidence indicating that the complex disorder of epilepsy may be linked to a deficiency of vitamin B_6 and an amino acid, GABA. The lowering of GABA in the system of animals results in seizures which bear a strong resemblance to epileptic convulsions in humans.

Are not the B vitamins and proteins we receive in the brewer's yeast and lean meats we eat extra insurance against contracting such a disease as epilepsy? Perhaps a strong concentration on such foods could keep someone with strong tendencies toward epilepsy from actually having seizures. If one were already epileptic, wouldn't it be sensible to make certain of a good supply of these two nutrients?

Malt Extract

Malt extract, another of those so-called fad foods that are good for a laugh, no doubt has earned the eternal gratitude of one group of patients suffering from pruritus ani. This problem of rectal itching is extremely distressing and often difficult to treat. Of a group of patients who had been suffering from this ailment for as long as 10 years, 80 per cent found relief within 2 or 3 days on one or two tablespoonfuls of malt extract daily. The article in *Diseases of the Colon* (Vol. 1, p. 372) goes on to say that this extract has been used in infants and older persons to relieve constipation. Wouldn't a natural product such as this seem worth trying in preference to the suppositories and laxatives we see advertised and which can have serious and harmful effects?

Vitamin A Aids Hearing

For relief of deafness, vitamins A and the B complex are mentioned as effective treatment in the *British Medical Journal* (August 15, 1959). In the question and answer section, these vitamins are described as "extensively used" in deafness due to changes in the end organ or nerve of hearing. Vitamin A is not only suggested as an improver of hearing, but it may also protect against the overstimulation of loud noises. Vitamin B_{12} receives special mention by the writer for its effectiveness. He says he has found, on several occasions, that vitamin B_{12} by injection has been followed by a slight improvement in hearing in certain types of deafness.

How many persons with nerve deafness have been told that there is nothing to be done? How many cases of nerve deafness would never have developed if the victims had been properly supplied with vitamins A and B complex in their diets?

Calcium for Bee Stings

Allergy to bee stings has proven fatal often enough to alarm anyone who might have such a tendency. The experience of Dr. D. G. Miller, Jr., a lecturer in medicine at the University of Louisville in Kentucky, has shown that calcium helps combat shock reactions to stings.

It began when a 3-year-old boy was brought to Dr. Miller on the verge of death—his parents thought he was dead. The boy had been playing in the high weeds when suddenly he ran to his mother and cried that a wasp had stung him on the head. Then he fell to the floor and turned blue. There was no pulse, no heartbeat, no apparent breathing. The parents didn't know whether to take the boy to the doctor or the undertaker. They took him to Dr. Miller.

The doctor tried the usual medications, cold compresses and histamines. A stimulant drug was added, but the response was extremely slight. Dr. Miller then recalled the use of calcium for neutralizing the poison of a black widow spider. He gave the boy a shot of calcium lactate. The improvement was dramatic and immediate, but did not last long. Another dose of calcium lactate was given. This time, the child recovered completely, while the mineral was still running into his arm, and he had no more relapse.

Some time later, a similar occurrence involved the dean of the Louisville School of Medicine, and he, too, responded to the calcium treatment at once. Dr. Miller now recommends that all physicians keep calcium lactate on their office shelves and in their bags ready for any emergency. We hope America's physicians have seen Dr. Miller's story. It would indeed be tragic to lose a life due to ignorance of this simple treatment. A good supply of calcium in the body would be a good protection against such an experience, and bone meal, for one, offers an excellent supplementary supply.

Seaweed for Ulcers

In January, 1960, *International Record of Medicine* printed the report made to the American Chemical Society, Division of Medicinal Chemistry, which told of a substance, carrageenin, which composes 60 per cent to 70 per cent of dried seaweed. This substance has given encouraging results in the treatment of peptic ulcers. It apparently interferes with the development of ulcers by blocking the action of pepsin, it was found in animal experiments.

The *Associated Press* sent a dispatch which appeared in papers January 11, 1960, which told of two Japanese surgeons reporting in the *Journal of the International College of Surgeons* on the use of a chemical from seaweed with water as a successful substitute for whole blood in emergency transfusions. This mixture has shown itself to be superior to salt water or sugared water in preventing shock during operations or after severe burns, because it does not break down in the blood stream.

It is plain, from these two pieces of information, that seaweed contains still unknown nutritional elements that we should take advantage of.

Rh Factor Dangers Reduced

Nutritional means of lessening the dangers of childbirth in cases in which the Rh factor is present, were described in *Newsweek* (February 29, 1960). Dr. Warren Jacobs of Baylor University, Houston, Texas, has been using CVP (natural citrus flavonoid, vitamin P complex and ascorbic acid) tablets to prevent the mixing of the infant's Rh positive blood with the mother's Rh negative blood, a mixture which often results in stillborn infants or infants who die shortly after birth.

In a controlled group of Rh negative women, all of whom had previously delivered stillborn children or suffered serious birth emergencies, 32 who received CVP (600 milligrams daily) from early pregnancy produced 24 healthy children—a showing of 75 per cent success; while 71 women who did not receive CVP had only 22 surviving infants—a success rate of only 30.9 per cent.

Can such striking results be ignored? Everyone, especially pregnant women, with or without the unfavorable Rh factor, should make the bioflavonoids and vitamin C a daily "must" in the diet.

Medical research is, at last, beginning to take advantage of the foods they've been calling fad foods all these years. We will be happy to see this attitude filter down to the practicing physicians who still think food supplements are laughable, largely because little is done in the medical schools and in the trade journals they read, to convince them otherwise. The notes on nutritional treatments are often buried in the back pages of the journals, while stories on drugs get prime space. Talk to your doctor about nutrition. Call his attention to new developments he may not have read about. When he knows, he will be a better doctor, and you will be a safer, healthier patient.

The Value of Food Supplements

A point of view which is commonly held by many incompletely informed professional men is reflected in the advice, "Nutrition comes from food. Eat good, wholesome food and nutrition takes care of itself."

Has your doctor or some friend or neighbor ever said that to you? It's another way of saying "get your vitamins with your knife and fork." A totally different opinion is found in the pages of the *Journal of Chemical Education* for April, 1960—an article written by Roger J. Williams of the University of Texas. Dr. Williams, a leading authority in the field of nutrition and the discoverer of the

B vitamin, pantothenic acid, shows in the article why it is necessary to take food supplements in modern America. We think his arguments are convincing. Try them on the doubters who tell you to get your vitamins with your knife and fork.

Dr. Williams says first that refinement and processing of food, which must be done so that it can be transported and stored for long periods of time, may make it lose much of its nutritive value. "No one can claim," he says, "that our food is of exactly as high a quality as it would be if we lived closer to nature."

2. Individuals may not possess effective regulating mechanisms which make it possible for them to choose food wisely—they eat too generously. "Sedentary lives, which are commonly led, probably contribute to transform 'body wisdom' into 'body foolishness,'" says Dr. Williams. In addition, nutrition is far more complicated than we know. Certain substances in food are needed by all the body cells. Others are needed by only some cells. How can one be sure that all the cells and tissues are getting, directly or indirectly, plenty of everything they need? "This is a large order," says Dr. Williams, "and one can have no assurance that maximum bodily health can always be maintained simply by more or less haphazard consumption of what is regarded as 'good, wholesome food.'"

3. Individuals (you and I) are often subjected to various poisons, to infections, to emotional stress. These may increase your need for some or all of the important things like vitamins. In individual cases, there is often a need for special attention.

4. Dr. Williams raises the important point (and he is a world-renowned expert in this field) that people are different. "Different individuals have nutritional needs, including those for vitamins, which are quantitatively different and distinctive. Some individuals, it follows, have unusually high requirements for specific nutrients. For these individuals 'good wholesome food' may not be enough. Their diets may require special attention in order that all the operating cells and tissues of their bodies shall not only be nourished, but well nourished."

Just How Different Are We?

He gives, as an example of this "biochemical individuality," a number of rats in his laboratory which were allowed to eat and exercise as they wished. They had a choice of different kinds of food and drink and they could exercise much or little as they wished. These were all "uniform" rats, whose parents and grandparents for many generations had lived under similar conditions, whose environment was otherwise completely similar. Yet, among these "uniform" rats, it was found that one rat ate 7 times as much butter as another; one rat ate 17 times as much sugar as another; one rat drank 15 times as much alcohol as another; one rat ate 45 times as much fortified yeast as another; one rat excreted 10 times as much urine as another; one rat excreted 1,000 times as much phosphate as another; one rat's exercise was the equivalent of traveling 150 feet a day while another averaged 6 miles per day.

Says Dr. Williams, "If experimental rats vary this much, it seems that human beings, with far more diverse genetics, vary much more."

5. We are all growing older and the process of aging causes individuals to develop nutritional needs which they did not have when they were young. "Those who prosper on 'good, wholesome food' during their younger years may need to pay more strict attention to their special needs as they age," says Dr. Williams.

In another article entitled "Available But Not Simple," which appeared in *Chemical and Engineering News* for March 9, 1959, Dr. Williams discusses further the needs for supplementing the diet with vitamins and minerals. He reminds us that "a deceptive but valid observation, which soothes many into regarding nutrition as unimportant, is that a death-producing diet may be eaten, especially by an adult, for a considerable period of time without obvious outward harm."

And, once again, he points out that differences in individuals are sometimes enormous. He says, "It is found that the amounts of individual enzymes often vary from individual to individual over a three- to tenfold range. Sometimes, the range may be a hundredfold or more; each individual exhibits a distinctive pattern . . . so-called normal, healthy people do vary greatly in their need for calcium . . . and in their requirements for each of the individual essential amino acids. . . . There is a great deal of direct and indirect evidence that the needs of unselected individual human beings for vitamin A, vitamin C, vitamin D and several of the B vitamins, vary not just a little, but several fold."

So the next time somebody tells you he is getting along all right on "good, wholesome food" and no supplements, remind him that maybe *he* can, but other members of his family may not fare so well on such a program.

Are You Deficient in Vitamins?

How can you tell if you are deficient in vitamins? Here, too, there are several pitfalls, according to Dr. Williams. Of course, there are classic symptoms of vitamin deficiency—you bruise easily if you lack vitamin C, you suffer from night blindness (inability to see at night) if you lack vitamin A and so forth. But, says Dr. Williams, a deficiency in pantothenic acid (a B vitamin) weakens *all* the tissues, instead of giving rise to some single dramatic symptom. And you need, in a food supplement, he says, about 5 times as much pantothenic acid as you need of thiamin, another, better-known vitamin. Most all-in-one food supplements contain not nearly enough pantothenic acid, if you are going to depend on the supplement to correct any deficiency. Zinc is a trace mineral of which we need, says Dr. Williams, about 12 milligrams a day. We should be getting in food supplements far more than the average all-in-one tablet or capsule gives us.

We think this is one of the strongest possible arguments not only for taking food supplements, but for taking desiccated liver, yeast, rose hips, bone meal in separate supplements. You will, of course, get far more of each of these valuable things than you could get in an all-in-one, simply because there just isn't room in one tablet to include enough of all of them.

Quotes from Researchers

An article by H. B. McWilliams in *Experimental Medicine and Surgery,* (Volume 16, 1958) speaks eloquently of the necessity of taking food supplements. Says Mr. McWilliams, "There are those who would have the American public believe that present-day foods are adequate in their vitamin and mineral content and that vitamin deficiency diseases and subclinical deficiencies are too rare to be a threat to public health." He then reviews a survey of 6,000 households in the United States conducted by the Department of Agriculture, in which it was found that 29 per cent of the diets did not furnish enough calcium, 10 per cent not enough iron, 16 per cent not enough vitamin A, 17 per cent not enough vitamin B_1, 19 per cent not enough vitamin B_2, 7 per cent not enough vitamin B_3, 25 per cent not enough vitamin C.

He quotes Dr. Robert Harris of the Massachusetts Institute of Technology as saying, before the New England Conference on Human Nutrition, March 22-23, 1956, that in surveys of this kind, the percentages may be even greater, for no investigator knows how much of the vitamins are lost by cooking, how much of the prepared food goes uneaten and what the actual vitamin content of food is from place to place. He tells of a very expensive survey in which the actual meals were taken from the table and analyzed, with the finding that there might be as much as 40 per cent error in simply getting a housewife's report on food eaten and actually testing it.

He quotes Dr. Martha Potgeiter of the University of Connecticut, speaking before the same conference, as saying, "Deficiency states are present on a large scale. Much more knowledge of the relation of nutrition to health is desirable." He quotes Otis W. Wells of Agricultural Marketing Service in a symposium sponsored by Michigan State University as saying that the nutrients most likely to be short in American diets are calcium, vitamin C and the B vitamins.

He quotes Dr. Frederick Stare of Harvard, whose current syndicated column in many daily papers consistently ridicules the idea that there is any necessity for food supplements. Dr. Stare said, in the preface to *Nutrition Education in Elementary and Secondary Schools,* "the need for better nutrition has been established by surveys of many types and is emphasized by the fact that poor food habits exist in varying, but sometimes large, proportions among all races and groups throughout the world. This is true even in areas in which the standard of living is high and essential foods are readily available."

He quotes Drs. J. I. Goodman and William Dowdell, in *Annals of Internal Medicine* (Vol. 43, 1955), as saying, "The great prevalence of malnutrition among chronically disabled persons, as revealed by this study, in a country as well stocked with food as the United States, is frustrating and irksome, if not actually shocking. The importance of the present observations is further accentuated by recent study showing that malnutrition, per se, is the sixth highest cause of prolonged disability. In other words, these malnourished individuals could have remained well and normally active if they had not failed to consume an adequate diet.

"Undernutrition, it can be stressed, with its various manifestations, is not a disease of the chronically ill and aged, but occurs in the so-called normal populations as well. Actually . . . the incidence of undernutrition and underweight among so-called 'healthy' individuals is almost as great as the incidence of this condition among sick people."

Dangers of Deficient Diet

Dr. J. F. Rinehart and Dr. L. D. Greenberg of the University of California, writing in *American Journal of Clinical Nutrition* (Volume 4, 1956), say that, while acute deficiency in pyridoxine, a B vitamin, may not be a contributing reason for hardening of the arteries and cirrhosis of the liver, "it may be that these diseases represent the toll of a smoldering, disordered metabolism resulting in part from years of pyridoxine deficiency."

The reason why nutritional deficiencies are allowed to go unchecked and unnoticed, says Dorothy G. Wiehl of the Milbank Memorial Fund, is that doctors don't know how to test for such deficiencies. The *Journal of the American Medical Association* (Vol. 164, 1957) states editorially that, although we know the symptoms of severe deficiencies in vitamins and protein, the effects of "subclinical" or slighter deficiencies are still not clear.

James M. Hundley, of the National Institute of Health, speaking at the New England Conference on Human Nutrition, 1956, stated that "We must be honest and admit that we don't know, in all respects, just what consumption of this type of diet (the deficient one) over long periods of time does in terms of health and disease."

There is a great deal of evidence available in scientific journals along these same lines. It is time, once and for all, to refute the theory that all of us are eating the right amounts of "good, wholesome food" and hence don't need food supplements!

Reasons for Taking Natural Food Supplements

In the abundance of misinformation, at present being widely broadcast in newspapers and magazines, on the subject of food and nutrition, there is one constant steady threat of propaganda—modern American food can't be improved upon. It's nutritious, it's healthgiving. No one needs food supplements (vitamins or minerals) so long as he eats a "good diet."

The "good diet" is not spelled out. One is given a list of general categories of food. "Eat some of these every day and you can't help but be healthy," say the nutrition columnists, the syndicated M.D. columns, the women's magazines and the TV commercials. Since most of the cost of these avenues of expression is paid by advertising for the very foods recommended, it is not surprising that the misinformation should continue unchallenged, except by a few "faddists."

The columnists give no explanation for the steadily rising incidence of degenerative disease (arthritis, diabetes, heart trouble, cancer, multiple sclerosis, etc.). If, indeed, the American diet is everything one needs, how can you account for this astounding incidence of chronic disease?

A resounding answer to the claim, "you don't need food supplements!" including a reasonable scientific argument for natural versus synthetic food supplements, appeared in the *American Journal of Digestive Diseases* for March, 1953. Written by Morton S. Biskind, M.D., a careful researcher and a practicing physician, this article makes very clear the great complexity of the problem of supplementing diet with vitamins.

All Important Food Elements Not Isolated

"Several misconceptions . . . have become increasingly prevalent," says Dr. Biskind. "One common misconception is that all the important nutritional elements have already been isolated and indeed, that a number of those currently available are not significant in human nutrition. The extremely conservative attitude of the Food and Drug Administration, which requires disclaimers on labels of vitamin preparations for the vitamins they consider not adequately studied in human nutrition, has further fostered the assumption that administration of only the pure factors thus far considered 'important' is sufficient for satisfactory nutritional therapy."

Many people often ask us why, beside many of the vitamins

and minerals listed on their food supplements, this statement appears: "Need for, in human nutrition is not established." This is what Dr. Biskind means. Any substance not studied for years and not officially accepted as being necessary to life in certain minimum amounts must be listed on labels as being "not established" as a necessary part of human nutrition.

A Single Deficiency Is Impossible

Furthermore, says Dr. Biskind, experts talking about nutrition are inclined to speak of deficiency of one or another vitamin— "thiamin deficiency," "riboflavin deficiency," etc. This is entirely incorrect, for such a thing simply never happens. In a laboratory, an animal may be put on a diet completely free of vitamins. Then all known vitamins except thiamin are added. Whatever symptoms are produced in the animal are then said to be due to deficiency of thiamin. But, of course, they are due to lack of thiamin, and all the other *unknown* vitamins as well!

Once thiamin is lacking, other food elements are lost from the body stores, so the condition finally produced involves the loss of all these known and unknown substances.

"In the human being, how much more unlikely that deficiencies of single factors should occur," says Dr. Biskind . . . "Not only are deficiencies multiple, but the administration of single nutritional factors or even of a combination of a few of them may actually lead to serious disturbance of a tenuous nutritional equilibrium and precipitation of new avitaminotic lesions"—that is, new symptoms of deficiency.

For many years, he goes on, investigators have stressed the need for complete therapy—which includes, of course, giving the deficient patient a source of all those as yet unidentified essential food factors. Dr. Tom Spies, a famous worker in nutritional fields, suggested many years ago that a "basic formula" be worked out which would include all those B vitamins discovered up to that time, which could be given to patients, *along with a natural source of the unknown vitamins.* But somehow, says Dr. Biskind, people began to think of this as a "complete formula" and soon it was given to patients as the only source of nutritional elements aside from their meals. The impression rapidly spread that this basic formula contained *all* the important vitamins. He tells us that, time and again, conditions which do not respond at all to the taking of such a synthetic preparation improve overnight when a natural source of the other, as yet undiscovered, vitamins is given.

"Simply adding desiccated liver or suitable liver fraction to the regime invariably has resulted in a dramatic and lasting improvement, often evident within a few days," he says.

A final misconception occurs, he continues—that the average

American diet contains all the necessary nutritional elements; that nutritional deficiency, when it does occur, results only from deficiency in the diet and that all that is necessary to cure such a deficiency is a "good diet."

Nourishment from Our Food

Dr. Biskind's answer to the first misconception includes these 6 points:

1. Depletion of much of the soil on which food is grown has produced crops that are nutritionally inferior. Since this statement is attacked so often in the press by such writers as Dr. Frederick Stare of Harvard, we give a reference for this statement—M. J. Rowlands and B. Wilkinson, writing in the *Biochemical Journal,* (Vol. 24, p. 1, 1930).

2. The increasing use on crops of incredibly toxic insecticides, which leave harmful residues in and on food and further harm the soil by killing necessary microörganisms and earthworms.

3. The increasing tendency to pick and ship produce before it has ripened, so that there is less danger of loss from spoilage. These days, most of us eat few foods that have been ripened on the vine and this ripening is essential to the full nutritional value of the food.

4. The continuously increasing tendency toward processing and chemicalizing our food—dyes, waxes, detergents, emulsifiers, bleaches, etc.

5. The use of virtually pure, vitamin-free sugar for as much as one-fourth of the average caloric intake.

6. The use of many chemical additives which may be toxic and many of which replace essential food elements—artificial fats and things of this kind.

The fact that Americans now consume about 100 pounds of sugar per person per year indicates that, here alone, a deficiency of thiamin and riboflavin (B vitamins) occurs. This would be a deficit of about 90 milligrams of each of these two important B vitamins in the course of a year. For niacin, another of the B vitamins, the deficiency would be about 10 times this much. "And those who refrain from using sugar in coffee or sprinkling it on cereals and fruit in the belief that the intake is thus reduced to zero, are, of course, mistaken. Sucrose (sugar) is incorporated in so many staple foods today, including bread, that it can hardly be avoided," says Dr. Biskind.

Other Reasons for Deficiencies

But even if one were getting plenty of all the vitamins in one's daily food, one could still be nutritionally deficient, because there are many conditions and circumstances which either cause one to lose vitamins or cause one to need more than the normal day's require-

ments. Any difficulty with the digestive tract which impairs our
ability to absorb vitamins can result in deficiency—diarrhea, colitis,
liver or gall bladder trouble or many more disorders. Pregnancy and
lactation increase one's need for vitamins, as does hyperthyroidism,
excessive physical activity, infections, etc. Antibiotics, sulfa drugs,
industrial poisons, inhalation of toxic substances such as lead from
polluted air, insecticide residues and so forth—all cause the destruction of vitamins. Emotional disturbances, especially when they are
protracted or severe, can cause extremely serious nutritional difficulties. For all these reasons, and from his own observations, Dr. Biskind
believes that "gross lesions (disorders) of nutritional deficiency,
easily detectable to the naked eye, are extremely common."

He reminds us that, once tissues have become deficient, it is
necessary to take many times the usual amount of vitamins to make
up for the deficiency—as much as 10, 20 or even 50 times the
maintenance amounts for people who have not suffered from any
previous lack. It is also, unfortunately, true, he says, that many times,
the tissues have been so damaged, that no excess amount of vitamin
therapy can repair them. He gives as an example laboratory rats
who were made deficient in riboflavin. After the damage had been
done to the cornea of their eyes, no amount of riboflavin in the diet
would restore the eye to its normal healthy state.

Furthermore, he says, how can we speak of some standardized
amount of vitamins which each and every one of us must require?
Would we insist on giving the same amount of insulin to every
diabetic? The consequences might be fatal. So why should we assume
that any two of us have the same requirements, nutritionally speaking? One person may need ever so much more of the various vitamins
than another!

Other critics of vitamin therapy (and how many times have we
read this in some newspaper column or other!) insist that getting a
certain vitamin in a food supplement is useless, since one may get
that amount in daily food. But, says Dr. Biskind, what they seem to
forget is that the food supplement does not *substitute* for the food—
it simply *adds* vitamins to those already being eaten in food. "Even
in biology," he says, "a 100 per cent increase can usually be
considered significant."

Nutrients Work Together

A sample of the incorrect use of nutritional therapy, he says is
the treatment called "lipotropic" therapy, in which certain members
of the B vitamins are given, perhaps with methionine, an amino acid,
to prevent hardening of the arteries and heart disease. The doctor
who treats his patients thus has overlooked the fact that such a
disorder means there is a general nutritional disturbance and many

other things are lacking—not just one vitamin or one amino acid. "The damaged liver, unable properly to cope with lipoid (fat) metabolism is deficient not only in the known 'lipotropic' substances, but in numerous other factors as well, water-soluble, liposoluble and insoluble. Only by providing all the missing factors simultaneously can healthy, self-regulatory mechanisms be restored."

Another urgent reason for using natural rather than synthetic food supplements is the complexity of the ways the body uses vitamins. A vitamin is not just something that appears in food, which goes to a particular cell of the body to be consumed and then excreted. Vitamins can be used only if all the other necessary elements are present to carry out the chemical processes our bodies are equipped to handle. Vitamins need certain minerals and proteins *right there in the digestive tract along with them,* if proper use is to be made of the vitamins. Lack of any of these factors—the vitamin, the minerals or the protein—can disrupt the entire process.

The water soluble vitamins (B and C) are stored hardly at all in body tissues, so these must be supplied every day. While the fat soluble vitamins are usually well stored by healthy persons, they are lost readily once a severe deficiency has occurred. This is especially true when severe liver damage has taken place.

Principles of Nutritional Therapy

To continue with Dr. Biskind's theories, he states that there are 3 basic principles of nutritional therapy: it should be *complete;* it should be *intensive;* it should be *persistent.* No halfway measures will succeed. Vitamins, minerals, proteins, phosphates, fats and trace minerals are forever related like links in a chain, when one is considering the way the body uses them. It is useless to strengthen only one or several of these links. All must be equally strong or the chain will fail. "Yet current practices in nutritional therapy reveal how poorly understood is this simple fact," says Dr. Biskind.

"While the range of permissible dosage for essential nutrients is wide, owing to the numerous safety mechanisms available to the organism, and the therapeutic range is ordinarily at least 5 to 10 times the range for maintenance and often more, this does not mean that (as is often done) massive doses of certain factors should be combined with minimal doses of others," he goes on.

Large doses of vitamin A, prescribed by doctors to alleviate one condition or another, may bring about a deficiency in the B vitamins. Giving all the B vitamins appears to "save" vitamin A, so that one does not need so much. Giving large doses of one or another of the B vitamins may bring on the very symptom one is trying to cure, since it may cause deficiency in other B vitamins.

Large doses of thiamin, alone or in combination with other

synthetic B vitamins, may do very little for alleviating the symptoms of beriberi, in which we know deficiency of thiamin is concerned. But giving the entire B complex of vitamins causes prompt amelioration of this disorder.

Imbalances Created

Says Dr. Biskind, many doctors who scoff at the idea of giving vitamins, use some of the vitamins in massive doses like drugs, especially those concerned with the body's use of fat—choline, inositol, etc. They call these "lipotropics" and they give them in large doses like drugs to combat cholesterol deposits. Yet large doses of these B vitamins may actually aggravate the basic nutritional deficiency in the B vitamins, he says.

Giving all of the B vitamins, along with other substances that accompany them in foods such as liver, gets excellent results, according to Dr. Biskind's own experience. "This illustrates further," he says, "that the proper object of nutritional therapy is treatment of the whole organism with reasonably balanced preparations and not simply a pharmacological (drug-like) attack on the liver with massive doses of a single substance. . . . Liver preparations, especially desiccated liver, are in themselves a rich source of the lipotropic substances." He also points out that there is little use giving such supplements unless there is plenty of protein in the diet, for the B vitamins cannot function adequately without lots of protein.

So it seems evident that the average doctor, asking nothing whatever about his patient's diet or way of life except the routine "Do you eat a good diet?" would fail to promote good health, if he prescribed some isolated, synthetic vitamin and mineral preparations to be taken along with the patient's usual diet. This diet, of course, was at least partly responsible for putting him out of sorts to begin with, probably a typical American diet of which a large part is refined carbohydrates—products made chiefly of white sugar and white flour.

Interference with Nutrition

No matter how adequate the source of one's diet supplements, the complete repair of a nutritional deficiency may be impossible under certain conditions. "Thus a person continually exposed to a hepatoxin (liver poison), such as one of the industrial solvents or one of the new chlorinated hydrocarbon insecticides, can expect, at best, only partial relief, so long as the inciting agent continues to act. A patient who insists on consuming vast quantities of sugar and other refined carbohydrates to the detriment of protein intake, can similarly expect little benefit from nutritional therapy. Likewise, an individual under the stress of acute anxiety, which impairs absorption and utilization and increases destruction and excretion of the essential nutrients, will not respond even to massive doses of these substances, so long as the emotional disturbance continues to act," says Dr. Biskind.

Here are some other circumstances of life and health which may impair one's ability to use the vitamins and minerals in diet to maintain health: poor appetite, diarrhea, insomnia, muscular tension, spasm of the digestive tract, etc. In addition, says Dr. Biskind, "the list of chemicals and drugs which impair cellular enzyme systems and produce tissue anoxia (lack of oxygen) is very long indeed. An incredible number of them are in such indiscriminate use that daily exposure to them is almost unavoidable for many reasons. These range from a variety of chemicals used in industry to carbon monoxide, lead and other products of combustion in automobile exhaust, the . . . insecticides, . . . paint solvents and drugs such as sulfonamides, antibiotics and estrogens."

Continued exposure to any of these substances causes loss of B vitamins. So, no matter with what devotion one is engaged in a program of good nutrition, continual exposure to the above poisons would render it to some extent ineffective. In research with animals, the same thing is true, says Dr. Biskind. It is well known that even the faintest trace of DDT is stored in the body fat. This poisonous insecticide interferes with the oxidation of foods in every cell of the body. Yet no account is taken of this in planning experiments dealing with nutrition and no effort is made to secure feed that does not contain DDT. Since practically all of the commercially available feeds contain DDT, it is easy to see that nutrition experiments are distorted.

The Dangers of Chemicals

DDT in extremely low amounts affects a certain enzyme in the heart muscle, says Dr. Biskind. But almost everyone is exposed to DDT and it is stored tenaciously in the body fat, so how can one repair such damage? Sulfa drugs and antibiotics also destroy B vitamins. The hormones given to food animals for rapid fattening remain in the meat and we consume them. These, too, interfere with the regular and proper use of vitamins in the body.

It is essential, says Dr. Biskind, to question any patient very closely about his exposure to all these various chemicals when outlining a nutritional program for him. (Did your doctor ever even mention such items?)

The next time you read in a newspaper or magazine that Americans are well-fed and there is no need to eat any special diet or to take food supplements, ask yourself, "Which American is well fed? Doesn't it depend on what his individual body needs are, how well planned his diet is, where his food comes from and what kind of soil it grew in, what drugs he is taking and what poisonous chemicals he is exposed to?" All of these things are important and all of these things must be considered in regard to every individual, as an individual different from any one else. Now you see how meaningless are the articles, sponsored by the processed food and chemical companies, which attack as faddists anyone who protests against chemicalization and overprocessing of foods and name as a "crank" anyone who recommends the daily taking of natural food supplements, as a necessary addition to the best possible diet.

Questions and Answers on Food Supplements

1. *Why do twentieth century Americans need food supplements in order to be healthy? Grandpa didn't.*

Because refined and processed foods lack the vitamin and mineral elements that were eaten at meals 50 or 100 years ago. We must have them to avoid malnutrition. The exhausted state of our soil and the widespread use of chemical fertilizers, rather than natural fertilizers, are two other reasons why you must use food supplements. You are exposed to far more poisons and other forms of stress, and this makes extra vitamins essential. Many surveys have shown that vitamin deficiency is widespread among modern Americans, especially our young people.

2. *Is there any single food supplement that should or should not be taken by everyone?*

All are necessary for good health. You may have special needs, due to your diet or health background, but in general, you must have all the vitamins and minerals, since they work together to keep you feeling tops.

3. *What are capsules made of—anything that might be harmful?*

The supplements we recommend come in capsules made of gelatin, not only completely harmless, but quite rich in food value, especially protein.

4. *Is there any difference in the value of capsules or tablets?*

No. The only thing to watch for is the actual content of each perle, capsule or tablet, in terms of protein, vitamins, etc. This will be listed on the label. Tablets contain the same substances as perles, pressed together in a tabletting machine.

5. *What about powdered or flaked supplements—are they just as good?*

Of course. They may not be as convenient as tablets or perles; that is the only difference. Some people do not enjoy the taste of brewer's yeast or rose hip powder and for them, it may be difficult to find ways to use the powdered form in food.

6. *When should you take your food supplements?*

They are food, so, of course, you should take them with your meals—before, after or during. If you wish, you may take the day's quota with one meal, or divide it among all 3. In the case of the B vitamins and vitamin C, which are water-soluble and hence, more easily excreted, it seems best to take these with each meal, rather than taking all of them at one meal.

7. *Should you start with only one supplement or begin right off taking all of them?*

Supplements are food, not drugs. The vitamins and minerals they contain work together for health. You should take all of them.

8. *How should food supplements be stored?*

A cool, dark place is best—the refrigerator, if possible. Foods like sunflower seeds will keep well unless they have been powdered or ground. When any food is broken or pulverized in any way, vitamins disappear rapidly and rancidity occurs.

9. *If food supplements are advertised as having a given potency and as being from natural sources, does a difference in price mean a difference in quality?*

In food supplements, as in everything else, you get what you pay for. In some cases, close study will show that the less expensive supplement lacks or includes little of one or several elements which are plentiful in the more expensive one. In some cases, price is higher because of special packing or fast service, prepaid postage and so forth—the very same considerations that influence price when you buy any other product.

10. *Is it worthwhile to use powdered supplements in cooking or are too many of the vitamins and minerals lost?*

Many people use large quantities of supplements when they cook, thus giving their families additional nutriment in every dish— brewer's yeast or wheat germ is added to salads; rose hip powder is added to fruit salad, etc. Some of the vitamin content is lost, of course, if the food is heated. Tea made from rose hips, for instance, probably contains less vitamin C because the vitamin probably disappears in the steam from the boiling water. Bone meal and kelp, lecithin and soybean flour—things like this do not suffer much in cooking and contribute greatly to the healthfulness of food.

11. *How can you get children to take food supplements?*

Many mothers tell us their children love supplements, chewing rose hip and brewer's yeast tablets as if they were candy. You can use a powdered form and put it in their food; you can pierce oil capsules and drop the oil into eggs or hamburger. Don't forget that children judge food and food supplements by the reaction of their elders. If you shudder over your supplements, so will your children. If you enjoy them, the kids will think they are treats!

12. *Should you take the same supplements Editor Rodale takes?*

Not necessarily, for your preference and needs may be different. Mr. Rodale takes desiccated liver rather than brewer's yeast; he takes two kinds of vitamin C supplements—one with a higher vitamin potency, because he wants to get as well, more of the things that accompany vitamin C in the low potency tablet. He takes large amounts of vitamin E for his heart condition. Do you have a heart condition? If you eat many meals in restaurants, you may need more of some vitamins and minerals than Editor Rodale takes.

13. *What happens to the extra amount of vitamins if you take too much?*

If you are taking natural food supplements, it is almost impossible for you to get too much of the fat-soluble vitamins (A, D, K and E), provided you study your own requirements and the labels of the preparations you buy. Any excess of the water-soluble vitamins (B and C) will be excreted harmlessly and cannot possibly damage you. The only way to get into trouble with these is to take synthetic vitamin B preparations which can cause an imbalance among the B vitamins, producing unpleasant symptoms.

14. *How can you tell synthetic from natural vitamin preparations?*

You can't, unless you can depend on the integrity of the seller who tells you his preparations are from natural sources. This is another good reason for taking individual supplements rather than all-in-ones. There is no such thing as "synthetic" brewer's yeast. There is no such thing as "synthetic" bone meal. There is no such thing as "synthetic" fish liver oil. But drug stores all over the country sell synthetic preparations of B vitamins which are made from chemicals, not from brewer's yeast; mineral preparations are sold which have not been prepared from any natural substance such as bone meal, and vitamins A and D (so plentiful in fish liver oil) are regularly sold in a synthetic form. In an all-in-one supplement, if the source of the vitamins is listed (vitamin B_1 from yeast, etc.), you are fairly sure that the product has a natural base.

15. *How soon should you expect to see results from taking supplements?*

There is, of course, no general answer to this, and there is no very satisfactory individual answer either. If you have steadfastly abused your body for many years, it may take a long time to regain your health. If you eat improperly, you cannot hope to attain good health just by taking supplements. The right diet is essential as well. But don't expect to make up for a lifetime of errors in a few months.

16. *Should you take supplements while you are being treated by a doctor and/or taking medicine?*

Why not? Supplements are food, not medicine. Sick people need them much more than well people. We cannot think of a circumstance in which any natural food supplement you take could possibly interfere with any medical treatment or medicine. If you are taking medicine that contains forms of iron, you should take your vitamin E at a different time from the time you take the iron, for medicinal iron may destroy vitamin E in the digestive tract. So some of the vitamin E you are taking may be lost. But don't think this is a reason to discontinue vitamin E! If you have been taking medicinal iron, it has been regularly destroying whatever vitamin E accompanied it in your digestive tract, so you are perhaps more in need of vitamin E than the average person.

Foods, Vitamins in

Fine Fall Foods

With the last days of summer, most sections of the United States lose access to many of the fresh, homegrown fruits and vegetables. The vitamin-rich peaches and tomatoes that grow nearby are gone for another year, and we can only approximate their wonderful flavor and goodness in the super markets during the winter. How could one begin to compare chain-store cartons of winter tomatoes with those fresh from the garden? Are frozen peaches nearly so good as the fresh ones? Of course, comparisons of the other fruits and vegetables are the same. Not only do we lose the pleasure involved in eating them fresh from the vine, but the food value is minimized, too.

There are wonderfully healthful foods that make their appearance in fall, however, and some of these come in late enough to make the winter seem a little shorter. Concentrate on these for the cold months and you will be adding to your protection against colds, grippe and other winter pests. Let us list just a few of the best foods available in fall: fresh apples, pears, citrus fruits, grapes, pumpkins, squash, avocado, nuts, sunflower and pumpkin seeds. These, plus figs, dates and dried fruits are all good sources of nutrition and conscious use of them is a good way of avoiding commercially canned goods in the winter months.

Apples a Pet

Apples are one of our pet fall foods. The apple is one of the most satisfying low-calorie foods one can eat. As a snack or part of a salad, it is unmatched. It's one food that few people prefer to eat any way but raw, which is, of course, the best way.

Apples have been used through the years for their medicinal value. In cases of infant diarrhea, raw apple pulp, scraped from the apple or shredded and mashed fine, given alone and with no other foods, was a well-known and effective prescription. Scientists are puzzled as to whether it is the apple's acid which might detoxify the system, the pectin which might help to solidify the stools or some other undefined element. But whatever it is, apples are a measure worth trying in such cases, before resorting to harmful patent medicines or powerful and dangerous drugs. Doctors also find that the same apple which can conquer diarrhea in infants can relieve constipation in adults. Curiously, none of the ingredients in the apple tried separately has this effect; only when the raw apple is eaten as is, does one see results.

Another of the attractions the apple holds, healthwise, is its ability to aid the body in absorbing iron from other foods. This trait is believed by some to be due to the acid content of the fruit. Furthermore, the apple is a wonderful cleansing and firming agent for the teeth, and it helps to retain the body's supply of calcium.

The skin of the apple has more vitamin C than the pulp; that is why we regret having to recommend that apples be peeled before they are eaten. However, layer upon layer of poisonous spray is used in our apple orchards, and as a result, the fruit has a peel that is impregnated with dangerous poisons which cannot be washed off. Make an effort to find a farmer who does not spray his apples, so that you can eat them as they come right off the tree, vitamin-rich skin and all.

Storage Improves Squash and Pumpkins

Vegetables of the pumpkin-squash family come into their own in the fall. They all have a high vitamin A content, with appreciable vitamin C, protein and minerals. Pumpkins are useful in ways other than the traditional pumpkin pie, always to be avoided by the health-conscious diner. They can be used just as squash is, or we have seen a recipe for a mid-European pumpkin soup which is worth trying.

The thing that has appealed to us most about these foods is their seeds. Pumpkin and squash seeds are very rich in protein. In a publication of the Massachusetts Agricultural Experimental Station (February, 1954), there appeared a paper which discussed the protein value of butternut squash seeds. The seeds were completely untreated after removal from butternut squashes which had been stored for various lengths of time, up to 221 days. It was extremely interesting to find that storage improved both the protein content of the squash themselves, and the protein value of their seeds. Squash that was fresh showed the protein percentage of the flesh to be 5.1, and the seeds were 28.3 per cent protein. After 221 days of storage, the protein value of the flesh was 15.2 per cent, and of the seeds, 32.7 per cent (that is, raw flesh and seeds). Cooked squash would probably lose some vitamin and mineral value, and toasted seeds (they are merely put on thick brown paper and set in a warm oven) would also have less value than sun-dried fresh ones. These facts are probably true of pumpkin seeds, too. Storage is not recommended for other foods.

In the past few years, several reports have been written on the therapeutic value of pumpkin seeds. One researcher suggested that they might be of value in the treatment of prostate gland disorders. Dr. W. Devrient, of Berlin, Germany, wrote an article in which he said, in certain countries where pumpkin seeds are eaten in great quantity throughout life, there is almost no incidence of enlarged prostate or other prostate disorders. The answer to this phenomenon lies in certain materials contained in the seeds which, says Dr. Devrient, are the building stones of the male hormones. These hormones help to keep the prostate healthy and allow it to continue its functions on its own. This is far more preferable than an attempt to by-pass the prostate by substituting for its function.

What it is in the seeds that has this most desirable effect, no one knows exactly. It is known that the pumpkin seed is very high in phosphorus; it has the highest iron content of any seed. The B vitamins are plentiful, and there is some small vitamin A content. With this, pumpkin seeds contain about 30 per cent protein and 40 per cent fat. The protein content could be responsible for the favorable action pumpkin seeds seem to have on the prostate.

While we're on the subject of seeds, we must mention sunflower seeds, those delicious snacks available all year round, which are storehouses of nutrition. They are wonderfully rich in B vitamins, especially thiamin. In 100 grams of sunflower seeds, there is 250 per cent of the minimum daily requirement of thiamin. That amount —about a cupful—also offers 50 per cent of the MDR (minimum daily requirement) of niacin, 5 times the MDR of vitamin E, large amounts of phosphorus and iron and 70 per cent of the MDR of iodine. The protein value, 25 per cent, puts sunflower seeds in the same league with meat, and valuable unsaturated fatty acids make up 90 per cent of the high fat content of these seeds.

Luxurious Grapes

Another of fall's luxuries is grapes. In the United States, we are told, 25 different varieties are grown. Each of us has his favorite— the sweet pale-green seedless, the large round, firm Tokays, the rich blue Concords, etc. There are few more luscious snacks than a bunch of grapes. And in each of them is contained vitamins A, B and C, plus the minerals potassium, iron, calcium, phosphorus, sulfur and others. Grapes contain, on the average, 80 per cent water and are considered essentially an alkaline food. They are said to be one of the greatest aids in the elimination of uric acid from the system. They stimulate secretion of digestive juices, and grapes are known to be helpful in combating constipation.

Unfortunately, we are faced with the vexing problem of sprays on the grapes we buy. Few of us have access to a grower who uses the organic method in raising his crop. Removing the skins on some types of grapes is easy—we are told that it is a good rule of thumb to remove all skins that come off easily, as they are not readily digested—but usually the job of peeling a grape is more trouble than it's worth. To avoid grapes that are sprayed, try raising your own in the back yard. They require a minimum of cultivation and give a bountiful harvest. If you cannot do this, and also have no way of ascertaining the source of the grapes you buy, at least wash them very carefully before eating them. While we do not believe that washing can eliminate all of the spray residues, it is of some small help in lessening their full effect.

Avocados and Pears

Avocado is a fall and winter fruit that is increasing in popularity. It is an unusual food, both in appearance (a dark green, pear-shaped, thick-skinned fruit) and taste, with a soft, oily pulp that enhances just about any other fresh fruit or vegetable with which it is served. Avocados have an abundance of unsaturated fatty acids, plus vitamins A and C. The B vitamins, especially thiamin and riboflavin, are well represented, and because no preparation is involved, all of the food values are left intact when the avocado is eaten.

Because avocado is so rich in unsaturated fatty acids, Dr. Wilson Grant of Veterans Administration Hospital in Coral Gables, Florida, set out to see if the fruit could affect the cholesterol levels in the blood of selected patients. The patients were given ½ to 1½ avocados per day as a substitute for part of their dietary fat consumption. The result was that the cholesterol level stayed the same in half of the subjects, and was significantly reduced in the other half.

Pears come in quite a few varieties, and fall is their season, too. The pear is actually a relative of the apple, and has a similar chemical composition, with more sugar. It is considered to be one of the best sweet fruits for diabetics, and is digestible by most persons even those who have digestive problems. They are an excellent aid to elimination, especially when eaten with the skin when soft, ripe and juicy. But again, we must urge our readers to peel this fruit before eating, unless you can be certain that the pears you buy have not been sprayed.

A Bowl of Nuts Appeals to All

A bowl of nuts on the dining room table is one of fall's trademarks in many homes. And what could be better? As a dessert with fruit or as a snack throughout the days, nuts offer a pleasurable means of acquiring nutrients that are all too often missing from our daily diet.

Nuts, like seeds, are rich in phosphorus, but unlike seeds, they contain plenty of calcium, too. They are an energy food, high in calories for a quick spurt when ambition lags, and a pound of nuts offers one almost half the protein needed for a day. (This is not complete protein as found in meat, or other animal foods, so one cannot depend exclusively on nuts for all necessary protein.)

Most nuts offer plenty of vitamin A and the B vitamins, especially thiamin. (The red skin of the peanut is especially rich in thiamin.) Some contain vitamin E. Nuts must be chewed thoroughly for proper digestion, for the digestive juices simply cannot break down the kernels unless they are broken by chewing.

Nuts are actually in season in fall, but they are readily available anytime. Sad to say, the people of the United States are not avid nut eaters, in spite of how easily nuts are acquired. We eat an average of about 1½ pounds of nuts per person per year, even though they are contained in candies and pastries, as well as eaten alone. We consume well over 100 pounds of sugar per person per year.

If we had to name the nut most popularly eaten in the United States, we would probably have to say the peanut. It is actually not a nut at all, in the botanical sense, but a plant whose nut-like roots ripen under the ground. Peanuts are a supremely nutritious food, and because of their value, flour made from peanuts has become a very important product for those who are interested in good nutrition. This flour contains over 4 times the protein, 8 times the fat and 9 times the minerals that appear in an equal amount of wheat flour. People use it in recipes as a substitute for the wheat flour called for, with great success. For those with allergies to cereals, peanut flour is the perfect answer. Then, too, peanut butter—actually nothing but ground peanuts with oil added to maintain some moisture—is a popular and wholesome food. Care should be observed in buying peanut butter, to be certain that it is not hydrogenated, a measure which counteracts much of the good to be gotten from eating peanut butter.

We say, without qualification, that all edible nuts are desirable as a nutritious food. If you can eat them raw, they are best. Roasting cuts into their nutritional value. Do not buy salted nuts or nuts fried in deep fat, as they often are. Eat them as close to the way they come from the tree as possible.

Space does not permit a complete review of all fall foods. These few should help you to plan more nutritious meals and snacks. Whole citrus, eaten occasionally, will enhance your vitamin C supply; and dried fruits, plus figs and dates, are the next best thing to fresh fruits. There's plenty of good food available in the cold months before one resorts to the commercial canned products.

The Search for High-Vitamin Foods

By Robert Rodale

The average fresh tomato sold in stores contains 23 milligrams of vitamin C in each 100 grams. But there is one variety of tomato —Doublerich—whose fruit has over twice that much vitamin C.

The average strawberry contains 62 milligrams of vitamin C per 100 grams, but if you can find Fairfax strawberries, you will get berries with as much as 96 milligrams of vitamin C.

Apples vary also. Delicious, one of the largest selling varieties of apple, is just about the lowest in vitamin C. McIntosh is also very low. But Northern Spy, Baldwin and Winesap can have 4 times as much vitamin C.

There are many other cases of produce sold in stores that is far from the best nutritionally. I will describe them later. But you are probably wondering *why* grocers handle food that is low in vitamin content. There is positive scientific evidence that some varieties of fruits and vegetables have much greater amounts of vitamins than others. And that vitamin superiority is constant, regardless of what kind of soil the food is grown on.

It is easy to explain this lack of interest in vitamin content. In selecting fruit and vegetable varieties for commercial use, growers give first consideration to factors affecting their pocketbook—yield, shipping quality, appearance, adaptability to processing, disease resistance and many others. Nutritional quality is usually the last factor considered when new varieties are bred. Consider the Fairfax strawberry, an old variety that has been grown in gardens across the country for many years. People who know strawberries are almost unanimous in their opinion that it is not only the best tasting strawberry, but the most attractive looking as well. And laboratory tests confirm that it is among the richest in vitamin C. But it has one serious defect, from the point of view of the wholesale fruit companies. Fairfax doesn't hold up under shipment. It must be eaten within a day or two of being picked. If super markets tried to handle it, their loss from wastage would be almost complete. So, when you next buy strawberries, you will be buying fruit that is of inferior color, taste and food value, but which is able to stay two weeks or more in a little wooden box without rotting.

Now, let's venture into the subject of blueberries. There is hardly any food grown on American farms that has been changed as much by plant breeding as blueberries. The blueberries sold in stores today are quite unlike the wild fruit. Mainly, they are much larger. It is not hard to grow blueberries, today, as large as a quarter. But, like strawberries, much of the selection of new varieties is based on shipping quality. The critical part of a blueberry, from the point of view of the commercial grower, is the picking scar, the point at which the berry is severed from the stem when picked. A "good" blueberry has a clean picking scar which will not allow any decay-causing bacteria to enter the berry and cause rapid spoilage. A "bad" berry ruptures when picked and spoils quickly.

There are other tests that a new blueberry variety must hurdle. Do the berries all ripen at the same time, thus simplifying picking? Are the berries the proper color? Are the plants resistant to disease and insects? Do the berries have a good flavor? By the time the plant breeder produces a plant that meets all these qualifications, he can hardly afford to apply the additional test of nutritional quality.

Interest Must Be Aroused

Unfortunately, even the very human quality of inertia mitigates against food of high nutrient value. Four or 5 years ago, the Oklahoma Experiment Station introduced Allgold, a new variety of sweet potato with 3 times the vitamin A content of Puerto Rico, the variety which is grown by practically all sweet potato farmers. Allgold turned out to be a wonderful plant. It yields just as well as Puerto Rico and its tubers are just as large. The average person probably couldn't tell the difference between the two types, but laboratory tests show the amazing difference in vitamin A content. What has happened in the years since Allgold was developed? Relatively little! It is used by many home gardeners, but the commercial growers are still growing Puerto Rico. Perhaps they feel that improved nutritional value isn't sufficient reason for changing a variety they have grown all their lives. Perhaps they just don't care.

Despite the inertia on the farm and in the market place, there are a few horticulturists who are making good use of the gene structure of plants to create types that consistently produce food of superior vitamin content. One of the most productive of these men is Professor A. F. Yeager, now retired from the University of New Hampshire. One of his most notable creations is the Doublerich tomato. He did it by crossing standard varieties with strains of the tiny wild tomatoes from Peru. These "cherry tomatoes" are the richest of all in vitamin C, but because of their size, they are not acceptable to consumers.

Another remarkable achievement with tomatoes was the development of Caro Red by Purdue University. This orange-colored tomato is very rich in vitamin A—and has superior flavor, too. A single fruit of Caro Red supplies more than one and one-half times the daily adult requirement of vitamin A. The high carotene content of the fruit is the inspiration for the name Caro Red. We grew a number of plants of Caro Red on the Organic Gardening Experimental Farm last summer, and many who sampled the fruit proclaimed it the most flavorsome they had ever tasted. Good health and good flavor go together.

Choosing High-Nutrient Foods

I hope that by now I have aroused your interest in the field of high-nutrient plants. I personally feel that they represent a most important challenge to farmers, food processors and consumers. They are a dream come true for health-minded people, and a secret weapon in the battle against hunger and malnutrition for all people in the future. The question now to be answered is—how can you get them?

Thousands of people all across the country, who live in the suburbs and the country, are growing them in their gardens. Gardening, especially by the organic method, is the best way to achieve a source of the finest, most nutritious fruits and vegetables. Not only can you select the high-vitamin types and varieties, but you can fertilize the soil properly and pick your produce at its peak of quality. Much vitamin content is lost in the time that elapses between the picking of commercial produce and its sale in super markets. Home gardeners avoid that loss.

Gardening—Gateway to Healthiest Diet

Gardening is the gateway to the healthiest possible diet, but in our urban-centered society, not everyone can be a gardener. I am primarily concerned about the many people who are missing these superior foods because they can't grow them nor can they buy them in stores. What shall they do?

Step number one is to be selective in purchasing. As I said above, Delicious apples are low in vitamin C. So are McIntosh. Look for the higher vitamin types when you shop. When buying lettuce, look for Romaine and Black Seeded Simpson. They are much higher in vitamin C than other varieties. Summer varieties of cabbage, such as Early Copenhagen, Golden Acre and Peerless, contain nearly double the vitamin C of fall and winter types. Taste is often a good guide to vitamin quality. The bland-tasting, shipped-in head lettuce you buy in the winter has only a fraction of the vitamin value of loose-headed lettuce and endive, whose leaves are more exposed to the sun. Their stronger taste indicates more food value. Apples that taste mealy and bland have little food value compared to tart, fresh apples.

You Don't Have to Buy the Biggest Varieties

Another secret to selective purchasing of high-nutrient foods is to free yourself of the compulsion to buy the biggest of everything. Frequently, fruits and vegetables have most of their vitamins and minerals concentrated in and near the skin. Smaller fruits not only cost less, but they have a much larger skin area per pound.

So, chances are they are more nutritious. Also, smaller fruits and vegetables are less likely to have been forced through excess fertilizing. Hereditary considerations are important, too. Some of the large hybrid tomatoes now being widely grown have been selected by plant breeders primarily for the size of their fruit. The ability of the genes of those hybrid tomatoes to produce vitamins may never even have been checked. So if you stick to the smaller tomatoes, you are more likely to get higher-nutrient types. Another place where smallness pays off is in eggs. The Colorado State University recently issued a statement advising people to buy pullet eggs in preference to hen eggs. "Because shells of pullet eggs are small and the volume of materials that goes into making an egg is small," stated the university, "a young hen is able to produce the highest quality of her laying career."

Up to the American Public

If the American public will learn to appreciate nutrient value in foods and begin to demand such foods, there is a chance that the farmers, food processors and storekeepers will put more emphasis on quality rather than quantity. There has to *be* a demand before a demand can be fulfilled. For example, a plant breeder working for the Department of Agriculture wrote that it would be very simple to produce a new type of potato that would be high in vitamin C. The only hitch is that the flesh would be yellowish rather than white, and this agricultural worker knew that the American housewife would not buy a "white" potato with yellow flesh. Unfortunately, he probably is right. How many people think of vitamins when they buy potatoes? Very few!

Another hope for better food is—believe it or not—an electronic device. I predict that, at some time in the future, there will be developed machines that will automatically sort foods according to their vitamin and mineral value. Eggs, for example, will move along a conveyor belt through an electronic machine that will quickly analyze them and sort them into high-nutrient and low-nutrient lots. The poultry man will be paid not by the case, but by the total amount of food value his chickens produce. The customer will pay for the eggs according to their food value, and not simply by size. Today, the farmer who produces high-vitamin food gets paid not a penny more for his labor than the farmer who produces low-quality food. The price per bushel is the same. If that situation can be changed, the consumer will begin to get better food.

A Change in Attitude Recommended

There will also have to be a change in the attitude of the top government and business leaders of the food industry. Today, they state firmly that "America is the best fed nation on earth," basing that opinion entirely on *quantity* considerations. They can't be standing behind the vitamin content of American foods, because there is no doubt that their vitamin content could be greatly increased. It may take quite a while for the food experts to wake up to the value of high-vitamin plants, but I am sure that they will eventually. The thing that will make them wake up is the population explosion that will soon begin to crowd our cities and tax the productive capacity of our land. When that happens, it will be absolutely necessary to make each acre produce the maximum in vitamins and minerals that it is capable of. We will no longer be able to afford the luxury of producing large tomatoes, if the same land will produce much more food value in the form of small tomatoes.

Garlic

Learning from the Baboons

Maybe it's too much to hope that an ape will turn out a great painting or a memorable piece of prose, but if you think we can't learn anything from them, think again. In the *Atlantic Monthly* (March, 1961), we learn that baboons suffering from gastric ulcer, rheumatism, influenza and malnutrition have taught medical men several remedies. In 1918, when a flu epidemic was raging in Cape Town, Africa, baboons, sick with the disease, were to be seen tottering from their mountain caves to burrow for wild garlic and gorge on it. When humans who were stricken with the disease ate the same bulbs, they found that both congestion and fever were relieved.

After this enlightening experience, Cape Town householders who witnessed other baboons who were suffering from rheumatism stuffing themselves with certain willow leaves were quick to try a strong tea brewed of the same willow leaves to bring relief to their own rheumatic pains. It was later that these very leaves were accepted as the basis for a commonly used rheumatism medication. (The *Atlantic* article does not say just what the medication is.)

Try Natural Treatment First

How wise of us it would be to profit by the innate intelligence and instinct of the animals who seem to know what is best for them. Scientists use animals for all sorts of experiments which are intended to show the efficacy of this or that newly developed drug. If the effect is the one that is hoped for, the drug is headed for human consumption, because it seems to have worked on animals. But when one mentions garlic as a treatment for flu or tea made from willow leaves as a treatment for rheumatism, and offers the fact that these were effective for baboons stricken with these very illnesses, as evidence that they are worth trying, doctors are either horrified or amused at such naive conclusions.

We believe that such remedies should be tried. We believe that the safety factor alone, as opposed to that of some popular drugs, is reason enough for giving them a chance. If eating a garlic bulb will reduce the fever and congestion of flu, why use aspirin or antibiotics? If the garlic doesn't do the job, nothing is lost; the antibiotics can still be used. But we say, try the safe treatment first. If it doesn't work, the more radical treatment is still available. Maybe monkeys have more sense than we give them credit for.

Gasoline Fumes

Getting Drunk on Gasoline Fumes

In the *Journal of the American Medical Association* (December 26, 1959), we find notice that nutmeg, plastic glue and gasoline are being sniffed to give the effect of intoxication. Teen-agers are often guilty of trying for a new thrill by doing such things as spiking beer with nutmeg. Of special interest to the corresponding doctor, Maurice Pruitt, M.D., was a 6-year-old child who was brought to his office so drunk the child could not stand. His mother said he had been addicted to sniffing gas from the age of 18 months. He concluded by saying that this practice was a common craze among the young children of his community.

We don't know how one can keep these things from teen-agers (though good nutritional training should deter them from such pastimes). But no such items should be within reach of small children. Accidents caused by children's having access to cleaning materials are more frequent than any others. Why should an 18-month-old child or even a 6-year-old child be able to become intoxicated with gasoline? It shows a shocking disregard for safety on the part of the parent. Be careful of what is in the reach of your small children. The caustic cleaners and disinfectants can be the cause of tragic, irreversible consequences.

Girdles

Rubber Girdles and Thrombophlebitis

If you ladies must wear a girdle, plan to stand as much as possible when you have it on. In *Scope* (April 13, 1960), Dr. William T. Foley, Chief of the Vascular Clinic at New York Hospital, was quoted as the source of a statement saying that women who sit in rubber girdles for many hours may run an increased risk of thrombophlebitis. He also noted that circular garters act as a tourniquet on the flow of venous blood in the legs.

We have argued against the use of girdles, so common among American women, for years. The close restriction caused by girdles pushes the vital organs out of their proper position and certainly interferes with proper blood flow. But aside from these deterrents to their use, girdles encourage sloppy posture and loss of tone in abdominal and gluteal muscles. While the girdle is holding a woman together, she looks well enough, but without the girdle, a woman who is used to it literally falls apart. Her stomach muscles don't ever have to work, because the girdle does their work. The muscles which hold her upper thighs taut and her derriére firm are like jelly. They can't do the job anymore, because they're not used to working. This eventually affects the lady's posture, her strength, her well-being—everything!

Avoid wearing girdles. Exercise will give you the muscular power to do what a girdle does, and much more comfortably. If you must wear a girdle, make it a point to do exercises regularly which will help maintain the tone of your abdominal and gluteal muscles.

Glaucoma

Check for Glaucoma

Myopia is one of the leading complaints among eye patients. In the *Journal of the American Medical Association* (August 20, 1960), we see an interesting warning to doctors concerning the diagnosis of myopia. The author uses 4 case histories to demonstrate that the recognition of glaucoma may be readily missed in myopic patients. When the causes of a lessening of vision are sought, glaucoma definitely should be taken into account, as well as myopia and cataract.

When glaucoma is discovered too late, or not at all, the removal of a cataract present or the initiation of any other treatment, is of little or no use in improving the sight of the eye.

When you have your eyes examined, if you have noticed any irregularities in your vision, ask the doctor to make absolutely certain that glaucoma is not present. This disease, caused by inner pressure on the eyeball, is not as readily apparent, as are some others, on superficial examination. The examiner must have it specifically in mind, so your suggestion that your doctor do so may save you grave consequences in the future.

Habits

How to Form a Habit

Can you actually make a habit of healthful living? Why not? Surely you can think of less important things you do that are the result of deliberately ingrained habit. Have you trained yourself to wash the dishes immediately after dinner, instead of letting them wait? Do you waken at a certain hour every morning because you know you need that much time to get to the office? Is it a habit for you to get the car greased or the oil changed? Are any of these activities more important than maintaining good health? Of course not; and if you learned these good habits, you can learn other more valuable ones.

Why We Form Habits

Just why one forms a habit is an interesting psychological question. A closer examination of the habits you have will tell you the answer. Take, for example, washing the dishes immediately after dinner, even though you'd like to postpone it 'till later. You've found, however, that your enjoyment of the rest of the evening is clouded by the realization that the dishes are still waiting to be washed. You might end up doing them at midnight, when you'd rather be in bed, or be faced by them in the morning before breakfast. Neither of these alternatives is preferable to the slight chore of washing the dishes immediately after the meal. Experience has taught you all of this so that you don't have to think it over each time there are dishes to be done. You've learned the lesson so well that it has become a habit.

What about getting up at a certain hour? Of course, you didn't always wake at 6:30 in the morning. But you soon discovered that getting up any later meant a scramble for the bathroom, a rushed breakfast and, possibly, a missed bus. You made up your mind to get up at 6:30 whether you felt like it or not, because you knew it made things easier for you. You got used to hearing the alarm at the same time each day and eventually, you were waking before the alarm went off. You didn't need the alarm—you had a habit!

Your habits with the car are the same. You keep it oiled and greased because you have been convinced, perhaps painfully, that it will break down otherwise. You don't want to suffer the consequences involved in that, so you've become accustomed to doing what must be done to keep the car running.

Forming a Habit

Each of these cases illustrates a basic factor in the development of a habit. You must really have a reason for forming a habit and the reason must make sense to you. It must be clear to you that you are basically dissatisfied without the action you wish to turn into a habit.

If you will examine your actions closely, you will find that your whole personality is the sum of your habits. Do you make it a habit to smile at people you see? Is it your habit to give acquaintances the benefit of the doubt? Do you habitually fly into a temper when things go wrong? Do you *always* put two spoonfuls of sugar in your coffee? Have you *never* eaten a certain type of fruit? You can think of hundreds more. Things that make you *you*—and mark you as different, in some way, from anyone else.

You Are Performing under a Handicap

In addition to really wanting to form a certain habit, there are several other rules for forming habits which one should apply. These are taken from the book, *Habits, Their Making and Unmaking,* by Knight Dunlap, Professor of Experimental Psychology at Johns Hopkins University, published by Liveright Publishing Corporation. Professor Dunlap says that one must analyze and understand his situation without the habit one wishes to acquire, and realize that one is performing under a handicap. (Without the habit of getting up on time, I must rush uncomfortably and might not get to my job on time. Why undergo this discomfort?)

One must also think of the advantages of having the good habit; these will be an incentive for working harder at it. (If the car is well maintained, the specter of a breakdown is eliminated and I can travel with confidence.)

Finally, Dr. Dunlap tells us that one must engage in the activity consistently, bearing in mind the reasons, that make the new habit worthwhile.

Acquiring a Good Health Habit

Now let us see how these points can be applied in acquiring a specific health habit. For example, you want to acquire the habit of daily exercise. You realize that you never have done any physical exercise that will keep your body's tone as high as it should be. You come home from work and throw yourself into a chair for the evening. Week ends are the same, except that you don't even have the exercise you get from walking to the garage for the car which you use to ride to work. You decide that you need 15 minutes of knee bends and deep breathing each morning, plus a half hour's walk in the afternoon.

Here is how you go about acquiring the exercise habit, applying Professor Dunlap's principles. First, you must really *want* to start exercising. You can't be indefinite or wishy-washy about your desire to start the exercise habit, or you simply won't keep doing it. Next, you must make yourself realize what a handicap you have been living under without the proposed daily exercise. Remind yourself that you've been gaining weight, you've become sluggish and lack pep and the ambition to do things. Your endurance is nil when you are called upon for some physical effort in sports or in rearranging furniture around the house. You don't even look as well as you once did. Your skin is lacking in color. Your circulation seems poor. Even your appetite has been poor lately. You'll be able to notice other symptoms of a lack of exercise activity that are peculiar to you alone. Keep these in mind when you're tempted to skip a session.

Remember What Exercise Will Do for You

The third point to remember is what this exercising will do for you. It will increase your pep and make you feel like doing more. You'll soon find that you tire less easily, both during your exercise periods and in other strenuous activities. Your circulation will im-

---

Harvey, William

William Harvey, discoverer of the circulation of the blood, was born at Folkestone, England, on April 1, 1578. Upon receipt of his Bachelor of Arts degree from the Caius College, Cam- 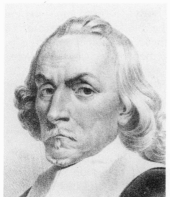 *bridge, Harvey entered the University of Padua to begin study toward his medical degree which he received in 1602. That same year he was admitted as a fellow to the Royal College of Physicians and in 1607 was granted the post of physician at St. Bartholomew's Hospital. It was here that he began his preliminary studies which resulted in the discovery of how blood circulates through the body. Before his time, scientists and physicians attempted to study the human circulatory system through the decrees of philosophers. Harvey, after studying thoroughly the Galenical theory of circulation, went on to show that only through actual observation of the human parts in movement, could the secrets of the heart and blood be learned. Thus through his painstaking observations of these movements in test animals, Harvey was able to present the true picture of the circulatory system—the movement of blood from the left side of the heart by the aorta and its subdivisions to the right side by the veins.*

prove and so will your color and the tone of your skin. Your appetite will increase, but you'll notice that excess poundage will melt away. This regular exercise will do wonders for you!

Acquiring a habit depends strongly on repetition. You must keep at it, otherwise you haven't a chance of successfully forming any kind of a habit. Make a schedule for your daily exercise and stick to it no matter what comes up. It is easy to find excuses for postponing a session, but don't be tempted. If you slide a little bit, you will soon find all of the good work you have done up to that time being wasted. You will soon be back where you started. When you are tempted, remind yourself strongly of how you felt before you began to exercise and how you feel now. Make yourself realize what exercise will do for your health and your spirit.

These suggestions can be applied to any habit you might wish to form. They are all sound ideas that will definitely be of help to you in your efforts.

Physiological Problems Sometimes Involved

In the case of certain habits you might wish to break, you will probably need more than these points to work with. There is more than a psychological problem involved in giving up tobacco, coffee, sugar, salt and other substances that are druglike in their effects. The use of these things forces the body to rearrange its entire metabolism to accommodate them. The blood sugar operates on a new level when falsely stimulated by these substances, and the body becomes used to this high-gear arrangement. It has no resources of its own to fall back on when the caffeine or nicotine is not forthcoming. Then, the dizziness and nausea—the general craving—often experienced by those who try to eliminate the use of these unhealthful items, takes hold. Addicts (for that is what they are) find that their resolve melts under the physical need they feel for a cigarette or a candy bar.

If you should find that you give in to such temptation, in spite of your efforts to apply Professor Dunlap's rules, you need the help you can get from good nutrition. If your system has a sufficient nutritional supply from wholesome food and food supplements to keep the blood sugar at a proper level, the sag in blood sugar that creates the craving for a smoke, coffee, sweets, etc., will not occur. Then the habit is strictly a matter of will power once again and you can apply the rules above with confidence.

Satisfaction in a Good Habit

There is something very satisfying about deliberately forming a new habit that will be of benefit to us. It is essential that we sometimes prove to ourselves that we can exercise such discipline over inclinations that we know are harmful to health. Those who do not are asking for ill health and misery.

Try it now. Do you have a bad health habit you want to break, or is there a good habit you wish you could acquire? Don't postpone it another minute! Resolve now to get going on the road to better health. You will be surprised at what a month of serious application can do. If you can get through the first month without backsliding, your new habit is as good as formed.

Another hint psychologists offer is this: get through a day at a time. Don't think of the months stretched out before you. Such thoughts are defeating. Wake up each morning and promise yourself, *"Today,* I will do my exercise without fail," or "I am determined not to smoke *today."* You will notice very soon that the days with your new routine begin to pass without the need to think about keeping to your resolve. It becomes automatic. You've got a habit!

Hair Sprays

Temporary Deafness from Hair Sprays

John Troan, science writer for the *Indianapolis* (Indiana) *Times* (January 30, 1960) quotes ear specialist, Dr. Albert P. Seltzer, as saying that hair sprays may cause temporary deafness in young children. If the spray gets into the ear canal, it may set off an inflammation which can block out sound. Dr. Seltzer suggests that parents using hair spray plug the child's ears with cotton or gauze before using. If one insists on using these sprays, certainly the ear plugs would be a wise precaution. However, we think that all sprays of this type should be banned in the home. The air around the user is bound to become saturated with unhealthful chemicals which he will inhale with every breath. Inhaling them is every bit as dangerous as swallowing them in foods.

Hardening of the Arteries

New Findings on Hardening of the Arteries

Three researchers of London, Ontario, Canada, report on their findings about cholesterol in patients with hardening of the arteries. In the *Canadian Medical Association Journal* for January 2, 1960, they review first the general theory that cholesterol (a fatty substance in the blood) is responsible for hardening of the arteries. They go on to tell us that, over the years, strong arguments have piled up, based on studies of people in hospitals, on laboratory experiments with animals and on studies of the dietary habits of various groups of people in one nation or another—arguments seeming to show that cholesterol is responsible for hardening of the arteries. Yet, they say, it is important to note that no one has proved that high levels of fat or cholesterol in the blood are associated with more hardening of the arteries than are low levels.

For 6 years before writing this article, these 3 researchers, J. C. Paterson, Lucy Dyer and E. C. Armstrong, had been testing the cholesterol levels of the blood of patients in a veterans hospital. These patients were permanently confined, and hence, could be followed closely. When any of the patients died, the severity of their artery hardening was determined and a comparison made with the tests made during their lifetime.

Results of Tests

The authors state that, taken at face value, the results of their tests offer little or no evidence of a relationship between either the severity or incidence of hardening of the arteries symptoms and the cholesterol level of the blood, when this level was between 150 and 300 milligrams. These are the levels that are found in 90 per cent of the people of our nation. It seems possible, they say, that very high levels of cholesterol may hasten the process of artery hardening.

Many of the patients studied were mental patients. The authors fear that arguments may be used to show that the cholesterol level of the blood of mental patients is perhaps different from that of normal persons. However, they point out that they are studying the relationship between the amount of cholesterol in the blood and the hardening of the arteries. So what they studied was the effect of cholesterol, badly used by the body, on the arteries. What the reason for this unhealthful use of cholesterol is should not affect the results. If, in the case of mental illness, the cause is different than with normal persons, it does not matter. All of the patients studied were in good physical health, up to the illness that caused their death.

During the 6 years of tests, they found that the level of cholesterol in the blood of their selected patients was remarkably stable. Other researchers, too, have reported that the amount of cholesterol in the blood of healthy young adults, measured over 28 months and repeated 12 years later, appeared to be maintained at a level which was typical of the individual and did not change.

The authors conclude that the results of their tests seem to show that the severity of hardening of the arteries is *not* related to the level of cholesterol in the blood except when the level is exceptionally high—that is, higher than 300 milligrams. Furthermore, they say that the complications of hardening of the arteries were just as frequent in cases with low cholesterol levels as in cases with moderately high levels—that is, from 250 to 299 milligrams.

Such research as this leads us to believe that all of us may have been stressing too much, over the past few years, the importance of cholesterol, the need to control the amount of animal fat in the diet and the need for getting large quantities of vegetable fat. Perhaps it doesn't matter so much whether you have high cholesterol levels. Perhaps other things having to do with nutrition and health are just as important.

Thyroid Deficiencies

We want to remind readers of other ideas along these lines. Dr. Murray Israel of New York has done valuable work giving thyroid preparations, along with a vitamin and mineral supplement,

---

Hippocrates

Hippocrates is the man whose works, research and teachings are responsible for the medical theory which has developed through the ages into what we know as modern medicine. Hippo-

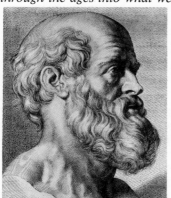

crates was born on the Greek island of Coss, about 400 years before the birth of Christ. Early in life he began to display the questioning attitude which later in life caused him to investigate and disprove the common beliefs of the day. He disagreed with his contemporaries on the causation of disease. Rejecting the theories of superstition, religion and magic, Hippocrates taught that medicine could only be practiced scientifically, based on facts, observation and study. He was the first physician to use diet, fresh air, medicinal waters and exercise in the treatment of diseases. Other profound innovations were his theories on the effect of climate on human health and his conviction that Nature alone can heal, the physician only assisting the natural processes. All of these ideas are found in his writings, which have shaped the historical progress of medicine. In addition, these writings were used as the chief reference for the preparation of the famous Hippocratic oath, used in the graduating ceremonies of our medical schools and ethical guide to the professional life of the physician. Hippocrates truly deserves the honor bestowed upon him— Father of Modern Medicine.

which was designed to lower cholesterol, as well as to provide those vitamins that we know are necessary for the body to use fat properly. Dr. Israel's article appeared in the *American Journal of Digestive Diseases* for June, 1955. Dr. Israel worked to eliminate these symptoms in his patients: fatigue, nervousness, depression, irritability, weakness, forgetfulness, inability to concentrate, coolness, drowsiness, insomnia, headache, dizziness, shortness of breath, heart palpitation, leg pains, numbness, backache, etc.

He believes that the hormones produced by the thyroid gland decrease with age, sometimes becoming so scanty that the body's needs are not met. His theory is backed up by other researchers. A Finnish doctor, writing in the *Lancet,* for July, 1959, stated that patients of his who died of hardening of the arteries often have goiter; in fact, goiters are significantly more frequent in such cases than in those dying from other causes. Dr. W. C. Hueper of the National Cancer Institute believes, too, that there is an important connection between the thyroid and hardening of the arteries. He theorizes that it is the failure of the body's metabolism that causes cholesterol to collect in blood vessels. Metabolism is the word for the body's process for using food. The thyroid gland regulates this process to a large extent. Including kelp and plenty of iodine-rich food in the diet helps keep the thyroid gland in good health, for it needs much iodine to manufacture its hormone.

More evidence on the importance of the thyroid gland to cholesterol in the blood comes from the University of California Medical School. Three researchers there are quoted in the *New York Times* for June 10, 1960, as saying that cholesterol in heart patients can be effectively lowered by giving them thyroid hormone, without stimulating their diseased hearts. They believe that people with sluggish thyroid glands do not produce enough of the hormone thyroxin which helps to regulate the way the body uses cholesterol. By using a special gland preparation which does not increase the heart rate, they have been able to lower the cholesterol in 40 out of 49 patients for a year's time.

Vitamin E Reduces Cholesterol

There is another suggestion that inclusion of vitamin E may play a big part in holding the cholesterol level low. An article in the *American Journal of the Medical Sciences* for November, 1958, indicates that vitamin E, combined with vegetable oils, may be an extremely effective method for controlling cholesterol.

Dr. Lawrence E. Meltzer, Albert A. Bochman and George H. Berryman, write of their experiment with 28 heart patients (suffering from myocardial infarction) who had high cholesterol levels in their blood. All the patients were eager to cooperate because they wanted to avoid further heart trouble. The patients were divided into 3 groups—those who ate less than 50 grams of fat daily, those who ate 50 to 100 grams and those who ate 100 to 150 grams of fat. All the patients had been studied for months before this experiment began and a careful record had been kept of their cholesterol levels, so it was easy to determine whether this was raised or lowered during the time the study was made.

It was found that every subject showed a decrease in blood cholesterol at the end of 3 months. The decrease was maintained or additionally lowered during another 3-month period when the dose of vegetable oil was lowered. The overall change over 6 months was important for everyone in Group I (low-fat diet), in 7 out of 8 of those in Group II (medium-fat) and in 7 out of 10 in the group eating a high-fat diet.

The substance tested consisted of safflower oil plus pyridoxine (a B vitamin) plus sterols (a kind of fat found in plants). One tablespoonful of the mixture contained 20 milligrams of vitamin E. Four tablespoonfuls were taken daily—one during each meal, one at bedtime. This would add 80 milligrams of vitamin E to whatever the patient was already getting in his diet, which might, of course, be very little.

No mention is made of any restrictions in the daily diet or any other food supplement used, so we must assume that these patients ate their usual diets—good or bad, as the case might be—and got reductions in blood cholesterol, even in Group III, when they were eating diets high in fat. Notice that one of the B vitamins was also given. Certain of the B vitamins are mentioned frequently in connection with the way the body uses fats. One must have them in ample quantities—and they are scarce in American diets.

Some Recommendations

It seems to us, with all this evidence at hand, that no one need any longer fear hardening of the arteries. To be on the safe side, we can go easy on animal fats and processed fats (the hydrogenated ones—solid at room temperature). We can use lots of natural vegetable fats (nuts, salad oils, avocados, seeds of all kinds). We can take food supplements that will help keep our thyroid glands healthy (kelp, especially). We can reduce our intake of starchy and sugary foods (especially those that have been refined like white flour and white sugar) to a minimum. And, finally, we can take vitamin E and make sure we are getting plenty of all the B vitamins in food supplements like brewer's yeast and desiccated liver.

Health-Conscious

Is It a Disgrace to be Health-Conscious?

By J. I. Rodale

The fact that one asks such a question shows that many persons are *not* health-conscious. In fact, the common attitude toward health seems to be that it is a *disgrace* to be health-conscious, and that a person who *is* that way is a hypochondriac. But there is a vast difference between these two classifications. Actually, the hypochondriac is a pathetic fool, while the health-conscious person usually is a very intelligent individual.

I had a friend whom I tried to guide in the ways of good health, because I saw that he was shortening his life. But one day he got angry and he suddenly blurted out, "Look! You take care of your cancer and I'll take care of mine!" Poor soul, he died a few years later of a heart attack at the age of 56. He could have lived much longer if he had been only mildly health-conscious.

This man was beginning to taste a delightful power in community affairs. His business had just developed to the point where it was making a lot of money. Then came some petty family problem which worried him sick and he got a heart attack. His body had been weakened by his reckless eating and drinking habits. He did not have the resistance that could have conditioned him against trouble. So he got mowed down by the grim reaper long, long before his allotted time, all because of an unforgivable ignorance of the simple basic facts of health. He had depended on medical checkups which had lulled him into a false sense of security. From various causes, millions of people die young, whose medical checkups showed that there was nothing wrong with them. No, sir . . . medical checkups are not all there is to health consciousness. But I don't advise you *not* to have your health checked from time to time. These tests indicate important things, though they are not the whole story, as you shall see if you follow our program regularly.

Many People Misinformed

Now . . . there are millions of people like my friend, who are terribly misinformed about health. There is the woman who appeared on a television program, holding aloft the can opener which she said she had been using since her honeymoon. She hugged that can opener to her bosom as if it were a precious symbol of a most wonderful way of life, not realizing that it represented a sorrowful degeneration in our eating habits, that we are digging our graves with our can openers—which reminds me of a story.

418

On a visit to Toronto, Canada, a few years ago, we took a bus tour of the city. The bus stopped before a girls' college which specialized in home economics, and the guide said, "This is a school that when a girl graduates, she comes out with a diploma in one hand and a can opener in the other." That was a smart old guide. You can be sure *he* was not using can openers.

Our schools are not everything we think they are. They are known to teach a kind of nutrition that is one of the causes of so many heart attacks, and this defective nutrition is at the bottom of the fact that one out of four persons living today will get cancer. And experts predict, that at the rate cancer is increasing, it will soon be one out of every three. Not a bright prospect to look forward to, is it?

Thoughts on Health Consciousness

Then there is the person who wants to be normal. Health consciousness to him is something abnormal. According to him, to be health-conscious is to be some sort of square . . . a nut, some sort of crackpot, or food faddist. But when you consider that the average person over 50 suffers from some kind of chronic condition of ill health, which would make it appear that disease is normal, then to be health conscious *must* be abnormal.

Then there is the person who thinks that health consciousness is a joke. A friend of mine was drinking some cola drinks on the grandstand at the Allentown Fair and, seeing me and knowing that I am *not* in favor of soda drinking, asked, "Is this all right, Mr. Rodale?" I replied, "You know it is *not* all right." Then he said, "Is it all right if I take a deep breath?" Actually, I knew that man's history. He was a heavy cigarette smoker, and really couldn't take a deep breath without pain. I know the signs. He had the beginning of a lung condition. He is the type who wants to run with the herd and be normal. He's the kind that fills our hospitals. I'll bet he knows the batting average of every baseball player, but not one thing about vitamins or how important protein is in the diet and such things.

Then there is the lady who once wrote me, "I think of health only when I'm sick." That about sums up the general attitude. But people don't realize that health habits can easily become established in the course of time. These habits soon become automatic and easy to follow, enabling people to be health-conscious in a painless, pleasant sort of way.

Philosophy of Living Dangerously

Somewhere, way back on the American scene, there developed a philosophy that living dangerously was brave and glamorous, like a soldier in a war, but that to watch one's health was a sign of weakness. It was a way of life that had captured the popular imagination.

It represented something brashly bold and chivalric, probably harking back to the days when knights were bold and people did not live to be old. For example, some years ago, it was the fashion among American factory workers to take all kinds of chances to impress their fellow workers. In a steel mill, a man would be looked up to if he walked teeteringly on the narrow ledge of a big pot of hot metal. Workers would hop about on precarious places high up on a building under construction.

But when the insurance companies saw what it was costing them, they took a hand and began a campaign of education to teach common sense to these workers, and soon they took an entirely new slant on the subject. Not only did the amount of accidents go down drastically, but it became unfashionable to take one's life in one's hands in a factory. Now, if a worker were seen needlessly taking chances, he would be considered a fool and his fellow workers would not hesitate to tell him so. It was a long program of accident prevention that accomplished marvelous results.

But why didn't the insurance companies go further and do the same with human health? I'll never know. They make stabs at it, here and there, but evidently what they teach is not doing the job, because while the accident rate in factories has been going down, the rate of chronic disease in factory workers has been going up.

Perhaps there is a subtle psychology to it. When a factory worker gets hurt, it costs the insurance company money in an immediate direct payment. But the payment for death is far in the distance. The factory worker has an immediate economic value like a cow, so a certain care is bestowed upon him.

A Cartoon

A man will take constant care of his car and his household equipment. He will use the right kind of gas and oil for fear of hurting his car's engine. But his own engine? Anything goes as far as that is concerned. There was a very interesting cartoon by Jimmy Hatlo in the *They'll Do It Every Time* series (King Features), which showed a businessman talking to a coal salesman and saying. "We're very particular about what kind of coal we put into our boilers, and before we could consider using your coal, we'd want an analysis of it. Can't go ruining our furnaces with shale, clinkers and sulphur." The next picture shows the same businessman eating at home and stuffing all sorts of unhealthful foods into himself with the statement, "But his own vitamin boiler he'll stoke with anything and everything."

Health and Cleanliness

If the average person could experience the wonderful pleasure of being healthy, I know he would become health-conscious. The average person is not health-conscious because he hasn't the slightest inkling of the pleasures it will give him. What a wonderful feeling it is to wake up some fine morning, to realize that you haven't had a cold or a headache for a year, that you have been free of pains, that you have more energy, that you are more cheerful! What a feeling of pleasurable achievement it will give you! Your body will feel cleaner internally. Cleanliness is next to godliness. Inner filth is not godlike cleanliness. Think about that when you go to your church. Disease and pain indicate that there are toxic substances in your body that are filth, and that shouldn't be there. They represent bodily uncleanliness.

When Rudolph Valentino, the old-time movie idol of the silent days, was opened up at autopsy at a rather young age, the examining doctors found a condition of bodily filth that was shocking. They said it was the worst they had ever seen. How about *your* body? Is it clean with good health? If it isn't, perhaps we can show you how to clean it up.

If you become actively health-conscious, you will look better and younger. You will be able to look forward to a future of old age in which you will not be senile. You will not only live much longer, but you will find it a pleasure to be old without having the ceaseless pains and aches of old age. With our method, your mind will retain a keen edge to the end of your life. There will be no doddering in mind or body.

Many people say, "Who wants to live too long?" They are thinking of the usual senility and unhappiness of old people that they know. These people are paying the penalty for not knowing how to live healthfully or they never cared. But the day of reckoning comes. They find it difficult to walk with comfort. Half the time they are dizzy, or fall down very easily and break bones. They cannot think deeply and are looked down on with contempt in their own family. Their opinion is not sought. They are actually in the way, and many of them wind up in homes for the aged. This does not have to happen to you. You can control your own health destiny.

There are many angles to this subject. For example, the older you get, the more you should be looked up to—not only among your family and relatives, but in public meetings and in your social life, provided, of course, that your mind keeps pace with your body, through good health practices. You may not think it possible, but there is much medical evidence that points to the fact that there is a close relation between our diets and our mentality. Actually, if we took people from childhood on and carefully controlled their diet, we could produce a race of people with super mentalities.

The Loss of Talented People

We were talking about the dividends that come with old age, if it is a healthy old age. How about what a person with certain skills and talents owes to his community? Think about the golden voice of Mario Lanza, cut off at the age of 40. Doesn't such a gift belong to the world? Isn't a man with such a voice selfish if he doesn't try to live in such a way that he will reach at least 80 years of age? There are many painters and engineers and writers and actors and scholars, men of extraordinary genius, dying in their fifties and depriving the world of their specialized knowledge.

Some great leaders of our gigantic corporations, Congressmen and statesmen, who are so badly needed in this modern world of ours, are cut off long before their time. Most of these are men who depend solely on medical checkups, and would not go out of their way to learn the basic facts of health.

I once saw a photograph of Einstein eating an ice cream cone, taken in the streets of Princeton. He was also obese. Einstein, with all his genius, did not know the facts of health. But if he did, he did not practice them and therefore, died at age 70, although he could have gone on to 80 or 90 or even more, if he had done a few things, including the cutting of sugar out of his diet and bringing his weight down. This is the age of specialization. Einstein specialized in the science of relativity and left health to doctors. But the doctors are specialists in disease, not health. As a class, they are dying younger than the average person in the population. So how can they teach us how to live long?

Isn't it strange that men who are geniuses, men who are brilliant in their own fields, do not seem to be aware that something is radically wrong with the way the public is being instructed in health matters. If some of these brains were turned toward the prevention of disease, we would all be amazed how simple it could be. But they say that is not their function.

Patriotic to Be Health-Conscious

Looking at it from another point of view: Is it patriotic *not* to be health-conscious? You never thought of it that way, did you? Do you know that a lot of your tax money goes towards building hospitals and to medical research, much of which is wantonly wasted? Your illness can contribute to a higher tax rate. Is it patriotic to follow habits that will weaken you as a citizen of our country? Where is your love of your fellow man? We all mean something to each other in a collective sense. A sick nation is a weak nation. Is it honest, is it patriotic to live so poorly, to weaken your body so much that you will pass on a poor physical heritage to the next generation? The sins of the parents are visited upon their children. For example, over 25,000 babies are born each year with heart disease, which no doubt is due to some deficiency or bad health habit of the mother, including smoking and drinking. Is it any wonder that Dr. Samuel Johnson said that a sick man was a rascal. If you look at it properly, he really is.

Take the case of a newly elected Congressman of about 50 years of age. He is elected at great cost to his party. He sits in Congress for two years and slowly learns the legislative ropes. Then he goes through another costly election and is re-elected. In the meantime, he eats any old thing, and takes no exercise. Suddenly, he dies of a heart attack at age 53. Is it patriotic to die just when his hard-bought skill could be put to use?

Congressmen should be in training like football players. All important people—executives, doctors and skilled people—should be in training so as to preserve their skills into a ripe old age. They owe it to their country to do this, because we are entering into a new phase in history, a battle of wits between one nation and another, and anything that will preserve our skills, in quality and amount, will be of great value in the war of wits on which the world is embarking.

Economic Implications

When a man dies young, he does not realize what a mess he is creating, what a heavy economic burden he is throwing on his survivors. If he has money and a business, there comes the destructive inheritance taxes which sometimes force many well-established businesses to be sold to obtain the cash for the taxes, and in many cases, they are sold for the low dollar. The government is hungry for your money when you're alive, but brother, when you die, you've seen nothing like it. They search safety deposit boxes and seek out every jewel hidden away, because all personal property is death taxable. They tax everything but the shroud. It's best to stave this day off as long as possible.

Many women live in a dream world as far as their husband's business or income is concerned. Then comes the day of death—the man of the house dies and the poor woman has to go to work. I was amazed some time ago to be waited on in a department store by one of these women. I thought they had been extremely wealthy. But death settled all that.

Life Is Pleasant

It's a tragedy to die. It's so pleasant to live. Think of the high cost of funerals these days. Your family will be in a much better economic condition if you remain alive. So, if you do not want to be health-conscious for yourself, do it for the sake of the family. Wouldn't it be better if you remained on the scene and watched over your children? Wouldn't it even be nice to be a grandfather or a great-grandfather, but not a doddering, senile great-grandfather. At family gatherings, a bright, sparkling old grandpa, dancing attendance on his grandchildren, could be a wonderful influence in the clan, could make its gathering a happy one. I know this pleasure, for I have 8 grandchildren. I must tell you that grandfatherhood is one of the greatest pleasures that I have experienced in life thus far, and can hardly wait for great-grandfatherhood. Man, life . . . healthy life is wonderful. So? Is it a disgrace to be health-conscious?

Hearing

What Drugs Can Do to Your Hearing

There are certain drugs which can cause an undeniable loss of hearing in susceptible persons. There appears to be no way of predicting who will and who will not suffer an impairment of hearing due to the intake of some antibiotic or another, or a sulfa drug, or even aspirin. It is obvious, then, that avoidance of the use of any and all of these drugs whenever possible should be the policy of every health-conscious person. Of course, when certain disease conditions exist which call for the drastic measures involved with the use of antibiotics and sulfas, the risks involved may be worth taking. However, we feel sure that many readers will recognize the names of drugs they use which could be substituted by a safer medication. It would certainly be the intelligent thing to make sure that the risk you are taking is unavoidable.

Aspirin May Cause Deafness

Aspirin has figured as an unsuspected villain in several types of disability. The myth of aspirin as a harmless pain reliever has been exploded before, but did you know that it is possible for the drug to cause deafness? It can indeed, according to an entry in the Question and Answer section of the *Journal of the American Medical Association* (April 25, 1953). The questioner asks if salicylates (aspirin) have any lasting effect on the hearing mechanism. Then, "If so, does this mean it would be unwise to give adequate doses of salicylates to a patient with acute rheumatic fever who has had some hearing loss as the result of a previous middle ear infection?"

The answer is one of those rather surprising replies one sees in this magazine, when the use of a favorite medication is questioned: "Impaired hearing due to large doses of salicylates of quinine is preceded by ringing in the ears . . . A safe rule to follow is to give salicylates as long as ringing in the ears does not occur. Slight degrees of auditory nerve damage from salicylates and quinine are reversible, so that prompt withdrawal of the drug, should ringing occur, should result in a return of the hearing to the present level."

Detecting the Warning

The doctor is apparently on his own, as is the patient, until the ears begin ringing. How can this be classed as a safe rule? One must assume that all doctors and patients are aware of what to look for, so the aspirin can be stopped before complete deafness takes over. What is happening to the rest of the body when confronted with a drug strong enough to cause deafness? No word on that. Why the calm attitude toward such a serious side effect? Don't doctors care that a course of aspirin therapy—a course so commonly prescribed—could make the patient deaf? And what about the patient who uses aspirin by the box on his own for headaches, muscular pain, colds, etc? Have any of the aspirin makers warned users about possible deafness due to the use of their product? How is a heavy user of aspirin to know that the ringing in the ears he experiences is a warning of impending deafness, and that, unless he stops using the aspirin, the deafness can be irreversible? We are appalled anew at the abandon with which aspirin is used in this country, and at the dangers presented by its use.

An Old Story

The story of the toxicity of streptomycin is an old one. In the November 2, 1950, issue of the *New England Journal of Medicine,* we saw this statement: "Deafness due to streptomycin toxicity has occurred sporadically, in contrast to the widespread vestibular (central portion of the middle ear) damage from the drug. Wallner reported on 93 tuberculosis patients receiving either one or two grams a day for 4 months . . . the majority receiving two grams a day and about half of those receiving one gram a day had some degree of vestibular damage . . ."

However, in spite of such reports, things got worse instead of better. A new and even more dangerous streptomycin compound, dihydrostreptomycin, was introduced. The deafness incidence became even greater with the use of this new drug. The *British Medical Journal* (November 17, 1951) carried a letter, signed P. E. Roland, which began, "I should like to support Dr. R. W. Biagi's plea to return to the use of streptomycin instead of the dihydro compound, as the latter appears to be more likely to cause deafness. Within the past few weeks I have seen 4 cases of severe deafness following prolonged therapy with dihydrostreptomycin. They affected 3 out of 4 children under treatment for tuberculosis meningitis and miliary (characterized by sores resembling millet seeds) tuberculosis. The fourth case was an adult suffering from renal (kidney) tuberculosis. All these cases showed marked nerve deafness and the last case was totally deaf in one ear."

On the same day, the *Journal of the American Medical Association* published this statement: "It was found that dihydrostreptomycin, whether hydrochloride or sulfate, is toxic to the auditory division of the eighth nerve in doses of two or three grams per day, when given for 3 months or more. It was far more toxic to the auditory mechanism than streptomycin, but less toxic to the vestibular apparatus. Streptomycin is, therefore, probably the drug of choice where long-term treatment is indicated. Loss of vestibular function is preferable to loss of cochlear (a spiral tube in the inner ear) function. The hearing loss from dihydrostreptomycin is progressive in many cases, even after the drug has been discontinued."

An Unheeded Summary

After reading in medical literature of several more damaging experiences with streptomycin compounds through the intervening years, this caught our eye in the *British Medical Journal* (June 22, 1957): "The curious and damaging affinity of streptomycin for the eighth nerve system was recognized by Hinshaw and Feldman (1945) soon after its introduction into clinical practice." Imagine, from the time this drug was introduced it was known as a danger to hearing, and still it was and is allowed to be widely used!

The authors of the article, T. Cawthorne and D. Ranger, of the British National Hospital for Nervous Diseases, wrote: "As we have seen a number of patients crippled by streptomycin therapy, some after small doses, we feel that the time has come to consider the toxic properties of streptomycin." And consider them they do. They summarize their findings at the end of the article and note that, in spite of the common impression among doctors that a daily dose of one gram will not cause toxic symptoms, they were able to give several instances in which poisoning occurred, even though this dosage was not exceeded. They also found that the number of cases of serious side effects from the use of streptomycin is on the increase, possibly due to a wider use of the drug. There was also a likelihood that any kidney damage present could cause stronger reactions to streptomycin drugs, because a retention of urine would allow the drug to pile up unduly in the blood stream.

Drug Still Used

Then, after 15 years of streptomycin use, after 15 years of warning by scientists and practitioners, the *New York Times* (September 27, 1959), as though it were big news, printed the headline, "Doctors Warned on Use of Drug." The article opened with the sentence, "The complete withdrawal of the *widely used* (italics ours) antibiotic dihydrostreptomycin has been urged in an editorial in the *New England Journal of Medicine.*" Then, in another paragraph: "The drug is frequently prescribed for illnesses ranging from the common cold to simple bacterial infections." Just think of the risks these patients took, without even knowing it! How many patients with simple colds were deafened by treatment with streptomycin? If it were only one in all the years of the drug's use, the fact would be deplorable.

The *Times* article went on to say that the drug, dihydrostreptomycin, is generally included in fixed combinations with penicillin. This means that patients under penicillin treatment for long periods (as many are) could suffer as serious a side effect as deafness from a drug they don't even need, an auxiliary drug the doctor might not even care to use! The reason for the inclusion of the streptomycin in the penicillin dosage was "that it may be preventing infections and that it is innocuous."

Streptomycin is still on the list of acceptable drugs for most physicians. Probably the *Journal's* plea has resulted in no changes in its use alone or with penicillin, just as all the other warnings since 1945 have meant nothing. Ask your doctor what drug he is giving you. If it is streptomycin, ask him if another drug can do the job and, if so, ask him to use it instead.

Other Drugs Can Cause Deafness

Other drugs can affect the hearing, too. How many we don't know, but in the *Journal of the American Medical Association* (June 1, 1957), a clue to why some deafness cases are caused by drugs appears. "Antibiotic deafness is due to the retention of fluid in the middle ear after acute otitis media (inflammation of the middle ear) treated with antibiotics. Conductive deafness may be caused by the large doses of antibiotics, which act rapidly (within 24 hours), arresting inflammation. The retained fluid becomes sterile and the capillaries are not stimulated to dilate and absorb this fluid. This is likely to become reinfected."

Terramycin is one antibiotic (aside from streptomycin and its compounds) named as a cause of deafness. In a summary of a Swedish paper on the subject, the *Journal of the American Medical Association* (October 16, 1954) carried the story of a woman of 48, who developed a rapidly increasing roaring in the ears in addition to other side effects, and her hearing continued to deteriorate for many months. She was expected to have a permanent severe hearing loss, and the cause was considered to be terramycin.

These are some of the pieces of evidence we have on the way some drugs can affect the hearing. We are inclined to suspect that any drug might have a similar effect on a susceptible patient. How does one discover who is susceptible? There is no way but to wait for the symptoms to appear. We say, avoid taking the chance. Don't use drugs unless you must! Keep yourself healthy enough through proper diet and food supplementation (vitamin A is frequently mentioned with its beneficial effect on the hearing apparatus) so that treatment with drugs will not be necessary. If you must use drugs, try to avoid those that are definitely known to cause deafness—and stay clear of aspirin unless your doctor *insists* on its use.

Some Rules for Better Hearing

The reason an elderly person does not hear is frequently owing to hearing loss of the nerve type, but occasionally, local or middle ear involvement may be at fault. At times, however, it is the speaker and not the listener who is responsible for the latter not hearing. According to Hoople (*Geriatrics,* 15:160, 1960), very few hearing losses in older persons can be overcome by medical treatment or surgery, but total deafness is almost never seen as the end result of these hearing deficits. "Rehabilitation in such patients consists primarily of instruction in the use of their residual hearing. Patients should be taught to acquire a new habit." Instead of saying, "What?" "I didn't hear you," or even "Please repeat that," they should say, "Please repeat that slowly and distinctly." Hoople continued: "The speaker should be asked to speak slowly, because in most elderly patients, there is some slowing of the mental processes. Slower speech is comprehended better. Secondly, the listener often is confronted with the problem of distinguishing between words that sound very similar. Slow speech can give him time to resolve this puzzle and he will be ready to listen to—and understand—the words that follow." (The *Eye, Ear, Nose and Throat Monthly,* November, 1960.)

Hiccups

Hiccups Can Be Serious

Occurring without any warning, hiccups have been responsible for a great deal of social embarrassment as well as a great deal of amusement. Actually, a hiccup is a sign that something has disturbed the nervous system and, until the disturbance is eliminated, you hiccup. A hiccup begins with any one of a number of factors, according to Dr. Charles Mayo in *Health,* October, 1957. An infection by certain organisms, mechanical pressure anywhere along the involved portions of the nervous system, hysteria (oddly enough, this type of hiccups occurs almost exclusively in women between the ages of 18 and 35) and chemical irritation of the stomach, intestine or breathing apparatus may disturb the nervous system.

There are other causes, too. Dr. J. D. Laycock, in the Letters to the Editor column of the *Lancet,* May, 1951, reports, "During the siege of Imphal in 1944, I saw a large number of severe cases of hiccup in men who had received penetrating wounds in the region of the diaphragm." Brain tumors, meningitis, encephalitis (inflammation of the brain) and advanced hardening of the cerebral arteries may also cause hiccups. In 1919, 1922 and 1924, epidemics of hiccups occurred in Winnipeg, Canada, which doctors at first blamed on mass hysteria. They soon discovered that a virus was causing the hiccups and was similar to the one which was creating an encephalitis in Winnipeg at the same time. Since then, physicians have noted that both encephalitis and hiccups may occur in the same patient at the same time.

Hiccups may also occur after surgery on the pelvis or upper abdomen. This condition, says *International Medical Digest,* April, 1953, often follows an operation on the bladder or prostate, but Baily reported in the *Practitioner* in March, 1943, that he had never seen even one case of hiccups in over 1,500 patients who had operations on stomach, gall bladder or repair of perforated stomach ulcer.

Hiccups Complicate Surgery

A dangerous complication of heart attack is the hiccup. It is most disturbing to the patient's mental state, because he is unable to get his proper rest and his general condition may deteriorate enough to bring on death. The *Journal of the American Medical Association,* August 11, 1957, carries the report of a case, observed by 4 doctors, who had to resort to crushing a nerve to save their patient's life. The patient, treated by Doctors Rubin, Albright, Bornstein, and Schwimmer, was a 70-year-old man admitted to the hospital with a stroke. Two days after admission, he developed hiccups so severe that he could barely eat or drink. Despite treatment with sedatives, his condition continued to grow worse, until it was deemed necessary to crush the phrenic nerve. The phrenic nerve is involved in an attack of hiccups because it causes the diaphragm to contract, forcing the lungs to suddenly expel any air in them. The abrupt closing of the vocal cords causes the "hic."

Patients who contract hiccups following surgery risk the ripping open of their surgical wounds which, of course, cannot heal until the hiccuping ceases or at least subsides. In addition, the patient is prevented from ingesting sufficient fluid to maintain a proper body-fluid balance.

An extended bout of hiccups may entail a serious weight loss. The case of Jack O'Leary of Los Angeles, California, is an example. After undergoing an operation for a ruptured appendix in June of 1948, Mr. O'Leary began to hiccup. For 8 long years, he hiccuped once a second, day and night, until 1956, when the hiccups occurred less frequently and finally stopped altogether. During the 8-year siege, Mr. O'Leary's weight dropped from 136 to 77 pounds.

Common "Cures" for Hiccups

Few cases of hiccups are as severe as this, but an attack of hiccups can be annoying. To combat these situations, there are countless remedies. Every family seems to have its own "sure cure" for hiccups. Among the most widely practiced, is the idea of holding the breath as long as possible. Another common remedy is that of breathing into a paper bag. This type of treatment must be continued until the patient reaches the point of mild discomfort, for he is really breathing in carbon dioxide, which will stimulate his respiratory center.

Other common treatments involve the use of products readily available in the average American home. We would recommend trying any of these simple treatments for hiccups, such as drinking a teaspoonful of cider vinegar. Compressing the eyeballs for 30 or 40 seconds may help, as well as applying pressure just above the collarbone or on the upper lip.

If the hiccups persist, see your doctor and he will recommend some of the more clinical treatments for hiccups. Doctors Albert Gigot and Paul Flynn in the *Journal of the American Medical Association,* October 25, 1952, recommend that the treatment of hiccups be carried out in this order: "Counterirritation, gastric lavage, atropine, heavy sedation, carbon dioxide, phrenic nerve block and phrenic nerve crush." There are drugs which have halted hiccups almost immediately, but their side effects range from nausea and sensitivity to light to breast engorgement.

It would certainly seem easier to avoid hiccups rather than try to cure them. The most usual cause of hiccups is overeating. Also, chemical irritants can bring on an attack of hiccups. It is interesting to note that, apparently, the chemicals taken in by a pregnant woman can give her unborn child hiccups. Two doctors have discovered that hiccups in the fetus are probably due to the movement of a chemical substance through the placenta. (*International Medical Journal,* April, 1953.) Certain poisons in the blood stream can produce hiccups.

You can avoid overeating. You can avoid irritating your digestive tract with chemicals. You can avoid putting poisons into your blood stream. You can do all these things by following a program of natural foods and supplements. If you are following such a program, you should never be a victim of hiccups.

Hormone Drugs

The Danger-Laden Hormone Drugs

A look at the medical literature of the late 1940's and early 1950's would leave little doubt that a way had been discovered to perform miracles. The excitement centered around two new hormone drugs, cortisone and ACTH (the corticosteroids or, for short, steroids). At that time, they were in scarce supply, for no way had yet been discovered for manufacturing them synthetically. For example, ACTH came originally from the pituitary gland of hogs, and in 1950, to make a pound of this hormone, pituitaries from 400,000 hogs were required. But, no matter what it cost, ACTH and its twin, cortisone, were in high demand. Could it have been otherwise when it seemed that every doctor who could take pen in hand was writing of his phenomenal experience in using these drugs for treating just about everything? Here are some, not all, of the diseases that were said to bow before the steroids: Addison's disease, arthritis, asthma, gout, hay fever, Hodgkin's disease, lymphatic leukemia, myasthenia gravis, ivy poison, rheumatic fever, tetanus, ulcerative colitis, conjunctivitis, burns, shock, fractures—even skin disease and baldness.

Quick Response

When the initial injection or tablets of cortisone or ACTH were administered, in many of these cases, the results were astounding. Patients who had been unable to move due to arthritic pains and stiffness were shopping downtown on the fourth day of treatment; the progressive muscular debilitation of myasthenia gravis seemed to be spontaneously arrested. In such cases, cortisone and ACTH were indeed miraculous. They prolonged lives where life was seriously threatened and they made life bearable where it had been unbearable. But it soon became clear that whatever activity these drugs possessed was temporary. To lessen the dosage, or stop it altogether, was to lessen the results or stop them altogether. Without the cortisone the arthritis victim was soon back to immobile agony, the myasthenia gravis once again depleted the strength of the muscles. The hormones were a relief, a crutch, a way of staving off the inevitable for a while. They were not—are not—a cure.

Like a Brush Fire

Tales of the powers of the two drugs spread like a brush fire. Everyone wanted to try them, and everyone who could afford it, did. Why wait for arthritis to get bad? Take a shot of cortisone now for that occasional twinge. Don't sneeze through hayfever season, try ACTH! Poison ivy? Get a few shots of cortisone. It was the story of sulfa and penicillin all over again.

431

Now, from the very first announcements of the production of these drugs, the possibility of side effects was always well known. They were usually mentioned, however obliquely, in publicity releases and interviews. The sample packets of the steroid drugs, received by physicians everywhere, contained the usual pamphlets describing the drug and its suggested dosage, and even these noted side effects to be expected. To be sure, the ones described in these pamphlets were optimistically calculated, but there was no use denying that something physiologically unsound could happen in the course of treatment. The nature of the drugs practically guaranteed it.

What the Steroids Do

The steroid or corticotropic compounds are based on an attempt to imitate, and replace or augment, the secreted hormone of the adrenal gland. This hormone is normally released in moments of stress; a sudden shock, an infection, intense cold or heat and the body gets a necessary shot of the adrenal hormone to defend itself, as it were. The mechanism of the body is expert in gauging just how much of this substance can be released without upsetting the delicate hormonal balance of the rest of the body. In injecting the body with even more of this hormone, science is, in effect, telling the body that its controls are out of date and inadequate to the situation. Soon, the artificial hormone begins to exceed the amount the adrenal gland would ever produce. The adrenal gland sees no further need for its services and dries up in inactivity.

However, the cortisone or ACTH being given is there to relieve one ailment, be it arthritis or Addison's disease. The body becomes used to this large dosage and learns to use all of it. Now, when something new turns up, in addition to the chronic ailment, there's nothing there to fight it. The adrenal glands don't secrete a hormone anymore and the drug the patient's been getting is not available for any new duties. The new infection, shock or stress has a free field in which to operate with no interference from the body's defenses.

Dazzle Obscured Side Effects

The drama of the early results with the steroids so bedazzled many of the doctors who administered them and all of the patients who received them, that side effects were seldom even considered. And where serious pain or complete incapacity were relieved, it is understandable. But for relief of ivy poison or allergy, the risk was hardly worthwhile, and it is hard to imagine just why a competent physician would have let his patients chance it.

As early as 1952, the apprehension of responsible scientists was reflected in an evaluation of cortisone's action by Dr. Philip Hench (one of the earliest experimenters) when he said, it is "a riddle wrapped in a mystery inside an enigma." (*Medical Journal of Australia,* July 19, 1952.) Even those who worked most closely with this new drug were puzzled by it.

In that same year, Dr. Jerome Conn, of the University of Michigan, was moved to tell the American Academy of General Practice of the "tremendous", complications occurring in arthritis patients who had been given two years continuous treatment with cortisone or ACTH. He said that some nations' chief arthritis specialists were of the opinion, even then, that it would be better not to give the drug at all (*Detroit Free Press,* March 28, 1952).

Obviously, this opinion was not taken seriously, for the use of cortisone and ACTH, once they were available from cheaper, synthetic sources, became almost as common as the use of aspirin. One could obtain them by injection, tablet, capsule, salve or ointment from almost any doctor who didn't want to be classed as old-fashioned.

A Representative List

The deluge followed soon after. An article in *The New Yorker* magazine (September 10, 1955) gives a representative list of the ways in which cortisone and ACTH can react. Streptococci infection is encouraged, as well as staphylococci, pneumonococci, brucellae, typhoid bacilli, spirochetes, influenza virus, polio and TB. They can revive infections already thought dead and can excite latent ones into activity. They can transform harmless viruses into dangerous ones and can even unhinge the mind.

There is plenty of evidence to substantiate the claims in that list, and there are other consequences of hormone treatment that are not even mentioned there.

For example, when you read that these drugs can cause mental problems, are you aware of the degree of these problems? Are you prepared for a letter referred to in the *Digest of Treatment* (October, 1951) in which a physician attributes the suicide of one of his patients to nothing but cortisone treatments? Certainly we don't mean to say that all patients using these hormone drugs kill themselves, or are tempted to do so, but who knows what could happen to one subjected to the effects described by *Modern Medicine* in its May, 1954, issue. We read that, in general, within a few hours after ACTH or cortisone therapy begins, nearly all patients experience a "ready state," a feeling of irritability, restlessness, tension or emotional instability. From this state, about half progress to normal reactions and relief of symptoms. In the rest, abnormal mental changes appear, usually by the fourth day. They may have thinking and behavioral disturbances. Relief of these symptoms usually occurs on withdrawal of the drug.

Subtle Effects

So much for the more observable mental effects. There are more subtle ones that can have even more serious consequences. Consider euphoria, a feeling that everything is wonderful, which is characteristic in cortisone-treated patients. It is suggested that this condition breaks down the usual critical control exercised by the cortex of the brain. This joyful attitude in a patient can translate itself into a conviction that normally painful or alarming symptoms of disease do not exist for him. The *Journal of the American Geriatrics Society* (November, 1955) tells of two cases in which the symptoms of active pneumonia were completely suppressed during treatment with cortisone and corticotropin. Both patients insisted that they never felt better, in spite of the fact that they both had severe pneumonia. The illness put no limit on the physical activities and might not have been discovered at all until it was too late, if the doctor in charge had not instituted regular physical examinations for his hormone-treated patients. The author concludes with this statement, "It cannot be stressed too often that these drugs should be used under close supervision, for, in their present form, there are too many side effects of fatal consequence."

In *Chemical Week* (January 26, 1957), the Food and Drug Administration seemed to concur with this opinion when it announced that hydrocortisone products should not be sold over the counter, because "available evidence fails to prove that hydrocortisone (steroid) products are safe to use without medical supervision."

It is difficult to reconcile these statements and others like them with the calm pronouncement in the publication, *Recent Advances in Medicine #2,* offered by the Upjohn Drug Company, which states that "Self-injection with ACTH over long periods is a practical and effective mode of treatment in severe rheumatoid arthritis . . ." Such a measure could actually be suicidal.

Hormones and Children

One of the most appalling files on cortisone and ACTH therapy concerns the effects of these drugs on children. The very idea of youngsters needing such drastic treatment is bad enough, but how does a child get through life afterwards if the expected atrophy of his adrenal glands has taken place? It is to be hoped that doctors prescribing such medication have considered this question.

The more immediate risks are enough to give anyone pause. *Modern Medicine* (April 15, 1957) carries the observations of 3 doctors on what ACTH can do to a child, and the prospect is as grim as can be. One frequent reaction is "overwhelming infection," with no noticeable manifestations until it is far advanced. The central nervous system is another target ACTH often hits, by way of convulsions, psychoses in unstable and in well-adjusted adolescents and blinding clots in the retinal artery. In the gastrointestinal area, the drugs can produce new ulcers or reactivate healed ones. Children given therapeutic doses of ACTH or cortisone are taking a drug that may induce or aggravate diabetes mellitus. Doctors are inviting demineralization of their bones in extended treatment with cortical agents and a generally lowered resistance to stress of all kinds.

While on the subject of children and corticotropic hormones, we must mention a frightening statement in a letter to the *Journal of the American Medical Association* (November 7, 1956). It says that chickenpox, that simple childhood disease, is thought to be fatal in children undergoing such therapy. Fatal!

Same Effects on Adults

Most of the reactions suffered by children plague adults who are taking these hormones. The ulcers and infections that crop up during cortisone and ACTH therapy are mentioned again and again in the medical journals. The damage to bones that results in easy breakage is mentioned in the *Scottish Medical Journal* (1958, 3:450). An asthma patient being treated with corticosteroids reported a spontaneous fracture of the femur. In the *Journal of the American Medical Association* (October 2, 1954), it is reported that 4 male patients receiving cortisone developed multiple fractures of the spine. Knowing that demineralization of the bone is a recognized complication of cortisone therapy, it is a wonder that doctors do not give large doses of bone meal to compensate for these lost minerals while such treatment is in progress.

By the same token it is known that the vitamin C content of the blood is lowered during the time these hormone drugs are in use, and *Munchener Medizinische Wochenschrift* (94:339-342, February 22, 1952) carries a recommendation by Dr. H. Schroeder that vitamin C be administered in conjunction with this therapy, but we have not seen a single report that this is done by our doctors.

Pregnancy Affected by Hormone Drugs

Women in the delicate condition of pregnancy are warned in the *New York State Journal of Medicine* (November 1, 1953) that large amounts of cortisone given early in pregnancy may cause abnormalities in the fetus and/or miscarriages. There was also some inconclusive evidence that babies delivered of mothers who had received large doses of cortisone were born with depressed function of the adrenal glands. It was concluded that pregnant women would do well to avoid such medication.

The *Lancet* (June 1, 1957) bluntly affirmed the fact that steroids could be a direct cause of death in themselves. Of 18 deaths associated with such therapy, the drugs were considered directly responsible in 11 cases, and probably hastened death in 3 or 4 more.

Evidence of the dangers involved in the use of hormone drugs is piling up, and few physicians could exist without becoming aware of it. One would expect to see a decline in the use of such risky materials, but the reverse is actually true. *Chemical Week* (January 31, 1959) laid bare the business expectations of the hormone drugs in a lengthy article. The hormones are currently fourth on the list of drug "best sellers," topped in sales only by antibiotics, vitamins and tranquilizers, and they cost the American public 120,000,000 dollars in 1958. This popularity is not accidental. Says *Chemical Week*, "More time, money and manpower is probably expended on steroid research, process development, clinical study and sales promotion than on any other single group of ethical drugs." The article lamented the fact that these hormone drugs are not yet used as freely as antibiotics are, but, ever optimistic, it promises that "Time and education will inevitably expand the steroid hormone market."

Like penicillin, the hormone drugs have been responsible for saving lives. And like penicillin, they have cost lives, too. In using these drugs, a tremendous responsibility resides in the attending physician. He should be aware of the possible consequences of their use; he should be alert to the first signs of such reactions and, finally, he should continually ask himself if the illness he is treating is serious enough to warrant the risk involved in hormone therapy. We think that very few courses of cortisone and ACTH treatment would survive such soul-searching on the part of the physician.

The Disaster of the Sex Hormone Fad

So many people are getting sex hormones of one kind or another these days, that it is time to set the record straight on some of the dangers one faces in using them. Of course, hormones are necessary for proper body function (especially where the enzyme system is concerned), but the dosage is carefully measured by nature, and the body's glands release no more or no less than it takes to do the job at hand. When the amount is not exact, trouble starts and we can soon tell that the body is out of kilter due to a hormonal imbalance. Luckily, thyroxin is available, cortisone is available, as are testosterone and the estrogens. When a hormone is necessary, it can be had, but meanwhile, the reason for its need should be investigated, rather than to continue giving the hormone indefinitely.

We do not object to such uses of hormones, but American medicine has so abused the power of hormones that they have become more of a menace than a help. Aspirin is hardly used more recklessly than hormones today. We have already discussed the irresponsible use of cortisone and ACTH. Thyroid hormones have gotten quite a play, too. But none has been more disgracefully abused than the sex hormones, estrogen and testosterone. Every complaint from acne to facial wrinkles has been treated with sex hormones, and the results in many cases have been tragic. These hormones are meant to act in an extremely subtle manner. When an imbalance is encouraged through injections, pills and creams, especially for cases in which good diet, simple hygiene or natural body processes would correct the problem in time, sudden, unintended results can far outweigh the original problem.

Hormones Important

The importance of hormones in the body cannot be exaggerated, for without them, the body processes would surely break down. They act as catalysts which are released to facilitate and activate the workings of the body's organs. In general, the effects of hormones on the body are these: (1) they produce changes in the concentration of enzymes in the tissues; (2) they may act as a component of an enzyme system; (3) they affect accelerators and inhibitors of the enzyme systems.

The body's glands—pituitary, adrenal, thyroid, etc.—manufacture these vital hormones, and they are always available in the proper amounts when needed, provided the glands which produce them are healthy and properly nourished. In recent years, the problem of insufficient hormone secretion has been met, not by investigating the reason for the gland's inability to do its job and correcting the disorder, but by manufacturing facsimiles of the hormones or using hormones from animals and injecting them into the body. Thus, many persons whose hormone problem could be solved by careful observation and treatment of the source of the problem, must instead be subjected to continual use of artificial hormones, which could easily result in a dangerous imbalance.

Results of Treatment

An unfortunate instance of such an imbalance was reported by *United Press* on October 17, 1957. The report told of a Brooklyn, New York, boy, of 9 years of age, who had been treated for enlarged tonsils, allergies and continuous colds. Now, many children are regular customers at doctors' offices for just such ailments. But this lad was being treated for these complaints with a male sex hormone! The results, as set forth in a million dollar lawsuit against the physician, filed by the boy's parents, were "the boy has acquired all the characteristics and sex attributes of a mature male and has since then been afflicted by a strong sex urge." Will the boy ever recover his normal appetites, viewpoints, feelings? Even if the hormone treatments were effective in relieving the conditions mentioned (and the 4 years of treatment required would indicate that they were not), the accompanying results of the treatments far outweighed any good that might have been done by them.

Perhaps, if more had been made of the work of scientists at the University of California and Rutgers University concerning the use of male hormones, the doctor in question might have gone easy in his hormone treatment. These men found that male hormones often used on infants for a variety of reasons, including underweight, might cause sterility in later life. The conclusions were based on experiments with 5-day-old mice (about equivalent in development to a one-year-old child) in which injections with male hormones caused complete sterility in adulthood. In 10-day-old mice, some infertility also developed.

Science News Letter (June 19, 1954) remarked that, while results with mice might not be directly applicable to humans, "the scientists feel they are significant enough to warrant extreme caution in the use of male hormones during formative years."

Effect upon Infants

Of further concern in the use of sex hormones, is their effect upon new-born infants whose mothers have been treated with large doses of estrogens in the early stages of pregnancy. In the *Journal of the American Medical Association* (August 8, 1959), we see a report from a German medical magazine describing 3 such cases of developmental disorders. The malformations involved the brain and spinal cord, the lungs, liver, spleen, intestine, muscles and bones. It was determined through careful calculations that the abnormal fetal development began at the same time as the estrogen treatment. Experiments with pregnant rats, showing severe fetal damage after the administration of estrogens, support this view.

The power of the sex hormones is evidenced further in the changes they can cause in the sex of an unborn child. Physiologists tell us that the true sex of a child is determined very early after conception, but that the external genital organs do not begin to appear until after the first 10 weeks of pregnancy. However, during this time, these organs are highly susceptible to the influence of hormones. The basic neutral structure is female, but the final differentiation is directed by the testis through its testosterone secretion. All of this normally happens through the secretions of the expectant mother.

Now, if androgens are given at this crucial point in the pregnancy, any excess may induce changes in the sensitive external organs of the fetus. Particularly is this so if the "true" sex of the fetus is female, for the treatment may easily simulate the hormonal effects of normal male development. The result is a female child born with both male and female characteristics. Only laboratory tests can then determine the "true" sex of the infant. Progesterone may cause the same effect through its partial conversion into testosterone. Pregnant women who take large amounts of testosterones—particularly during the third and fourth months—may deliver babies with abnormal genitalia. The *British Medical Journal* (July 26, 1958), in which this material appeared, ended the article with this warning, "Such treatment (hormonal) is anyway of doubtful therapeutic value, and in view of the inherent dangers, it is probably unwise in any circumstances during early pregnancy."

In the April 23, 1960, issue of the *Journal of the American Medical Association,* another alarming report appeared. The French Society of Gynecology was told of the occurrence of acute abdominal complications in 25 women, ranging in age from 13 to 25 years, who were given excessive doses (10,000 to 13,000 units) of chlorionic gonadotropin for sterility or amenorrhea (interruption of menstrual cycle). Detailed examinations of these women revealed a large amount of blood-stained fluid in the peritoneal cavity formed by the lining of the abdominal wall and large tumors of the ovaries, some of which had ruptured.

Dangers of Self Treatment

Some years ago, the mail-order business jumped on the hormone bandwagon. Before the courts stepped in, men from coast to coast were treating themselves with mail-order testosterone, the male sex hormone. Dr. Erwin E. Nelson, then medical director of the Food and Drug Administration, pointed out that sterility and even cancer of the prostate, due to the stimulation of dormant cancer cells present in the prostate glands of many men, are potential dangers from the misuse of testosterone.

Women were warned by Dr. Nelson of the danger lying in the unsupervised use of the female sex hormone, estrogen. This hormone was, and still is, used unscrupulously as an ingredient of "bust creams" and face creams. In sufficient dosage, these hormones can have a profound systemic effect. Prolonged use may bring about sterility, especially in women whose natural hormone secretion is normal. The use of such drugs, in pill, liquid or even cosmetic lotion or cream form, is extremely hazardous, especially when used without responsible supervision and without a true need. When the body is not producing sufficient sex hormones for normal function, proper nutrition might be the only answer necessary. Wheat germ oil contains valuable amounts of the male hormones and female hormones appear naturally in some animal fats.

The use of hormones has indeed become widespread in medical practice. Of course, they are not always used with as little discretion as in the cases above. Sometimes, their use is the only possible answer, and the most conservative medical authorities are grateful for their availability. But the question keeps recurring: Do the medical doctors you and I consult know what potential dynamite they are prescribing? Do they know that each capsule or injection of a hormonal substance as a treatment presents a calculated risk that, if figured wrong, can mean even more serious illness for the patient and even less chance for recovery?

Hospitals

An Exciting Concept in Hospital Planning

Two of the main problems faced by hospitals in the confinement of small children are cross-infection and homesickness. Cross-infection has especially caused concern, for it has happened several times in recent years that whole nurseries have been wiped out, because a deadly infection has been passed from one child to another. The danger is compounded by the current existence of staphylococcus germs which do not yield to conventional forms of treatment or commonly used antibiotics. It seems that small children are even more susceptible to transmitted disease than adults, so the start of such an infection in an infant's ward can have tragic consequences.

When Mother Is Most Needed

It is generally agreed that the mother's presence almost always has a tonic effect on the hospitalized child. Experts bewail the fact that a child is often deprived of the comforting, reassuring presence of his mother at a time when he needs her most, those terrifying hours which immediately precede and follow surgery. It is known that the anxiety the patient feels slows his recovery, lessens his willingness to cooperate and can create whole new physical and psychological problems which did not exist before.

In the *Lancet* (February 27, 1954), the solution to both of these problems is offered in an article by Cecily M. Pickerill and H. P. Pickerill. The Pickerills run a hospital which specializes in plastic surgery for infants and small children. They had been maintaining this institution for 11 years at the time of this report, and had had no single case of transferred infection, nor of homesickness in all of that time. Further, their mortality rate was phenomenally low, 0.3 per cent. The answer lay in their system of a separate room for each patient, with provisions for his mother to remain with him there as his nurse.

Bacteria Control a Problem

It was the Pickerill's reasoning that the exchange of bacteria in open wards is impossible to control. The oiling of floors and blankets, the use of sprays and ultraviolet lights, restricting visitors, using masks and the best antiseptic techniques—none of these is the complete answer to controlling cross-infections. These precautions cannot discount the strong possibility of a nurse's spreading contamination due to the many jobs she does in many places, the strenuousness and haste involved and the obvious fact that she simply can't take the time to scrub up after each minor duty she performs.

The mother-nurse system provides each patient with a nurse to whose bacterial organisms he is immune from birth, since mother's antibodies are known to be transferred to the child through the umbilical cord. She touches no one but him, has no duties outside his room and puts him into the hands of others only at the time of surgery.

Feeding is usually a problem in the nursery wards of hospitals. Aside from the time it takes for even a hungry child to be fed, few busy nurses have the patience to coax a child to eat as he should. Mothers are expert in this. They not only see that the child has enough to eat to maintain proper weight, but most of the patients at the Pickerill's hospital actually gain weight.

A Stroll in the Sunshine

Did you ever hear of a stroll in the sun for a hospitalized baby? It's hardly likely that a nurse could take the time to give any of her charges a sunning. It's different when the mother is the nurse. She can walk him in the fresh air which will increase his well-being and heighten his resistance to infection.

The mother-nurse system allows for other safeguards against cross-infection which are impossible any other way. The mother changes the child, using his own diapers brought from home. She handles only his diapers, so can bring no infection from the excretory matter of other patients. If the child uses formula, the mother makes it in bottles brought from home. If it's dishes she needs, she has brought them, too. She keeps the room clean and changes the linen as necessary. There is no need for any outside contact which might result in the transmission of infections to or from the patient.

Every ward, sooner or later, acquires the type of bacteria that cannot be removed by routine cleaning and soon becomes residential. Because the ward is so rarely empty, they survive, and are often of the type that are resistant to penicillin and streptomycin. In the system of separate rooms, the room can be completely cleaned and aired after the discharge of each patient. The germs can't hide in other parts of a ward that can't be thoroughly cleaned because they are still occupied by patients. The new patient coming into the room has no leftover infectious bacteria to contend with.

One of the Greatest Benefits

One of the greatest benefits of the mother-nurse arrangement is the psychological effect on the child. Who can have a more soothing effect on a child than his mother? What sedative is more effective than that of patting or stroking of her hand and the sound of her voice? Who knows better how to make him laugh and forget pain and confinement? The psychological effect on the mother is also worthy of note. She knows her child is getting the attention he needs. She knows how well he is responding to treatments and she learns how to encourage proper response. The lessons she learns in changing dressings, preparation of medications and proper exercise of affected muscles, are carried home with her and applied with greater dedication and with the confidence that she is acting properly.

Mothers Happy to Be with Children

It has been suggested by critics that mothers cannot, and will not, take the time away from their homes and other children to spend a week or 10 days with one child in a hospital. The *Lancet* article refutes this objection completely. The Pickerills write that refusal of a mother to accompany her child has not occurred even once. Mothers always manage to have a relative come to the house to care for the family or farm out the children to different relatives or friends for this short period. Those involved say it is a wonderful change for the children, the father and the mother.

Too Expensive?

"It sounds wonderful," say some administrators, "but who can afford to erect such a plant? There is trouble in keeping up with the demand for hospital space without any fancy extras." The Pickerills say that such administrators are laboring under a misapprehension. While it is true that the single room system requires more floor space, and more walls and doors, the space is actually twice as efficient as in the usual type of hospital. Patients require only half of the average time for hospitalization, so that two patients can use a bed in the same time that one patient would take up a ward bed. Also, the mother-nurse policy saves floor space and rooms that would be required for staff members normally needed in a ward.

Other Hospitals Might Adopt the Pickerills' Plan

The plan the Pickerills present appears to be an excellent one for other hospitals to adopt. It is economical in the long run and efficient. The child is protected from the contamination of others at a time when his resistance is lowered and he is most susceptible. He is allowed close contact with his mother at the time he most needs it. Hospitals who have such difficult problems in acquiring help would have a good part of their problems solved by adopting the mother-nurse system. They could cut down on both nursing and maintenance staffs. We hope serious consideration of this system will be given by those influential in forming construction plans of projected hospitals.

Injections

Why Not Use Disposable Hypodermic Needles?

The spread of infectious diseases such as hepatitis, the increased incidence of encephalitis (an inflammation of the brain), unexplained allergic reactions and staphylococcus infections have all been tied to injections. Often, the use of a contaminated needle or syringe is the cause of the problem. Time and again, we have seen warnings in professional journals urging the use of sterilization techniques which include high heat and steam for at least 15 minutes. Doctors are repeatedly warned that chemical solutions are not to be trusted to do a thorough job of disinfecting. They are also warned that syringes, as well as needles, must be sterilized before re-use if the patient is to be fully protected. That these injunctions are not scrupulously followed is evident in the large number of cases of infection due to injections we see reported.

Dentists run into the same risks, perhaps even greater, when they inject pain-killing substances into the gums. The mouth is a wonderful breeding place for germs, so that contamination of instruments used there is quite likely. In *Dental Abstracts* (June, 1961), we saw one solution offered. There are available disposable, sterile dental hypodermic needles.

These needles would eliminate the need for autoclaving of hypodermic needles, the only sure way of cleansing them of all infectious organisms. Many dentists do not have an autoclave (steam heat sterilizer) and merely chance the patient's escape from infection.

Aside from the obvious advantage of disposability, the article noted that, on these toss-out needles (Monoject is the trade name), the lancet point of the needle is so sharp, that trauma damage to tissue is at the lowest level and healing at the highest. Also, allergens are often present in some hypodermic needles when they are re-used. This needle eliminates that problem, too. Monoject has been tested successfully in Massachusetts General Hospital, Johns Hopkins Medical School and Texas Medical Center. The article also pointed out that the time and expense of having conventional hypodermic needles resharpened makes the cost of such a needle greater than that of the disposable needle.

We see no reason why disposable needles should not be universally adopted for all types of injections, if needles are to be used at all. Perhaps, even legislation requiring their use could be passed, in the interests of halting possible contagion. The fact that the difference in actual cost is minimal makes such a law feasible and worth serious consideration. The wonder is that physicians of all types, and dentists, too, would not voluntarily begin using disposable hypodermic needles exclusively, just to protect their patients and themselves.

The Dangerous Site for Injection

In the *Journal of the American Medical Association* (March 25, 1961), in an abstract from *Journal of Pediatrics* (February, 1961), F. H. Gilles and J. H. French review observations on 21 pediatric patients in whom sciatic palsy was associated with intragluteal (buttocks) injections. The palsies began after single or multiple injections of antibiotic medications, either alone or in combination with other materials. Penicillin and tetracycline are the only two antibiotics directly implicated, although multiple drugs were involved by association.

The results of these injections are interesting. In one child, the complaint was diminished leg movement. The other 20 children had "conspicuous foot drop." Six of these eventually required bracing and physiotherapy and 3 others had a limited gait as the final result. "It is suggested that the buttock be abandoned as a site of injection in infants and children. The lateral distal third of the thigh is recommended as a preferable injection site."

Here we have just two clinicians who, between them, have seen 21 cases in which the results of buttocks injection were most unfortunate. Who knows how many more occurred across the country and have been missed or badly diagnosed? The number could be very large. But still the injections go on, given in the same dangerous location. Doctors don't know or they don't care. They feel the possibility too remote, perhaps.

It is up to you, then, to insist that the injections your child receives be given in the recommended area of the leg. Show your doctor these facts and ask him if he ever knew of this before. Then request that he use this preferable site, not only on your child, but on all of his other patients. Your action could save some child a serious physical handicap.

Insecticides

The Hazards of Insecticides

Midsummer means insecticides to most people. This is the time of year when the gnats, the grasshoppers, the mosquitoes become most troublesome and it seems as if a whiff from the aerosol can which lays them low, is the only thing that will help. Towns and cities are busy laying down choking screens of bug killers; ponds are sprayed; gardeners douse the beans and tomatoes with evil-smelling poisons.

Our large file on insecticides contains much material so frightening that we can hardly bring ourself to leaf through it, these days. The *New York Times* for November 11, 1959, tells us that it is conceivable that man could commit species suicide and that there might not be a historian left a century from now to look back on today's events—if we continue our present program of insecticide spraying.

In our files we have a number of scientific articles which point out that insecticides are killing microbes as well as insects. Microbes are our scavengers. They destroy garbage, manure and all other organic matter. If this stuff piles up and accumulates, life on this planet would soon cease.

A folder labeled Birmingham, Alabama, tells the story of an attempt to spray that city with dieldrin to control fire ants. It has been shown that this kind of spray kills not only ants, but also practically everything else living that is exposed, up to the size of raccoons. It has been shown that the fire ant is beneficial since it destroys some of the most destructive insects, including the boll weevil. It has been shown that the fire ant can be destroyed easily and cheaply without harming any other life by distributing poison pellets in such a way that no other form of life will get them. Nevertheless, spurred on by the state and federal departments of agriculture, plans went forward to spread this deadly insecticide over 10,000 acres of the city. We are glad to report that the plan fell through and that we had a part in this decision.

Proof of Toxicity

Most frightening, perhaps, of all our current material on insecticides is a booklet from the United States Department of Agriculture, *The Nature and Fate of Chemicals Applied to Soils, Plants and Animals.* Prepared by the greatest experts in this field, this book gives details of experiments performed over the years to determine just what happens to these deadly substances when farmers use them.

Two researchers from the United States Department of Agriculture, Kerrville, Texas, contributed an article entitled "The Toxicity of Pesticides for Livestock." They say some things which should interest farmers who regularly use insecticides. They should also interest those of us who are not farmers, for our world is polluted with insecticides to such an extent that not a mouthful of commercially bought food is free from them and, for many of us, the air we breathe every minute and every mouthful of water we drink also carry their quota of these poisons.

The discovery of DDT as an insecticide by Muller in 1939 was a great advancement of our potential for insect control, and for it he received a Nobel prize. The low acute toxicity of DDT for most mammals suggested there would be no problems associated with its use. Several developments caused a revision of scientific attitudes toward the safety of DDT and toward several similar compounds then under development," say the Texas scientists.

The authors go on to relate the finding of DDT in the milk of cattle sprayed with DDT. Experts believed that this occurred because of contamination of the cows' udders with the insecticide, because "at the time, it was not an acceptable theory that such compounds could pass through the unbroken skin to the blood and be circulated."

So the researchers at Kerrville devised tests whereby they could collect milk in completely closed systems so that no contamination of the milk from the udders could possibly occur. DDT was still found in the milk. Then it was argued that the cows were licking themselves and thus getting the DDT into their bodies. So the cows were restrained in stalls which did not allow them to lick themselves. DDT still appeared in the milk.

"From the beginning, none of us dealing with the toxicity of these compounds for livestock had any doubts concerning the speedy absorption of insecticides from any of the body surfaces, either external or internal. One does not doubt when animals are poisoned and die within 30 minutes of treatment without having licked themselves," say our authors. However, note what follows. There was no possibility of getting the final authorities to agree that the tests showed the dangers of DDT, for, as the article goes on, "Although the evidence was overwhelming, even the Council on Pharmacy of the American Medical Association insisted that the tests must have been done by inept people and should be repeated by competent persons without delay. As we now realize, these early studies were sound and have stood the test of time."

So the experts in the American Medical Association refused to believe the "overwhelming" evidence of the way DDT acts in the bodies of cattle. The researchers were "inept," they said. Doesn't this sound familiar? Researchers presenting "overwhelming" evidence of the harmfulness of chemicals in food, water fluoridation, vaccination or dosing with drugs get the same treatment from the official "experts." The research is "inept," they tell us.

Who Is Harmed Most?

Continuing with their discussion of experiments on the toxicity of insecticides, Radeleff and Bushland tell us they found that calves one to two weeks old were the most susceptible to harm and that resistance to poisoning increased as the animals grew older. They found that emaciation and lactation predisposed animals to poisoning by certain of the newer insecticides. They also found that conditions of stress made a great difference in the susceptibility of animals to poisoning.

"When the same material is given to sick animals, to those castrated, dehorned, vaccinated and drenched in the same day, the results may be far different. It is not possible to determine all the possible combinations animal owners may devise; therefore, we suggest that pesticide usage should follow or precede such drastic stress by several days."

These experimenters are speaking of animals, not human beings. Animals have market value, so their health must be protected no matter what. Therefore, say the authors, be careful not to subject your animals to poisons at the same time they are under stress of one kind or another, and vaccination is mentioned as one significant form of stress. It is not possible to determine, they tell us, all the various combinations of stressful situations that might arise with animals.

How much less possible is it to determine all the conceivable combinations of stress to which a human being might be subject at the same time he gets a whopping dose of poison from insecticides in his food, combined with other chemical food additives, air pollution, drugs, injections, fluoridated water; combined, of course, with sundry psychological stresses such as worries about his family life, his job, his finances. Yet here is scientific evidence showing clearly that stress—both physical and psychological—predisposes one to additional harm from insecticide poisoning.

The Texas researchers then take up the special problems posed by systemic insecticides. These are poisons which are injected or fed to animals or plants, making the entire animal or plant poisonous to insects.

It is probably surprising to know that it is necessary to do investigations to see if such preparations are poisonous to the human beings who eat the animal or vegetable thus poisoned. How could they not be? However, in doing this kind of research, it has been found that the systemic insecticide is changed into something else by the tissues of the plant or animal after it has been injected, so that tests of the original insecticide proved nothing. The substance which is formed inside the plant or animal must be tested, too. Does this not immediately suggest that the metabolism of an entirely different kind of living thing—a human being—may also change insecticides and other poisons into something infinitely more poisonous?

An Extremely Complex Problem

Radeleff and Bushland give us some interesting information on the complete impossibility of assessing the hazards involved in spraying insecticides on bodies of water for control of mosquitoes, etc. They say, "we may treat a body of water for insect control and accomplish the objective, but organisms not killed by the treatment may absorb and store the chemical. They, in turn, according to their biological position, may be consumed as food by other species, and these, in turn, by others, until there is ultimately a removal from that water of a species serving as food for mammals and birds, or man. The cycle is then continued outside the original environment." So the "harmless" spray program on marshes and lakes, rivers and streams may show its poisonous effects many miles away and many months later in food you buy at your market.

Several paragraphs dealing with the symptoms of insecticide poisoning are something to stand your hair on end. Some of these are: muscular twitching and spasms; convulsive seizures, with trembling, depression and violence; appearance of disorientation; loss of appetite; abdominal pain; diarrhea; shortness of breath; difficulty in walking. The nervous system of the animal has been poisoned.

How can a veterinarian tell whether or not symptoms like these are the result of insecticide poisoning or arise from some other cause? There is no way to tell, according to these researchers, who have, remember, devoted full time to study of the insecticides for many years. They are writing this article for veterinarians and stock farmers whose livelihoods are vitally concerned with the answer to this problem—how can you tell whether or not the symptoms of illness your animal shows are the result of insecticide poisoning? The answer is clear and unequivocal—there is no way of knowing.

Use This Information to Protest Spraying

We have here, we believe, one of the best weapons against the use of insecticides. Documented with a bibliography of 122 references to scientific literature, the article shows clearly and irrefutably the following:

1. Scientific facts presented with complete scientific accuracy showing the dangers of the newer chemicals, especially insecticides, are simply not accepted as facts by the very persons who should be warning us against these poisons. Exactly the same thing is happening in regard to chemicals in food and water fluoridation.

2. There is wide variation in the response of individuals to poisons—some react one way, others another. Some die within

moments, others not for days. Sick animals, animals under stresses of one kind or another and young animals are especially sensitive to harm from insecticides. There is no such thing, then, as declaring that "tests prove" no one will be harmed by such-and-such an insecticide. *The only thing we are sure of is that some people will be more harmed than others.*

3. How will you know if you have been harmed by an insecticide? You won't. There is no way to tell whether the symptoms you experience have been caused by the insecticide, so your doctor cannot know how to treat you. Nor can you sue anyone for insecticide damage, for you cannot prove that this is what it is.

4. Finally, here is the statement made in the conclusion of this article: "No matter how carefully the product may have been prepared and labeled and no matter how complete the scientific background may be, the consumer or user may nullify these totally and completely and produce a catastrophic result to his animals, plants or himself. It seems silly to say that the most important consideration in the safe use of pesticides is the ability of the user to read and follow the label instructions; yet we are constantly reminded that this is the weak link in our safety chain, and that by far the majority of cases of poisoning of all kinds of people, animals and plants are due simply to carelessness or unwillingness to follow the directions."

So there you have it. If that distant farmer or his farmhands who grew the lettuce you have for dinner tonight followed the instructions on the label of the perhaps 7 or 8 insecticides he used in the growing process, perhaps the dose it contains may not harm you. This is the only safeguard you have. If the pilot flying the spray plane that drenches your county, city or town with insecticide mixed the stuff according to directions and flew at exactly the correct distance from the ground, with the right kind of wind prevailing, perhaps you may not suffer immediate damage from the spraying.

Protecting Yourself from Harm

We recommend: protest against insecticides whenever and wherever they are used. Every mouthful of commercially bought food contains them. Every drop of drinking water that comes from a river, lake or stream contains them. They are cumulative in your flesh. They are stored in the fatty tissue of all of our bodies. The only reason insecticides are necessary is that we have destroyed with chemicals the balance of nature in which every harmful insect has its natural enemy. Our insecticides have killed the beneficial insects along with the destructive ones. As more and more insects become resistant to our poisons, stronger and stronger poisons must be invented. Everyone of them is deadly and every new one becomes more deadly.

Don't ever use insecticides yourself. Garden organically, screen your homes, endure with complacency the minor irritations of insects outside. They can't possibly harm you as insecticides can. Write your Congressman, the Food and Drug Administration in Washington, the Department of Agriculture in Washington. Protest the ever-increasing use of insecticides.

Here is an excerpt from a letter from a manufacturer of insecticides who decided, in 1957, to give up his insecticide business:

"There is beginning to pile up a great deal of incomplete data which appear to make out a sound case against the general use of the current broad spectrum toxic organic insecticides. Our decision, however, was based on our own study over a 12-year period. We saw the Louisiana cotton area welcome the new insecticides a very few years ago. Today, for practical purposes, no cotton area can control any of the cotton insects with any known insecticide. From a position of losing part of their crop from insect infestation, they are now faced with going out of cotton entirely. At least, until a natural balance is again developed. The Washington and Oregon apple people started spraying for coddling moth a few years ago. Today they are spraying up to 15 times to control mites and this is a losing battle. I could cite many more.

"Examination of the milk supply and food animal flesh is showing a relatively high reading for DDT and other organic toxicants. Although the USDA claims this is below a toxic level, they also say the chemicals are cumulative. Many cars of lettuce have recently been confiscated in the New York market for high concentrations of parathion.

"In the handling of parathion, for example, 25 milligrams on the skin can be fatal. Frankly the whole thing began to cause us all so much concern I decided to discontinue any connection with such production.

"Sincerely,

WM. T. THOMPSON,
Thompson Chemicals Corporation"

Pesticides Condemned by a Mayo Clinic Doctor

The struggle against becoming completely saturated with insecticides, now called pesticides, since the target has long ago widened to include more than insects, is becoming monumental. Already there are few stores or public buildings one can enter without being overwhelmed with the clouds of pesticide being sprayed or otherwise disseminated everywhere. Fruit counters, theaters, restaurants, barber shops and beauty parlors, trains, buses and planes, banks, tourist cabins—there isn't a place you can go to be free of them. As you drive home, fields you pass are being sprayed. When you arrive at your house, it is likely that the city has just sprayed your tree out front. Your neighbors are spraying their roses as you sit out back on a summer evening. You've been forced to inhale some pesticide everywhere you've been.

The people who favor the use of pesticides point out this very fact. You've gotten all of that spray into you, why worry? You're still here. Yes, but for how long, if it continues?

The concern over the prevalence of pesticides is shared by many thinking scientists and medical men. Among these is Dr. M. M. Hargraves, of the Mayo Clinic, Rochester, Minnesota. Dr. Hargraves gave his views on the subject in a speech to the Twenty-third Annual Convention of the National Wildlife Federation in New York City on February 27, 1959.

He began by pointing out the basic danger involved in manipulating man's environment. For hundreds, even thousands, of years, man has gradually adjusted to the existing world around him. He changed those things he found undesirable, when possible, and got used to those things which he could not change. In time, there evolved a balance of Nature which is just as manifest in the coming of the gypsy moths and Japanese beetles, as it is in the death and birth of human beings. To upset and readjust this balance is to tamper with something of which we are essentially ignorant, to set in motion a chain reaction, the conclusion of which we cannot possibly foresee.

Petroleum Products Are Deadly Pesticides

So much for the ultimate problem we invite in the use of pesticides. Of more immediate concern is the health hazard presented by pesticides. Here Dr. Hargraves speaks with logic, knowledgeability and persuasion. Pesticides may be made, he says, of arsenic, lead, sulfur, mercury, hydrocarbons and other substances. In recent years, the hydrocarbons, petroleum derivatives, have far surpassed the others. It all began a hundred years ago when coal oil was mixed with soap suds to make a pesticide. Many will recall that this was the standard treatment for body lice. Since then, refinements in petroleum have been made so that more than 200 hydrocarbons are presently obtainable from crude oil. In the refining of oils, efforts are made to retain an increased percentage of the efficient aromatic hydrocarbons (benzol series). These aromatic hydrocarbons, many of which are used as pesticides, are known to produce such diseases as aplastic anemia, leukemia and lymphomas (tumors of the lymph glands, or Hodgkin's disease).

Many More Dangerous Than DDT

It is interesting, says Dr. Hargraves, to note that the newer pesticides, such as Lindane or DDT are seldom pure compounds. A look at the label of a spray can will tell you that it contains 2.5 per cent of one or more of these deadly hydrocarbons, suspended in 10 to 14 per cent petroleum distillate (more deadly hydrocarbon), plus some dispersing agent. It is possible, therefore, that the accompanying hydrocarbons may be more dangerous, when inhaled by humans, than the DDT or Lindane!

The gypsy moth spray is a concrete example. The standard formula is: one pound of DDT suspended in one gallon of petrol distillate (light oil) plus one quart of zylene (dimethyl benzene). Inhaling the DDT is certainly dangerous, but the droplets of hydrocarbons one gets with it are known to cause leukemia, asplastic anemia and lymphoma.

Tolerances Useless for Sensitive Persons

Dr. Hargraves deplores the practice of setting tolerances for exposure to pesticides. True, humans and animals are exposed, in experiment, to doses likely to be used, and the physical effect upon them is noted. However, not every human being has average sensitivity to such poisons. What does not affect a normal person might easily kill an extremely sensitive one. The situation parallels the testing and use of modern medical drugs. A test including 500 individuals who have no adverse effects from a drug gives no guarantee that all future administrations of the drug will be equally free of undesirable effects. The 501st or the 100,000th person to use it may be so sensitive that it will kill him. The same is true of pesticide sprays, but they are probably the last thing the coroner would think of in looking for a cause of death.

Repeated exposure is another neglected factor. While one or two exposures to hydrocarbons might not have a deadly effect, continual exposure may lead the sensitive individual to the point at which one more inhalation will result in serious consequences. Periodic spraying programs are tragically effective in bringing on such a disaster.

Multiple Sources

Consider, too, that sources of exposure to chlorinated hydrocarbons do not stop with spray pesticides. They occur in many processed foods to be stored, as eaten, in body fats; they occur in gasolines, fuel oils, paints, varnishes, thinners, as solvents in rubber and metal industries, and in the atmosphere as industrial vapors and smog.

To compound, even more, the problem of multiple exposure, Dr. Hargraves reminds us that one hydrocarbon often enhances the effect of another. He gives, as an example, Piperine, an insecticide, which has also been used as a flavor booster in brandy, and is somewhat more toxic to house flies than Pyrethrum. Yet, a mixture of .05 Piperine and .01 Pyrethrum is more deadly than 10 times the amount of Pyrethrum alone.

Some pesticides have the ability to block the body's protective mechanism, warns Dr. Hargraves. While the body is thus prevented by one agent from using its defenses, a second agent can invade and kill. Dr. Hargraves believes that such mechanisms are in operation when pesticides impair health.

A Housewife Sprays against Spiders

The most impressive part of Dr. Hargraves' speech lay in a series of cases he described, in which the illness of the patient could hardly have resulted from anything but exposure to pesticides. One of the most frightening cases concerned a housewife who had a strong aversion to spiders, and, in mid-August, used an insecticide aerosprayer (DDT and petroleum distillates) to spray thoroughly throughout the kitchen and basement. She became nauseated and ill immediately after using it, but recovered in a few days. In September, she repeated the process twice, and got ill each time. She began to develop fever, joint pains and a general sick feeling. Acute phlebitis flared up in her left leg. She was hospitalized and diagnosed as acute leukemia. *She was dead in less than a month.*

A Puerto Rican entered the clinic with multiple abdominal masses and Hodgkin's disease. For most of his life, the man had slept under mosquito netting. Then, three years prior to his admission, the netting was displaced by chlorinated hydrocarbon-petroleum distillate spray several times a week. The bedroom was sprayed and closed for a period of time, before the patient retired. Is it surprising that Hodgkin's disease, a common result of hydrocarbon poisoning, came about?

Then there was the 10-year-old boy who developed acute leukemia shortly after using an entire "bug bomb" fighting wasps in a closed garage. Also, there is the case of a farmer admitted to the Mayo Clinic with acute leukemia. He had spent a great deal of time the preceding winter refinishing his furniture, using a varnish remover containing "less than 49 per cent benzol, plus paint and varnish." Another case involved acute leukemia in a tile setter who washed the excess adhesive off with gasoline after the job of setting was complete. He had two "big jobs" with formica the year before with a great deal of gasoline exposure; then, after another big job, he contracted flu, followed by leukemic symptoms from which he never recovered.

The cases are numerous and all are characterized by an exposure to large amounts of pesticide before the onset of a deadly blood or lymph disease. There is no pattern in the choice of victims. Dr. Hargraves tells of doctors, businessmen, farmers, children, old folks, housewives, all types of people. All of them had been exposed to pesticides in a way that would seem quite natural and harmless to most persons. They became deathly ill, and most of them died.

Do you know of any reason why the same thing couldn't happen to you? Don't use pesticides—ever! Protest the spraying of public lands. You might save yourself from serious illness, even death, in this way.

Spray Bombs Are Deadly for You

By way of warning to those who plan to use poison spray bombs for cleaning out garages and cellars or for discouraging the bugs of summer, may we call attention to the case of Rudolph Apelt, as reported in the *Cleveland* (Ohio) *News* (December 9, 1959). Mr. Apelt, apparently quite healthy, spent the afternoon spraying the vegetables of a greenhouse near his home with an aerosol bomb containing the chemical insecticide, Phosdrin. Not one to do such things carelessly, Mr. Apelt had covered himself completely, even to wearing a gas mask. Only his ears were uncovered. Shortly after the job was done, Mr. Apelt lapsed into a coma. The condition persisted and the victim never regained consciousness, but died at the end of 3 months' hospitalization.

The obituary notice ended with the information that the sale and use of Phosdrin has officially been halted by the Ohio State Extension Service. If inhaled, the experts said, Phosdrin attacks the nervous system.

It is not clear from the newspaper whether Phosdrin was generally used by the public or only by greenhouse operators. We are reasonably sure that anyone could have bought it, and still can in other states that have not banned its sale. We wonder why the manufacture of so dangerous an item is permitted. Will each state have to wait for an Apelt tragedy before its extension service will call a halt to the distribution of Phosdrin?

What about the Phosdrin that stayed in the plants? Who can categorically assure us that none of that stuff will be on the vegetables that reach our tables? If inhaling it can kill a man, what will eating it do to us? Again we are faced with the decision: do we want perfect-looking fruits and vegetables that might be coated with poison, or can we put up with the natural imperfections an insect might cause on the skins and feel safe in eating them?

Above all, don't use poison sprays for anything. The process that makes them sprayable also makes them light enough to hang in the air you breathe. Inhaling these fumes has been deadly to more than a few isolated cases. Perhaps one spraying will not kill you—or even two or three—but the fourth exposure might, or the sixth, or the tenth. The point is that you can't know. Even the so-called "harmless" poison sprays have not been tested on *you,* if they have been tested at all on humans, and their reaction on *you* could be fatal.

Death by Spray

The fatal poisoning of two young boys, 14 months and 3 years of age, puzzled Wisconsin authorities (*Appleton* [Wisconsin] *Post Crescent,* July 25, 1960). The boys lived in separate homes on adjoining farms, but had been poisoned at the same time by the same chemical. The riddle was unravelled when it was disclosed that 14-month-old Ronald was playing in his sandbox and his father drove by with a crop-spraying machine which was shooting highly toxic parathion onto the potato crop. The boy inhaled the air-borne fumes as he played. Conrad, the 3-year-old, handled the pressure sprayer his father had used to spray the inside of the barn with the same parathion. The chemical contamination on his skin was great enough to pass from hand to mouth and he was poisoned.

The boys became ill at about 6 o'clock in the evening, and were both dead within two hours. Doctors said that even a small amount of the chemical could be fatal to children.

We Are Led Like Sheep

Medical Press (January 18, 1961) printed an interesting story which carried a potential far greater than man would surmise on reading it. The article tells of an outbreak of chronic copper poisoning in sheep following the use of copper sulfate as a spray in their grazing grass to control a pest. The fields (about 40 acres) were sprayed with one per cent copper sulfate—about 50 gallons per acre. Three weeks later, a flock of nearly 100 ewes was put out to graze on the area.

About one month later, two of the ewes died and the flock was immediately withdrawn from the treated area, and given supplements of hay and concentrates. Nevertheless, 4 more ewes died and the symptoms were: abnormal blood condition, liver and kidney inflammations. Several of the sheep, when examined, showed, understandably, extremely high levels of copper in the blood. Up to 5 months after the spraying, the grass of the area was found to contain copper in the range of 220 parts per million, as contrasted with the count of untreated pastures: 10 to 20 parts per million of copper.

Copper sulfate is not a rare kind of spray. Farmers use it all the time as a pesticide and the crops that grow as the result of no bugs in the field, are plump and beautiful. They also contain 20 times as much copper as is natural and safe. You and I are the sheep who eat this contaminated fruit. *We* eat the copper sulfate, *we* eat the DDT, the arsenates, etc., and we aren't put on unsprayed food and given concentrates. Our nephritis (kidney disease) rate rises, hepatitis hits a new high and blood diseases multiply. We have drives to find a cure for these and other diseases, but we don't seem much interested in finding the causes. We buy more pesticides, invent more pesticides and consume more pesticides. We read labels of pesticides which warn that contents are deadly if inhaled. We are careful not to inhale them, but we eat them without a qualm. We read reports such as this one, which tells us that animals when exposed to a common pesticide, are affected with the very diseases which plague us and we go right on using the stuff, unable or unwilling to put two and two together. Talk about lambs being led to slaughter!

We Need the Fire Ant

The United States has done everything but call out the marines against the fire ant. The destruction by powerful insecticides of vast areas of land and wild life has left the problem far from solved and, in spite of many suggested alternatives, still more land and wild life is being sacrificed to this senseless effort to stamp out the fire ant.

As with the lowest of living things, the fire ant has a valuable function in the scheme of nature. *Science News Letter* (August 12, 1961) tells us that 15 of 21 fungus organisms, most of which infect humans, can be held in check by fire ant venom. Studies have shown that, though it is painful, the bite of the fire ant injects venom that could repress some bacterial infections. The venom also inhibits the growth of fungus infections.

Do we know what problems have been let loose on us as the result of the extermination of the fire ant? Will fungus infections attack our plants or us? Will infectious bacteria multiply and invade us since the fire ants are no longer there to intercept the problem?

Again we see that an insecticide existence may be letting us in for more trouble than we had before. We exterminate a bug we can see and fall prey to 15 less obvious ones that not only make us ill, but can be fatal. The bug we exterminated was our only protection, we now discover.

Ions

Ionization: the Therapy of Tomorrow?

"The increased negative ionization, it is claimed, relieves hay fever and asthma, and destroys air-borne bacteria and viruses, thus supposedly preventing the spread of such infections (to quote one of the more flamboyant claims) as 'poliomyelitis, tuberculosis, common cold, influenza, meningococci infection, German measles, scarlet fever, etc.'

"The most charitable thing that can be said about such claims is that they are premature and exaggerated, based on scattered, poorly controlled studies."

This is the opinion of *Consumer Reports* magazine (April, 1961) on the newly prominent and controversial science of negative ionization as a medical treatment. It is grudgingly admitted in the article that "the impression was created that negative ions were beneficial to human well-being, and positive ions were harmful." It is clear, from what the editors say, that *they* were not impressed. Nothing they have seen has convinced them that negative ions are objectively beneficial.

We have been asked now and again for our opinion on ionization. Is there something to it or is it a quack, get-rich scheme? Well, we do not believe it is a quack scheme. That there is a scientific basis for the theory behind the therapeutic value of negative ionization cannot be denied. The question we are trying to answer is: is it practical? Can you confidently plug in a commercial ionization machine and expect it to work for you? Will you get a more exuberant feeling? Will your sunburned back be more comfortable? Will your headache disappear? We would like to share with you the material on ionization that is in our files, and let you decide on the merits of this discovery.

The Theory of Ionization

First, perhaps a quick rundown on the theory behind ionization will help. You see, every cell of the body can be classed as a form of electrical battery, according to *Associated Press* science editor, Howard Blakeslee. The electrical field of these "batteries" is changed when the nature of the ions, or charged atomic particles that are always in the air, are changed, and this change affects the way you feel. Positive ions have a tendency to dominate the atmosphere, generally, with a smaller number of negatively charged ions present. However, the number of negative ions is increased by such natural phenomena as thunderstorms. For most persons, breathing a high concentration of these negative ions is mildly exhilarating. For asthma sufferers, however, the effect of breathing such air is almost miraculous—within minutes, bronchial tubes clear and most symptoms of distress disappear.

The idea is, of course, to duplicate, if possible, this effect at will by means of a machine that will do to the air what thunderstorms do to it. Giant electrical manufacturers such as Philco, General Electric and Emerson Electric claim to have done it. The currently manufactured machines use electrical energy to knock electrons loose from a metal sheet in the device. These electrons then combine with molecules in the air to form negative ions. As can readily be imagined, such a system allows for no definite planning as to the exact number of ions that will be formed. The hope is that some means of definite control can be achieved, so that the minimum number of ions and their effect can be accurately predicted.

Russians Are Pushing Ahead

In Russia, for some reason, the value of ionized air is taken very seriously. As long as 40 years ago, a Soviet scientist, Alexander Chizhewsky, began research in this field (*Soviet Union* magazine, #109, 1959). He proved that test animals kept in air completely lacking in negative ions of oxygen would die, no matter how "fresh" the air might seem. But still more important, he found that animals living in air that is constantly saturated with negative ions do not get sick and they grow much faster. Birds treated with ionized air lay more eggs, cows give more milk, suckling pigs gain weight faster. Furthermore, they live longer.

The article in *Soviet Union* told of ion "chandeliers used by medical men to combat fatigue and bring relief to patients suffering from high blood pressure, bronchial asthma and rheumatism." Then there was a survey conducted at a Russian coal mine which showed that the illness rate among workers who used an ionization device was much lower than among those who did not. So impressive have been the results up to now that so-called "pure air machines" have been introduced into factories, hospitals and other public buildings and have won great praise. Dr. Chizhewsky has become renowned throughout Russia, and has had diplomas conferred upon him by 40 universities, academies, etc., in recognition of his ionization discoveries. *Soviet Union* predicted that it won't be long before the city dweller will take street ionizers for granted. Fountains to saturate the air with negative ions will be in city squares.

Is this the kind of write-up *Consumer Reports* has in mind when it says there is no data given to support these favorable opinions of ionization? One must admit that there are no tables or charts in the article, but the question of just what the magazine would have to gain by making untrue statements about ionization remains unanswered. They have no commercial ionization machines to advertise in Russia.

More Evidence

In the *Journal of the American Pharmaceutical Association* (scientific edition) for October, 1960, there was an article on the effects of negatively ionized air on penicillin production. The authors trace the study of air ionization back 200 years. Several reports have stated that an excess of negative ions existing in the atmosphere at some of the most famous spas in Europe, is partly responsible for the supposed health-restoring qualities of those resorts. Then—"In our own time, negative air ions have been reliably reported to relieve and positive ions to aggravate sinusitis, rhinitis (inflammation of the nasal passages), asthma and pollenosis (allergy to pollen) in humans, and positive air ionization has been reputed to induce headache, dizziness, fatigue and malaise, while negative air ions have been said to ease the breathing and induce a sense of well-being. These reports deal with subjective clinical response.

"Objective laboratory research has revealed significant qualitatively measurable effects of ionized air on various biologic systems. For example, exposure to positively ionized air causes a reduction in the succinoxidase content of the adrenal gland of the intact rat, both positive and negative air ions are lethal to staphylococci and negative air ions increase and positive air ions decrease or abolish ciliary movement (that is, movement of the thousands of very fine hairs which are intended to sweep harmful invaders away from the vulnerable parts of the body) in mammalian trachea (that is, the windpipe of animals, such as humans, who are physically equipped to nurse their young)."

A *Reader's Digest* article (October, 1960), by Robert O'Brien, discussed the subject of ionization. He mentioned the results achieved by Dr. Igho H. Kornblueh, at the University of Pennsylvania's Graduate Hospital and at Frankford Hospital in Philadelphia. He and his associates have administered negative ion treatments to hundreds of patients suffering from hay fever or bronchial asthma. Of the total, 63 per cent have experienced partial to total relief. "They come in sneezing, eyes watering, noses itching, worn out from lack of sleep, so miserable they can hardly walk. Fifteen minutes in front of the negative ion machine and they feel so much better they don't want to leave," said one doctor.

Ions Relieve Pain

Dr. Kornblueh studied brain-wave patterns and found evidence that negative ions tranquilized persons in severe pain. Mr. O'Brien writes of one of the doctor's experiences in which he held a negative ionizer to the nose and mouth of a factory worker who had been rushed to the hospital suffering from second-degree steam burns on his back and legs. In minutes, the pain was gone. Morphine, usually administered in such cases, was not necessary. Now, all burn cases at that Philadelphia hospital (Northeastern) are immediately put in a windowless, ion-conditioned room. They are left there for 30 minutes every 8 hours. In 85 per cent of the cases, no pain-killing narcotics are needed. A spokesman for the hospital was quoted by Mr. O'Brien as saying, "Negative ions make burns dry out faster, heal faster and with less scarring. They also reduce the need for skin grafting."

What About Dosage?

How much of a dose of negative ions does one need for proper results? *House Beautiful* (February, 1961), in an article on ions, quoted the same Dr. Kornblueh as recommending 600 to 1,000 negative ions per cubic centimeter in the breathing zone for climate control ion replacement. For therapy, as in hay fever, 8,000 to 10,000 negative ions per cubic centimeter are needed.

Apparently, the problem of an overdose of negative ions does not exist. Dr. Kornblueh has done repeated tests showing no harmful effects from large amounts of negative ions. Others exposed 300 infants and children to high negative ion counts and, again, no harmful effects.

It is of interest that many persons—about 35 per cent of us— are insensitive to negative ions. And it has been found that long-time exposure to concentrations of negative ions tends to create an insensitivity to further effects from the ions.

The difficulty in making a scientific evaluation of negative ionization lies in the fact that the results are primarily subjective. You can't show a patient's relief of pain with numbers on a chart. If he says he is feeling more comfortable, you must believe him. This is true of a hay fever or a rheumatism patient also. The fact that there are so many favorable, if subjective, responses to negative ions, causes us to sympathize with those who have been attempting to promote this form of therapy. Certainly, if 30 minutes exposure several times a day will help a burn victim more easily and safely than other means, it is worth doing. If breathing before an ionization machine will relieve hay fever when other things can't, we can see no reason for not doing so, if such a machine is available to you.

Cost of Machines

We are told that the ionization machines being sold commercially range in price from 75 dollars to 250 dollars. This would appear to be quite an investment for a machine which may or may not be effective for you, and for one which some medical men and some scientists are reluctant to endorse. However, if the cost is not a major consideration for you and if you know you are not one of the 35 per cent upon whom negative ionization has no effect, we see no real objection to trying an ionization device to relieve a physical problem. There is plenty of opinion, and some rather convincing evidence, making us believe that we will be learning much more about the therapeutic value of negative air ionization in the coming years.

Iron Dextran

Iron Injections Found Dangerous

Many women, children and older people suffer from iron-deficiency anemia. A report in *Scope Weekly* for February 13, 1957, stated that a group of blood specialists announced that such anemia is widespread among children 6 to 18 months old. It is also prevalent among pregnant women and women who have had several children or more. It is likely, too, to be an aggravating factor in any condition that results in loss of blood. Such conditions are more frequent among older folks.

Studies reported by Dr. Philip Sturgeon of the University of Southern California Medical School showed that iron-deficiency anemia was present in 22 per cent of the children in families which could and did provide generally good diets. A similar group made up of families in lower income brackets who paid little attention to diet showed 78 per cent of its children in the borderline anemia class.

It would seem that solving the problem of iron-deficiency anemia should be simple—you simply give the patient concentrated iron in the form of a pill or a liquid.

But it's not quite so simple as it sounds. No agreement has been reached as to which is the best kind of iron to give and, sadly enough, it has been found that many iron preparations, given by mouth, are unacceptable because of the frequent ill effects they produce.

The *Lancet* for May 31, 1958, states, "There are many recommended iron preparations, and the fact that new ones keep appearing indicates that we still lack one that is completely satisfactory. One of the main difficulties is that iron preparations to be taken by mouth are liable to cause troublesome digestive side effects, such as nausea, heartburn, diarrhea or constipation. These side effects often cause the patient to stop taking their pills."

Ferrous sulfate is the most commonly used iron preparation. This is iron combined with a form of sulfur. Medical literature is full of references to children who have died or have been almost fatally poisoned by eating quantities of such pills. In some cases, the quantities were not large. Medical articles always stress the fact that such preparations should be given out in extremely small quantities and plastered with warnings to keep out of reach of small children.

How Can a Poisonous Drug Be Good?

The question naturally arises in the mind of a health-conscious person—how can such a preparation be good for anyone? This is the iron medicine that has the worst record where unpleasant side effects are concerned. Ferrous gluconate (a combination of iron and

461

glucose) is much less irritating to the patient and this form is used by many doctors.

However, it is only to be expected that, since there is difficulty in giving iron preparations and disagreement about which kind is best, injections of iron should have some popularity. Chief among these is a compound called iron dextran. In the May, 1958, issue of the *American Journal of Medical Sciences,* two doctors found that this preparation, injected into the muscles, was nonirritating, relatively easily absorbed and effective in producing more red blood cells, which is the important thing in iron-deficiency anemia. They report that "no local or general bad effects were noticed." They suggested that this preparation be used for patients who show poor iron absorption from food, have ailments in the stomach or digestive tract which may be aggravated by iron given by mouth or who need to get a lot of iron in a short time. Eighteen patients were studied.

Tumors Develop

In England, the iron dextran preparation was popular. Then, in the April 11, 1959, issue of the *British Medical Journal* appeared an article titled "Induction of Sarcoma in the Rat by Iron Dextran Complex," by H. G. Richmond of the University of Aberdeen. Now, sarcoma is cancer. Dr. Richmond tells us that, although iron preparations have caused trouble in the past, no one has ever before linked any medicinal iron with cancer. So this iron dextran preparation was used in a lab experiment to test for something else, and it was specifically chosen because there was no reason to believe that it could cause cancer. None of the animals used in the experiment had ever developed spontaneous tumors, so nothing but the iron compound could have been responsible.

In one of the experiments, tumors developed in 22 rats, at the site of the injection, from 6 to 8 months after the end of the treatment. Rats which received injections of dextran alone showed no tumors. So the iron seemed to be responsible.

"From these observations," says Dr. Richmond, "it is clear that intramuscular injection of iron dextran complex is carcinogenic (cancer-causing) in the rat." He says, further, that the dose given to the rats was massive, when compared with dosage given to human patients. He also points out that lung cancer is increasing among miners who work with hematite (rich in iron) and he believes that the evidence he has submitted suggests that iron may be the most important cause of this.

Vitamin E and Iron

We think that Dr. Richmond's theory as to how iron preparations produce such effects is most interesting. He says that certain compounds produced at the site of the injection are similar to those produced throughout the body in a deficiency of vitamin E. It is also true, he says, that the compound which develops as a result of getting too much iron can be largely prevented by giving vitamin E. Therefore, he believes that one way in which iron acts inside a cell is to block the action of vitamin E. This results in the formation of the compound mentioned above. Whether or not this has anything to do with the formation of the cancer is not known.

However, we think the above theory is especially important. The form of iron used in medicine destroys large amounts of vitamin E in the digestive tract, so we advise taking iron medication at a different time from the time you take vitamin E, if at all possible. That is, take the iron first thing in the morning and the vitamin E last thing at night, or some such arrangement as that.

Is it not "wasteful" to take vitamin E at the same time you are taking iron preparations, since the iron may destroy or inactivate the vitamin E? Of course it is, but in the light of the information given above, doesn't it seem wise to take the vitamin E so that one's body will have *some* of this important vitamin even though some is destroyed?

Some people have asked us whether they should take food supplements rich in iron (kelp, liver, etc.) when they are taking vitamin E. Aren't the two things working at cross-purposes, they ask. We have the word of Dr. Evan Shute, a world authority on vitamin E, for the answer to that one. Dr. Shute reminds us that, if iron in food destroyed vitamin E, then everyone who has ever lived would have been deficient in vitamin E, for iron is widely distributed in food—and often in the very food that is richest in vitamin E— wheat germ, for instance, and other seed foods, green leafy vegetables and liver. Of course, the iron present in these foods has not destroyed the vitamin E that is there and hence, it will certainly not destroy any vitamin E that goes "down the hatch" with the food.

But medicinal iron is something else—and a quite mysterious "something else"—that even the most experienced researchers understand imperfectly.

What Is Going to Be Done?

To get back to iron dextran and cancer, *Medical News* for March 9, 1960, reports on another researcher's work, Professor Alexander Haddow of a research institute in London. "The British investigator underscores the need for closer scrutiny of the effects of iron compounds widely used for anemias and of the involvement of industrial iron oxides in lung cancers." Dr. Haddow produced cancers in different kinds of laboratory animals with iron dextran.

An article in the April 9, 1960, issue of the *Medical Journal of Australia,* comments on the iron dextran matter asking "whether the product concerned should continue to be prescribed and whether its manufacturers should continue to make it available for sale."

They quote the manufacturers of the drug who state that, over 7 years, their researchers have carried out experiments and are convinced that, "in clinical practice, the drug is harmless. Over a period of 6 years, more than one million patients are estimated to have been treated with this drug. It is widely recognized as a highly effective treatment for iron deficiency. About 100 published scientific papers pay tribute to its value." However, the company suspended sale of iron dextran "pending an independent re-examination of all the available evidence."

Injections Should Be Avoided

The editorial in the Australian *Journal* then went on to point out that no reports of cancer had occurred in man, and that several other species of animals did not show cancer when given injections. Furthermore, in another laboratory study, when the dosage given was lowered to only about 50 times what would be given to a human being, the rats got *no more cancers than they would get from injections of glucose, fructose, arachis oil and many other 'innocuous' materials."*

We think this last statement is most interesting. A number of perfectly harmless substances may produce cancer when *injected* into the body. Doesn't this seem to be weighty evidence showing that injections of anything are just plain not good for you?

Now, finally, the Australian *Journal* points out that the iron dextran preparation has not been withdrawn from sale in Australia and counsels doctors to decide for themselves whether or not they wish to use it. They say that the risk, "like the risks associated with the use of many effective drugs, needs to be balanced against the therapeutic needs of the individual patient."

Here is a frank admission by the editor of a medical journal that many drugs are toxic and the doctor must decide whether the chance the drugged patient takes is worth it. Iron dextran has also been withdrawn from sale in the United States.

Prevention of Anemia Is the Only Answer

The lesson to be learned from this grim story is, we believe, to avoid injections whenever you possibly can. Injections of even harmless substances are dangerous. Injections are completely unnatural. The human body is purposely enclosed in a skin which is very effective in keeping foreign matter out of the blood stream and the body cells. An injection is an insult to this integrity.

To avoid iron-deficiency anemia, the best plan is to make certain you are eating foods that contain plenty of iron and that you are not suffering from any kind of hidden bleeding. Women are especially susceptible to anemia because of their loss of blood in the menstrual flow each month. This must be replaced. Pregnant women lose iron to the child they are carrying. This iron must be replaced. Persons suffering from infections, from bleeding piles, ulcers, diarrhea, may become anemic.

Here are some foods rich in iron. Do you and your family eat plenty of them? Wheat germ, liver, meat, eggs, heart, kidney, lentils, dried mushrooms, blackstrap molasses, soybeans, sunflower seeds. Milk contains extremely little iron; cereals contain phytic acid which tends to destroy iron in the digestive tract; so, the milk and processed cereal which form the backbone of many American children's diets could readily lead to anemia.

Itch

Treatment of the Itch

By J. I. Rodale

The *Wall Street Journal,* in a very comprehensive article about drug firms and itch remedies, says, "Medical researchers have conquered at least half a dozen dread diseases in the last 10 years, but they are still largely in the dark, they admit, in finding relief for one age-old ailment—the itch . . . Drug executives foresee a market of $35 million a year for potions and pills that would do away with the annoyance of the itch. Doctors estimate that as many as 20 million to 30 million people in the U.S. come down with some form of this affliction every year."

One drug firm struck a right note when it said recently that its product works by removing the desire to scratch, but that it would be better to eliminate the cause of the itch. The salves and ointments are only palliatives. A physician says that doctors are pretty much in agreement that most drug store medicines are worse than none at all. "In the majority of cases," he said, "these ointments and lotions are too harsh. Literally, they add insult to injury. As a matter of fact, in at least half of the cases of itching, the causative factor is not a skin disease, but a general medical problem."

Another physician: "During the past 5 years (before 1955), at least 60 different new preparations have been reported to be of aid in the treatment of pruritus (itch). Almost all of these have not been adequately controlled, and in the future will probably be relegated to obscurity, like so many medications of the past."

A doctor refers to the usual treatment for the itch as being wholly empiric. Empiric means experimental, based on experience, rather than by reasoning or theory. But at best it is a case of guessing, or trial . . . and error.

When the patient becomes frantic with itching, one authority gives reserpine and chlorpromazine, both high-powered tranquilizing drugs. They calm the patient and make it easier for him to bear the itching. This, according to the authority, gives the doctor a chance to focus his attention on "treating" the skin trouble, but rarely to remove the cause.

Anesthetic Type Drugs

A local anesthetic type of salve called dyclonine gave relief in most of 200 cases of itching, but some of them reported irritation and other signs of sensitivity. I wouldn't want to take this drug, because it might just be my luck to be sensitive to it.

Another anesthetic type of drug for the itch is procaine and it is advised to be taken either by mouth, injected into the veins or applied on the itching skin. One would be foolish to swallow this stuff for an itch when there are sensible ways to go about discovering and eliminating the cause of it. Incidentally, a medical article says that procaine is about one-fourth as toxic as cocaine.

How does procaine act? "It affects all living cells, but its main action is on the nerve fibers, where it produces an attenuation in the conduction of impulses." In other words, the effect is to fool you, to get you to stick your head in the ground. The itch is still there, but it is kept from your nerves which would ordinarily dispatch the message to your brain, telling you that you itch and that you should begin scratching. For my money, I'll take prevention. This article says, "A patient highly sensitive to procaine will develop untoward symptoms within a few moments after its use." And they reassure us that they "were unable to find any report of fatality, due to the oral administration of procaine." But some of the symptoms resulting from oral administration were headache, dizziness, weakness, nervousness, nausea, drowsiness, flushing, heartburn, vomiting, fatigue, cramps, diarrhea, abdominal pain, frequency (of urination), belching, visual disturbance, and palpitation. No, thank you. Not for my money.

Here is another statement from a different journal: "In general, cortisone, hydrocortisone and ACTH given systemically tend to relieve itching, but these are powerful drugs, and if the underlying cause of the pruritus is not removed, then prolonged administration is necessary, with its subsequent dangers."

There are Burow's solution, camomile extract, Lassar's paste, amino acid ointments, amphetamine, methyltestosterone, injections of alcohol, and tattooing of the involved skin with mercuric chloride in the case of pruritus vulva (the female organs) and a thousand other drugs and procedures.

Dangerous to Interior of Body

But the use of ointments can be dangerous to the interior of the body. One imagines that they remain only on the surface of the skin. But that is not so. They can be absorbed into the blood stream. Take a case reported in the *Archives of Dermatology and Syphilology* (29: 382, 1934). A dentist, aged 52, suffered from a pruritic condition diagnosed as scabies and a sulfur ointment was used on 6 successive days, applied over his entire body, including the face. The condition became much worse. He had had a normal heart condition. He became very uncomfortable. His entire skin became brownish red and he was given colloidal tub baths with various soothing remedies. He went from bad to worse and died of acute interstitial myocarditis within a few days. Myocarditis is an inflammation of the muscular walls of the heart. Interstitial pertains to the interstices or interspaces of a tissue.

According to this article, this type of myocardial failure often comes after ointments are used on some skin condition. Cases demonstrating this fearful side effect are mentioned, such as a man with an infected burn, a carbuncle on the neck, an abrasion of the arm, a skin infection of the groin, etc. A typical case was an infection of the foot that was treated. Thirteen days later, there developed cardiac (heart) symptoms.

The article winds up with the following statement. "It seems timely to emphasize the disastrous results that may follow the indiscriminate use of proprietary remedies."

Overtreatment Dermatitis

In an article in the *Journal of the American Medical Association* (157: 720, 1955), the problem of the overtreatment of skin conditions is stressed. Many of these remedies produce other skin diseases which the author terms "overtreatment dermatitis," and the users "drug store physicians." One hundred and fifty thousand such cases are reported annually. L. E. Gaul, M.D., the author of the article, says that the statistics show that overtreatment dermatitis is in the top quarter of common skin diseases in the country.

When it was first announced that sulfonamides could be used in skin ointments, the incidence of overtreatment dermatitis increased greatly. But soon, reports began to appear, like that of the AMA Council on Pharmacy and Chemistry, which warned of the dangers following the external use of the sulfonamides. Reports like this seldom get much attention in the newspapers, so, although doctors knew of the warnings, the general public went right ahead rubbing the sulfa preparation into their skins, and overtreatment was the final result.

Other Drugs

Turning to local anesthetics, antihistamines and topical antibiotics, we find the same results. Local anesthetics reverse their intended effect; that is, instead of relieving itching, they cause it.

I found an advertisement of one drug product that is worth mentioning. This is Borcherdt's Malt Soup Extract, for use in cases of pruritus ani (rectum). A Dr. Louis H. Brooks is quoted in the advertisement as saying: "It was found that administration of Malt Soup Extract in dosages of one or two tablespoonfuls twice daily produced favorable results. Within two or three days after beginning this simple regimen, the itching and burning usually disappeared." The advertisement claims that the malt extract works by restoring the normal acid condition in the lower tract and by promoting the growth and development of aciduric bacteria. Whether this does the job or not, at least the malt extract is a rather bland substance and cannot do much harm.

A Doctor's Experience

Here is a letter sent by a physician to the editor of the *Journal of the Australian Medical Association* (June 28, 1958). He speaks of a case of pruritus vulvae. The vulva is the near-the-surface part of the organs of generation of the female.

"DEAR EDITOR:

"As a medical student, I eagerly frequented the houses of dermatologists and physicians in Macquarie Street and there, was prescribed for with a frankness that drove from my heart, the young and magic mystery of medicine. For my advisers would read the textbooks with me and between us we would pick a seeming-good prescription. And so, with the years, the pruritus continued on its own way and my patients derived some ever temporary benefit from my own sufferings and from the ointment and lotion sections of the various hospital pharmacopoeias and the dermatology books. Finally, I became convinced I was one of the great living experts on pruritus therapy. That was till I met my first case of pruritus vulvae in my then country practice. The red, swollen and irritable vulva appalled me, but I assured the lady she was being advised by a specialist—and the cocaine and its cogeners, the carbolic and the calamine, the hygiene, the rest and all the sedatives drove my patient to a dermatologist in Brisbane, and lo! to my surprise and chagrin (?), she was back in her country home in two weeks bright and cured, except, of course, for the little itch that is the pleasant reminder. The specialist was kind enough to let me have his secret: 3 per cent silver nitrate dissolved in nitrous spirits of ether—which I soon got going onto myself. Oh! The piquant agony of the application; the fiery, apneic, psyche-consuming, nerve-tingling, half minute. Then the glow! And then the ease! Paradise for days! With ensuing applications, ease for months; then forever—but ever with the remnant occasional prod to recall the intense rawness of other days.

"So my patients and I developed a technique—and they were keen to use the doctor's personal treatment—the 'silver ease.' Wash with cotton wool and soft soap and water after defecation. Clean underwear daily. Bath twice daily. No greases or lotions. Apply the nitrate solution with a soft brush—liberally—with the nates well spread. There is time for this swift liberal application before the silver burn arrests all activities. Finish off by applying a layer of witch-hazel vanishing cream—which seems to smooth off skin roughnesses and at least has a delicious cooling sensation. No more silver is applied till the pruritus again drives you to it.

"Any man who treats himself has a fool for a doctor—and if so, in this case we can agree with Pope: 'You think me cruel? Take it for a rule. No creature smarts so little as a fool.'

"Or with Ausonius: 'Mules may ease each other's itch.'

"Dr. Wilson, and you, sir, will, I trust, detect no hint in all this that pruritus ani may be associated with 'pruritus disputandi.'

"Yours, etc.
H.O.T."

Treatment without Drugs

Now on to the subject of how to treat itching without drugs.

Dr. Rolf Ulrich in his book, *Coffee and Caffeine,* says that, in an experiment with eczema cases who were given coffee, all reported that they felt warmer and that the affected part itched worse than before and showed a redness.

It is a known fact that pruritus is aggravated by heat. A physician states that itching is increased by the vasodilating effect of heat and decreased by cold. He states, however, that if the heat sensation is sufficiently intense, the resulting burning might abolish the itch. Vasodilation means the enlargement of the blood vessels. This, in the case of the application of heat, causes an inflammation.

One method is to diminish the symptom by replacing it with something else. Baths or soaks can accomplish this, or even the application of water with wash rags, preferably cool water. This doctor suggests putting starch in the water. He also suggests the application of calamine lotion.

Cooling the skin is one of the best ways to give relief. The cold dulls the nerves and produces an anemia in the skin. Menthol has also been used for this purpose, but it is only temporary in its relief. However, I would like to caution you against running cold water on the feet. They are a dangerously vulnerable spot for cold water. If you have to put cold water on them, follow it immediately with hot, alternating cold with hot.

Perspiring

Perspiring is one of the causes of pruritus. That is why it is desirable for an obese person to reduce, for the excess weight brings on excess perspiration. Such a person sweats heavily between the legs causing a pruritus there. Perspiration is healthy, but after a period of perspiring, one should wash it off the body. Recently I had an itch between the legs. I used to bathe once a day. But when I washed 3 times a day, I got it under control more or less . . . once in the morning after a night of perspiring, once after my daily walk in which I merely sit in the tub with water only covering the pruritic area, and again, the same position in the tub before going to bed. If it is not convenient to use 3 tub baths, one can use a wash rag or sponge.

To prevent too much perspiration, one should use the minimum of bedclothes and, if necessary, employ an electric heating device in winter under the bed sheets. One should wear loose underwear and clothes that are not too tight. I found in my case that I frequently sat in a narrow chair with side arms that kept my feet too close together, and this caused much perspiration in the midsection.

Cleanliness is of the greatest importance, especially in pruritus ani, and in women, in pruritus vulvae, which involves the sexual area. There must be cleaning after each urination and bowel movement and in doing this, there should be patting, not rubbing, with soft toilet paper, cotton or tissue. One should not scratch. One physician advises, "Scratching only aggravates the itching, and much greater relief can be obtained by pinching the portion of skin that itches or by applying firm continuous pressure on the involved parts with the closed fist or fingers."

Senile Pruritus

A dry, aging skin is another cause of pruritus, especially in people in the 50's and 60's. Sometimes it is referred to as senile pruritus. A panel of dermatologists at Columbia University recommended a mixture of 10 per cent olive oil, 70 per cent lanolin and 20 per cent water, applied directly to the skin to eliminate such dryness.

A Dr. Rein, of the above-mentioned panel, advises that showers be discontinued by persons suffering the itching skin that is so bothersome to many people, in winter especially. He tells us that colloidal baths can be valuable in softening and lubricating scaly and itchy skin. Such a bath can be made up in this way: a cup of oatmeal is put in a container with two teaspoonfuls of oil (olive, corn, cottonseed or peanut oil), mixed with a quart of milk, then poured into a tub of lukewarm water. The patient then soaks himself in this solution. The soothing warmth of the water, coupled with the fats and oils, is intended to restore softness and moisture to the skin. Greasing the skin with more of the same type of oil is recommended after the bath.

The entire panel of dermatologists was unanimous in its condemnation of the use of soap. They agreed that the skin is only irritated by the chemicals contained in soap, and each time it is used it introduces new dryness and itching to the skin. The panel also recommended that one avoid rubbing with a towel, but rather that one pat the skin dry, thus preserving the oils and avoiding added irritation.

Effect of Climate

One physician has found that a change of climate was very effective. Harold Eidinoff, M.D., reporting in the *Journal of Investigative Dermatology,* followed the record of 34 cases of intractable pruritus of various kinds who were living in a low-level, humid climate area. "When these patients left the low, humid climate and moved to a high, dry climate, all but 3 of the 34 were able to achieve a practically complete remission or improvement, some within a relatively short time. This was accomplished without any other treatment by some patients," while most of them had the effect of exposure of the parts to the natural sun. These patients went to El Paso, Texas.

Dr. Eidinoff goes on, "The patients who recovered remained generally well (except for occasional minor relapses) as long as they stayed in the high, dry climate." A return to a low, humid climate for any length of time often resulted in a severe recurrence of the disease. By returning to a high, dry climate the dermatitis again cleared, except in one case.

The climatic condition of El Paso is: altitude 3700 feet, average temperature 70 degrees Fahrenheit, average humidity 35 per cent, rainfall 10 inches per year. The effect of a high, dry climate is to increase the rate of water evaporation from the skin.

Once, when I had an itch in the midsection, I was able to get it nicely under control, but when we went to Palm Beach for the entire winter, it came back. This section of Florida is a low-level, high-humidity area and should be shunned by sufferers from any kind of pruritus. They should favor certain sections of Texas, Arizona, etc. What a lot of scratching must be going on in such places as Palm Beach, Miami, etc.!

Juvenile Delinquency

A Reason for Delinquency in Europe

The famous authority on juvenile delinquency, Judge Samuel S. Leibowitz of Kings County, New York, returned from a summer European trip and announced that juvenile delinquency "is sweeping like a holocaust all across Europe." He noted that the rise is sharpest in the prosperous countries, and that Europeans blame American movies and magazines for the rise in juvenile crime, according to the *New York Herald Tribune* (August 31, 1960).

Are Food Synthetics Responsible?

We have no doubt that some of the unwholesome influences we see in these media could have such an effect, or at least be responsible in part. We wonder, however, about the effects brought about by some of our less sensational exports—sodas, candy bars, refined flour, instant pudding, chocolate syrup, etc. None of the European countries were ever exposed to such a deluge of American foods as they have been in the past 10 years. The youth of these nations have grown up, as have our own, on the colas, candy bars and cake mixes of America. If diet has any influence over mentality whatsoever, and it has been proven that it is a very important factor, then certainly a measure of the new delinquency which so shocked Judge Leibowitz can be explained in that light.

The Effect Follows the Cause

European children don't rely on whole-grain breads; they can eat white bread just the way we do. They can eat American candy instead of fruit or honey-sweetened foods. They don't need fresh foods because we have given them our know-how in preserving foods for weeks and months. They eat our refined sugar, our lifeless wheat and our chemicals, too. If we have a juvenile delinquency problem, why shouldn't the Europeans? They're influenced by our movies, our publications and our food.

Kelp

Kelp Proves Itself as Food

It is a well-known fact that soil depleted of trace minerals produces food that is deficient in these minerals. For this reason, commercial fertilizers which contain only a few of the major minerals are insufficient. This is one of the main reasons why we recommend the use of food supplements—because they supply the extremely valuable trace minerals missing from much of our commercially produced food.

What are these trace minerals? They are referred to as "trace" because they exist in very small amounts—only a "trace" of them in most things. Some trace minerals are copper, cobalt, iodine, zirconium, titanium, zinc.

One of the richest sources of trace minerals is, of course, bone meal. Another is kelp—seaweed which contains minerals that are abundant in the depths of the sea. Although modern human beings have done much to deplete soil of trace minerals, by not replacing those which have been taken off the land in crops, the sea's riches in this field are still untapped. And, as a matter of fact, the sea is steadily becoming richer in minerals, as rivers carry away eroded soil from the land to the sea.

Kelp in Cattle Feed

An encouraging story on the value of kelp in cattle raising came to our attention recently. Sid Cox, writing in the *Fresno Bee,* Fresno, California (January 15, 1961), tells the story of dairymen in that neighborhood who use kelp regularly in their cattle feed. Many leading dairymen give kelp credit as a production booster, says this author, and also declare that it prevents foot rot during wet weather, improves conception rates in breeding, makes calves grow faster and cuts down on bills for hay.

One farmer, who has 200 head of cattle, stated that 20 of these had foot rot when he began to put kelp into their feed two years ago. The trouble is practically gone, the cows look better and have smoother coats. Just to make certain the kelp was responsible, he stopped giving it once for 6 weeks. The cows dropped off in their milk, he reported, and *"ate about ¾ ton more hay each day."*

Apparently, something about the kelp had enabled the cows to perform as milk cows should while eating far less rations. This is practical good news for a farmer. Isn't it also good news for those of us who are inclined to be overweight? Isn't it possible that not getting enough of the trace minerals might be one good reason for overeating?

473

Dr. Melvin Page of the Page Foundation, 2810 First Street, St. Petersburg, Florida, says, in his book, *Degeneration and Regeneration* (published by the Page Foundation), that we crave sweets because we are actually craving the minerals that go along with the sweets in nature—the minerals in fruit and sweet vegetables. He says that the sweet taste was placed there by nature to guide us to the valuable minerals. Is it possible that, in our hunger for minerals, we overeat on sweet things—especially white sugar from which all the minerals have been refined and thrown away?

Wins Praise of Dairymen

Here are some other experiences of the California farmers who fed kelp to their cattle. One dairyman with 500 milk cows has been using two per cent kelp in the feed of his cows. Production of butterfat has jumped by 1,000 pounds each month, he says, and his current crop of calves is the best he has had in 30 years.

Another farmer said his butterfat production has climbed steadily since his cows could have as much kelp as they wished. Conception rates among his cows have improved and his veterinary bill is practically nil.

Another farmer found that test calves which were put on kelp grew faster and were healthier than those given regular feed. In another herd, the 600.8 pounds of butterfat per cow jumped to 637.7 pounds, reportedly a national record for a herd this size. Indications are that this record will go to 650 pounds.

A 7-year-old cow fed on kelp recently set a state record of 1,434 pounds of butterfat in one lactation.

We are not suggesting that human beings who eat kelp will produce butterfat—far from it. The health and vigor of milk cows is judged largely by their production of milk. So it seems possible that a similar increase in well-being might occur in human beings who take kelp for its trace mineral content.

Some dairy scientists, we are told by Mr. Cox, are inclined to discredit kelp and point to an analysis of its contents to back up their position. They say there are more economical sources of calcium and iodine available. These are probably the same kind of people who disparage bone meal and rose hips as sources of vitamins and minerals. The very idea of getting food elements in a purely natural food, untouched by laboratories or processors, is something that many specialists feel they must oppose—it's just too simple. They are convinced that chemists know better what people should eat than nature herself and that mineral supplements concocted in a laboratory are preferable to natural foods.

All the California dairymen have to do is point out the eagerness with which their cows gulp down their kelp ration and ask for more, plus the astonishing increase in good health which follows when kelp is being given.

Some Further Facts on Kelp

From *Science News Letter* for May 2, 1959, comes the information that, in an experiment with 200 Royal Pastel mink, Dr. John A. Miller and Thomas F. Daly of Ohio State University reported that the addition of one per cent kelp meal to a standard ranch ration resulted in a savings of 1,228 pounds of food per mink over a 135-day period—a 9 per cent saving.

Here is some information about seaweed in general from a publication of the Fish and Wildlife Service, Washington, D. C., *Seaweeds and Their Uses:*

"The Oriental peoples, particularly the Japanese, have long

Koch, Robert

Robert Koch, the German bacteriologist whose experiments laid a foundation for the modern germ theory of disease, was born in Clausthal, Hanover, December 11, 1843. His career in

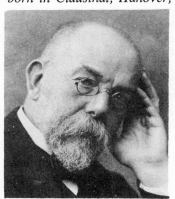

bacteriological research began with the isolation of the anthrax bacillus. Realizing that he was being stifled by improper facilities for research, Koch, in 1880, went to Berlin where he became a member of the Imperial Board of Health. Here, utilizing his new found laboratory facilities, Koch, in collaboration with Karl Joseph Eberth, isolated the typhoid bacillus. However, it was not until two years later (1882) that Koch made his most important discovery—the isolation of the tubercle bacillus. This scientific finding virtually revolutionized the treatment of tuberculosis. Koch's genius did not stop here. He went on in the following years to discover the bacilli of two kinds of infectious conjunctivitis, identified the comma bacillus as the cause of Asiatic cholera, found and improved methods for the purifying of public water supplies by the filtration process and proved that the tsetse fly was the carrier of the dread sleeping sickness. For all these triumphs Koch received the Nobel Prize in physiology and medicine in 1905, just five years before his death.

used seaweeds for human food. This use in the United States, however, has been quite limited . . . Irish moss is used, mostly in the New England states, for making blancmange. Dulse is used commercially as a thickener in soups, sauces and gravies. It is also used in salads and relishes. . . .

"Inasmuch as seaweeds are not as digestible and palatable for most Western people as are vegetables, the seaweeds are not likely soon to become as popular a food item in the United States as they are in the Orient. . . .

"Seaweed has found considerable use in Europe as an animal food. On the coast of Ireland, sheep are said to eat seaweed even when grass is available. . . .

"From 10 to 20 per cent of seaweed meal can be included in the diet of sheep, pigs and horses, and up to 10 per cent of the meal can be included in the diet of poultry."

The booklet reminds us that all seaweeds are high in potassium, a mineral which is of utmost importance for good health. Its chief source in daily diet is fresh vegetables and fruits. If you feel you are not getting enough of these, kelp is an excellent supplementary source.

People sometimes ask us how much kelp they should eat. We cannot recommend any special amount, any more than we could recommend how many apples you should eat or how many nuts. Kelp is a food, rich in minerals. In some parts of the world, it is eaten by the dishful as we eat salad greens.

Could it be harmful? We have a clipping from a newspaper, whose name and date are unknown, stating that Japanese surgeons report they have successfully used a seaweed compound mixed with water as a substitute for whole blood in transfusions. It doesn't seem that anything so nearly like our own blood in composition could possibly be harmful, now does it?

What About Salt in Kelp?

It is true that kelp contains sodium chloride along with its other minerals—it's salty in taste, like the ocean water it comes from. People on a low-salt diet should probably not take kelp in great quantity. However, the sodium chloride in kelp, like the sugar in fresh fruits, comes combined with many other completely natural substances, so that it could never be accused of doing the harm done by refined table salt or refined white sugar—which are almost "pure" substances, from which all other natural elements have been removed. Chemically "pure" substances don't exist in nature. This makes them drugs to our way of thinking.

We think that some one trying to cut down on salt would find kelp a welcome substitute. Its chief value, of course, especially for people who live far from sea water and eat little seafood, is its iodine content. It is richer in iodine than any other food. Iodine is a most important element which may be completely lacking in foods grown in soil deficient in iodine. There is no way for you to know whether the foods you eat are grown this way, so your best assurance for getting plenty of iodine is to take kelp as a daily food supplement.

Iodine is used by the body chiefly as the most important ingredient of the hormone made by the thyroid gland—thyroxine. The thyroid gland plays an important part in regulating many body functions—the sex glands, the pituitary gland, the body's use of calcium and phosphorus and many other important activities. Lack of iodine can lead to goiter.

Here is a chart of the minerals contained in kelp. Note the very high content of iodine (which usually is measured in parts per million) and potassium.

	Per Cent		Per Cent
Iodine	.18	Magnesium	.740
Calcium	1.05	Sodium	3.98
Phosphorus	.339	Chlorine	13.07
Iron	.37	Manganese	.0015
Copper	.0008	Sulfur	1.
Potassium	11.15		

Trace Minerals: barium, boron, chromium, lithium, nickel, silicon, silver, strontium, titanium, vanadium.

Kidney

The Kidney—a Remarkable Filter

The kidneys and the liver have one very important function in common. They each filter waste from the body. For the liver, this is one of many jobs, and the function is largely chemical. In the case of the kidneys, the filtering action is purely a physical one. As the blood circulates through the kidney, waste products are strained out of the blood—much as a sieve would do—and dissolved in water. This mixture of solid material and water is called urine and is accumulated in the bladder for release.

The kidney is dark reddish brown and is shaped like a lima bean. The normal human body has a pair of these, situated to the rear of the trunk, one on each side of the spinal column, just below the rib cage. From each kidney, there is suspended a sort of tube, the ureter, which conveys the waste, or urine, to the bladder for release from the body.

Impossible to Duplicate Kidney's Efficiency

As is the case with most of the body's organs, the efficiency of the kidneys is difficult to analyze and impossible to duplicate entirely. An artificial kidney has been developed, and was used to great advantage many times in helping damaged kidneys to do their job in an emergency. However, the machine is as large as a gallon paint can, its exterior exhibits several plastic tubes whose function and connection can only be applied by experts and the artificial kidney is totally impractical for use anywhere but in an operating room under carefully controlled conditions. Even so, the machine doesn't perform many of the functions the natural kidneys perform automatically.

Subtle Actions of the Kidney

For example, the kidneys react to bodily stress by working even harder. The kidneys maintain the balance of water and salts in the body, even retrieving certain normally discarded proteins for the blood stream in emergency. The *New York State Medical Journal* (July 1, 1955) tells us that the action of the kidney is affected by anxiety, fear, anger and other emotions. In 400 tests run on 5 persons leading normal lives, it was shown that, when they needed increased alertness and readiness for action, the kidneys helped by damming up reservoirs of water and mineral salts in the body. Once the crisis was past, the kidneys flushed out the extra water and salt in urine. The same accommodation is made for illness. In cases of pneumonia, the kidneys also hold extra salts and water in the body during the danger period, and flush it out once the crisis is over. Tension can make the kidneys hold back and relaxation or excitement can cause them to release. Can you imagine a machine that could be made sensitive to such subtleties? The article concludes by saying that difficulties that food and drink can cause are slight compared with those incurred by emotional changes.

Transplanting a Kidney

In *Science Digest* (June, 1951), Dr. L. Newburgh, of the University of Michigan, is quoted as saying that 5 per cent of the kidney will do the entire job required of it, complicated though its functions are. We can be comfortably served by as much kidney function as is found in a white rat.

The body can manage quite well with only one of its two kidneys, and many persons whose one kidney has been removed, live normally. However, one kidney must be functioning. Transplanting of a kidney has been attempted, but it is rarely successful. The only possibility exists in identical twins, one donating to the other. In other cases, the body treats the new organ as an invader and ets up antibodies against it, resulting soon in the patient's death.

Cause of Severe Strain on Kidneys

When illness sets in or when fevers and infections occur, the strain on the kidneys can be severe. Fevered blood is full of tissue waste which is caught by the kidneys and can clog them. When such clogging occurs, protein and blood cells leak into the urine. It is for this reason that the presence of red corpuscles and albumin (protein) in a urine specimen, alerts the doctor to the possibility of kidney trouble. Other signs of possible kidney disorder are swollen face or ankles, puffy eyes or urine that looks cloudy, bloody or wine-colored over a period of time. The swelling is, of course, a sign that the kidneys are not maintaining a proper water balance in the system. The discolored urine can mean that filtering is not being properly accomplished.

In the *New York Times* (March 14, 1957), an interesting representation of what happens to kidneys when serious, chronic disease strikes was given by Dr. Daniel Pease. He visualizes kidney cells as having "arms." These arm-like protrusions end in extensions, rather like fingers, which surround the blood vessels of the kidney. When disease occurs, these "fingers" swell, squeezing the blood vessels and cutting off the circulation to the cells.

Kidney Stones Most Common Kidney Disease

Of all kidney diseases, the most common is kidney stones. These stones are calcium deposits which occur due to a misuse of calcium by the body, so that too much of this mineral is poured out through the urinary tract. The calcium in quantity forms into tiny pebbles, too large to pass through the kidneys and, in time, the function of the kidneys becomes blocked. Sometimes, the small "stones" can be passed through the urethra, but for the larger ones, surgical removal is usually the only answer. Unfortunately, persons who have suffered with kidney stones once are likely to be subjected to the problem again. *Science News Letter* (March 29, 1958) carries statistics showing that the rate of recurrence of small stones, passed by patients, is 15 to 20 per cent. For stones removed by surgery, the rate is 60 to 70 per cent. Obviously, the reason for this record of return of the unwanted calcium deposits lies in the fact that surgery removes only the result of the body's improper use of calcium and does not remedy this improper use. Of course, the calcium deposits will continue to be formed just as before. An assessment of the body's metabolism is in order to find out why the calcium is misused and it is the only sensible move toward a complete cure.

There are many guesses concerning the reason for the calcium formations. In *Capper's Farmer* (May, 1957), the work of Harvard Medical School researcher, Dr. Philip Hanneman, using phytin, a calcium magnesium salt occurring in seeds and tubers, to treat kidney stones is discussed. He gave regular dosages of phytic acid to 41 test patients and found that their urinary levels of calcium returned to normal and all new stone formation was stopped. These results continued up to the time the report was written—more than a year.

Vitamin C and Urinary Tract Deposits

Dr. W. J. McCormick, writing in the *Journal of the Canadian Dental Association* (August, 1946), tells us that people whose diet is low in vitamin C are often victims of heavy tartar deposits on the teeth. He suggests that this might happen because a shortage of vitamin C leads to a breakdown of body tissues, including those of the mouth. The mucous lining scales off and mixes with remnants of food particles, creating the unsightly deposit which clings to the teeth.

Could this same action be taking place in the urinary tract, asks Dr. McCormick? With a shortage of vitamin C, the mucous lining of this area might scale off and form the nucleus of stones. In observing his patients, Dr. McCormick found that cloudy urine, containing phosphates (which constitute some kinds of kidney stones) and pieces of sloughed off mucus from the walls of the urinary canal, went hand in hand with a shortage of vitamin C. Giving large doses of vitamin C (we would imagine he means 500 to 1,000 milligrams per day), Dr. McCormick could clear the urine in a matter of hours. The patients using this same treatment reported not only that their urine cleared, but that tartar deposits were clearing from their teeth and dentures. Nurses in hospitals reported that patients whose urine had formerly caused calcium deposits on the urinary utensils now found that the utensils remained free from deposits.

These patients were all on high-protein, vitamin-rich diets, but vitamin C proved to be the nutrient which prevented the accumulation of the unwelcome deposits.

Who Gets Kidney Stones

In the *Times-Picayune* of New Orleans, Louisiana (April 20, 1958), Dr. Edwin L. Prien remarked that, statistically, people of the south are more likely to suffer from kidney stones than northerners. Soil in the deep South, particularly along the Gulf Coast (southern Florida excepted), is deficient in magnesium. It was Dr. Prien's guess that the absence of magnesium might be a factor.

The *Journal of Pediatrics* (October, 1957) says kidney stones are rare among dairy-farming people, but frequently seen among those living on monotonous diets or those for whom whole cereals form a staple food. (Further support for Editor Rodale's opinions against grain foods.) The *Journal of the American Medical Association* (December 11, 1954) prints the account of experiments begun in 1917, and repeated successfully since, in which kidney stones were induced in rats by diets deficient in vitamin A. So-called "stone areas" are the hot, dry sections of the world: Mesopotamia, North India, South China. The people have scanty urine output and high concentrations of urinary salts. They are often from the poorest strata of society and subsist on inadequate diets of largely rice and grain, with no vegetables, fruit or meat. A lack of vitamin A is a common denominator among these people.

Kidney stones occur in all age and social groups. They occur most frequently in persons between the ages of 20 and 45 years. Also, men are more frequent victims than women.

Many times, a doctor will advise a patient to reduce his intake of calcium-rich foods. Unfortunately, this does not solve the problem, for it is impossible to avoid all calcium in foods, and if the body is misusing calcium, the stone formations will occur eventually, regardless of efforts to avoid calcium in foods. Further, calcium is vital to our good health, and we all need a certain amount of this mineral in our diets.

Nephrosis—Kidney Disease in Children

A heart-breaking type of kidney disease is known as nephrosis. It is most common in children ranging between one and four years of age. Adult cases are rare. Nephrosis lasts anywhere from a few months to 5 years. It involves a basic loss of kidney function and shows itself in loss of appetite, no pep, swelling of the face around the eyes and swelling of the abdomen and lower extremities. A child stricken in this way becomes literally waterlogged and is severely handicapped. Chances for recovery are 50-50. He may recover and return to normal spontaneously. He may be left with permanent kidney damage. He may die. The cause of nephrosis is still unknown. It is not due to infection and it is not inherited.

One diet, given with encouraging results to children suffering from nephrosis, is outlined in the *American Journal of the Diseases of Children* (February, 1950). Fifteen children were involved. They were given liberal fluids to help flush out accumulated sodium; acid-ash fruit juices (cranberry, plum and prune) were used to establish the acidification of fluids and an acid-ash, high-protein diet (meat, eggs and cereal foods) was adhered to. The entire diet was salt-free. *Modern Medicine* (January 15, 1956) recommends a diet high in protein and calories and low in salt.

High Blood Pressure and the Kidneys

High blood pressure can be the result of kidney trouble. In the *Journal of the American Medical Association* (no date), Drs. Witman Walters and Nelson W. Barber cite 5 cases in which high blood pressure readings returned to normal after an affected kidney was removed. In the diseased kidney, as pointed out above, the arteries of the organ may be obstructed. In 57 cases of chronic kidney inflammation, seen by the same doctors, 26 were seen to have an elevation of blood pressure. Kidney extract has even been used experimentally to lower blood pressure.

Dangerous Effects of Drugs and Poisons

No one really seems to know what brings kidney trouble. Why should kidney stones hit one person and not another, why does nephrosis fell one child and skip his brother? Aside from the guesses logged above, *Time* magazine (March 2, 1959) says kidney disease can be caused by shock with heavy blood loss (after a severe accident or surgery), some severe infections, mismatched blood transfusions and many poisons. Carbon tetrachloride attacks the kidneys directly. Overdoses of aspirin and barbiturates affect the kidneys by overloading them, so that the victim can't void quickly enough. Streptomycin has an adverse effect, and doctors are warned against its use unless it is specifically needed. The sulfa drugs have also shown themselves deadly enemies of the kidneys.

Other drugs can have serious effects on the kidneys, too. For example, *Science News Letter* (July 2, 1955) printed the story of a 57-year-old woman being treated for high blood pressure with potassium thiocyanate, a quite powerful drug. After 6 weeks of treatment, the woman began to act oddly and neglect her personal appearance. Eventually, hospitalization was found necessary, and once there, the patient became assaultive and showed a persecution complex with suicidal tendencies. The condition was traced to the medication, which the kidneys could not remove from the body. An artificial kidney was required to do the job. The medication was immediately stopped and, luckily, the woman recovered. The medication in her system might have driven the woman hopelessly out of her mind or blocked the kidneys entirely, thus insuring death.

The *Practitioner* (March, 1953) says that acute respiratory infections often lead to kidney complications. Tonsillitis, scarlet fever and pneumonia are most common. The kidney complication does not occur immediately, at the height of infection, but later. So if one is longer than expected in recovering from a sore throat, cold or the like, a kidney infection should be watched for. The best policy is to avoid respiratory infections from the start. Keep a good supply of all vitamins, especially vitamins C and A, in the system, and get plenty of rest.

Lead Poisoning

Unsuspected Causes of Lead Poisoning

The *Journal of the American Medical Association* (January 21, 1961) described the case of 7 scrap metal workers who suffered lead poisoning while using torches to cut heavily painted steel bridge girders. All of them showed the classical symptoms of lead poisoning, including gagging, nausea, loss of appetite, muscular weakness, generalized aching and fatigability.

It was discovered, in due course, that the paint chipped from the girders contained 21.6 per cent lead. Samples of the air taken where the men were working contained 20 times the maximum allowable concentration of lead. Several of the men became ill after one week on the job, and all 7 were poisoned within 5 weeks.

Of course, none of these men knew he was being poisoned at the time. If only one of the men had actually become ill, the project might have gone on indefinitely, with lesser bits of the poison entering the bodies of the other workers, and perhaps not affecting them until some other weakness showed up in later years. It's only because so many were hit at exactly the same time that something was done. Cause and effect were obvious. But how often is it so obvious?

Do you recall the case of Clare Boothe Luce when she was ambassador to Italy? Twice, during her tenure, she returned to America for treatment of a mysterious ailment, which showed itself in symptoms such as nausea, loss of appetite, loosening of teeth, general weakness, etc. At long last, it was discovered to be arsenic poisoning from invisible flakes of paint falling from Mrs. Luce's bedroom ceiling into her morning cup of coffee.

These are two instances of unsuspected sources of poisoning. There are probably dozens which each of us faces every day. The exposure may not be long, it may not be concentrated enough to cause downright illness that can be observed. But who of us doesn't breathe the lead of gas fumes from car exhausts or inhale a mixture of a dozen industrial smokes which blanket almost every city or drink the chlorine and fluoride in our city water or eat the preservatives in our foods? We're being poisoned, in a more subtle way, just as surely as the steel workers or Mrs. Luce were. The sad and dangerous thing is that we aren't fully aware of what is happening to us. We don't get sick enough to do anything about it. We don't get stomach aches or loose teeth. In later years, we get the quiet cancers, the liver trouble, the poor circulation, the bad kidneys— things that we presume just happen.

Our only defense is a body healthy enough to fight when these poisonous invaders appear. This takes plenty of ammunition, in the form of vitamins and minerals in good supply when they are needed. The B complex and vitamin C are especially important in fighting such invaders. Fresh fruit, vegetables and rose hips are your best sources of vitamin C. The B vitamins occur plentifully in desiccated liver, brewer's yeast, wheat germ and the organ meats.

Lead Poisoning of Children

The ghost of lead poisoning due to children's eating painted plaster and woodwork is still very much alive. The *Chicago Daily News* of July 27, 1960, reported that the city health department recorded 193 cases and 17 deaths. Of course, the count must be similar in other big cities and proportionate everywhere.

The paint companies of the country long ago stopped using lead in their interior paints, because youngsters often chew on painted surfaces and sometimes eat fallen plaster that has been painted. However, many of the older homes and tenements in run-down districts still have walls and woodwork painted with these deadly paints. When the plaster falls or chips and sills splinter, the problem is acute if small children are around.

Parents moving into different quarters should pay particular attention to painted walls and sills. If they are badly worn, they should be patched or replaced and painted with the harmless paints that are available today.

A child who is experiencing lead poisoning shows symptoms of tiredness, vomiting and convulsions, and the reaction of the lead usually takes place in the summer in response to the action of ultraviolet rays of the sun. If your child should show such symptoms in summer, ask the doctor to check for lead poisoning. It could save his life.

Leukemia

Are We Progressing against Leukemia?

The blood disease which has created the greatest wave of fear and panic in modern man is leukemia. "Blood disease" is not exactly the accurate term. Leukemia is actually a disease of the organs which make the elements of the blood. However, it is identified in the minds of laymen as cancer of the blood, and the association is close enough to be considered applicable.

As explained in *Today's Health* (January, 1958), the body organs that manufacture the blood—the spleen, the lymph nodes, the liver and the bone marrow—"go on a frenzied spree, wildly producing white cells, many of which are abnormal, and reducing the elements needed for making red cells and the tiny platelets that prevent and stop bleeding. . . . Overworking the blood organs to achieve this superproduction results in swelling and tenderness around the liver, spleen and lymph glands of the neck, armpits, chest, abdomen and groin. . . ."

The white cells, usually the body's defense against infection, are utterly inefficient in leukemia patients, in spite of the great numbers of these cells which characterize the disease. Easy bruising and bleeding from delicate tissues in the nostrils and the gums occur because of the inefficiency of the platelets, which are supposed to halt such bleeding or prevent it entirely. Because of the red cell supply being inadequate, the duty red cells perform, that of transporting oxygen to the tissues, is never fully accomplished. As a result, the leukemia patient grows progressively paler, more tired and short of breath.

The Types of Leukemia

Children are attacked most frequently by a type of leukemia known as acute lymphatic leukemia. When the white cells are immature, the term "acute" is applied, and "lymphatic" leukemia means that the disease originates in the lymph glands. This type of leukemia has an extremely high mortality rate.

This same leukemia, when chronic (fully developed white cells), ordinarily strikes older persons and, in them, is more benign than other types of leukemia. Conversely, myelocytic leukemias, a type of "adult leukemia" which has its root in the bone marrow, resists treatment and appears quite hopeless.

The accepted treatments for leukemia are radiation, blood transfusions and chemicals. None of these is presumed to be a true cure.

How Science Is Meeting the Challenge

A sad fact about the currently attempted treatment of leukemia is that the radiation and chemotherapy, which are held to be most promising, are tied to the destruction principle. Instead of developing in the body a new strength which will help it to defend itself, these modes of therapy merely aim to destroy the leukemic cells. However, if the chemical or radiation dosage used is to be effective against the leukemia, it must also be so powerful that it destroys the ability of the bone marrow to manufacture blood cells. This being so, such treatment can only end in death to the victim—if not from the leukemia, then from the treatment. Time is the only advantage to be gained. If the damaged bone marrow can manage to produce new blood fast enough to keep up with or surpass leukemic cells' survival rate, the patient continues to live, but as this ability diminishes, the patient weakens toward death. Unquestionably, since the very tool for survival—the bone marrow—is being attacked by the treatment, the cards are stacked against the patient. He might gain a few more months or so, but will not recover.

Bone Marrow Removed

An effort to evade what appears to be the inevitable, lies in the work done by the New England Center Hospital and Tufts University Medical School. Experimentation there has aimed at a technique for removing a good part of the bone marrow while superdoses of nitrogen mustard (deadly poison used as a leukemia treatment) are given to kill cancerous cells. Then the marrow is injected back into the patient after the series of treatments has been completed, the hope being that the undamaged bone marrow will begin once more, once inside the patient, to manufacture wholesome red blood cells.

In an experiment with 5 patients described in the *New York Times* (February 22, 1955), the bone marrow was injected into the veins as described above. Three of the patients were said to have had brief remissions, but all 5 were dead as the report was made.

In the case of corticosteroids used to treat leukemia, the destructive principle is again employed. Here, the plan is to force acute leukemic blood cells into maturity and death by accelerating their old age, as it were. Leukemic cells are known to be slow to mature and hence have a greater staying power in the blood stream. They frequently divide before maturity, forming new, young leukemic cells, and these never really grow old.

Cortisone used effectively to mature these cells is necessary in such great amounts that it will force the normal cells to maturity and death much faster than it can do so to the leukemic ones. *Science News Letter* (April 7, 1956) estimated the difference in speed in this way: "The normal cells start to show the effects of the hormone in about 3 minutes. The leukemic cells are not visibly affected for about 45 minutes." It is apparently another losing fight.

Methyl GAG Can Kill as It Cures

Methyl GAG is another of this type of therapeutic measure which can kill as it cures. In this case, Dr. Emil Freireich, of the National Cancer Institute, spoke with hope of leukemic remissions of from 4 to 14 weeks (*Drug Trade News,* November 13, 1961). The rub is that, in patients with advanced neoplasms, clinical evaluation of methyl GAG revealed "impressive gastrointestinal and hemotological toxicity and in a few patients, severe hypoglycemia (low blood sugar)." A chemist producing the drug stated that the obvious goal is to produce similar drugs which would retain potency, but would have less toxicity.

A process which offered a different approach to the treatment of leukemia was reported in the February 22, 1955, issue of the

New York Times. A Toronto, Ontario, doctor, Charles Bardawill, M.D., piloted a project which used a hormone extracted from the pituitary glands of hogs, sheep and horses. The treatment was intended, through the injection of this hormone, to correct the normal body supply of alkaline phosphate, thrown out of balance by leukemia. Dr. Bardawill's treatment fought to restore body processes to their normal function, rather than to destroy, by other means, the white blood cells produced uncontrollably by leukemia victims.

During a 10-day course of treatment with this method, the usual tests are reported to have shown a trend toward recovery of the patients. There is no indication as to how long the trend continued. However, this attempt at positive therapy has apparently been short-lived. The above-described treatments are still preferred.

Laënnec, Rene Theophile Hyacinthe

One of the greatest aides to the science of physical diagnosis is the stethescope. Its developer was the French physician, Rene Theophile Hyacinthe Laënnec. Laënnec, born at Quimper, Brittany on February 17, 1781, re-

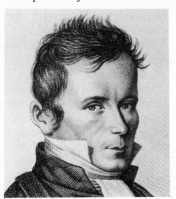

ceived his medical education from his uncle and such noted physicians of the time as Corvesart and Guillaume Dupuytren. After receiving his M. D. in 1804, his professional reputation began to grow with such force that in 1814 he was appointed editor-in-chief of the Journal de Medecine *and two years later became chief surgeon at the Hospital Necker. It was here that he first hit upon the idea for the device which was to make him famous. While examining a female patient, he discovered that he could not fully hear her heart beat due to her unusual stoutness. Folding a piece of paper into the form of a tube, and putting one end to his ear and the other on the chest of the patient, Laënnec found that he could now distinctly hear her heart beat. Further development of this crude instrument led to the modern-day stethescope and the auscultation (the act of listening to sounds within the body) method of physical diagnosis. Laënnec died in 1826, having contributed to medicine, in addition to the stethescope, much knowledge concerning the diseases of the thoracic cavity.*

There is talk of a vaccine against leukemia, but the very scientists who propose it are the first to admit that they are not sure what causes leukemia, and consequently, can't be sure that a vaccine can be made, nor that it would be effective. Meanwhile, the leukemia rate makes spectacular rises. The *New York Herald Tribune* (May 27, 1959) quoted the American Cancer Society as reporting a 300 per cent increase from 1930 to 1959. Only lung cancer has the edge on incidence and the hope of a cure for that disease is equally vague, it seems.

The Many Guesses

Guesses are numerous as to the actual cause of leukemia. *Scope* (November 19, 1958) headlined the proposition that a lack of an enzyme essential for normal growth is responsible when leukemia occurs. In the absence of this controlling enzyme, a new and metabolically different race of cells grows. If this be true, the answer suggested by Dr. William Dameshek, Chief of Hemotology at New England Center Hospital, Boston, is to modify, somehow, the metabolism of these cells and to replace the missing enzyme. Apparently, this job takes some time in the translation from theory to fact. Leukemia we still have with us, and no word since 1958 on the development of the missing enzyme or a means of modifying the metabolism of these cells.

In *Medical Science* (May 10, 1960), appeared Dr. Daniel Stowens' guess that diabetes and leukemia might be related. He found an insulin deficiency in the pancreas of leukemic children. Of 285 observed cases of leukemia in children, there was a 25 per cent incidence of diabetes in the family (in contrast to only 4 per cent in non-leukemic children), and the presence of abnormal amounts of sugar in the urine.

Dr. W. J. McCormick wrote in the *Journal of Applied Nutrition* (Vol. 14, No. 1, 2) of his conviction that smoking by pregnant women is a factor in the rising rate of leukemia in children. In support of his contention, Dr. McCormick quoted two cancer workers, Lawrence and Donlan (*Cancer Research,* 12: 900-904, December, 1952): ". . . The acute leukemias are an example of disease that may have such an origin (embryonic tissue damaged by carcinogenic agents). Leukemia seems to be increasing in recent years, especially in children under 5 years, suggestively due to carcinogenic stimulation in prenatal life."

Dr. McCormick believes that the carcinogenic factor mentioned is the neutralizing effect tobacco has on vitamin C. The fetus needs vitamin C and without it, malformation of the blood-making system in prenatal existence is quite possible.

A short squib in *Today's Health* (December, 1961) told of a virus present in the blood streams of leukemic rats infected with what is termed "virus-caused leukemia." The question now is whether one can pinpoint viruses as the cause of human leukemia. Some support of the virus theory appeared in the *British Medical Bulletin* (no date) where authors Stewart and Hewitt noted the very real increase in the leukemia rate and remarked that environmental factors must be considered. Virus is included among these.

Is It Modern Living?

A leukemia article, which appeared in the *Chicago Daily News* (December 7, 1960), cited a study in New York state which seems to show that "the modern way of life has something to do with it (leukemia). It increases in families as economic standards increase." Does this point to increased luxuries (so-called) in diet for the children, such as more sweets, more highly processed foods? Does it point to a greater alcohol consumption, greater cigarette consumption in teen-agers and adults? What do people who have enough money for more than the bare essentials, do with it that might influence the blood manufacturing process?

The most likely of all guesses on the cause of the current rise in leukemia is radiation. It might be from therapeutic X-ray as well as from fall-out after nuclear blasts. There are strong arguments which point to this possible cause as the most formidable one we will ever have to contend with. The *Journal of the American Medical Association* (January 16, 1960) carried a story which told of a survey of 6,473 children who had been given X-ray treatments since 1930, and "in agreement with previous investigations, the incidence of leukemia was higher among irradiated than among non-irradiated children."

Expectant mothers have long been warned against submitting to X-ray, especially in the pelvic area, either for treatment or diagnosis, unless there is a medical reason so urgent that waiting until the birth of the child is not practical. Much evidence has been published in medical journals showing the link between leukemia in children, as well as other congenital defects in newborn babies, and prenatal use of radiation.

The Rise Is World-Wide

The rise in leukemia has been world-wide and Dr. Shields Warren, Professor of Pathology at Harvard Medical School, cited this rise as a possible result of greater radiation exposures all over the world (*Scope,* February 12, 1958). Dr. Warren stated that he believed, "there is a threshold of radiation necessary to produce leukemia . . . above 50 to 100 Roentgens for adults . . . probably less for infants in utero (in the womb)."

Studies of cities in Japan which were bombed with nuclear explosives, show that increases of leukemia have been induced by this radiation, according to Dr. Warren. He said that two per cent of those exposed to a single dose of 100 to 500 Roentgens (a large amount) would become leukemic. He added that, ". . . there seems to be a wave of such leukemia 5 to 10 years after exposure."

There is no sure way to know if the genetic effects of radiation exposure due to fall-out and direct exposure to nuclear explosions will afflict future generations with serious blood disorders until several generations have had time to be born. We do not know what dosage could have such effects. We do know that strontium 90, for one, is a radioactive element of fall-out which seeks the blood-manufacturing bone marrow and can disrupt that entire process by the changes in the cells that it can cause. Increased fall-out can only enhance the danger.

Are We Completely Helpless?

As we see the leukemia picture at present, the outlook is grim. One can only do one's best to avoid the suspected causes of this terrible disease, for once it takes hold, recovery through currently recognized medical implements is not very promising. Studiously avoid any unnecessary radiation, insure a generous calcium intake through calcium-rich foods and food supplements, including bone meal both as a decoy for strontium 90 and a means of growing healthy strong bones; keep a high vitamin C level in the system, and eliminate the foods which are processed with possible leukemiogenic substances.

We are also on record, once more, as favoring—no, urging!—the thorough and serious investigation of all unorthodox treatments for all types of cancer. We can see no real basis for organized medicine's ridiculing the Gerson treatment or Krebiozen or the Drosnes-Lazenby theories, when nothing demonstrably better has been produced, in spite of the millions invested in approved cancer research throughout the country.

A Dangerously Narrow Attitude

Considering the admitted puzzle leukemia presents to medical researchers, we cannot suppress some irritation and dismay at the typical attitude of the medical men, described in a story by Eldon Roark, which appeared in the *Memphis* (Tennessee) *Press Scimitar* (November 17, 1960). Mr. Roark told of a friend, Robert L. Miller, who was suddenly and seriously afflicted with leukemia. One diagnosis after another confirmed that fact. He was in a most critical condition, exhibiting some of the worst symptoms of leukemia.

Because he was so desperately ill, a new experimental drug was used on him—cyclophosphamide. In 10 days, Robert was much better—well enough to go home. Once there, he began to read about leukemia and became convinced of the value of diet in preventing a recurrence. He took to eating raw, fresh vegetables because, "Those writers convinced me that cooking destroys vitamins." He also ate plenty of meat. That, of course, was cooked.

Meanwhile, he kept taking the cyclophosphamide pills, along with the good diet. After 3 months, he checked out as normal. The leukemia appeared to be gone!

The columnist friend was astounded by the story. He checked it out at the hospital. It was all true. Robért had had leukemia and it did appear to be arrested—the doctor wouldn't say "cured." Aside from the new drug, the doctor credited Robert's "attitude." He was unafraid. He kept working and remained cheerful.

"Yes, but what about the importance of raw vegetables?" asked the columnist of the attending physicians. "The doctors smile and shake their heads. They say Robert has become a food faddist. They don't think raw vegetables have played an important part in the case. 'Oh, food is important,' one of them said. 'You must have a balanced diet. But beyond that . . .' he shrugged."

Leeuwenhoek, Anton Van

Anton Van Leeuwenhoek, the Dutch biologist recognized as the Father of Microscopy, was born at Delft, Netherlands, on October 24, 1632, and died at his birthplace on August 26,

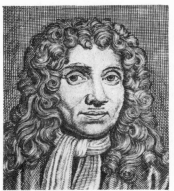

1723. The work of Leeuwenhoek can best be evaluated if one considers what a loss modern science and medicine would be at without the use of the microscope. Although Leeuwenhoek is not credited with the actual discovery of the microscope, his development of the early instruments which could be held close to the eye and could magnify objects up to 160 times their actual size, paved the way for the construction of the modern-day microscope. Yet his greatest contribution does not lie in this gift to scientific investigation. The reason for his fame is credited to his investigations of those objects eluding detection by the human eye. Thus through his perfection of the microscope he was able to make important advances in the observation and description of the development of bacteria and such organisms as the ant and mussels. Of equal importance are his profound findings on human and animal blood cells and the flow of blood through the capillaries.

How long Robert will continue to be well, we can't say. We can't say for certain whether it was the pills, the diet or both that brought him back to apparent health. But neither can his doctors!

How can they say with such assurance that diet was not a factor in his recovery? If cyclophosphamide were solely responsible, there should be no talk of leukemia drugs being deadly and only mildly palliative. Here is a man who had the worst symptoms. He took a drug and the results were astounding. It was followed by a remission that had already lasted a year when the story was written. Why should researchers be fooling with bone marrow extracts if a drug they already have can do this!

We object to the doctor's slotting of Robert Miller in a food faddist pigeonhole because he began to eat raw vegetables. He believes that cooking destroys vitamins. Well, it does, and any of the doctors who snickered at his eating habits would have to agree with Robert on this point. Furthermore, vitamins and minerals are essential to good tissues and bones—the tissues of the organs and the bones that make healthy blood. Is it faddism for Robert Miller to take the obvious precautions for saving himself from a relapse? We can only hope others stricken with leukemia, who are so fortunate as to have some improvement in their condition, will have the good sense to do the same. To those who are well and healthy, we think Robert Miller's story is an excellent clue to a preventive course against leukemia's ever striking.

We are also convinced of the likelihood that the answer to leukemia's rise lies in some new development or usage of modern living. True, radioactive fall-out is a strong factor, but that doesn't account for the big rise, and what was raising the rate before the first nuclear explosion?

Prevention of leukemia seems to us to be the most important and the most promising course to follow. Let us check out, one at a time, even the slightest possibility that the things we eat and the way we prepare them, the air we breathe, the jobs we have, the habits we are advertised into adopting, the polluted waters we are given to drink, are free of suspicion. Time enough then to seek some exotic factor. Let's start with basics. We are convinced that we will have to go no further.

While waiting for this kind of research to be done, eat foods as close as possible to their natural occurrence. Take brewer's yeast, desiccated liver and wheat germ for maintaining healthy blood-manufacturing organs, and maintain your overall health with good diet as your best protection against all ailments.

Light

What Is the Effect of Daylight on Health?

Have you ever stopped to think that living behind glass, as most of us do (spectacles and windows in houses and cars) might have a very important effect on daily health? Has it ever occurred to you that possibly, plain, unfiltered daylight taken in through your eyes (with no glass intervening) has a lot to do with other organs of your body in addition to your eyes?

We recently saw an article about a man who is building a house in which all windows will be made of plastic rather than glass. We discovered that this man is a well-known photographer, and surely a photographer should know more than the rest of us about the effect of light. We discovered that this man, John Ott, had written a book explaining his ideas. The name of it is *My Ivory Cellar,* and it is published by Twentieth Century Press, Chicago.

Mr. Ott shares so many of our ideas on gardening and the environmental causes of things like plant disease, that we were immediately fascinated by the story of his work, which is time-lapse photography. For those who have never seen any of the films made by Mr. Ott, we will explain very simply what time-lapse photography is. It consists of taking a series of motion pictures spaced at intervals throughout a day, a week, a month or longer depending upon what you want to photograph. If you want to photograph the opening of a morning glory bud into a flower, you set your time-lapse camera so that it automatically takes a picture of the bud every minute or every 5 minutes or whatever time you decide upon. After the flower is fully open, you turn off the camera and develop the film. When you run it in a movie projector, you see the bud opening before your eyes, very rapidly, for all the movement involved is concentrated in the few minutes which it takes to run off the film. So, what actually took perhaps an hour or several hours or several days, flashes briefly before your eyes.

Mr. Ott's breath-taking pictures of flowers and plants have been widely used in advertising and films, for the sight of a flower unfolding or a leaf growing or a root descending slowly but surely into the ground are inspiring and dramatic pictures. So far as science is concerned, the hitherto unknown facts that can be learned from time-lapse photography are almost limitless.

Photography Yields Clues to Hay Fever

For instance, Mr. Ott was troubled with hay fever. He decided to study ragweed pollen—the worst offender. Doctor friends told him that irritation of the nose membranes causing hay fever arises

493

from simple contact with the outer surfaces of a grain of ragweed pollen. With his time-lapse camera, Mr. Ott discovered that, by adding some nasal secretion from a person with hay fever, he could make the ragweed pollen grains exude drops of water. Nasal secretion from persons not susceptible to hay fever would not produce this result.

"In all," he says, "I made approximately 12 such experiments, half hay fever and half non-hay fever samples, and in each specimen from a person *not* subject to hay fever, the results were completely negative—no droplets given off. The ragweed pollen was from exactly the same source of supply in each instance.

"What does this mean?" he goes on. "It is hard to say definitely, but I am hopeful that it may show that the body chemistry of people who suffer from hay fever is just right to cause ragweed pollen to give off these little droplets of fluid, which in turn might possibly be the irritating factor to the nasal membranes, rather than the mere contact with the outer surface of the dormant grains of pollen themselves. If this is so, then the exact chemical balance of the particular individual that causes this activity might be altered by raising or lowering such things as the sugar ratio or acidity (pH) or something else vital to ragweed pollen. Possibly, hay fever could then be prevented, rather than trying to cure it or counteract it with medicines after the irritation has set in."

As might be expected, experts on hay fever ridiculed Mr. Ott's findings, declared that they could not possibly have any significance for hay fever, reminded him that they had read all the books on hay fever and had not found such comment, so obviously it couldn't be true. However, there is much evidence which shows that hay fever, along with asthma and many other disorders, are undoubtedly the result of an unbalance in blood chemistry.

Light Important to Flowers

To come back to the morning glory bud which was to be photographed as it opened, there were endless difficulties. No matter in what background Mr. Ott placed his morning glory plants for photographing, the buds dropped before they opened.

The morning glories outside bloomed fine. But the ones inside his greenhouse would not open. One morning, when he was up well before sunrise, he noticed that the morning glory flowers outside were already open. So they were not morning-bloomers after all—but, instead, opened their flowers during the night! Perhaps this had something to do with his failure. That night, Mr. Ott took all the lights he used to photograph flowers outside and hung them around the outside morning glories. Next morning, all these buds had dropped, too!

The answer was the light used for taking the time-lapse pictures. Morning glories buds must have a night of total darkness, it seems, if they are going to open. Since the pictures had to be taken, Mr. Ott experimented with different lights and found that, if he used a blue light, the morning glories would open properly. So not only was the amount of light important, but the kind of light!

This is just one sample of the many fascinating details of his work with plants. His thinking naturally led him to speculate on the possible effects the different kinds, intensities and exposures to light might have on animal life.

Growing a pumpkin under fluorescent lights, he discovered that the *female flowers* of the pumpkin vine turned brown and dropped off. The male flowers grew vigorously, but no pumpkin could be produced, since there must be pollination from one flower to the other. The next year, he used a different kind of fluorescent light (a daylight kind) and found that all the *male flowers* of the pumpkin vine dropped off and only the female ones remained. In later experi-

---

Lister, Joseph

Joseph Lister, an English surgeon and founder of antiseptic surgery was born at Upton, Essex on April 5, 1827. Upon graduation from the University College Hospital in London, Lister

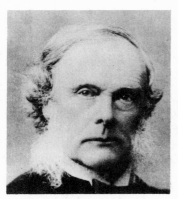

turned his attentions to the study of a way of combating the infections which would occur as a consequence of the surgical operations of his day. Even the most minor operations resulted in infection and in many cases death followed. Such was the plight of surgical patients before Lister's discovery that these infections were being caused by bacteria. Using various types of carbolic-acid spray, Lister was able to prevent the germs in the air from invading the open wounds. He later learned that this antiseptic procedure also had to be applied to the personnel and instruments in the operating room. Strict adherence to Lister's antiseptic methods reduced the stigma of infection associated not only with surgery but also with the cleansing of minor wounds and abrasions. This highly significant contribution to medicine earned for Joseph Lister the title of Father of Modern Surgery.

ments with chinchillas, he found that, by varying the kind of light the mother chinchilla lived in before the birth of her litters, one could control the sex of the babies.

Effect of Light on the Body's Glands

Such discoveries could mean only one thing—that light has a powerful effect on the body's glands. Sure enough, Mr. Ott tells us, "It is now known that the lengthening night periods cause certain glandular changes in birds that are responsible for their seasonal migration. People in the poultry business turn lights on in the hen houses at night to lengthen the daylight period, so the hens lay more eggs. Originally, it was thought this merely kept the hens awake longer, but more recent research has proven that increased egg production is attained *as a result of the light reacting through the chicken's eye on its pituitary gland.*"

So light coming through the eyes reacts on the pituitary gland! In the hen, at least. The pituitary gland is the master gland in the body which controls all the others. Hence, says Mr. Ott, "Different types of light and lighting conditions, ranging from natural unfiltered sunlight to various kinds of artificial light or natural sunlight filtered through different kinds of glass or light reflected from different colored interior decorations in a room, could affect the physical well-being of an individual."

Applying His Theories to Living

In the last chapter of his book, Mr. Ott tells us about the astonishing results he got when he began to apply to his own life some of the facts he had turned up about the relation of light to life! For many years an arthritic, he discovered that his arthritis improved when he spent long hours in the outside daylight *without his glasses.* This meant that there was no glass or other man-made shield between his eyes and the light. (He avoided getting sunburned.) Later, he found that the condition of his eyes had improved greatly. Sore throats and colds became less frequent. Friends who tried his experiment reported beneficial results for disorders ranging from bursitis to bleeding gums.

"One day, I met a man who had previously taken a number of still photographs for me," he writes. "He had meanwhile been on an assignment that required an intense amount of artificial lighting in a large interior area. He was an extreme diabetic and, while on this job, had a severe attack of his diabetes, which resulted in the bursting of some blood vessels in the retina of both eyes. As a result, he became almost totally blind and could just distinguish the difference between day and night. He had been in this condition for approximately 4 years, during which time he had numerous additional blood vessels burst in his eyes. He continued to work for the same company, but in the photographic darkroom where he was put in charge of processing film."

Friend's Eyes Achieved Miraculous Improvement

Mr. Ott goes on to tell us that he explained his theory to this friend, who arranged to spend as much time as possible outside from then on. Six months later, he had not had a single blood vessel burst and could see enough to follow the vague outline of the sidewalk when he was walking.

"If the theory of the importance of the full spectrum of sunlight energy proves to be true, it will necessitate some changes in our present way of living," says Mr. Ott. "However, it certainly will not mean that everybody will have to go back to living in caves or grass huts. It will mean using certain types of plastic or glass that will permit the transmission of ultraviolet and shorter wave lengths of light energy. Unfortunately, at the present time, the trend on the part of manufacturers of plastic has been to add a substance that stops the transmission of ultraviolet light, so that the light-transmission qualities of plastic will be as nearly like glass as possible. This substance also reduces the deterioration of plastic from ultraviolet radiation. It will also mean that artificial lights will have to be developed that more closely give off the same distribution of wave length energy as natural sunlight. . . .

"It will mean the reappraisement of the possible usefulness of such glands and organs of the body as the appendix, tonsils, adenoids, gall bladder and others often removed with the thought of good riddance when there has been something wrong with any of them.

"New interest and enthusiasm should be stimulated in all outdoor activities and sports. It should emphasize the importance of such organizations as the Boy Scouts, Girl Scouts, Campfire Girls, Isaac Walton League and others devoted to outdoor activities. It should encourage people to be outdoors as much as possible and without eyeglasses or dark glasses. Some companies might even want to consider changing the regular working hours in order to lengthen the lunch hour and permit employees to get outdoors during the daylight hours, particularly during the winter season. The general attitude toward walking a mile or more to school or to work may change so that such a walk could be looked on as a pleasure, rather than a terrific hardship. More people may find it fun to eat their meals on an open porch or use the backyard barbecue. Winter vacations for people living in colder climates will undoubtedly become less undesirable, particularly if it is possible to go to the sunny southland for a midwinter outdoor break. It should not be too difficult to find many more ways for outdoor living."

Liver Extract

The Value of Applying Liver Externally

There are few foods we eat that claim to be superior to liver for nutritional value. Its importance as an arsenal of B vitamins alone would be enough to put it high on a list of desirables. However, new discoveries on the therapeutic value of liver and its various forms (liver extract, desiccated liver) are constantly being made. Here is some of the most exciting information we have on the subject. We are certain that it will encourage you to add more liver to the week's menu at your house.

For no reason known to us, researchers are beginning to experiment with the application of nutrients directly upon the site of infection or irritation. Salves and sprays have been made of vitamin E and vitamin C, and their effects have been remarkably good. Wounds and skin ulcers that have not responded to any treatment over periods of months and even years, yield quickly to topical application of these vitamins. Now they're using liver extract topically and the results are equally impressive.

In an article which appeared in a German medical journal, *Hautarzt* (11:86, 2, 1960), by W. K. Meyerhoff, we read of one clinician's experience with this form of therapy. We think Dr. Meyerhoff's findings can be of immense value to doctors and patients everywhere, and we hope that readers will call their doctors' attention to this article in the hope that the news of this therapy might spread.

Accidental Discovery

Dr. Meyerhoff discovered the value of topically applied liver extract quite by accident. He tells of how, in 1954, he read of the value of liver extract, given by injection, in treating acute thrombophlebitis. He was looking for some treatment which would be beneficial in treating surface ulcerations, so he wondered if the liver extract might not be the measure he was seeking.

A 69-year-old woman with a 10-year history of an ulcerated left leg, which became progressively worse, was seen by Dr. Meyerhoff. She also suffered recurrent paralysis of the entire left side and heart muscle weakness. The ulceration resulted in severe pain which necessitated light pain killers. The ulcer at the tibia (the big bone between the knee and the ankle) was the size of the palm of a man's hand and another, just above the side of the ankle, was the size of an egg. There was also an ulcer at the heel. All gave off abundant putrid secretion. Applying the liver extract directly to the ulcers was decided upon, due to the patient's severe dropsy, which made the buttock injection, usually used to administer liver extract, inappropriate in this case. Dr. Meyerhoff cleansed the ulcers with 3 per cent solution of hydrogen peroxide. Then, a dressing which was saturated with liver extract was applied. The extract had been diluted in a saline solution in the proportion of one part extract to four parts saline. (The doctor says he hit on the idea of diluting the liver extract for strictly economic reasons. Luckily, the ratio proved to be just right and has been used by him ever since.) The surrounding area was covered with zinc ointment, and the dressing itself was covered with "lawn" (gauze bandage) which acted as a moist chamber. This was left on for 24 hours.

At the first change of dressing, an extensive clearing of the injured area was observed and the severe pain which had previously been present was practically gone! (This remission of pain has since come to be characteristic of the treatment, though the reason for it is not known.) After 48 hours, the surface was completely clean and covered over with fresh "blood flecks." After 14 days, granulation came up to skin level. A complete cure was attained in 21 days. In the beginning of the treatment, the dressing was changed every day, then every other day.

After this first experience, Dr. Meyerhoff decided to try a controlled experiment to test more fully the value of externally applied liver extract. Three of 6 cases of skin ulcer were treated with injections of liver extract and 3 by application of the extract directly onto the sore. The 3 who were treated locally were cured quickly, just as in the case described above. Those treated by injection were not affected (except for a clearing of the area and some slight, loose granulation), even though every other phase of the local treatment, excepting the application of the liver to the sore itself, was followed.

Severe Osteomyelitis Responds

Dr. Meyerhoff then described several illustrative cases in which the power of externally applied liver extract could be shown. One involved a 54-year-old miner. The man had suffered a fracture of the tibia 12 years before consulting Dr. Meyerhoff. Osteomyelitis (inflammation of the bone) had developed, with an ulcer of the skin about 4 inches long by an inch wide, which showed no signs of healing in spite of several attempted skin grafts. The patient could not walk on the leg due to the severe pain involved. He became an invalid. The case was diagnosed as hopeless, and it was recommended that the leg be amputated.

Dr. Meyerhoff followed the previously described course of treatment beginning in May of 1955. The effect of the liver extract was, at first, rapid, then slower, but steady. By March, 1956, the 4-inch sore was the size of a dime. By September, it was the size of a pea.

The patient's pain diminished almost from the first days of treatment. After about 4 weeks, being free from pain, he had fully regained his ability to move about. During the entire period of treatment, the surface of the ulcer was kept entirely free from infection. The patient, who had been a complete invalid for 12 years, was able to resume light agricultural work. No other treatment was used, only the liver extract.

From 1954 to the time the article was written, Dr. Meyerhoff treated 40 such cases, varying, of course, in degrees of seriousness. Without exception, all cases responded to the treatment and were completely cured.

Liver Extract for Burns and Acne

Burns responded very well to the application of liver extract. Healing of large injured areas which formerly needed many weeks to heal, was accomplished within a few days. The scarring commonly associated with such burns was eliminated almost completely. The case history given to support this assertion concerned a 6½-year-old child. He received second and third degree burns of the left buttock, in an area about 4 inches by 3 inches. About two-thirds of the area was a third degree burn. Within 72 hours of the application of liver extract 3 times to the area, total healing took place. Only one small, light scar, the size of a dried pea, remained.

In treating serious eczema, liver extract proved to be almost miraculous. A 4½-year-old girl who, since birth, had suffered with chronic oozing eczema was brought to Dr. Meyerhoff. She had undergone almost constant treatment at a university skin clinic, without success. She had been given several series of internal and external treatments with cortisone. Her lack of success was apparent in the severe oozing eczema of her face, body and all extremities.

At first, Dr. Meyerhoff tried cortisone salve for 24 days. No effect. He then used the dressing with liver extract, and there was *complete clearing after two dressings!* At the same time, there was rapid improvement in her formerly poor health condition.

For the treatment of burns, eczema and other skin problems, such as acne (a favorable response, with skin clearance within 3 weeks, as a rule), an ointment can be used—liver extract mixed into a nonirritant base. It is more convenient, but no less effective. The ointment is sold in Germany under the trade name Hepaderm, but we do not know if it is available in the United States at this time.

Rarely Fails

Dr. Meyerhoff points out that his paper does not discuss failure in the use of topical liver extract. The fact is that it rarely fails—only once in his experience did healing fail to take place, and that was a case of acne vulgaris. The treatment depends entirely upon the activation of the tissues, so that they can repulse the invasion of infection naturally. The liver extract does not kill the bacteria which cause the problem. Actually, healthy tissue growing rapidly merely forces the infection from the site.

The problem of toxicity does not exist with topically applied liver extract. It is a natural medication which can do no harm. No need to worry about dosage (except that there must be enough) nor side effects. Whatever amount you use is safe and cannot cause any side effects. It is the type of medication we advocate whenever its use is possible or feasible.

If we are given a choice, however, between using a safe medication for curing an ailment and using a healthful food to prevent an ailment, we will certainly choose the latter every time. If using liver extract on a sore spot will help it to heal, may not frequent inclusion of the same liver in the diet prevent the problem in the first place? We believe it will. The same elements that make liver extract capable of stimulating tissue growth and blood quality are available in the piece of beef liver that you can broil as the main course at any of the day's 3 meals. These valuable elements are also present in desiccated liver.

Desiccated Liver and Liver Extract

The difference between liver extract and desiccated liver is small. Liver extract is the result of several filtration processes after the fresh liver has been ground with water, then mixed with various percentages of alcohol, then dried, or dehydrated, and mixed with about one-tenth of its weight of sodium chloride (salt). Desiccated liver is liver, pure and simple, nothing added or taken away. The fresh livers are dried in a vacuum, not exceeding 60°, and that's all. Desiccated liver equals about one-fourth, by weight, of the fresh liver from which it was made.

Many of our readers tell us of the problems they have in treating ailments such as those described by Dr. Meyerhoff. They complain of years of doctoring with no result, and of unfortunate side effects from medications such as cortisone, aspirin, X-ray, etc. We think these people, and any others who have skin diseases or sores that won't heal, due to osteomyelitis or a similar ailment, should ask their doctors to try liver extract as a therapeutic agent locally applied.

If, for some reason, the doctor should refuse to use liver extract in this way, you might try powdered desiccated liver, made into a paste with water, on your own. It can't do any harm, and its similarity to liver extract should make it just as effective.

Meantime, if such problems do not affect you, continue to get all the liver you can—fresh and desiccated—to help keep yourself in good health and free from skin disorders of all types.

Margarine

Our Answer to the Margarine Question

A question we frequently hear is how do we feel about margarines, since there are many new margarine products on the market, advertised as making the earlier products obsolete? We feel the same about margarines as we did before: they are hydrogenated, contain synthetic preservatives, synthetic colorings, synthetic flavorings and synthetic nutrients. We oppose additives in processed foods, especially synthetic additives, so our objections to the use of margarine by the health-conscious person still stand. If you must use a spread or solid shortening, "the 70-cent spread" is certainly to be preferred.

Probably the greatest factor in increasing margarine sales was the decision in most state legislatures to permit the coloring of margarine at the factory. For many years, margarine came to the housewife looking like cold cream, with a perle or envelope of coloring that was intended to be mixed by the housewife until the whole thing looked just like butter. The inconvenience and the unappetizing look of the white margarine took their toll in margarine sales. It was worth the few extra cents to have butter, rather than go through all of that mess.

In the post-World War I years, the battle began in earnest to allow the sale of colored margarine in every state. The fight was bitter in New York state, where dairymen saw an end to butter profits and a chain reaction ending in lowered revenues all the way around. In spite of all their efforts, in 1952, colored margarine sales were legalized in New York. Soon every state but Minnesota and Wisconsin was allowing butter-colored margarine to be sold.

Margarine Outsold Butter

It's no wonder that the dairymen were worried. The margarine price was attractive, and so was the packaging. Margarine packages looked just like butter packages, only better. And the margarine was always spreadable. By 1958, *Chemical Week* (April 19, 1958) estimated that margarine was outselling butter by more than 100 million pounds per year.

With such a fat goose to lay profitable eggs, it is not surprising that legislation allowing colored margarine was pushed through. The dairymen were fighting all alone, but there are many groups who get a slice of the margarine pie. They all lobbied and influenced as best they could to cash in on the margarine profits. Remember, for the 1,500 million pounds of margarine sold, somebody had to supply: 24 trillion units of synthetic vitamins A and D, 3 million pounds of

502

mono- and di-glycerides, 37.5 million pounds of salt, 300,000 pounds of artificial flavor and coloring agents, 1.05 million pounds of sodium benzoate and 2.5 million pounds of lecithin. Regardless of the reasons given by legislatures for allowing colored margarine into our lives, no one can deny that somebody is making plenty of money from the scheme. Even before 1958, that same magazine (February 27, 1954) noted that "nearly 25 per cent of all soybean oil produced in the United States and a slightly lower percentage of the cottonseed oil output—winds up in oleo."

To make vegetable oils stand firm, as they do in margarine, and keep them from spoiling, as they are kept in margarines, they must be hydrogenated. This process calls for infusing the unsaturated fat molecules in the oil with hydrogen, which turns them into saturated fats. The body cannot use the fats in this saturated form. Increased consumption of saturated fats is, indeed, blamed by many for the increase in heart ailments in the United States. Cholesterol and margarine had almost become interchangeable terms.

The Corn Oil Margarines

To alter this concept, it was decided to incorporate unsaturated fats into the final product and take due notice of their salutary effect on the heart. The *Wall Street Journal* (October 19, 1960) told the story of the new scramble to shake off the cholesterol label. One company, upon introducing its corn oil product, wrote this in its stockholders report: "Some medical findings support the opinion that corn oil is especially effective in reducing blood cholesterol levels and, since a high blood cholesterol level is believed by many to be an important factor associated with coronary heart disease, corn oil is expected to play a more prominent role in the American diet."

What the reader was not likely to realize was that the corn oil must be unsaturated to avoid this cholesterol tie-in. Hydrogenated corn oil is as dangerous to good health as any other hydrogenated oil. The manufacturer did not make it clear how much of the corn oil used would be unsaturated, if any.

Later, other products were introduced, with their packages bearing life-like pictures of golden corn. One product advertises that the corn oil in its margarine "has never been hardened by hydrogenation." However, one discovers, upon careful investigation, that, while the claim is true about the corn oil, cottonseed and soybean oils are also present, and *they have been hydrogenated.*

Another product has an even more subtle gimmick. It claims to be "100 per cent corn oil," and it is—but part of the corn oil in it has been hydrogenated to make it solid. The shape of margarine is a dead giveaway. If oil is not hydrogenated, it is liquid, not solid. Unhydrogenated corn oil comes in a bottle, not a stick.

Other Gimmicks

Not to overlook the sales potential to be had in hinting at the health value of the new margarines, without actually claiming such a value, one company advertised, "your doctor can tell you about the special nutritional benefit of liquid corn oil in your daily meals." The implication being, of course, that your doctor will extend and elaborate the statements made on the health value of the margarine product.

Still intent on catching the brass ring of the good-health-margarine tie-in, in *Today's Health* (June, 1959), an American Medical Association publication, a manufacturer ran an ad for a new margarine product that could only, it was advertised, be bought in a drug store. The name was so designed as to be inevitably linked with the medical profession and the advertising copy was intended to reassure the public that the needs of those who have special diet problems would be met by this product. "If your doctor has advised a change in your diet, you and your whole family will welcome (it). . . . eliminates the chore of preparing special dishes for one member of the family." Actually, few, if any, special diet problems would be solved by this or any other margarine product.

The Objectionable Additives

Almost all margarines have added salt in them. One or two offer an unsalted alternate, but they sell salted margarine as the prime product. If one is to eat salted margarine, one might as well eat hydrogenated margarine, if heart trouble is involved. The salt is as dangerous as hydrogenated fats would be.

The just-right corn-yellow of the margarines is no accident, nor is it a natural phenomenon. It's due to dyes. *Food Technology* (May, 1954) carried a report which said: "Although carotene is the principal natural pigment in butter, it is quite common practice to supplement the natural coloring with annato extract, the 'certified' coal-tar colors F, D, C_3 and C_4, or carotene. Margarine is colored principally with coal-tar dyes or carotene." Coal-tar dyes have been found to be cancer-causing. Avoidance of any product which uses them is the least one can do to preserve one's health. Margarine would be off our list on this count alone, even if there were no other objectionable contents.

But, of course, there are other ingredients to which we object. Artificial flavorings are sheer chemical approximations of what the product should taste like. How they react in the body is anybody's guess. The same holds true for emulsifiers, texture agents, preservatives, etc. One would have as hard a time breaking down the individual synthetic components of margarine as one would those of commercial white bread. The processes by which these other additives are manufactured involves still more synthetics, and to unscramble them would involve the services of an extremely capable biochemist.

The Anti-Spatter Agent Epidemic

We cannot begin to consider individual companies who include in their formulae gimmicks intended to attract wavering consumers to their specific margarine product. For example, a British-Dutch margarine manufacturer thought he really had something in his anti-spatter ingredient. His salt-free margarine would not subject the housewife to the annoying and dangerous fat-spattering during frying. It was discovered that this relatively new development was responsible for a mysterious skin disease that hit thousands of Dutchmen in August and September of 1960. "The patients showed an extensive rash, frequently involving the mucosae, accompanied by fever and severe itching . . . The similarity of the epidemic with the one described in West Germany in 1958 . . . was noted," said *Archives of Dermatology* (May, 1961).

The article goes on to say: "The factory immediately stopped the production of the margarine, and all packages with the new margarine were taken back from the stores and the consumers . . . In the following weeks, thousands of cases were reported by general practitioners who had been requested to do so by radio. In Rotter-

---

Mendel, Gregor Johann

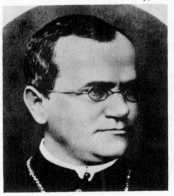

    The man responsible for our present day understanding of the fundamental laws of heredity is Gregor Johann Mendel. He was born in Heinzendorf, Czechoslovakia on July 22, 1822, and in 1843 entered the Augustinian Order of Monks. His education in mathematics and natural science was gained at the University of Vienna and after completion of this training, he returned to his Order to become a teacher at the Realschule at Brünn. It was here that Mendel carried on his famous breeding experiments with peas and beans showing how living organisms inherit certain characteristics and features from their parents and direct ancestors. Through these experiments, Mendel formulated his "Mendelian Laws"— the foundation for the science of genetics.

dam, 44 of the 1,200 cases were hospitalized. In the entire country, 16,250 cases were reported, although the total number of patients was probably over 50,000." When the anti-spatter agent (called an emulgator, "ME18") was removed, the epidemic disappeared within a few weeks.

No One Knows Exactly Why

It was not known exactly why this reaction should have occurred. As the *Archives* article put it, "The explanation of the pathogenesis is probably as far off as that of many drugs causing skin rashes, although nobody doubts their causative role."

Many of the processed foods we eat contain strange, and probably dangerous, compounds. Who knows whether the heart disease, the diabetes, the ulcer, the arthritis in this or that individual is the result of a food additive taken in daily for years and years? Those Dutchmen and Germans were lucky that their problem turned up as an epidemic. If a few isolated citizens had come down with a skin disease, chances are that no investigation would have been forthcoming, no one would have checked the anti-spatter agent. The margarine would still be on the market with its dangerous formula intact. The few people adversely affected by it, might go on using it, wondering what strange malady they'd contacted, never linking their favorite margarine to their problem.

We Americans operate that way. We get one cold after the other and call it virus. We blame it on weather, or on personal contact, or anything but our food. Heart disease goes up and we blame that on tension and fast living. Heart patients give up a lot of things before they change their diet. Kids get shots against polio. Their parents refuse to believe that the high sugar intake of American children could be responsible for the polio rate.

Does our enormous consumption of margarine have anything to do with increased disease? Who can say? We know that many of margarine's ingredients are unhealthful. They could be responsible, but unless we have an epidemic, or unless someone is actually stricken fatally immediately upon consumption of the product, margarine will never be indicted as a cause of ill health. But more than many other foods, margarine bears the earmarks of an undesirable product: it is made up of many synthetic ingredients and is put through a great deal of processing which has an even more adverse effect on its final form. Speaking from a health point of view, we can see no excuse for the use of margarine, let alone any advantage to it.

Meats

How Red Should Hamburger Be?

The *Pi Beta Phi* sorority of Northwestern University had an interesting dinner on November 7, 1960. It was so interesting that it made the *Chicago* (Illinois) *Sunday Tribune* (November 27, 1960) under the headline: "Sorority Food Poisons 44 at N.U.; Plan Suit." Who was suing whom? The city of Evanston, Illinois, sued the meat company which supplied the hamburger for the sorority's meatballs. As the gang sat munching away, 39 coeds and 5 waiters began to experience a flushing of the arms and legs, face and neck. They were treated at the student health center and two were overnight patients at Evanston Hospital.

A checkup revealed that the cause of all this was sodium nicotinate, a chemical sometimes added to meat to make it more red in color. It was added to the meatballs. Dr. Edward Press, Evanston public health director, said that more of the 121 persons who ate the meal might have become ill, except that people have different tolerances to the chemical, and that the chemical probably was spread unevenly throughout the meat.

There is an important point illustrated here in the effect of a B vitamin (nicotinic acid or niacin) made synthetically and mixed with an element foreign to its nature. It has a toxic effect when it is presented as sodium nicotinate. We have said before that any B vitamin, with the possible exception of vitamin B_{12}, can create a dangerous imbalance in the body when taken out of its natural context. Natural vitamins, because they are actually natural foods, eliminate this danger. Niacin occurs in brewer's yeast, desiccated liver, wheat germ and organ meats, in perfectly safe amounts.

The other reason Dr. Press gave for this episode is that people have different tolerances to the chemical. This means, of course, that there are probably those who have almost no tolerance to it. It could make them seriously ill, so that 44 out of such a group could have made a real tragedy out of the sorority dinner.

Chemical Not Needed

At last we come to the question: who needs sodium nicotinate in his meat? Certainly not the consumer. It's another of those gimmicks the producer and the retailer use to cover the inadequacies in their product. The consumer buys meat that is fresh on his own when he is not duped by such measures as the use of sodium nicotinate. We don't need "oranged" oranges, dyed cherries, plumped and hormoned chickens or freshened bread. In the dear, dead days of long ago, when one knew what one was buying, because there were no chemicals to add, the bread was fresh or one didn't buy it; one bought a fresh chicken, not one made to look fresh; a Florida orange had a green tinge to the skin—so what?

We got along quite well without additives then, and we still could—especially without additives known to be harmful, such as sodium nicotinate, Red #32 and stilbestrol. Does your state public health department allow the use of sodium nicotinate? Why? Certainly not for your advantage. Demand that, as a taxpayer, you be spared this dangerous exposure. If the meat seller wants his meat to look fresh, let him try selling fresh meat!

Menopause

Vitamins Aid in Relieving Menopause Problems

Among the classic problems presented by menopause for many women are leg cramps at night, frequent bruises and nosebleed. Ann Horoschak, M.D., writing in the *Delaware State Medical Journal* (January, 1959), stated that each of these symptoms could be traced to capillary weaknesses. That is, weaknesses in the walls of the capillaries, which are the tiniest of the blood vessels.

In the case of leg cramps, Dr. Horoschak believes that the pain could be caused by a shortage of oxygen in the muscles, due to poor functioning of the capillaries supplying those muscles. High susceptibility to bruising, usually found in women of fair complexion and thin-textured skin, is probably caused, she says, by the thinness of the skin, abnormal fragility of the smaller blood vessels and defective cushioning of the deep vascular bed. Concerning the spontaneous nosebleed, Dr. Horoschak is convinced that such nosebleeds are the result of a capillary system not properly strengthened by needed nutrients.

Resistance to Stress and Injury

The answer to these problems, then, is to reinforce the capillary resistance to stress and injury. Long known as active agents in this area are vitamin C, the bioflavonoids, hesperidin and rutin. The bioflavonoids are known to act in connection with vitamin C and to help the body retain this quickly lost vitamin for longer periods of time. Aside from the increased fragility of the capillaries in deficiency cases of the bioflavonoids, pain in the extremities at any effort and laziness, also follow as a result of a shortage of this nutrient.

As A. Szent-Gyorgi states (*Annals of the New York Academy of Sciences*, 61: 732, 1955), "There can be little doubt that flavonoids are not only useful therapeutic agents in conditions of capillary fragility, but have many diverse actions in the animal body." G. J.

Martin adds this, in *Experimental Medicine and Surgery* (12: 570, 1954): "It (combination of bioflavonoids and vitamin C) is to be regarded as supplemental therapy of value in virtually all disease states and specific in action with respect to some."

It was with such opinions in mind that Dr. Horoschak entered into an experiment to determine the effect of a mixture of hesperidin (a bioflavonoid) and vitamin C on 40 patients with various of the 3 symptoms outlined above: 14 had leg cramps at night, 15 showed easy bruisability and 11, spontaneous nosebleeds. The patients were an average of 51 years old, and none had any diseases which might have caused the complaints. Most of them had been "doctoring" and had received various medications, but with no apparent effect. All of the symptoms were more pronounced during the time when the patients would have had their menstrual period.

Some Psychology Involved

The treatment was divided into two phases. The first consisted in nothing other than establishing an amicable relationship between the doctor and the patient. It was considered important that the patients understand that such ailments are frequent in menopause and can be remedied, and that a full and productive life can and should continue through, and follow after, menopause. The patients discussed their problems freely and received advice when they asked for it. The whole procedure was intended to relax tension and relieve anxiety, and as a result, cooperation of the patients was freely given.

The hesperidin-ascorbic acid (vitamin C) capsules contained 100 milligrams of each. At the beginning, all patients received two capsules after each meal and two at bedtime for two weeks, then one capsule 4 times a day for 4 weeks. As improvement was noted, the patient was directed to lower the dose. When all symptoms disappeared, the patient took a maintenance dose of two capsules a day, then none.

Of the 14 suffering from nocturnal leg cramps, 4 were under control within two weeks, and the rest within an average of 7 weeks.

Of the easily-bruised patients, 11 out of the 15 showed a resistance to bruises after only 8 weeks of treatment with 8 capsules, then with two capsules daily. The remaining 4 took 8 capsules a day for 16 weeks before their resistance was evident.

Nosebleed, a source of concern to 11 patients, stopped within 6 to 11 weeks in the 8 moderate cases. They began with the regular 8 capsules, and then went on a maintenance dose of two capsules a day for a year.

Three of these 11 patients had severe nosebleed, and they responded less positively. One of the 3 was under control in 3 months, and stayed that way on a maintenance dose of two capsules a day.

The condition was lessened in the other two patients, but never completely controlled, until it stopped suddenly in the fourth year.

Effectiveness Not Surprising

It is not surprising to us that so simple a device as vitamin C and the bioflavonoids in a capsule would be effective in treating these problems. A shortage of these and other nutrients is most likely to occur during the menopause. The female system receives a tremendous shock at this time, for the body shuts down a set of hormones which have been operating, and affecting every part of the body by their operation, for 30 or more years. Now a shifting of gears is required. The body must learn to operate without the intimate influence of these hormones. This new learning places a stress on the body and such stress uses nutrients from everywhere else to keep the body going. These nutrients must be replaced by diet and supplements. When they are not, things go wrong—the things that many doctors simply designate as "menopause problems," for which they have no cure. So many middle-aged women find themselves condemned to 3 or 4 years of headache, cold sweat, cramps, backache, irritability, nervousness, etc. All this because no one considered replacing the nutrients used so extravagantly in meeting the needs of these stressful years.

Prevent Deficiencies

If a disease can be cured with nutrients, it is only logical to assume that a deficiency existed. Such deficiency can be prevented by a more careful intake of all the nutrients, and the disease is automatically prevented, too. Special attention should be paid to food supplements at the time of menopause. Extra amounts of vitamin C —the stress vitamin—should be added to keep the skin healthy and well supplied with nutrients, through strong arteries and capillaries. Easy and long-lasting bruise marks are the result of little else than a shortage of this vitamin. It also prevents infections at a time when the body is most susceptible to them due to lowered resistance.

Vitamin E, to keep needed oxygen in the blood longer, is essential to treating many menopause symptoms, including leg cramps, hot flashes, etc. The B complex vitamins also deserve special attention, for they are most active in preserving the full health of the nerves—the nerves which are often the cause of headaches and irritability at this time.

Menopause is a perfectly natural process and should cause no more difficulty than any other basic bodily function. The key is, of course, a healthy body to begin with. Such a body can only result from healthful eating, proper rest and exercise. The time to prepare for menopause is long, long before it arrives!

Menstruation

Have You Tried Vitamins for Menstrual Difficulties?

If homes aren't actually broken due to menstrual tension, they are certainly sorely tried because of it. The wife can't explain her irritation at little things and her husband is likely to tire of putting up with her irritability. The result is a loud argument and a strained household for a few days.

Generally, symptoms of premenstrual tension may appear as early as two weeks before menstruation (the bleeding phase of the menstrual cycle), increasing in intensity until they reach a peak shortly before menstruation begins, then disappear completely with the beginning of the flow.

Symptoms vary through mild depression, irritability, anxiety, nausea, headache, tiredness or agitation, abdominal bloating, swelling of extremities, dizziness, blurred vision, swelling and tenderness of the breasts, cravings for certain foods, etc. The list is endless and can be extended by almost every woman who notices a change in her emotions and physiological make-up prior to menstruation. It is important to make it clear, however, that such mental stresses and physiological manifestations are not necessarily the normal pattern to be expected in a healthy woman. Women should not be willing to resign themselves to physical discomfort and psychological tension just because they are due to have their monthly period. In many cases, premenstrual and menstrual problems can and should be treated.

The Mechanics of Menstruation

Science has tried to discover just what it is about the natural process of menstruation that should create such difficulties for so many—not all—women. To understand the proposed treatments, perhaps it would be best to start with an analysis of the actual mechanics of the menstrual cycle. What actually occurs in menstruation, and why?

The average menstrual cycle lasts about 28 days. The schedule of just what occurs in this time runs approximately like this:

The first day of bleeding begins slowly and builds to a maximum flow on about the second or third day. By the fifth day, menstruation usually ends. The blood which flows carries with it the lining of the uterus, which was intended to act as a bed for the egg, should it have become fertilized. The unfertilized egg is ejected, too. Meanwhile, the ovary begins to produce a follicle containing a new egg.

As the follicle matures, it produces a hormone, estrogen, which stimulates the growth of a new lining for the uterus—a lining intended once more for implantation of a fertilized egg. This process goes on for about 14 days, at which time the egg follicle bursts, discharging the fully developed egg into the Fallopian tube. Now, the egg waits for possible fertilization by a male sperm. If this should occur, the fertilized egg implants itself in the wall of the uterus to grow for the 9 months of gestation. If fertilization does not occur, the egg travels down the uterus to be expelled when the menstrual flow begins again.

In the meantime, the follicle which held the egg has been transformed into a solid yellowish ball which secretes two hormones: estrogen and progesterone. (The latter produces a swelling of the lining of the uterus intended to prepare for the development of a fertilized egg.) If pregnancy has taken place, the egg has implanted itself on the wall of the uterus and the uterine wall will not slough off. This means, of course, that menstruation will not occur. If the egg has not been fertilized, uterine bleeding, characteristic of menstruation, begins again.

The Troublesome Stage

The stage of the menstrual cycle that takes place between the 14th and the 28th day is the one which seems to create most problems for women. It is during this time that the previously described distressing symptoms appear. It is suspected that the cause lies in the fact that two very powerful hormones, estrogen and progesterone, are secreted in irregular patterns of supply. These supply patterns are, as yet, little understood by scientists. Both of these hormones affect a number of glands and organs in the body and, should there be any deviation from the proper ratios of secretions, it would undoubtedly show itself in some kind of discomfort.

The emotional problems of menstruation, say some doctors, are aligned with a varying degree of basic emotional instability in the individual woman. It is not the direct cause of the problem of premenstrual tension, but unstable emotions may act to make one woman react more violently than another to the monthly menstrual stress. Women who react emotionally to ordinary situations with which they are confronted, can be expected to react in the same way to the physical strain presented by the menstrual cycle. This emotional reaction to the physical symptoms may result in increased output of the very hormones which caused the original physical discomfort.

The treatments offered by most doctors take cognizance of the hormonal factor. They either treat to step up or decrease bodily hormone secretions. They use sedatives, pain killers, tranquilizers, diuretics, etc. Even psychiatry is resorted to in cases of extreme emotional upset.

Why Should a Natural Process Be Painful?

As might be expected, we are allied to the fact that premenstrual tension is not a necessary and normal part of the menstrual cycle. The fact that the problem is so common, has convinced many suffering women that they might as well resign themselves to the pain and stress they experience and consider it as a part of the unfair burden of their sex. The fact that many women do not suffer at all is enough to dispose of that theory. Why should suffering be involved with a natural bodily process? We believe the answer to menstrual difficulties lies in our nutrition and environment.

In March, 1955, the *Medical Journal of Australia* carried a summary of the work done by A. P. Hudgins in which he showed the relationship between nutrients and premenstrual pains. He used, in his research, only those patients who had cramps severe enough to require bedrest, heavy sedation or time loss from work. The test included 220 women who suffered in this way. Each was given a basic dosage of 100 milligrams of niacin every morning and evening and 100 milligrams of the same every two or three hours during the period of actual cramps. Dr. Hudgins stated that each dose may be increased by 50 to 100 milligrams or more to maintain flushing for maximum effect.

The effectiveness of niacin, the B vitamin, was improved by adding a combination of rutin (60 milligrams) with 300 milligrams of ascorbic acid (vitamin C). The theory was that the blood vessel-dilating effect of the niacin was made more effective by the improvement in capillary permeability brought about by the two added nutrients.

In most cases, the niacin was effective if it had been taken 7 to 10 days before the onset of the menstrual flow. The effectiveness of the therapy continued for several months after therapy was discontinued. This led Dr. Hudgins to conclude that the problem is nutritional in origin. The effectiveness of the therapy is evident in the fact that 90 per cent of the patients studied were relieved of cramps.

Vitamin A Found Effective against Tension

As far back as June, 1951, the *American Journal of Obstetrics and Gynecology* carried a report on the role played by vitamin A in menstruation. Dr. Allesandro Pou of Uruguay told of using a solution of vitamin A in olive oil on patients with premenstrual tension and delay of the menstrual period. The tension was characterized by edema, nervousness, tenderness of breasts, etc.

The patients received 150,000 International Units of vitamin A per day, orally, for 15 days prior to menstruation. The treatment was followed for from 3 to 6 months. In 13 of 24 patients thus treated (54.17 per cent), the results were termed "very good." The symptoms had completely disappeared.

In 7 of the remaining 11 patients, the results were termed "fairly good." Symptoms were partially relieved in 4 of them, but in 3, though there was remarkable improvement, there was still some discomfort.

The last 4 patients could discern no change and one of the women showed a remarkable intolerance to vitamin A.

Over all, it was concluded that improvement was obtained in 83.34 per cent of the patients. Further, it was seen that stopping the administration of vitamin A led to an immediate reappearance of the symptoms in 8 of the 20 patients, 40 per cent, who had shown improvement.

Vitamin K for Cramps and Prolonged Flow

Vitamin K was employed to regulate the menstrual cycle by Richard Gubner and Harry E. Ungerleider, and they wrote of their experiments in *Transcript of the American Therapeutic Society* (April 9, 1954).

A synthetic vitamin K preparation was employed and was given to a total of 43 patients. These people were employees at an insurance company's home office who regularly presented themselves at the infirmary for treatment and rest periods due to chronic prolonged menstrual flow, some with clotting and some with severe menstrual cramps.

The authors theorized that prolonged bleeding could be due to an impairment of the clotting mechanism. It was suggested that there is a malfunction of the liver that is indicated when profuse bleeding occurs in menstruation. The liver is the original site of the prothrombin mechanism, the tool for blood clotting. Vitamin K is intimately involved with prothrombin formation and its administration is indicated where a prothrombin deficiency exists. In view of this possibility, vitamin K was given to these patients in dosages averaging about 25 milligrams over a 5-day period. The vitamin was given one or two days before menstruation began or on the first day of the menstrual period. This was the only medication given.

Of 12 cases with a history of prolonged menstrual flow, lasting 6 days or longer, the duration of the flow was reduced by one or more days in 8 cases and was unchanged in 4 cases. Twenty-six of the cases studied usually had clots in the menstrual discharge. Of these, the clots disappeared or diminished in 16 cases, were unchanged in 8 cases and increased in 2 cases.

All of the 43 patients studied by Drs. Gubner and Ungerleider suffered from moderate to severe menstrual cramps. Of that total, the cramps were lessened or abolished in 28 cases, and unaffected in 15 cases.

Vitamins E and A Combine to Give Relief

The *Bulletin de la Federation des Societes de Gynecologie et d'Obstetrique de Langue Francaise* (10, 3-7, 1958) carried a report on 54 patients experiencing chronic premenstrual tension. They were each given 90,000 International Units of Vitamin A plus 210 milligrams of vitamin E daily. Results were termed "good" (i.e., complete disappearance of symptoms) in 73 per cent of the cases, "intermediate" (i.e., symptoms were lessened) in 10 per cent of the cases. The most frequently observed symptoms—breast congestion, depression, abdominal tension—disappeared in 80 per cent of the cases. Nervous agitation and premenstrual pain were markedly relieved.

This is some of the evidence that convinces us of the need for a healthful diet as a preventive against menstrual problems. We feel that, if one's diet contains sufficient of the B vitamins and vitamins K, E and A, there will be no need for treatment during menses. And, of course, fresh, unprocessed foods, properly prepared, are one's best guarantee that one's meals will supply the proper intake of nutrients.

If one is already suffering with a difficult menstrual cycle, we believe that the above-quoted experiments should act as an excellent guide to possible therapeutic measures to be taken. Consult your doctor, and ask him to try, at least, vitamin therapy before resorting to hormones and tranquilizers as a means of relieving the distress. These can have dangerous side effects which are as bad or worse than the original distress. The nutrients, on the other hand, pose no such problem. The possible exception is vitamin A, which if taken in amounts of more than 100,000 International Units per day, should be taken under doctor's supervision.

Above all, don't suffer in resignation when plagued with menstrual disorders. Check your diet and your natural food supplementation. If you are certain that you are getting the nutrients you need, see a doctor to make sure yours is not a serious physiological problem.

Mental Health

Mental Illness and Poison Sprays

Mental illness is the target for a thousand theories on cause and effect. In the final analysis, one can only guess at the reason for the tremendous increase in the number of inhabitants of mental hospitals and psychiatrists' couches. Some people blame modern civilization's pressures, others say it is rejection or overprotection in childhood; we have evidence showing that poor diet can cause mental problems, just as improved diet can cure them.

In view of the uncertainty which surrounds the causes of mental illness, we feel that there is room for more consideration of yet another point. It is that modern insecticides lead to mental illness. An article in the *Lancet* (June 24, 1961) prompted us to look at the problem in more detail. Two researchers, S. Gershon and F. H. Shaw, documented observations involving 16 subjects in which the psychiatric aftermaths of exposure to insecticides were recorded. None of the subjects had ever given any indication of mental illness prior to exposure, nor did any have a history of mental illness in the family. Of the 16 persons observed, 3 were scientific officers studying the effects of sprays, 8 worked in greenhouses and 5 were farm workers. Two types of reaction were seen—schizophrenic and depressive.

The history of Case 4 is significant: A man of 43, a greenhouse technician, had been exposed to insecticides, including parathion and malathion, for 10 years and had complained, from time to time, of nausea and vomiting, as well as giddiness, excessive perspiration and muscular incoordination. He became progressively tired, but had difficulty in sleeping. He was very worried about the impairment of his mental ability.

Psychiatrist Consulted

He consulted a psychiatrist because of severe depression—he was restless, irritable, cried occasionally and felt unable to continue at home or at work. Sedatives and anti-depressants were given with little improvement.

Although he was not exposed to the insecticides for 4 months, he still complained of headache, digestive troubles, impaired mental ability and lack of ability to concentrate. He could not remember the names of plants under his care and found difficulty in understanding anything he read. It took another 6 months away from exposure before the man lost his depression, could sleep and had regained his memory and normal ability to concentrate.

Case 8 was that of a man of 30 who was actually admitted to a mental hospital in March, 1960. Several weeks prior to admission he had been poisoned by an insecticide he was spraying. He had recovered, physically, from the classic symptoms of such poisoning within 24 hours.

His friends noticed psychotic behavior for only a few days before his admission to an institution, but he said he had been persecuted for months. He stated that he had felt for some time that there was a movement afoot to have him transferred to another division. Some were against him, others on his side; but someone intended to shoot him. Even when he was alone he had heard voices talking about him. He'd heard it on the radio and people on the street stared at him, and this terrified him.

Diagnosed, on admission to a mental hospital, as a paranoid schizophrenic, the man was treated and released as apparently well one month later.

Testing a Theory

The range of patients treated in this paper was somewhat similar to the two detailed above—some a little more, some a little less severe. It was deemed important to check on whether these psychiatric disturbances were commoner in areas in which insecticides were used frequently, than in other areas. Two separate fruit-growing areas were chosen, and 16 local physicians were asked their opinions as to whether or not mental ill health had increased, and if so, whether those in the country were more affected than the town dwellers.

Most of the physicians questioned believed that it had not increased; three, however, thought that depression, at any rate, was commoner in orchardists and two supported this by case records. Further inquiries among orchard supervisors, police and pharmacists revealed that, in hot weather, safety precautions are almost entirely neglected. It appeared to be a general rule that, if a worker is acutely poisoned, the experience is so distressing that he either takes more precautions or refuses thereafter to handle the material at all.

The Question Is Debated

In a succeeding issue of the *Lancet* (July 8, 1961), J. M. Barnes took exception to the above paper, saying that it was inconclusive, and that it might influence, adversely, the use of the newer insecticides in areas where they were badly needed to control mosquitoes, and where the mosquitoes had already become resistant to the commonly used sprays. Aside from this, Dr. Barnes held that no ill effects had come from using similar compounds in the past, how could one object to the newer ones as being unsafe?

The *Lancet* (July 15, 1961) printed two more opinions on the insecticide question. Dr. Franklin Bicknell, author of a book on the subject of environmental poisons, *Chemicals in Food,* argued that it is illogical to expect that new compounds will have only those effects experienced and recognized with old compounds. If such a supposition were valid, argues Dr. Bicknell, "then we should still be using and being permanently paralyzed by the o. p. (organophosphorus) insecticide, mipafax, which, in 1951, was new, 'and above all, safe for even the amateur to use,' and which was immediately withdrawn when its new and particular effect of causing demyelination (destruction of the protective sheath over the nerves) of the central nervous system in man was recognized."

The Lump and the Brick

In further support of the argument against insecticides, Dr. J. G. Davis wrote, in the same issue of the *Lancet:* "I have myself seen cases of malaise, headache, dry mouth, sore eyes, etc., simply from the drift of agricultural sprays. Certainly I have done no 'survey' nor drawn up any 'statistics,' but one needs no great diagnostic powers to connect the lump on the forehead with the brick that has just fallen on it. Especially when the lumps and bricks crop up continually among different people in different areas. We have moved into farce if we pretend insecticides, pesticides, etc., are (a) not poisons and (b) have not poisoned people."

We have much evidence in our files which establishes, pretty well, the fact that insecticides are poisonous to the human body, but let us look some more at the evidence which shows this damage to take the form of mental illness. In April, 1949, Drs. Morton Biskind and Irving Bieber had their paper, "DDT Poisoning—A New Syndrome with Neuropsychiatric Manifestations," printed in the *American Journal of Psychotherapy.*

They described the feeling after being poisoned as one of unbearable emotional turbulence. There are, at various times, excitement, hyper-irritability, anxiety, confusion, inability to concentrate, inattentiveness, forgetfulness and depression. Perhaps one common phenomenon is extreme apprehensiveness. These episodes can easily be confused with anxiety attacks . . . disturbances of equilibrium may occur . . . intractable headache and insomnia are frequent."

Now, although this paper was written more than 10 years ago, the symptoms it describes—the depression, confusion, inability to concentrate, fright—are the very ones described in the 16 patients seen by Gershon and Shaw in 1961! If anything, since 1949, the insecticides have become more potent and their adverse effects on the human body even more deadly.

Sources of the Poisons

So much for those who work with these poisonous sprays. One can understand that these people might be dangerously exposed to pesticides, but what has that to do with the great majority of Americans who never go near a field or see a bag of pesticide?

Drs. Biskind and Bieber remind us that we all get a dose of pesticide just about every day, and can hardly hope to avoid it. If we live anywhere near a rural area, it's in the air. Unless we eat foods absolutely organically grown, we eat pesticides. How much? It depends on your luck. Did the farmer who sprayed read the directions on the label? Did he pay attention to them? There is no way to be sure. Some farmers are careful and conscientious and others think they have no obligation whatsoever to the anonymous millions who will consume the foods they grow.

Are We Protected?

Those who depend upon the law to step in and protect us from spray residues which might be present in toxic amounts, should know these facts:

1. While we are given the impression that all foods are checked for excessive residues of pesticides, and if found contaminated, are removed from the market by federal court order, the impression is not quite accurate. Only spot checks are made, covering only a small portion of the vast amount of produce being shipped to market every day. A proper, thorough check would take armies of additional personnel.

2. The Food and Drug Administration inspects only that food which is intended for shipment across state lines. What regulations the state provides are entirely up to the individual states.

You might be fortunate enough to get produce raised by a careful farmer and checked by government agents as it passed across state lines or by state authorities in your own state, and, therefore, produce carrying pesticide residues that are within set tolerances. However, it is also possible that you might buy produce raised by a farmer who pays no attention to directions on the labels of the pesticides he uses, who disregards the law's directions on their use (or is perhaps unaware of them) and who has never been caught in a spot check or who ships inside his own state, where laws might not even have any effect on his operation.

If you believe that some use of pesticides is necessary, you owe it to yourself to appeal to the state and federal governments for adequate policing of the produce offered to you in the stores. Even the most optimistic user of sprayed and processed foods is aware that there is a limit to how much poison he can take before it kills him. Make sure you get at least the minimal protection the law offers. Tell your Congressman that you would prefer to see an increase in the number of food inspectors before an increase in the new highways or the number of space scientists.

Organically Grown Foods

To many people, the answer to pesticide-ridden foods is organically raised foods. They prefer not to take chances on how much spray residue they can handle. Nobody can say that a sprayed tomato, or a basket of them, will cause physical ill effects. But no one can be sure it won't. How will the pesticide from the tomatoes mix with the pesticides from the lettuce, the apples, the grapes? How much poison have you already stored from years of sprayed foods? Which tiny bit more of poison spray will affect your liver, your spleen? Which tiny bit more of poison will affect your nerves, your mentality?

We've been using pesticides and insecticides on our crops, in earnest, for close to 20 years. Some of us have had a cumulative dose of this stuff that would kill a cow. We know that the body doesn't throw off all insecticides and pesticides; it stores some. No one knows just how much it stores. No one knows how much more one can take without ill effect. Why take a chance? Try to use organically grown foods whenever possible. Use the B complex and vitamin C regularly to counteract the poisons in the sprayed foods you can't avoid. It's one way to avoid being poisoned.

What Do Our Mental Patients Eat?

By far the most populated of all hospitals in the United States are those devoted to the care of the mentally ill. Each year, about 250,000 new patients are admitted, with nowhere near that number being released. Consequently, the patient load increases year after year, requiring more and more personnel, more buildings and other facilities. It is a sad fact that few of these needs are being met. Unless a mentally ill person has the means for a stay in a private institution (and only about two per cent do), he is likely to be housed inadequately, treated by a minimal professional staff and fed a diet that is desperately lacking in the basic nutrients required for maintenance of health in even a perfectly well person.

Nutritional Therapy

The food served in these institutions is, we believe, a vital factor in restoring the mental health of these patients. As Drs. L. Owens and G. White of the Department of Mental Hygiene of the State of California wrote, "Food is one therapy in a mental hospital that is available to all patients 3 times a day." We see this therapy to be especially important in the light of our research which proved the importance of vitamin-rich foods, especially those high in B vitamins, where mental illness is concerned.

It is sad, then, to note the secondhand part the mental hospitals play in state and federal money grants. On April 21, 1959, Arthur Flemming, then Secretary of Health, Education and Welfare, was quoted in the *New York Times* as saying, that the 217 state and county mental institutions are "inadequate for even the simplest methods of treatment." He also stated that the average money spent per patient each day in such a place is a miserable 4 dollars and 7 cents. This covers everything—medication, linens, therapy, doctors' fees and food. The shabby inadequacy of this expenditure is evident when one learns that the average cost per day of a patient in a general hospital is 26 dollars.

Carbohydrates and Starches

With this slim budget they have, dieticians in these hospitals aim at menus which will be filling, whether they are especially nutritious or not. The trays are heavy with carbohydrates and starches that satisfy easily and contribute little to the repair of the body. In the *Lancet* (June 11, 1955), Dr. D. Hanes gives some idea of the meals served in English mental hospitals, and we are certain that conditions in United States hospitals parallel those he describes. He speaks of preparing meals for 2,500 to 3,000 inmates in space hardly adequate for preparing half that number. The help is inexperienced and often made up of a number of patients. To serve the meals at a specific hour, a large part of the cooking must be done in advance, thus much of the food has the chance to spoil and lose flavor as well as what few nutrients it contains.

The prepared food is then carted from the central kitchen to the buildings on the grounds which house various types of patients. These buildings are often separated by a block or more and the equipment for keeping food hot under such conditions often is not available.

What do the patients get to eat? Here is a sample day's menu at what is considered a large, well-equipped mental hospital in the London area: breakfast—porridge, marmalade, margarine and tea; dinner—meat pie, cauliflower, potatoes, stewed fruit, blancmange (a kind of custard) and French ice cream; tea (always served in English hospitals)—jam, buns, margarine, tea; supper—savory fish, pie, cocoa (or cheese, pickles and cocoa).

A quick look at this menu will show that economy is well served. There is no fresh fruit whatsoever and no salad. The only vegetable is cauliflower. Starch is plentiful, as seen in the pies served, the potatoes and buns. Protein is barely present in the bits of meat contained in meat pie and the fish or cheese. Sugar appears in large quantities at every meal (marmalade, jam, ice cream, pie, etc.), and this sugar uses any B vitamins the patient might have in his system as it is processed in the body. Any replacement of these B vitamins must occur away from the table set by this institution, for, with the possible exception of some few B vitamins in the porridge, the meat in the meat pie and the fish, these vitamins are totally neglected.

Remember, the B vitamins are proven to be a most important factor in the occurrence and cure of mental illness!

Expenditures in Mental and General Hospitals

We think the chart carried in the *Lancet* (table 6), showing the difference in food expenditures for mental hospitals and general hospitals, is worth reproducing. You will see that the mental patients are required to exist on about half the weekly food budget allotted to other hospital patients. In the light of this fact, there is no question as to why these people have such a low rate of recovery.

Table 6: COMPARISON OF EXPENDITURES

Item	Regular Hospital		Mental Hospital	
Milk	5s	(70 cents)	2s 6d	(35 cents)
Meat	3s 6d	(49 cents)	2s 6d	(35 cents)
Poultry	1s 1d	(15 cents)	1d	(1 cent)
Fish	1s 3d	(18 cents)	9d	(11 cents)
Fruit and Vegetables	4s 3d	(60 cents)	2s 6d	(35 cents)
Miscellaneous Groceries	11s	($1.54)	8s	($1.12)

Figures in parentheses are the American equivalents.

Is it surprising, then, to find a report, such as that made by Z. A. Leitner in the *Lancet* (June 25, 1955), of a survey of 2,500 mental patients, showing a definite shortage in them of both vitamins A and C?

Moody to Maniacal

The question of mental illness in relation to diet was forcefully illustrated in a story run by the *Chicago Daily News* (May 2, 1956). The staff science writer, Arthur J. Snider, reported on a statement to the American Psychiatric Association, in which it was said, that certain commonly eaten foods can produce mental symptoms in susceptible persons which range from moodiness and irritation to maniacal behavior. The foods labeled as the worst offenders are, in the order of effectiveness, corn, wheat, coffee, milk, eggs and potatoes. Doctors can induce strong symptoms right in their offices, within minutes or hours after the patient eats the food, depending upon dosage and frequency. The whole process is akin to the allergies, suffered by some persons, to specific foods—rashes, headaches, perspiration, abdominal cramps, etc.

It would seem that a test for such an allergic possibility should be worked out for each patient being treated for a mental problem that could be eliminated by the avoidance of a single type of food —a food which he might unwittingly eat every day.

The Present Situation

The conditions under which those suffering from this most disastrous of all diseases, mental illness, must live in our hospitals, grow worse each year. The numbers confined in these places are growing, with little provision being made for the increase. One of every 10 United States citizens will spend some time in a mental institution, and the average stay is 8 years. At present, 40 per cent of the beds for our mentally ill are contained in obsolete, deteriorated or condemned buildings, and new space is needed for an additional 290,000 beds. In the way of staff, 66 per cent more nurses are needed and 78 per cent more general help, not to mention doctors and technicians and therapists.

Where is there room for an adjustment of the food values mental patients need with all these other budget problems? Room must be made! The work of Dr. E. M. Abrahamson in the field of blood sugar level control through proper diet, has demonstrated the value of this treatment in mental disorders. Dr. George Watson showed dozens of instances of mental rehabilitation through the use of nutrition. Still more evidence along these lines is offered by the work of Joseph Wilder, M.D.

Is the mental hospital in your locality concerned with the overcrowded conditions? Are they trying for funds to put up new buildings? Write to your county mental health society, asking them to consider, as well, the nutritional needs of the patients there. Recommend that they read E. M. Abrahamson's *Body, Mind and Sugar,* a copy of Joseph Wilder's article on the subject in the *Nervous Child,* April, 1943-44, George Watson's findings as contained in *Journal of Psychology* (43, 47-63, 1957) or *The New Psychiatry* by Nathan Masor, M.D.

Perhaps this information will interest those who have the power to act in considering more carefully the dietary possibilities involved in mental rehabilitation. Any spark that can be ignited might spread into an awareness that would lead to a change in the whole approach to mental illness.

The Relation of Nutrition to Mental Health

From scientific laboratories, where investigators are discovering new things every day relating to nutrition, have come positive proofs of the relation between nutrition and mental health. This is not surprising when you consider that the brain and the nervous system, along with all other parts of the body, must do their work using whatever is available to them in the way of vitamins, minerals, proteins, etc. What is surprising is that physicians concerned chiefly with mental health seem to know so little about this relationship.

Medical and psychiatric treatment of mental disease seems to progress at a snail's pace. We don't keep mental patients in chains these days—aside from this one improvement, we don't seem to be much farther along than we were several centuries ago.

Or, at least, so it seems to anyone in whose family this problem has arisen—and this includes one American family in about every 5 or 6. Tranquilizers are the current vogue in treatment of mental disease and, while they certainly make life easier for doctors and attendants at mental hospitals, we have yet to see any evidence that their use has decreased at all the terrible incidence of mental disease, which continues to rise at a frightening rate.

We marvel, as we search through medical literature, at the wealth of material there, indicating how closely the welfare of the brain and nervous system are tied in with good nutrition. Why is this information gathering dust on library shelves? Why is not the first examination given to a mental patient an examination of his nutritional state and his eating habits?

Summary of Articles

An excellent summary of many scientific articles came to us recently from the author, Elizabeth C. Bell, Ph.D. The article was published in the *Journal of Psychology,* Vol. 45, 1958, pp. 47-74. Here are some brief notes from this very helpful review which includes consideration of 182 separate articles, books or communications on the subject.

*   *   *

D. G. Campbell, writing in *Modern Nutrition in Health and Disease,* claims that the nervous system is more sensitive to nutritional variance than any other part of the body. He emphasizes the great importance of the B vitamins in making carbohydrate food available to the nerves for energy. He points out the importance of minerals for nerve tissue.

*   *   *

Three researchers reported in the *Bulletin of the Staff Meetings of the Mayo Clinic* (Vol. 14, pp. 787-793, 1939) on an experiment with mental patients. They cut their intake of thiamin (one of the B vitamins) far below the necessary amount for 147 days. The patients developed changes in their behavior within 10 days to 5 weeks. That's as long as it took. There was inability to concentrate, confusion of thought, uncertainty of memory and weakness. All of them became irritable, depressed, quarrelsome, uncoöperative and fearful of some impending disaster. Two threatened suicide. All lost their manual dexterity, had headache, painful menstruation, insomnia and sensitivity to noise.

*   *   *

Four investigators at Elgin State Hospital, Illinois, put some of their patients on a restricted intake of thiamin. They tested them at monthly intervals. Attention span, interest, ambition, playfulness, sociability, speed and manual dexterity were all affected adversely. This report appears in a government publication, *National Research Council Bulletin, No. 116,* 1948.

* * *

Dr. Tom Spies, a worker in the field of nutrition who was honored by the AMA as their "man of the year," declared that a timid and depressed person can be transformed into a pleasant and coöperative individual with a dose of thiamin (a vitamin B fraction). All patients he treated, in a series of 115 cases, who were on a diet low in thiamin, reacted this way within 30 minutes to 20 hours of the time he gave them the vitamin. Wouldn't you say such a treatment might be called almost a miracle? This observation of Dr. Spies was reported in the *Association for Research on Nervous Disorders* publication, 1943, Vol. 22, pp. 122-140.

* * *

I. N. Kugelmass in the *American Journal of Digestive Diseases,* Vol. 11, pp. 368-373, 1944, reports that neurasthenia (mild mental disorder) is the symptom first observed in children who are not getting enough thiamin in their diets. They suffer from fatigue, anxiety, irritability, forgetfulness, headaches, impaired judgment, bodily complaints, hypersensitivity, frustration and sleeplessness. An adequate diet, reinforced with thiamin as a supplement, improves, even if it does not always cure, the condition. He says that he cannot see any difference between what these children are suffering from and real, diagnosed mental illness.

* * *

V. P. Sydenstricker, writing in the *Annals of Internal Medicine,* Vol. 14, pp. 1499-1517, states that, because nerve cells are more sensitive to disturbance of nutrition and oxygen supply than any other cells, deficiency in various nutritional elements produces many mental and nervous symptoms. He says that these symptoms may come first—long before there are any other indications that something is lacking in the diet. He mentions such symptoms as these: loss of memory for recent events (often seen in older folks who can remember well envents of bygone years), insomnia, anxiety, apprehension, distractability, also partial deafness, particularly for high tones, digestive disturbances, heartburn and flatulence.

* * *

Dr. Spies, whom we have quoted above, reported in 1939, in the *Journal of the American Medical Association,* Vol. 113, pp. 1481-1483, that, among 194 children suffering from pellagra (a disease of vitamin B deficiency), the chief symptoms noted were: that the children were irritable, easily frightened, fretful, crying a good deal, listless, tiring quickly, apprehensive, lacking in appetite and the normal interests of children. Dr. Spies gave them brewer's yeast and good diets, along with a supplement of niacin, one of the B vitamins, and they responded immediately.

*   *   *

Again, Dr. Spies, writing in *Clinical Nutrition,* stated that the nutritional deficiency which causes pellagra, along with the mental and nervous symptoms that accompany it, has, in most cases, existed for months or years in a mild form in any given patient. In another article, he stated that *most malnourished patients have some degree of mental disturbance which frequently is the only evidence of anything wrong early in the story.* During such time, a doctor may diagnose the trouble as hysteria, depression, neurasthenia or an anxiety state. Of course, since the condition is nothing more or less than nutritional deficiency, it can be alleviated quickly by giving the missing B vitamins, *along with a good, nourishing diet.* Dr. Spies never failed to insist upon this latter.

*   *   *

Here is a story from the *Proceedings of the Society of Experimental Biology,* Vol. 86, pp. 693-698, 1954. Four men were placed on a diet deficient in another of the B vitamins, pantothenic acid, for 35 days. After the second week, they began to complain of fatigue and the desire to sleep during the day. Loss of appetite and constipation plagued them by the third week. They were quarrelsome, discontented and irascible by the fourth week. They complained of burning feet—another symptom of a serious lack of this B vitamin. If such symptoms can appear after only 35 days on a deficient diet, what can happen to someone who lives on a diet only a little better than this over a whole lifetime?

*   *   *

Biotin is the B vitamin we often mention in connection with experiments on raw egg white. This vitamin is destroyed by a substance in the raw egg white. Depriving volunteers of biotin over a period of 5 weeks produced extreme lassitude, sleepiness and hallucinations in one subject and mild panic in two others. This was reported in the *Journal of the American Medical Association,* Vol. 118, pp. 1199-1200, 1942. It seems doubtful that anyone is going to eat so many raw eggs that he will bring such symptoms on himself, but what about the less serious deficiency that may haunt him for life, if he consistently does not eat foods that contain enough biotin?

*   *   *

Aside from B vitamins, what food elements are most important for good mental health? Researchers have found that phychological stress, or stress coming from one's surroundings, causes sudden and extremely great decreases in the blood levels of vitamin C and, in some instances, vitamin E. Other studies showed that alcoholics with mental symptoms had far too low a level of vitamin C in their blood. Another researcher found that elderly patients suffering from mental deterioration had low levels of vitamin C.

*　　*　　*

W. Clinibal, writing in *Hippokrates,* Vol. 22, pp. 481-482, 1951, told of giving vitamin E to children as a supplement for 3 years. He found that their nervousness and irritability decreased; they were able to sleep better and had increased sexual sensitivity. Dr. Spies noted that a deficiency in vitamin E could cause a form of nervous upset which responded to vitamin E therapy. A South American M.D. treated Mongoloid children and children with other mental handicaps with huge doses of vitamin E, and got excellent results.

*　　*　　*

We know that one of the direct effects of iodine deficiency is a poorly functioning thyroid gland. And this can bring mental symptoms of apathy and sluggishness. In extreme cases, retardation and even idiocy are found. Vitamin A is related to the well-being of the thyroid gland, too, according to several references given in Dr. Bell's article, so vitamin A, too, is essential for good mental health.

*　　*　　*

Anemia which results from lack of iron is described by Dr. Norman Jolliffe in *Clinical Nutrition.* Apathy, lassitude, anxiety, irritability are commonly observed. Difficulty in swallowing may be a symptom which, of course, causes great apprehension and tension. So we need plenty of iron in our food.

*　　*　　*

Calcium deficiency is almost always associated with instability of the nervous system. This important mineral is required for the transmission of impulses along nerves. According to *The Physiological Basis of Medical Practice,* by Best and Taylor, a calcium deficiency frequently occurs during the rapid growth of adolescence, at menstrual periods, during pregnancy and lactation. Taking calcium supplements relieves the nervous symptoms.

*　　*　　*

M. and G. Seham published in the *American Journal of Diseases of Children,* Vol. 37, pp. 1-38, 1929, the information that children who have mild nutritional deficiencies are restless; those with more serious deficiencies are quieter than they should be. Couldn't this one fact alone explain much of the restlessness among modern American children and adolescents which is widely excused by saying "It's a stage; they'll outgrow it"? In more primitive cultures than ours, such restlessness is not a characteristic of children and teen-agers—so one cannot possibly describe it as something that just always happens at this time of life.

How to Use These Facts

We have only scratched the surface of the material outlined in this article by Dr. Bell. She reminds us that there is no such thing as a deficiency in one vitamin; also that there may be many other reasons for mental disease, but certainly one of the first things to consider in treating mental illness is the state of nutrition. She admits that there is much still to learn about foods and their relation to health. These unknown aspects, however, in no way prevent us from improving symptoms by means of the best methods currently available for nutritional therapy.

How can you use the facts above to help protect yourself and your family from the horrors of mental illness and the (perhaps, in some ways, almost as horrible) lesser evil of daily maladjustment to life, as evidenced by fatigue, nervousness, irritability, instability, anxiety, inability to concentrate, sleeplessness and so forth?

We do not advise that you take massive doses of the vitamins, B vitamins or any others, as many of the patients did in the experiments and treatments described above. We think you should concentrate, instead, on all the aspects of good nutrition which are important for good mental health—and, of course, good physical health, too. The B vitamins are extremely important. They are almost completely lacking in many modern diets. If you eat white bread and refined cereals; if you shun fresh fruits and vegetables in favor of pastries, desserts and sweet between-meal snacks; if you disregard the importance of meat, fish, eggs, nuts and other seeds (for their fine protein content)—you most probably have a deficiency in B vitamins.

Take Natural Food Supplements

We suggest that you remedy this by revising your diet accordingly. And we think you should add natural food supplements, as did Dr. Spies and most of the other nutrition experts we quoted above —brewer's yeast and desiccated liver are the best sources of B vitamins. You should take them like food, not a medicine. They are rich, as well, in minerals, especially iron. And they contain lots of protein. Other foods which are rich in B vitamins are: meats (especially organ meats like liver and kidneys), eggs, seed food (like sunflower seeds, wheat germ and nuts, fresh fruits and vegetables.

Calcium, so necessary for the health of the nerves, is best supplied in fresh fruits and vegetables, eggs and nuts. Milk is a good source, but we do not recommend milk for adults. We think everyone should take bone meal as the food supplement for plenty of calcium.

If there is a case of real mental illness in your family which requires treatment, we think it would be very worthwhile for you to ask your doctor or psychiatrist to send for a copy of the excellent article we have reviewed above.

Prayer, Pretense and Perseverance

This is a reprint of a column by Mary Haworth which appeared in the Washington Post *for March 5, 1959.*

DEAR MARY HAWORTH:

Some time last spring, I wrote you, asking advice on deep depression. If you replied, I know your answer was wise and thoughtful—but I never saw it, as I went to the hospital in May and read no papers there.

However, you really had answered me many times, before and since, in your advice to others, to read *Body, Mind and Sugar* (Henry Holt) and investigate the possibility, outlined by Dr. E. M. Abrahamson, of emotional depression being due to hyperinsulinism.

How much suffering, expense and loss could be avoided, if only people would pursue this line of inquiry before trying other modes of treatment. If only I had heeded your advice! May I offer my experience—to help others?

About a year ago, under great financial strain, I began drinking much coffee, heavily sweetened, to clear my head and spur myself to longer, harder hours of writing. Result: more depression, worsening symptoms. Suicide beckoned, but I made a desperate search for help. I had simple surgery, blood transfusions, hormone therapy, sedatives, tonics. No improvement. A certain tranquilizer put me in lower spirits than ever. Finally psychiatry!

Electro-Shock: Excursion into Hell

A psychiatrist, after one brief interview—no physical or laboratory tests—told my scared husband that I must have electro-shock treatments. He consented; I wasn't informed of this, and entered the hospital, I was told, for rest. There I was locked up and forced to submit . . .

Dazed with the first electro-shock treatment and nearly inert—but with a strong will and constant silent prayer—I resolved to escape somehow. But you had to be docile, had to be a good actor, had to pretend optimism, had to hang on to reality somehow—even while wanting to scream out against this excursion into Hell.

Never once did the psychiatrist talk to me, or listen. Once, when I appealed to her, in the torture room before a treatment, she turned her back on me and said, "Be quiet and lie down." I am a timid person, so couldn't insist.

Eventually, giving a performance of pretense that would merit an "Oscar," I won out. After 10 shock treatments in two weeks, I was taken home—supposedly "well," but actually in much worse shape, I knew.

Now I was really lost, completely disoriented. I had forgotten how to cook, couldn't add. The dresses in my closet looked strange. I couldn't remember my neighbor's names. Friends called, many of whom I didn't recognize, saw my condition and wept openly, crying: "What have they done to you?"

Unknown Friend Answers Prayer

The dizziness was worse than ever; the blackouts more frequent. I remembered my earlier worries and started worrying again—but lacked the mentality to carry through a financial plan. I couldn't type, spell or write a check.

Now I felt I *had* to die; but first I went to a minister and asked his prayers. He prayed and also won my confidence. (I never expected to trust again.) I told him the whole story and he prayed again, that I would be guided to right help.

Next day's mail brought a book from an unknown donor: *Body, Mind and Sugar*. I read it, tried the diet, within a few days felt like new. Then a friend sent me to a doctor doing work with blood sugar cases and, though afraid of all doctors by this time, I went and found the answer to my long search for health.

A 6-hour glucose tolerance test disclosed a very serious condition of hyperinsulinism. I was put on a strict corrective diet and now, 3 months later, I have a wonderful sense of well-being and look 30 years younger than I did 8 months ago! So please keep up the good work.—P.Y.

Miss Haworth's Answer

DEAR P. Y.:

Sorry I've had to cut your fascinating story by one-third. But it still ought to curl the hair of a certain psychiatrist you have known! It reminds me of a pioneering analyst's sharp comment some years ago, to-wit: "The time is coming when we will look back on electro-shock treatments as the medical barbarism of the twentieth century."—M. H.

Glutamic Acid and Mental Health

A person's nutrition is a factor in his mentality. We will now become more specific and will discuss one item in our food setup that scientific evidence shows is closely connected with the functioning of the brain. This is called glutamic acid. It is one of the 20 or so amino acids of which protein is composed. When you eat an egg, about 12.8 per cent of it is protein. Eggs, of course, are an acid food, and important for a good diet. If we shunned acid foods and confined ourselves only to foods that have an alkaline effect on the body, we would not be long for this world. Glutamic acid occurs naturally in meat, eggs, beans, fish and the like, and we do not recommend its being taken as a separate supplement.

It is hard to believe that the quality of one's brain can be influenced by food, or food factors, but the evidence is clear. Glutamic acid is, however, only one of the many elements in our nutrition which add up to a good mental endowment.

Glutamic Acid for Retarded Children

Let us first consider an article in the *Journal of Nervous and Mental Diseases* for September, 1946, where Kathryn Albert, Paul Hoch, M.D. and Heinrich Waelsch, M.D., report on an experiment in giving glutamic acid to mentally retarded children. They tell us they first became interested when they read of giving glutamic acid to epileptic patients. According to this earlier report, the epileptic patients responded well, with a marked increase of mental and physical alertness. Two sets of investigators then experimented with rats, testing their ability to solve mazes and reason out other problems, with and without the addition of glutamic acid to their diets. It was found that the rats who received the glutamic acid learned the maze more rapidly and with far fewer mistakes than those which did not receive the glutamic acid. Solving a problem involving a certain series of plates that must be stepped on in order to get food, once again, the rats receiving glutamic acid responded with a higher score than those which did not. Since it is not possible to figure out what particular mental ability in human beings corresponds to these various skills in rats, no conclusions could be reached about the possible effect of glutamic acid on mental ability in human beings.

So, in 1946, researchers Albert, Hoch and Waelsch worked with 8 mentally retarded children to whom they gave, at various times in the testing period, glutamic acid in the form of tablets or placebos in similar tablets. Placebos are pills containing nothing of any physiological value. They are given in experiments so that there can be no possibility of the people involved responding in one way or another simply because they took pills. In this case, everyone was given pills that looked exactly alike, but some of the pills contained glutamic acid and others did not.

Results of the Tests

The various psychological and mental tests given to the children are not important to us. They were standard tests that are used regularly to determine intelligence quotient, mental age, manual dexterity and so forth. Here is a sample of one of the results. A boy of 13, whose mental age was that of a child of 3, was classified as an imbecile by the staff of the Psychiatric Institute to which he was taken. His speech was indistinct and he knew apparently only sentences of two or three words. He was given tests in intelligence, drawing, memory and skill with hands, and records were made of the results. His intelligence quotient was 42. Then he was given glutamic acid. Two months later, while he was still taking the glutamic acid, his score on one of the tests had gone up 9 points. At the end of 3 months, another score had gone up 8 points. In still other tests the increase was 6, 5 and 9 points. In the 7½ years prior to the tests, his mental age had increased two years and 5 months. During the two months on glutamic acid, he gained one year and 5 months in mental age. At the end of 3 months, the glutamic acid was withdrawn and placebos were given instead. He was tested a month later and it was found that his intelligence quotient had dropped to within one point of its original level.

In a second case, a child of 6 with an intelligence quotient of 71 was given placebos for two months. Then he was tested. The scores showed no change from the level of intelligence he had when he was admitted. Then he was given glutamic acid instead of the placebos. During the next 5 months his intelligence quotient in one test given rose 13 points. In another, it rose 19 points, and so on. After 5 months, he was given no more glutamic acid and within two months, his intelligence quotient had dropped to its original level.

A third patient, 20 years old with a mental age of 7, was given glutamic acid with similar results—a gain in mental ability of 17 points in 2½ months. After stopping the glutamic acid, the mental age dropped once again to the original level. The authors of this article are quick to point out that their evidence is certainly not conclusive. The group they worked with was small. A criticism might be made that the patients learned the tests and so were more efficient later on than at the beginning. But we must remember that, after the glutamic acid was stopped, this increase in learning did not go on, but dropped to the original level in spite of the fact that the patients were familiar with the tests.

The authors tell us that, "it appears possible that glutamic acid does not so much influence or increase the intellectual function as such, but only enables the patient to regain his intellectual function which was inhibited by other mechanisms." They do not know, they say, whether other amino acids might have the same effect or whether glutamic acid would have this same effect if it had been given in conjunction with other amino acids. So, they do not know whether they are dealing with a deficiency of glutamic acid. They point out that glutamic acid not only occurs in food, but that it can also be manufactured within the body.

Other Experiments

In *Psychosomatic Medicine* for May-June, 1947, another similar experiment is reported by Frederic T. Zimmerman, M.D., Bessie B. Burgemeister, Ph.D., and Tracy J. Putnam, M.D. Sixty-nine patients were tested, with a control group of 37 who received no glutamic acid. These were all patients with convulsive disorders, such as epilepsy, but a number of them were retarded mentally as well. Without going into the details of the tests, we can tell you that the conclusions reached were as follows: (1) that glutamic acid speeds up mental functioning in human beings; (2) that this is a general effect noticeable in a wide variety of tests; (3) that the most striking changes occurred in the group most seriously retarded; (4) that there was a greater improvement in tests of reasoning ability and abstract thought than in tests of physical skill or dexterity; (5) that in many cases, a greater degree of emotional stability resulted from taking the glutamic acid.

Reviewing the whole story of the experiments, Roger W. Clapp, M.D., of St. Louis, in the *Journal of the Missouri State Medical Association* for March, 1949, tells us that laboratory tests involving pieces of brain tissue show that glutamic acid has an important part in brain metabolism. In other words, there is some chemical basis for believing that a lack or an abundance of glutamic acid might affect the working of the brain. Speculating on how these reported good results might have occurred, Dr. Clapp reminds us that glutamic acid is contained in a number of foods—milk, wheat, corn, etc. He says, it is difficult to understand how such a substance could be beneficial as a supplement since it occurs so widely as food. Yet, he recalls, we did not know of the almost miraculous curative power of liver in cases of pernicious anemia, until we began to give massive doses of liver.

He tells us that, in the St. Louis Society for Crippled Children Cerebral Palsy Training Unit, glutamic acid is administered while the children are receiving physical, occupational and speech therapy. It appears, he tells us, that the glutamic acid results in a slightly higher achievement level in these children.

But in view of Dr. Clapp's findings that laboratory tests, involving pieces of brain tissue, show that glutamic acid has an important part in brain metabolism, we cannot rule out entirely the beneficial effect of this amino acid on the functioning of the brain. It is possible that the effect of glutamic acid will show up very graphically in mentally retarded cases, but will do little, if any, good as an added food supplement for normal people, but the lesson is clear. It is good insurance to eat a high-protein diet.

This Is Psychodrama

This article is reprinted, by permission of the publishers, from Picture Post, *London, England, July 10, 1954.*

A man of 62, above medium height, broad and somewhat bulky in proportion, is standing on a platform in Hampstead Town Hall. He is a dynamic and impressive figure with an air of hawk-like alertness about him.

His name is Dr. Jacob Levy Moreno and he is giving a public lecture on psychodrama—a novel system of psychiatric treatment, of which he is the inventor and master exponent.

But this is no ordinary lecture and he is no ordinary lecturer. For although Dr. Moreno is a psychiatrist, he does not speak in the now all-too-familiar jargon of the psychiatrist. You hear nothing from him about "transference, sublimation," and the like. There is no professional manner, no condescension. Only an air of great natural force, sincerity and conviction.

Mental or nervous sufferers are usually treated in isolation. Moreno, like Adler, insists that the patient must be treated as one of a group.

Patients are usually treated in the privacy of the consulting room. Moreno insists they must be treated in public.

Neurotic problems are usually evolved and resolved through long, protracted talks between the patient and his doctor, often extending over years. Moreno insists that talking by itself is useless. The patient must *act out* his problems. At once! On the spot!

These ideas are novel, revolutionary and difficult to convey. But Moreno, on the platform, makes no attempt to give a considered, or even coherent, account of them. There is no time for that. All he can do is throw out vivid hints and fragments.

He exerts himself to the utmost, physically and mentally. His message is too urgent to wait, even for the right word or phrase. His mood and expression change rapidly, to suit the argument. He uses every possible gesture, grimace, antic or improvised pantomime—serious or comic—to convey his meaning. His presence does not lose, but gains, in force and dignity by these seeming extravagances.

For instance, at the climax of his argument, he tends to stand almost on tiptoe and to spread out both arms horizontally and sideways from the shoulders, with the fingers of each hand fluttering rapidly and ceaselessly. He is then like an enormous hawk hovering above his audience; a benign hawk with intent, not to swoop and kill, but to help and heal.

He is trying to explain, by rapid word and gesture, that there is no clear dividing line between the insane and the neurotic, or between the neurotic and the normal; that neurotic troubles do not arise in isolation, but through contact with other human beings, whether insane, neurotic or normal; that neurotic troubles are universal and that normal people not only experience them in some degree, but take part in their creation.

If these troubles do not arise in isolation, they cannot be cured in isolation or by segregation. They must be acted out by the participants concerned, and in public. Sick and well can then both benefit from that emotional purge, or catharsis, which it is the special function of psychodrama to bring about.

If neurotic sufferers cannot be cured in isolation, neither can they be allowed to suffer in isolation.

At this point, he makes a direct appeal to his audience. Is there anyone in the hall suffering because of despair, fear, loneliness or any problem of any sort? Anybody? Any problem?

There is a silence. Moreno stands half on tiptoe, his arms stretched out full length sideways, his fingers fluttering ceaselessly. Anybody? Any problem?

A half-inaudible word comes from somewhere in the middle of the hall. The finger fluttering ceases! The arms drop! The hawk swoops! Moreno clambers down from the platform, walks towards a man in the audience and literally embraces his prey!

The psychodrama has begun!

SCENE I

They both climb up on to the platform. For the time being, Moreno forgets his audience and concentrates exclusively on the man standing beside him.

He holds him by both arms. There is a barrage of questions. "What's your name? What's your age? What do you do?" and so on; almost ceaselessly.

The man turns out to be a journalist in his early fifties. Let us call him David. His trouble, in one word, is alcohol.

"When was your worst drinking bout? Or the one you remember best? Where did it happen? When? How?"

David thinks slowly, and makes some hesitant reply.

"Yes! Yes! Where was it? Denning! Where is Denning? In Sussex! Whereabout in Denning? In a room in a house! What was the room like? How many windows were there? Where was the clock? The table? The chairs? The telephone?"

"You were alone in that room! Why were you there?"

"My mother was dying in the next room," says David.

"What did she look like when she died? What did you do?"

"I kissed her and came out!"

"What did you do then?"

"I sat down at the table!"

"Sit down!" says Moreno, pushing him into a chair at the table beside the chairman.

"What did you do then?"

"I started to drink!"

"What did you drink?"

"Brandy!"

"Here's your brandy!" says Moreno, pushing the chairman's drinking glass towards him. "Help yourself!"

"How long did you drink?"

"All night! Right through till morning!"

"What did you do then?"

"I had a wash and a shave."

"What then?"

"I had to make arrangements for the funeral!"

"Make the arrangements," says Moreno, pushing an imaginary telephone in front of him. David hesitates. "Go on!" says Moreno peremptorily.

Almost without thinking, David calls Denning 0811 and talks to the undertaker.

SCENE II

The first scene is cut short, and Moreno jumps to the second without a break.

"What was your mother like?" Again a barrage of questions. David describes her. Moreno nods to his own wife, who is sitting in the front row of the hall just beneath him. Mrs. Moreno climbs up on to the platform.

"There is your mother," says Moreno to David, pointing to Mrs. Moreno. "Talk to her!"

They sit down and talk together as if they were mother and son.

The conversation has gone on only for a minute or so when Moreno intervenes. The talkers get up. Moreno rearranges the chairs.

He turns to David and says: "Now, you, David, are your own mother. And," turning to his wife, "you are David. Talk to each other," he says. "Go on!"

David and Mrs. Moreno talk to each other with their roles reversed.

It transpires that David's mother had three sons, but that two of them are now married and away. Her husband is dead. She and David are living on alone in the house at Denning.

SCENE III

Moreno suddenly interrupts again. "Are you married?"

"No!"

"Was there ever any girl you might have married?"

"Yes!"

"What was she like?" Again a barrage of questions.

Let us say her name was Pamela. Moreno turns to his wife, still on the platform, and says to David: "There is Pamela. Talk to her!" David and Pamela sit down and talk.

Again the roles are changed. David becomes Pamela and Mrs. Moreno becomes David. They sit and talk again.

The time is now 9 or 10 years ago, and David's mother is still alive. It seems that David and Pamela both wish to get married, but that David is unwilling or unable to leave his mother. Pamela is a little impatient.

SCENE IV

The scene now shifts to the garden. Under Moreno's rapid questioning, David describes the surroundings in detail. He is now introducing Pamela to his mother in the garden. He then becomes Pamela and talks to Mrs. Moreno, who is now his mother. He then becomes his mother and talks to Mrs. Moreno, who is now Pamela.

It seems that the mother has no objection to the marriage. She approves of Pamela, but wants the couple to live with her at Denning. It is a pleasant house, and there is plenty of room. Pamela demurs.

Mrs. Moreno now becomes David's conscience, or "alter ego." David and his conscience sit down side by side and argue things out.

There is now a series of rapidly changing situations in which David is sometimes himself, sometimes his mother and sometimes Pamela.

It now appears that David promised his father on his deathbed that he would always look after his mother. He feels that he cannot break that promise. He does not marry Pamela.

David's mother died 8 years ago. David has no idea where Pamela is now. He lives alone. He has been drinking heavily ever since.

For the last 5 months, he has been in a hospital for curative treatment.

The psychodrama is ended. It was only an improvised fragment. There was no time for more.

It is here written up as a fragment—without comment. There is no space for more.

But this much can be said: that psychodrama, though entirely spontaneous and impromptu, is primed, and to some extent directed, by a great variety of specialized techniques developed by Dr. Moreno during long years of experience.

Further, that psychodrama is merely the means to the dramatic exposition of a philosophy of life, in which the guiding principles are dynamism, spontaneity and the breaking down of all barriers between human beings, whether of age, sex, nationality, custom, convention or creed.

It might seem that it was merely a case of the audience experiencing the demonstration at David's expense. The audience was certainly gripped by the drama as it unfolded. But David was not acting in retrospective agony, as might be supposed. Clearly, he was benefiting from that catharsis—which it was the function of the demonstration to produce. His voice and presence grew in weight and confidence as the drama moved on. And he certainly left the platform a livelier and happier man than when he climbed on to it.

Many members of the audience, as became evident in the short discussion which followed, had experienced this catharsis in special degree, because all, or parts, of the drama had touched on or crossed some profound and similar experience of their own.

This mutual participation strengthens both actor and audience. The drama brings out the causes, and thereby proceeds to the cure. Actors and onlookers automatically become their own psychiatrists.

Even Dr. Moreno himself, who, like David, participated in maximum degree and in full view of the audience, was not exhausted by his strenuous participations, as again might be expected, but invigorated.

Psychodrama

By J. I Rodale

A few years ago, when I began to write plays, I thought back to an article on psychodrama I had published in my old *Fact Digest* magazine, somewhere around 1938 to 1941. I recalled vaguely that it was about a psychiatrist who had given up the couch and was curing mentally disturbed people by getting them up on a stage and having them act out their difficulties. The fact that it involved acting interested me, but when I found that the psychodrama method had repudiated Freud and all the non-scientific mysticism of psychoanalysis, my interest was even greater.

I got in touch with Dr. J. L. Moreno, who is at the head of this psychodrama organization (Moreno Institute) at Beacon, New York, and was told that they had a place in New York City on 40th Street, where, on a few nights each week, the public was invited to see demonstrations of psychodrama. My wife and I attended a few of these meetings and found them utterly fascinating. In fact, when volunteers were called for, Anna took the part, pure improvisation, of a mother of a disturbed girl. For the moment, I had gone into Dr. Moreno's office, and when I came out, there was Anna on the stage talking away as if she had rehearsed the part for months.

What is psychodrama and how did it begin? Dr. Moreno is a psychiatrist, a sociologist, an educator and a great dramatist, who rediscovered the old truth that the word is not enough. "In the beginning was the act," he says. "We are all actors as infants long before we learn to speak. Therefore, we must turn our patients into actors and see them when they act."

Theatre of Spontaneity

How did he come to find this out? In the year 1921, Moreno opened a theatre on the Maisedergasse in Vienna. It was intended as a new art form in the theatre, a theatre of spontaneity in which the actors improvised a great deal. Dr. Moreno was groping, looking for a new social force in life, and he surrounded himself with actors and actresses who were equally dedicated. On some evenings, the performances were so outstanding that the audience could not believe it was spontaneous, and accused the director and players of "rigging" the show.

So Moreno hit upon an ingenious device to prove that the productions were truly spontaneous. He suggested that they use for their plots real and dramatic events, things which had just happened on the streets of Vienna. In this way, the audience could understand that their productions were genuinely spontaneous, since no one could anticipate the news of the day and they could come to the Theatre of Spontaneity to get the latest news, instead of waiting for their newspaper. Moreno sent his scouts throughout the city and these roving reporters called in their stories. Thus came about the Living Newspaper, a form of play taken up and developed by the great German dramatist, Bertolt Brecht, and during the depression in this country by the government subsidized American Federal Theatre.

A Case History

One of the youngest actresses of the Theatre of Spontaneity was married to a poet who came every night to watch his wife perform. One day, Moreno said to him, "George, you must certainly love your wife to come here every night for a whole month." The poet replied, "I hate her." The story as related by George was that in the theatre she acted out heoric parts, always being virtuous, kind and loving, but at home, alone with him, she changed into a virago and had violent temper tantrums during which she abused him verbally and physically, hitting, kicking and lashing him with her vile tongue. Informed of this, Moreno assured George that he would try a remedy. When Barbara appeared that evening, Moreno told her that her repertory should be broadened to include a wider range of roles, to avoid typecasting and becoming stale. Her role range should now include roles of the not so lady-like type. Barbara liked this idea and just then, one of the reporters flashed in a startling news item. A streetwalker in one of Vienna's red light districts had been killed by a man whom she had solicited. Barbara was given the role of the streetwalker and Richard, that of the murderer. On stage, Barbara rose to the occasion magnificently; she embodied the new role with great reality, getting into a heated argument with the accosted male, using abusive language and kicking him in the legs. George, her husband, became anxious while watching her, but could not intervene. Suddenly, the actor in the scene grabbed a knife, a rubber prop, from his pocket and began to chase Barbara. He ran after her while she ran away, by now truly afraid of what she had started; in circles they ran, closer and closer. The audience became so involved, it seemed so real, that they screamed, "Stop it, stop it!" But nothing could stop them until Barbara was "murdered."

This performance of Barbara's was the beginning of her "treatment" and thus, the Theatre of Spontaneity changed overnight into a treatment setting, what Moreno later called the Theatre of Psychodrama. From then on, Barbara was allowed to be that "other" Barbara, that person who no one believed existed within her, whom middle class society refused to accept, but who pushed herself into the foreground when her lady-like behavior could not contain itself any longer. The roles she portrayed on the stage, where they were accepted as suitable for the occasion, made it possible to cleanse herself of their pressures, reducing the need for expressing them in life itself. But not only Barbara was treated, George also became an actor on the stage, so that they could learn together and find different ways of living together. Gradually, they began to enact scenes from their own life, and this led to deeper understanding of their mutual needs and of the many ways in which they affected one another. They learned this in a setting which is closely patterned after life, but more inclusive and flexible, less threatening, without some of the consequences of life itself and offering ways of practicing new and different kinds of behavior.

Imagine that Barbara would have been treated on a couch, instead of on the psychodrama stage. The chances are that she would never have come to a psychoanalyst, although she certainly needed help. Remember that it was George who brought her difficult behavior to the attention of the therapist. But even if she would have come, she may have taken years to come to the realization that her behavior was not what it should be; this is true, because we do not see ourselves very clearly, and we can not easily objectify our world by mere talk. It was only when Barbara was seen in action as a veritable she-devil, that many of her deeper layers of self, of which she was largely unaware, came to the fore. Besides, it was in interaction with certain types of males, counter-roles, that these not so pleasant aspects of Barbara were brought into focus. Therefore, talking about herself, Barbara might have blamed George for her unpleasant reactions, rather than come to realize what her own contributions to the difficulties between them were. Indeed, Moreno discovered that it is the relationships *between* people which need clarification, and these can never be uncovered or treated by words alone. In order to understand this, both persons involved in the difficulty must be present, studied, treated and restrained in action. George learned to become more tolerant of Barbara and to know the ways in which she responded to certain things in him. They learned to laugh about their own shortcomings and to correct their most flagrant interpersonal mistakes before they became established habits. In other words, they found themselves with a larger repertoire of roles in life itself, and learned to apply greater spontaneity to the task of daily living.

From this point on, the Theatre of Spontaneity changed its character, Dr. Moreno's entire concept of the treatment of mental disturbance was remodeled.

Psychodrama for Children

Psychodrama has been used with children as a method of acquainting them with the world around them. One way in which children learn is through the experience of their parents. Taking this a step further, psychodrama makes it possible for people to take to each other's role. For example, it turns the parent into the child and the child into the parent; this is called role reversal. It makes good sense. How often have we not, in an argument, said to someone: "Put yourself in my position. What would you do if you were me?" In psychodrama, this is actually done, though in life, this is not possible. In role reversing with a parent, a child gets to "feel" what it might be like to be a parent, and to have to deal with a child such as he is, and thus to "grow up" a bit beyond what life itself would permit.

Dr. Moreno experienced a situation with his own son, Jonathan, who was then only 3 years old, which is worth retelling. Moreno was making a long-distance call, and Jonathan began to be very noisy, pushing around a small table, chair and other pieces of furniture. Moreno angrily demanded that Jonathan be quiet; then Mrs. Moreno entered the argument by defending the boy. Dr. Moreno decided to use a bit of psychodrama. He told Jonathan that they were going to play a game—a reversal of roles. Jonathan was to become his father. And vice versa.

"Now, Jonathan, take the phone and make a long-distance call to Munich."

Jonathan entered the spirit of the game and began to talk into the phone while Dr. Moreno began to cavort around, disturbing the furniture and cackling like a chicken. This, of course, disturbed Jonathan who shouted, "Can't you see I'm trying to get through to Munich? How can I hear if you make such noise, etc., etc., etc.?" Jonathan never again made noises while his father and mother were on the phone. Incidentally, I have used a role reversal in a children's play I have written called *Dr. Jingle and Little Jack Horner.*

It is interesting to note with what maturity a 3-year old is able to live the role of a responsible adult, to "borrow his status," and how this learning leads, in turn, to more responsible behavior on the part of the child. This psycho-dramatic role reversal is so important to children, because every child has to learn to absorb within himself these two adults who are central to him, who are outside of him, yet an intrinsic part of him and whom one day he has to digest, overcome and be able to leave, emerging as an entirely new entity himself, but with subtle bonds which tie him to these two people. They must become well-integrated parts of himself before he can be the adult he deserves to be. Yet, he is himself different from both and he must find out for himself who he is. Role reversal can help him find the way to his own self more completely.

Example of Role Reversal

Why does "role reversal" help us to understand ourselves and others better? A very large part of our life remains dormant, unexpressed, buried in a dream-like state in our minds. Life does not permit us to give free expression to everything we think, dream, expect, feel. If this is true about ourselves, how much more is it true about our experience of others. We form images of ourselves and others which are full of misconceptions. Often, it takes us a lifetime to correct them, some stay with us in their misshapen form forever. Imagine, for instance, if, when Khrushchev and Eisenhower met, they could have appeared in front of a forum, a group of interested spectators of both Russian and American delegates. First, they could have presented themselves, each one with his own particular "role," Eisenhower as the President of the United States of America, the man who, some 15 years ago, was the overall military head of the Allied forces which conquered Europe, a man who believes in the dignity of the individual, his rights and privileges and who has tried to embody this in his capacity as President of the greatest power in the world we know. Then Khrushchev presents himself, the man who embodies the communist idea, who is certain that his world will conquer the future, who has risen from the ranks of the peasantry through a hard school of training, unlike any we know, barely escaping death by several narrow margins, now symbolizing the hopes of his countrymen. Their personalities and their backgrounds are so different they could never understand each other. They dislike each other. But let them "reverse" roles and then you may see the difference: Khrushchev trying to act the part of Eisenhower and Eisenhower trying to act the part of Khrushchev. By reversing roles, they gain an insight into each other they never had before. Each is taking the role of the other and facing each other in a discussion. Khrushchev now enacted by Eisenhower; Eisenhower now enacted by Khrushchev. Each has now to use his perceptive powers to enter into the skin of the other, sense his burdens, responsibilities, aspirations and limitations, ideals and goals, and live them out, here, now, before the representatives of both sides. At the same time, he sees himself mirrored by the other, in the manner in which he is perceived, assessed, weighed and responded to. Each is given a sort of inverted double vision of himself and the other, and has to absorb these kaleidoscopic images and assemble them into a meaningful whole, all while interacting. Think what the United Nations might really have been able to achieve if, all along, this method were used at crucial, critical points. How much more we would be able to understand one another or, if not understand, at least appreciate each other's difficulties. New insights would be gained, which in turn would lead us to more mature handling of conflicts. Imagine, if you can, the next summit meeting, in which every participant would have to reverse roles with every other before final decisions are made!

The Marriage Question

One of the chief sources of difficulties in our everyday life today is that we make immature choices, for instance, in the matter of marriage partners. The increasing number of teen-age marriages points the need for methods of evaluating ourselves and others in terms of our potential growth, not merely to assuage immediate needs. The adolescent is but as old and inexperienced as he is; we can not expect him to make decisions at 18 which will do credit to a person 10 years older. We cannot let him get married without going through the process itself. But psychodrama offers several alternatives. On the one hand, the youngsters can explore their future together; on the other, they can learn to look at and evaluate the consequences of their actions, without first having to make what may become a dreadful mistake. Psychodrama takes them from the present situation, "we want to get married," into the "future." The psychodramatic director will say to such a young couple: "Very well, let us explore what it will be like in two or three years from now, when you are married."

He now asks the youngsters to set the scene for the future as they foresee it. Assuming that they are married, he turns to the wife and says: "Where are you? Take us into your home." Now Julie stands up and describes her home—it may be realistic or it may be way off. This is important; Fred, her fiancé, learns more about her expectations of him now than he ever could, even in discussing it with her. For instance, Julie knows he is going to be a teacher. Yet, in the "future projection" on the psychodrama stage, she describes a lavish home which would better befit a president of General Electric. He is learning all the time, while watching this, for somewhere it will sink in that this is not the future he foresees.

Now, Julie says: "We have 3 children and I'm not working."

Fred recalls that, in 5 years, he may still be getting his graduate degree in education and Julie may very well *have* to work to meet anticipated expenses and that they cannot possibly have 3 children. Now, Julie says: "This is a weekday evening and we are at home. It is after dinner and the children are in bed. Fred sits in his chair over there." The director motions to Fred to sit there, after he has asked Fred if he agrees with this. Fred is willing, though in his mind he knows he will not merely be cozily sitting, he will be marking papers of his students and studying for his exams. He wonders why Julie does not realize how much work a teacher has at night.

Julie and Fred now proceed to enact a quiet evening at home together. First, they are disturbed by one of the children—enacted by a trained therapeutic actor—who continuously makes one or the other get up to give him water, a cookie, a goodnight kiss, etc. Now both must show their capacity for dealing with the demanding child in the role of the parent, as well as to demonstrate to one another how their theories of education converge or depart. Julie is for giving in, Fred argues that she is too lenient and besides, he is too tired to get up himself to help her or to put a stop to the child's scenes. Friction immediately ensues. After they have argued for a few moments, the director says: "The telephone rings. Answer it." Fred is not too tired to do so, but is immediately disheartened when the caller turns out to be a former boy friend of Julie who tries to make a date with her. While Julie does not exactly encourage the other man, she is obviously flattered by his continued interest in her and this, in turn, fans Fred's irritation. Finally, he orders her to hang up and make an end to the conversation.

Finding the Truth

While Julie has been on the phone, the director has allowed Fred to turn his head away and say out loud what he thinks of this call and he conveys his unhappiness quite clearly, bringing up the fact that this Bill was the boy Julie dated before she fell in love with him. Now he tells Julie, "Hang up on him, why do you have to give him so much of your time and attention?" Julie gets rid of Bill, wanders over to Fred, looks at him as if she has never seen him before—which is probably the truth, she has never seen him *this way*—and declares firmly, while stepping off the stage, "Now I know I can never marry you."

She gives him back his ring and sits down in the audience. Shocked, Fred turns to the director who recalls Julie to the stage. Julie comes up, says, "I realize it would be a great mistake. Now I understand it better. You see, it is because my mother likes Fred so well that we became engaged. She is a widow and has a hard time making ends meet. It is she who likes Fred; in fact, she likes him better than I do. When I came here, I was sure this was the man I ought to marry, but now I know it would be very bad for us." The members in the group, and Fred, too, are unhappy. Why is psychodrama breaking up this beautiful romance?

The psychodramatist now has the responsibility towards Fred, to help him, to make sure that this is not just a decision of Julie's only. How does Fred feel? He does not know, he is bewildered by the speed with which things have happened, but somewhere the doubt has become bigger in his mind. He, too, is not as sure as he was when they came in together, that marriage is right for them. They decide to leave matters as they are and to return for another session if they cannot work it out together. As the events turned out, they did not marry; they broke the engagement and each married another person several years later. What has really happened: they had a chance to objectify their relationship in a way which, had it been left to chance in life, might have led to another divorce statistic or to a miserable marriage. They had a chance to taste marriage conflicts—without actually going through with it—to feel their way into each other and the kind of life they might expect with each other, and to realize that this was not what they wanted or dreamed about. In other words, they aligned their dreams with the actualities and felt it better to wait and see if either their dreams had to be altered or they themselves had to undergo changes. In most cases, it is a little bit of each that must occur for growth to take place, but how often can life offer such growth without bitter suffering and dire results which involve the marital partners as well as their families and children?

Used in Industry

A growing use of psychodrama is in the fields of education and industry, particularly in the area of human relations. For instance, the union leader who wants to unionize the employer's business and the employer who is opposed to a closed shop. In the industrial application, these two men are confronted with each other; they have to reach an agreement. Or take the problem of getting fired from a job. There is hardly any situation which is as traumatic or anxiety-causing as that. These, and many more, are being subjected to psychodramatic exploration. The fired employee, for instance, gets a chance to face his employer, enacted by a trained psychodramatist, so as to give him at least a chance to understand why this happened to him. And many who are in the audience may identify themselves with his predicament.

Therapy for Mental Patients

Thus far, I have described how psychodrama deals with the problem of the normal individual, who is able to live in the community, to earn and make his way there. But psychodrama is increasingly being applied in the treatment of the mentally disturbed. It is used in mental hospitals and clinics. Patients have an opportunity to explore, by means of psychodrama, how they got sick, what influences contributed to their breakdown and how to avoid these in the future when they return home. They learn about themselves as well as about other patients in the hospital. They discover that no one is entirely sick and that even those who are or have been sick, have some natural resources within them which can lead to a return of mental stability. They find that they are able to help each other, often before they can help themselves. They also discover that even the so-called well persons have areas in which they are disturbed, so that they cease to be overly sensitive to their own shortcomings.

The mental patient cannot be treated by analysis, largely because he does not realize that he is sick. He does not coöperate in the treatment or, at best, does so only partly. The therapist's job is, therefore, to enter into the world of the patient, no matter how confused, to accept it as real—which it is for the patient—and to become his assistant in the production of his inner drama. One may think of the mental patient as of a playwright who is unable to complete his drama by himself; he is in need of helpers. Psychodrama supplies him with these helpers who assist him in bringing his baby into the world.

Once it is born, completed, he can look at it, objectify it as something outside of himself and perhaps forget it. As long as it remains inside of him, half-unborn, he cannot free himself of it, it holds him enthralled. One of the most involved applications of psychodrama was that of the man who believed he was Adolf Hitler. With the assistance of several trained psychodramatic therapists who filled the roles of Göring, Goebbels, Hess, etc., he was gradually able to free himself from these ideas and to resume his former identity. He was able to befriend his helpers, at first, only because they befriended him, so to speak. He did not see them except as the people he wanted them to be, but as he began to trust and know them, they began to be able to influence and guide him until he could accept them in their private identity, and this in turn helped him again to accept his own.

Where to Use Psychodrama

The most important application of psychodrama is, however, not to the severely disturbed, no matter how laudable this may be in itself. Psychodrama, in the opinion of Dr. Moreno, finds its most valuable use in the guiding of personality, in training for professional roles, in the *prevention* of major personality disturbances. It should become a part of our everyday life, to purge us as we go from minor disturbances, which, left unchecked, might result in serious illness. He believes that an ounce of prevention must take the place of the pound of cure. It is the so-called normal, well-adjusted person who needs most help. He lives in the fullness of life, with all its continuous difficulties. The sick, the delinquent, the criminal—these are safely locked away, where they can do no harm. But you and I, our friends and neighbors, the normal persons—we make the wars and revolutions, the manifold troubles which rock our world. Even the sick, the criminal and the frightened were once considered well, before they showed their inability to live among us; they lived side by side with us, our world made them what they are now. It is our responsibility to keep each other well and as happy as we believe we are capable of being.

Milk

We Still Say "No!" to Milk

Editor Rodale's still being asked how he could ever have come to the conclusion that milk can be an undesirable element in the diet. There are a large number of references from medical literature upon which we based our position, the literature which doctors are supposed to be reading to keep current. These same doctors are the ones who can't understand where we get the impression that cow's milk is harmful for humans.

Perhaps they will recognize some of the sources for our anti-milk sentiments:

In *Modern Nutrition* (February, 1959), Dr. Irvine McQuarrie of the Department of Pediatrics at the University of Minnesota scuttles the idea that milk is necessary for infants and children. He reminds us that many civilizations simply do not have access to milk of any kind—the Eskimos, for one. They supply milk's important nutrients—calcium, phosphorus, some B vitamins and protein —with eggs from wild or domesticated birds, intestines, meat from warm-blooded animals and small-boned fish. He says the food values of milk, plus more, are there. Dr. McQuarrie offered an easily made formula as a substitute for milk: ½ cup strained beef, ½ teaspoonful of bone meal powder, 1 teaspoonful of soybean oil, 2 tablespoonfuls of honey, 1 heaping tablespoonful of rice. Mix enough water with this in a blender, or with an egg beater, to bring the volume to one pint. This is nutritionally equal to one pint of cow's milk.

Penicillin Sensitivity

Archives of Dermatology (January, 1959) carries an article by Murray C. Zimmerman, which warns of an increase in penicillin sensitivity in Americans, probably due to the large amounts of the drug we drink in our milk. Cows get sick (at any given time, 6½ million suffer from mastitis, a disease of the udder), Dr. Zimmerman says, and are treated with penicillin. In 1950, the standard dosage was 1,000,000 units "at any suspicion of mastitis." The estimate is that 49 per cent of this comes through in the milk. Are you getting any of this contaminated milk? Measurable quantities of penicillin were found in 96 per cent of the samples of commercial milk tested in a recent survey. If you or your children consume a quart of milk, it can mean a penicillin intake of 500 units. A highly allergic person can go into shock if exposed to .000003 units of penicillin. In a glass of milk, you are likely to get 100 million times more than that. Can every milk drinker be sure that his reaction to this much penicillin will be negative? Can you be sure your baby will not have a reaction?

Journal of Nutrition (no date) prints the conclusions of Dr. Joseph C. Muhler of Indiana University. He found that rats eating heated powdered milk had a caries incidence of 9.3, while the incidence of those on unheated powdered milk was 5.4. We heat most of the milk we drink in the pasteurization process.

These few will give some idea of the kind of authority upon which we have based our views on the allergenic properties of milk and the intensive (and proven undesirable) growth factor in milk. The frequent public statements by researchers, nutritionists, pediatricians and other specialists and general practitioners, admitting a disenchantment with milk or an actual opposition to its free use, lend credence to our views. Here are some samples from the current literature your doctors see in professional journals:

The *Lancet* (December 3, 1960) carries a short letter from a doctor in a Winchester Pathological Laboratory reminding the readers that infants fed on cow's milk develop antibodies to the proteins in the milk. This indicates that these proteins are not compatible with the blood stream and the body actually must defend itself against them. Some systems cannot muster such defense and then the milk proteins present a serious danger. It is presumed that breast-fed infants do not develop antibodies to mother's milk.

Consumer Bulletin (March, 1961) quotes Dr. Frances E. Camps of the London Hospital Medical College as saying that there is some evidence to indicate that the majority of all babies between the ages of 7 and 97 weeks are sensitive to cow's milk. He blames unexplained crib deaths, which occur mostly in this age bracket, on the normal healthy child's regurgitation (vomiting) of milk during sleep, at which time he could inhale sufficient material to cause allergenic reaction in the sensitized tissues of the lungs. In experiments with guinea pigs, such reactions were easily induced and a quiet death without struggle ensued.

In view of the above, it was with special interest that we read a story in the *Minneapolis* (Minnesota) *Sunday Tribune* (December 11, 1960). It detailed the report of two Minneapolis doctors concerning "sudden and unexpected death" of at least 50 infants a year in the Minneapolis area. Most of the infants are under 4 months of age. A "deceptively mild respiratory infection" is presumed to be the cause of death in most cases, but many times the cause is obscure.

In the state of Minnesota, it is estimated that 220 such deaths occur each year. In the entire United States, the figure is presumed to be 11,500. Officials call the situation "alarming" or "puzzling." The baby is put to bed at night and is found to be dead in the morning. In all but a few cases, no "bugs" or bacteria, no viruses have shown up. Smothering is also discounted by health officials. In some cases, an autopsy shows pneumonia (inflammation of the lungs), but such an inflammation must have some cause. A study of 84 infant deaths showed that only 5 were considered so ill that parents had called a doctor. In two cases, the babies were pronounced normal only hours before death. The entire story reads like a dramatization of the theory of Dr. Camps.

The Minneapolis team said they knew of Dr. Camps' milk theory, but couldn't imagine how a sudden reaction could occur, based upon past experience. Perhaps the changes in milk wrought by today's methods of animal husbandry and the drugs used for treating the animals and the milk are responsible.

Milk Encourages Tallness

One of the main pillars of our argument against the uncontrolled use of milk for children is the growth factor involved. Mr. Rodale has shown that tallness is not a desirable attribute from the standpoint of good health. For one thing, it creates circulatory problems which burden the heart with undue strain. What the growth factor in milk could be is not known, but we do know that it is not calcium, since calcium is a constituent of many foods, bone meal especially, which have been shown to have no recognizable influence upon growth, as milk definitely does.

To show that milk stimulates growth, let us refer to the most recent item we've seen on the subject. *Roche Report* (June 26, 1961), told of the work done by 3 researchers of Northwestern University Medical School. Ten undernourished children whose bones showed a retarded maturity due to dietary shortages, showed a definite increase in bone growth when a milk supplement was introduced into their diet. They received reconstituted non-fat dry milk 6 days a week for 6 months. Then, the supplement was discontinued for a time and begun again for another 6 months. The amount of non-fat dry milk was equivalent, nutritionally, to two quarts of skim milk per day.

The children averaged a growth rate of .8 inches in the 6 months preceding the introduction of the supplement to their diet. During the first 6 months of supplementation with milk, their growth rate doubled to 1.6 inches. In the next 6-month period, during which no supplement was given, the growth rate dropped to just above its earlier level: about .95 inches. The supplementation with milk began again for a 6-month period, and the rate of growth went up to 1.5 inches. When the milk was stopped again, the growth rate went down, too.

It is our conviction that Americans are, on the average, taller than people of other nations because we make such a fetish of drinking plenty of milk. We tend to think of milk as our only reliable source of calcium and try to get the children to drink a quart a day. We believe bone meal to be a richer source of calcium, without milk's drawbacks. Bone meal, supplemented by a good high-protein diet, with B vitamins-rich foods, will deliver all the calcium necessary and allow for normal, healthy growth.

Minerals

Check on Your Mineral Intake

We are all vaguely aware of the need for minerals in our diets, in order to maintain good health. Somehow, we do not attach the same degree of importance to minerals as we do to vitamins. We simply assume that the proper amount will come to us in our regular meals. We know that minerals are not so easily lost in food preparation as are vitamins, so we take them for granted. However, the need for minerals is not solved so automatically. What you eat, how it is prepared and *how and where it was grown* determine your mineral intake. It can fall short of what is necessary, and often does.

In a talk reported in the Spokane (Washington) *Daily Chronicle* (December 3, 1955), Dr. Harry Warren, Professor of Geology at the University of British Columbia, Vancouver, accented the fact that minerals in soil and water have a far greater effect on health than climate. Among the possible physiological effects of the mineral content of the soil, according to Dr. Warren, are a retarded birth rate, goiter, anemia and poor digestion.

He offered several instances to substantiate his views: In India, iron in a river bed filtered out so much of the river's iodine content that persons living downstream generally suffered from goiters. Cobalt added to salt ended a world-wide epidemic of "falling sickness" among sheep. Bacteria which digests food in a sheep's stomach need cobalt to function. Cobalt is also essential to humans.

A Delicate Balance

The delicate balance of mineral needs in animals was illustrated by Dr. Warren's story of a virus-like infection in Florida grapefruit trees which was cleared up by spraying the trees with a dilute solution of molybdenum, a mineral essential to animal life. Too much of this mineral, however, killed animals in Somerset County, England. The threat was overcome by feeding these animals copper. Apparently, it was the extra copper which the body needed to process the molybdenum.

While it is true that both plants and animals obtain minerals primarily from the soil, it is not true that plants require the same minerals as animals do. For example, plants do not need iodine, and that is why plants grown around the Great Lakes and in the Pacific Northwest (two "goiter belts") are deficient in iodine, yet grow well. Conversely, minerals which are essential for the growth of plants, are sometimes not necessary for humans. Boron and vanadium are two such elements. Also, the mineral values of similar plants vary by location.

These facts bring us to another conclusion. It does not follow, because a plant grows well—or appears to grow well—that it is as rich in mineral values as a similar plant, grown elsewhere. This is what causes us to differ with experimenters who blanket farming areas with chemical compounds which can change the character of the earth and the minerals it contains. The change cannot be guaranteed to be better for the consumer, merely because it makes the plants grow well.

It is true that, when a piece of land is tested and found wanting in a particular mineral element, a natural compound rich in that element can be added profitably. But when synthetic compounds are added haphazardly, merely to make good land into super-land that will burn itself out growing whopping tomatoes and giant potatoes, the consumer stands a strong chance of losing out. The fruit and vegetables grown in this way are very likely to be short on mineral and vitamin content.

Minerals as Catalysts

Borden's Review of Nutrition Research (Vol. XVII, No. 4) characterizes minerals as catalysts; that is, they are required to be present to allow a needed change to take place in other elements brought into the body, much as a fire changes logs into charcoal. The fire is not contained in the final result, nor is it changed in the process. Still, without fire, the transformation of the logs cannot take place.

Magnesium is extremely valuable as a catalyst, for without it, the carbohydrates we ingest cannot be properly assimilated. In rats and dogs, a deficiency of magnesium causes a series of convulsions and hyperemia (hemorrhages). Magnesium is necessary for the processing of many sugars in the body. In most cases, manganese will act as a substitute for magnesium and manganese is involved in the conversion of monosaccharides to ascorbic acid (vitamin C). This fact is offered as a possible explanation of the phenomenon which allows some animals to manufacture their own vitamin C. Humans are incapable of this remarkable ability.

Enzymes Depend upon Minerals

Zinc has been shown to be a constituent of the enzyme, carbonic anhydrase, which acts upon the combination of carbon dioxide and water in the tissues and the blood to form carbonic acid. This means that zinc plays an important part in the respiratory system and, for this reason, it must be included in the diet of animals every day.

Iron has a number of important jobs. It is well known that a deficiency in this mineral will produce anemia in animals, for 66 per cent of the iron in the body is contained in the hemoglobin of the blood, the remainder being located primarily in those sites where red blood cells are formed. One need only reflect on the essential character of the blood in proper body function to realize how vital a good iron supply is in the diet.

Cobalt and copper are also intimately connected with the formation of hemoglobin. Often, when iron does not bring results for anemic patients, copper alone, or in combination with vitamin B_{12}, can have the necessary effect when added to the diet.

Copper has been shown to be the specific metal component of the enzymes tyrosinase, laccase and ascorbic acid oxidase. Tyrosinase is involved in the transformation of the amino acid, tyrosine into a substance which is again converted into melanin pigments—skin coloring. Copper, as a trace mineral, may actually be involved in the disease (vitiligo) which results in complete loss of skin pigment in certain areas of the body. Perhaps albinos (those who lack skin pigment over the whole body from birth) are short of copper during the gestation period or, for some reason, are unable to utilize the trace metal properly.

In the *Canadian Journal of Public Health* (April, 1961), we read of trouble on farm land which contained less than one part per million of copper. In grazing areas definitely low in copper, many of the animals dependent upon the hay grown there had to be destroyed, because they were unhealthy. In another instance, cattle grazing on copper-deficient soil were unable to reproduce. Copper added to the feed solved the problem.

Jobs Minerals Do

In February, 1957, *Modern Nutrition* carried an article on trace elements by J. F. Wischhusen. In it, he touched on some of the many jobs minerals do:

Protein cannot be formed without calcium, nitrogen and sulfur.

The vagus nerve that controls stomach activity requires potassium to function properly.

Vitamins cannot be found in either plants or animals without minerals. (An excellent argument, we think, for the value of natural vitamin supplements.) For most vitamins, there is an intermediate nutrient. For example, cobalt is implicitly involved with vitamin B_{12}. There is reason to believe that vitamin B_{12} (also called cobalt amine) can be made by the body if given an adequate supply of cobalt.

The author tells us that cobalt, combined with vitamin B_{12}, serves to remove excessive amounts of carbon-hydrogen-nitrogen groups. It is known that multiple sclerosis victims suffer from damage to the covering of the nerves by a carbon-nitrogen compound. If cobalt normally removes such a detrimental compound, one could call multiple sclerosis, among other things, the result of a cobalt deficiency. Had sufficient cobalt been present, the nerve covering might not have been damaged, since this damaging element would have been removed.

Zinc is an important constituent of the insulin molecule. Here we are confronted with the possibility that a shortage of zinc might be involved with diabetes, which is the result of an insufficiency of insulin.

Minerals influence the contraction of muscle and the response of nerve.

Mineral concentration acts to control liquids in the body to allow nutrients to pass into the blood stream.

A mineral signal controls the coagulation of the blood.

Mental alertness is related to a group of trace elements: manganese, copper, cobalt, iodine, zinc, magnesium and phosphorus.

Certain metals in the blood stream exert a bactericidal action. The healthy body can, therefore, make its own antibiotics, provided the essential raw materials are present.

Of course, for body bone structure, calcium and phosphorus are essential. About 95 per cent of the skeleton and teeth are made up of this combination; about 18 other elements are also involved.

By the time the food you buy reaches your table, you have no way of knowing just what percentage of minerals is still intact, unless you have grown and cooked it yourself. This means that one is quite likely to struggle along on a minimal intake of some minerals. We would again quote Mr. Wischhusen from another article which appeared in the *Science Counselor* (March, 1957):

"Since all refined foodstuffs, whether in the carbohydrate or protein group, have minerals as well as vitamins removed, a general supplementation of these to the average diet is called for. This is readily possible . . . All in all, about 37 different inorganic elements have thus far been found to be in one or another way involved in the fabric of life, and 23 thereof have been shown to be invariably essential to all forms of life. . . ."

Table 7 is a partial list of the foods you can add to your diet for an immediate increase in mineral intake.

Table 7: FOODS HIGH IN MINERALS

Figures given below are, unless otherwise specified, in milligrams per 100 grams (average serving).

	Calcium	Phosphorus	Iron	Sodium	Potassium
BREWER'S YEAST	106	1893	18.2	150	1700
BLACKSTRAP MOLASSES	579	85	11.3	....	....
WHEAT GERM	84	1096	8.1	2	780
HONEY	5	16	.9	7	10
DESICCATED LIVER*	12	220-358	8.30	....	....
KELP	1.05%	.339%	.37%	3.98%	11.15%
SUNFLOWER SEEDS	57	860	6.0	.4	630
BONE MEAL	30.52%	22.52%	.004%	.46%	0.20%

Also contains 2.5 milligrams of copper per 100 grams.

Miscarriage

Miscarriage Is No Accident

Because recovery is usually rapid and there are seldom serious effects from miscarriage, there is a tendency in the medical profession to shrug it off when it happens and treat it as a bit of bad luck about which little or nothing can be done. But miscarriages do not occur without cause. Not only are they often a severe emotional shock to prospective parents suddenly deprived of the expected child, they also may well be an indication of a health problem in the mother that requires and deserves attention.

In any case, there is nothing pleasant about a miscarriage. It is something to be avoided and something that the prospective mother *can* avoid in most cases.

Let's take a look at this far too common occurrence and see what can be done about it.

Spontaneous Abortion

When we talk about a miscarriage (or spontaneous abortion), we mean the birth of a baby before it has developed enough to be able to live outside the womb. This usually means birth prior to the sixth month of pregnancy. After that time, it is usually possible for a child, even though premature, to be kept alive and to develop outside the womb.

"About two-thirds of all miscarriages occur in the first 3 months of pregnancy, and these early miscarriages are fairly common," according to *Prenatal Care,* a booklet written by Dr. Ann DeHuff Peters and published by the Children's Bureau of the Department of Health, Education and Welfare.

As with many health problems, doctors tend to regard miscarriage as something of a mystery, because they have not been able to pinpoint a single cause for it. To us, this seems about as wise as calling sneezing a mystery because it is sometimes caused by house dust, sometimes by pollen and sometimes by snuff. Miscarriage is obviously a health abnormality of either the mother or the fetus, and it is only reasonable to suppose that measures to insure good health in both will avert premature ejection of the embryo from the womb.

Influence of Poor Nutrition

Nutrition Reviews, in September, 1954, reported on many experimental studies made in various parts of the world to determine the influence of diet on the course of pregnancy. Ebbs, Tisdall and Scott, a group of researchers, gave food supplements to a group of 90 women who were pregnant and found to have lived on nutritionally poor diets. These women were compared with a second group, with an equally poor nutritional background, who were not given any supplements, and with a third group who had always eaten better. "The rates of occurrence of abortions, premature births, stillbirths and neonatal deaths were significantly higher in the group of women on the poor but unsupplemented diet," it was concluded.

In a remarkable book, titled *The Birth of Normal Babies,* Dr. Lyon P. Strean, a prominent researcher, points out the enormously important role of the B vitamins in pregnancies. "One out of every ten pregnancies usually ends in failure—miscarriages, stillbirths or congenital abnormalities," he states. He then goes on to show that the villain in many of these cases is cortisone, the hormone produced by the adrenal gland in times of stress. "Traumatic stress in the expectant mother in the first 3 months of her pregnancy will result in more than usual concentrations of cortisone in the circulation and, under certain conditions, this catabolic hormone may pass through the placental barrier and produce an abnormal intra-uterine environment."

B Complex Vitamins and Stress

Stresses, Dr. Strean points out, can be either physical or emotional. One can fall downstairs or be shocked by the death of a dear one. In either case, the stress induces greater adrenal activity, which serves the purpose, in times of crisis or danger, of speeding all the metabolic processes and making one stronger and faster-reacting. When the crisis is over, however, the body is left with excessive amounts of cortisone, according to Dr. Strean, which can do damage in the child-bearing uterus. As a basic protection against this kind of situation, Dr. Strean recommends the B complex vitamins, which are known to improve the health of the nerves and thus to prevent exaggerated reactions that lead to excessive adrenal stimulation. Dr. Strean strongly advises doctors to avoid prescribing cortisone or ACTH for pregnant women.

Remarkably, the avoidance of salt seems to have a definite effect in minimizing the danger of miscarriage. Professor K. DeSnoo of Utrecht points this out in the July 10, 1948 issue of the *Netherlands Medical Journal*. He shows that edema, swelling of the body tissues through accumulation of water, is epecially common in pregnancy. This condition can lead to high blood pressure and eclampsia (convulsions) in the pregnant woman that can have serious consequences. Dr. DeSnoo quotes figures to show that, when Dutch women consumed less salt during the war, they had far fewer abnormal pregnancies. He recommends that salt be avoided during pregnancy.

Dr. Peters, in her *Prenatal Care* booklet, confirms this viewpoint, also recommending the avoidance of foods that contain extra salt, such as bacon, ham, corned beef, smoked fish, salted nuts, popcorn and potato chips.

Of course, we have long advocated that table salt be eliminated from everyone's diet, there being enough sodium naturally present in food for the body's small requirements. This is recommended for everyone, but, as we have seen, in pregnancy, it becomes particularly important.

Vitamin C, as it occurs naturally in the bioflavonoids, is another enormously important food factor in a woman's ability to carry a child normally. Dr. Carl T. Javert of Cornell University, speaking at a symposium in 1955, described his method of treating pregnant women who had histories of chronic abortion. Giving them a diet rich in vitamin C, with additional supplements of flavonoids, for a total intake of 500 milligrams a day of vitamin C, Dr. Javert achieved successful pregnancies in 91 per cent of the women under his care.

At the same symposium, Dr. Robert Greenblatt of the Medical College of Georgia confirmed these results and pointed out that the habitually aborting women he had treated all had capillaries that burst easily, a condition that was corrected by the vitamin C.

Now, if, as we have seen, vitamins B and C are particularly important for the avoidance of miscarriage, then we are driven inevitably to the conclusion that smoking must play a large role in causing miscarriages. This is speculation. We can not find any experimental study specifically dealing with the relationship between smoking and inability to carry a child. But we *know* that smoking, by forcing our bodies to defend themselves against the poisons in the smoke, uses up vitamins B and C at an alarmingly fast rate. A single cigarette will remove 30 milligrams of vitamin C from the system. Therefore, we respectfully suggest to the medical profession that a study of the smoking habits of women who habitually abort may prove unusually fruitful.

Good Diet Is Best Safeguard

As we consider these matters, however, it is well to remember that the process of reproduction is a remarkably vigorous and tenacious one. There are many women who are chronically malnourished to some extent who still manage to keep their children and have normal births. Miscarriage is not an inevitable result of malnutrition, nor is it an inevitable result of illness during pregnancy (another common cause) or abnormality of the child. These things make miscarriage more likely and should be guarded against.

Miscarriage will sometimes come about because the fetus, for some reason, has failed to remain alive. In this occurrence, vitamin E is supposed to play a vital protective role, according to Woollam and Miller in the *British Medical Journal* (June 2, 1956). They attribute failures classified as "of unknown origin" to insufficiency of oxygen in the blood supply the embryo receives from the mother. Vitamin E is known to be a prime agent in preserving a higher oxygen content in the blood.

Dr. Evan Shute, writing in the *Canadian Medical Association Journal* (January 9, 1960), reports his experience in being able to anticipate spontaneous abortion in women with certain types of hormone deficiency, and to prevent it with vitamin E. Dr. Shute reports that, by routinely prescribing vitamin E for all obstetric patients, he has reduced the rate of threatened miscarriage from 10 per cent to 5 per cent, and then, with additional vitamin E therapy, has salvaged better than 80 per cent of the remainder.

Warning Signal

Frequently, before miscarriage occurs, there are warnings in time to do something about it. These consist of slight bleeding from the vagina and pain in the lower abdomen, according to Dr. Peters. "The bleeding may be only a slight spotting," she says, "or it may be a gush of blood with clots." The first means that a miscarriage is only threatening, and Dr. Peters advises the woman to whom it is happening to go to bed at once and stay there until her doctor has examined her and tells her it is safe to get up. Often, the doctor can determine the cause of the threatened miscarriage and prevent it.

A gush of blood, of course, indicates that a miscarriage is already happening. In such a case, all the doctor can do is prevent infection and attend to possible excessive hemorrhaging. In such a case, more careful attention to your general health will be found most helpful in making the next pregnancy successful.

Mouthwashes

Do Mouthwashes Really Work?

In an effort to eliminate, or at least to mask, bad breath, many Americans turn to the routine of mouthwashes. The sad fact seems to be that those who are most careful about using such preparations are the ones who have the most trouble keeping their breath pleasant. Do mouthwashes work? What do they do to eliminate unpleasant oral smells? Do you need one just to be on the safe side? Can a mouthwash do any harm?

To take first things first, there are many possible causes for bad breath. Most of them originate in the mouth—bad teeth, food particles, traces of pungent-smelling foods which remain in the mouth. These are the usual causes of bad breath. Then there are the physiological disorders which manifest themselves by odors in the mouth—liver malfunction, nervousness, psychological disturbances, poor metabolism and, sometimes, menstruation. Constipation is given as a possible cause of bad breath by some physiologists and completely discounted by others.

Another factor in the problem of maintaining a sweet breath lies in the powerful and lasting odors in some of the foods we eat. For example, it requires only a billionth of an ounce of onion oil to make enough of an odor to be detected by the normal sense of smell. Garlic, the other of the best known causes of bad breath, is so strong that it can be detected on the breath of a newborn baby if the mother has eaten it within a reasonably short time before delivery. There are many other such strong odors in the foods we eat, so that one is constantly exposed to the hazard of harboring unpleasant breath. But the fact remains that for most people, bad breath it not a problem, while others are almost unbearable because of their breath.

Bacteria Necessary

There is a reason for this. The mouth of a healthy individual should be generally free of odor. One researcher has likened the oral cavity to an aquarium which is filled with healthful bacteria, balanced by nature to stay sweet and clean. It is only when this balance is upset that mouth odors appear. Medication for long periods of time can break down the colonies.

Mouthwashes are often advertised as antiseptic and bactericidal. These products, if they kill any undesirable bacteria, also kill the bacteria necessary to maintain nature's balance in the mouth. One does not pour bactericides into an aquarium, because much of the bacteria there is necessary to the quality of the water and the health of the fish. In the same way, one must also be wary of destroying necessary elements in the mouth through the use of bactericides.

A full discussion of mouthwashes by Frederick M. Kraus, M.D., D.M.D., appeared in the *Bulletin of the National Dental Association* (April, 1958). He likens the claims of today's mouthwash preparations to those made in the eighteenth and nineteenth centuries, when promises of benefits from oral rinses included cure of headache and restoration of gum tone and solidity of the teeth. Says Dr. Kraus, "Not only do mouthwashes fail to live up to the advertised claims, but some may actually be harmful if used continually. A large number of medicated mouthwashes are toxic, even in dilution. For instance, those which contain organic mercurials are potential kidney poisons. Others containing antibiotics may lead to allergies, to the development of bacterial resistance and to the development of an unsightly black, hairy tongue. The latter condition has also been described as the result of continued use of mouthwashes containing or liberating hydrogen peroxide."

Some products are advertised as deodorants. They promise to "sweeten" breath and the ads give the impression that the sweetening action lasts all day. An evaluation by Dr. Kraus is as follows: ". . . Moreover, the quality of breath will also be improved more effectively by mechanical procedures (brushing) than by cosmetic preparations. It has been found that the use of a toothbrush lessens mouth odors for at least two hours, whereas the masking aroma of a dentifrice lingers on for one-half hour only."

Is Decay Inhibited?

The mouthwash advertisements would lead one to believe that the problem of dental caries will vanish with their use. Dr. Kraus writes that the requirements of such a mouthwash are so complex, that no one has ever been able to perfect one. He remarks that stannous fluoride (the type applied directly to the teeth by dentists) in solution has proven effective as an anti-enzyme in inhibiting the oral acid-forming systems. However, "Because the fluoride is likely also to inhibit other enzymes, *one may anticipate side effects.*" (Italics ours.) One of these, says Dr. Kraus in the *British Medical Journal* (July 1, 1961), is the breakdown of an oral defense mechanism against infection, particularly against diphtheria, found to exist in human saliva. It is suggested that resistance to influenza infection might also depend upon this mechanism. Is it possible that the recent yearly "flu" epidemics are somehow connected with fluoridation? These questions remain unanswered and in Dr. Kraus' view, the use of fluoride-containing preparations should be "discouraged until they can be proved to be entirely innocuous (harmless)."

We can be assured that these dangers will not prevent someone from introducing a fluoride-containing mouthwash. We already have toothbrushes which are intended to coat your teeth with fluoride as you brush; stannous fluoride is a component of at least one toothpaste and now, another manufacturer has put sodium fluoride in his toothpaste. No one seems able to explain how the use of fluoridated toothpastes, brushes and topically applied fluorides, in addition to drinking fluoridated water, will permit the ingestion of the optimum, one part per million of fluoride, that is supposed to be the safe dosage. Logically, it would appear that the child who drinks fluoridated water and has the fluoride topically applied, is getting more fluoride than he should have, unless the fluorides in the water were insufficient in the first place—which they are guaranteed not to be. Now, suppose the child also uses the toothpaste and brush. Is he getting enough fluoride to do him harm? No tests have been made. We know that sodium fluoride is a deadly, corrosive poison, but there is apparently no limit set on its use in oral hygiene. Dr. Kraus' worries over side effects from mouthwashes that contain fluorides would hold true for other fluoride-containing products in the same area, but it doesn't seem to bother the Food and Drug Administration. On receiving our inquiry about a toothpaste containing sodium fluoride, which has been on the market for several months, the Food and Drug Administration responded that it knew of no tests done to ascertain the product's safety, nor were they in any position to make a judgment on its safety. The sponsor of the product is under no legal obligation to clear his product with the department. It's a product that is being advertised on TV, in magazines and it is available in almost every store where such things are sold, but our federal agencies have done nothing about making sure it's safe for us to use!

Eliminating Bad Breath

If mouthwashes won't do the job of eliminating the effects of bad breath, what will? The positive action of brushing seems to do more than anything else to control bad breath. Brushing without any dentifrice or mouthwash is as effective and more healthful as if one is used. Eating what are called detergent foods—apples, carrots, celery, pears, etc.—also helps in cleansing the teeth and hence, removing odor-causing food particles from the mouth. Furthermore, these foods, rich in vitamins and minerals, are a great asset in maintaining the health of the gum tissues.

Outdoor exercise, especially walking, introduces more oxygen into the lungs, and this is believed by some to dilute the odorous elements in the system and thereby lessen bad breath.

It can be accepted as a truism that commercial dentifrices and mouthwashes only increase the problems of oral hygiene. Careful brushing with a toothbrush free of all pastes and powders is the best way to prevent unpleasant breath. Careful rinsing of the mouth with plain water is a help and so is the use of dental floss to cleanse food-trapping crevices. Aside from these efforts, we believe that careful diet is the answer to unpleasant breath. Eat foods that are rich in nutrients to protect the teeth and keep them healthy. Eat them raw when possible to provide hard chewing surfaces which will strengthen the gums and cleanse the teeth as well. Avoid foods that are soft and sticky, especially carbohydrates, for they do nothing that will benefit the teeth or the tissues of the oral cavity, but they do lodge in the crevices of the teeth and the inner surfaces where they can act as direct causes of tooth decay. The decay, of course, is a prime cause of bad breath.

There it is: the experts say skip the mouthwashes and use a plain toothbrush often, rinse frequently and eat proper foods. This is your best defense against bad breath.

Multiple Sclerosis

Current Picture of Multiple Sclerosis

Briefly, multiple sclerosis is a condition in which the protecting sheath (myelin) which surrounds the nerves and spinal cord is destroyed. This leaves these nerves exposed and the impulses from the brain center run into interference as they pass through this area. The MS victim's brain wills a hand to grasp an object, but the message from the brain is sidetracked and often doesn't reach the hand at all. The hand, of course, cannot grasp.

The key to multiple sclerosis lies in just what it is that causes this so-called insulation to disintegrate from around the nerves. What makes it last in most of us, but not in all? Some have suggested a hereditary factor, but, in the *British Medical Journal* (March 12,

1957), Dr. Douglas McAlpine expressed the opinion that any genetic factor would be extremely weak and would have to be reinforced by outside factors. Furthermore, MS occurs in persons who have absolutely no history of the disease in the family.

Climate was questioned as a cause, since multiple sclerosis appears more frequently in the north of Europe and America, than in the south of either of these continents. One doctor (R. L. Swank in the *American Journal of Medical Sciences,* October, 1950) advanced the possibility that, since the people of these regions have more fat in their diet, it could be a factor in the frequency of multiple sclerosis. However, two years later, in *Neurology* (September-October, 1952), it was reported that, in a test of 65 MS patients, 24 per cent were shown to have a lack of fat in their systems, rather than an overabundance.

MS and Certain Grain Foods

The article in *Neurology* did come up with some worthwhile information. It showed a definite relationship between multiple sclerosis and allergies to rye and wheat. The author noted that there is a high incidence of MS in countries where rye bread is one of the important food factors; also, there is a low incidence in countries in which rice is a staple food.

A diet free of all suspected allergens was given to all 65 of the subjects in the experiment. Favorable results were seen in 31 per cent of the cases. In 12 of the cases, temporary reintroduction of the allergens brought back the symptoms. Of these 65 patients, 50 per cent were shown to be short of calcium and iron and 36 per cent lacked the proper amount of protein.

An interesting finding was advanced by Drs. Adams and Gordon and reported in the *Kansas City Star* (January 4, 1954). They blamed MS on a kink in the body's metabolism. Normally, when food is processed in the body, ammonia is deposited in the nerve cells. This ammonia is quickly removed by the other body processes, thus eliminating any chance for poisoning of the nerve cells. In many multiple sclerosis patients, the process for removing the ammonia failed. It was discovered that a chemical normally present in the body, succinate, when injected into the body of an MS patient, made possible the removal of ammonia from the nerve tissues. The question is, of course, why do MS patients lack sufficient succinate? Does their supply not work properly? Is it less potent than it should be? Would regular injections of succinate alleviate the symptoms and progress of multiple sclerosis? We have seen no more information on this theory.

Supplements and Diet

The B vitamins (niacin, thiamin, pyridoxine and B_{12}) have been used to treat MS with varying success. For the most part, the progress the patients made was not permanent, though there was definite brief improvement.

Dr. E. M. Abrahamson saw 126 multiple sclerosis patients in 18 months, and found high or low blood sugar in each of them, as well as a lack of calcium (*New York State Medical Journal,* June 1, 1954). With a diet correcting the sugar level and injections of calcium, Dr. Abrahamson had remarkable results in treating MS.

On October 6, 1960, a newspaper in Fort Dodge, Iowa, carried the syndicated column of Earl Ubell, science writer for the *New York Herald Tribune,* in which he wrote of the use of a drug, Orinase, normally used to control diabetes, against multiple sclerosis. The trial of the drug by a University of Minnesota neurologist, Glen T. Sawyer, was accidental. A veteran was admitted to a veterans hospital with rapidly progressive MS. Dr. Sawyer noticed that the man had severe acne on his back, and because he had heard that acne responded to treatment with Orinase, he tried using it. To Dr. Sawyer's complete surprise, the veteran "showed remarkable improvement" in his multiple sclerosis condition. Fearing that the remission might be the temporary type that is characteristic of multiple sclerosis, with or without treatment, Dr. Sawyer tried withholding the drug and substituting a look-alike pill with no drug value, a placebo. In 3 days, the patient began to have the same MS symptoms. Six more MS patients responded to the drug in the same manner.

High-Carbohydrate Diet Suspected

Dr. Sawyer reasoned that, since the drug is intended to be active against diabetes and since diabetes is aggravated by a high-carbohydrate diet, multiple sclerosis might be aggravated by a high-carbohydrate diet. He found this supposition to be true. On a high sugar and starch diet, the conditions of the multiple sclerosis victims worsened. This leads us to surmise that a diet low in sugar and starch, without the drug, would be effective as a treatment for multiple sclerosis. If, as was suggested by another researcher, multiple sclerosis is a disease caused by poor metabolism, the bodies of multiple sclerosis patients may not be able to handle the sugars and starches even in normal amounts. Further, we feel that the avoidance of any drug is best, if it is possible, since the side effects of the drugs are often as dangerous as the disease against which they are used. Orinase is one of the drugs which has perilous side effects.

In *A Biochemical Basis of Multiple Sclerosis,* Roy L. Swank, M.D., Ph.S., of the University of Oregon Medical School, seeks to give a comprehensive picture of multiple sclerosis, what is being done and what can be done for those who are stricken with the disease, and to protect the rest of us from falling victim to it.

Dr. Swank feels that blood values are a primary factor in multiple sclerosis. But there are various changes at various times, and this is the fact that puzzles researchers who are looking for one consistent abnormal condition in the blood of all MS victims. As Dr. Swank writes:

"It seems evident that changes do occur in the circulating blood, although the nature of these changes is not clear. Periodic changes in the pattern of plasma proteins, periodic fluctuations in the amount of fibrinogen, periodic fluctuations in the number of platelets and reduced ability of the plasma to hold neutral fats in stable suspension —all suggest an altered suspension stability of blood. The exact degree and perhaps reliability of these reported changes is still open to discussion. In any event, there is ample reason to suspect that changes in the blood itself do occur."

As can be readily seen, the question of just which of these blood abnormalities is basic to the onset or aggravation of MS is difficult to ascertain. Furthermore, in such a situation, the treatment of one problem could lead to the establishment of another.

Low Tolerance to Heat

Researchers have done surveys on "Factors Which Influence the Frequency and Severity of Multiple Sclerosis," the title of a chapter in this book. Some interesting facts come to light here. An MS patient is sensitive to temperature changes. He has a low tolerance to heat. Warm, humid weather—even a hot bath—leaves many patients with increased disability. Immersion of patients in cold water while they are suffering the effects of immersion in hot water, abolished the increased disability quickly. It is believed that this unfortunate reaction is due to the diverting of the effective circulating blood to the surface of the body and away from the nervous system when the body is heated, as is seen in the reddened skin. With cooling, the reverse is true, and even more blood reverts to the nervous system as a result of the narrowing of the blood vessels of the extremities.

Other situations which create increased symptoms for MS victims, says Dr. Swank, are pregnancy, surgery, hemorrhaging of any kind and certain diagnostic procedures, especially spinal punctures and myelograms. Fatigue, especially when deep and prolonged, means trouble to patients with multiple sclerosis.

Fat in Diet a Factor

Surveys of many areas of the world, with careful attention to the type of diet eaten by the people in each place, convinced Swank that the amount of fat in the diet is an important factor in the development of multiple sclerosis. A graph is offered which shows the number of multiple sclerosis cases per 100,000 to rise in direct proportion to the amount of animal and butterfat consumed in the country. This theory is an extremely controversial one, however, with many scientists presenting figures to prove just the opposite. Swank insists, though, that patients treated by low-fat diet benefited significantly. About 95 per cent remained the same or improved during a period averaging nearly 8 years.

It has been shown that red blood cells in patients with MS are larger than those observed in normal subjects. Dr. Swank observed enlarged blood cells in animals after fat meals. Is it possible, as the author suggests, that the large cells in the MS victim and in the animals were due to the same cause, namely, high-fat intake?

The course of multiple sclerosis is a complex one. There seem to be no clear-cut answers to how it can best be treated or how it can be prevented. Diet somehow seems to hold the key. More fat, less fat? No one is sure, but Dr. Swank does seem to have successful results on his side, after using a low-fat diet. The Abrahamson Diet also has its successes. Whatever system is used, certainly, food supplements and avoidance of processed foods, can only aid in bringing about a return to good health.

Mushrooms

Mushrooms Are a Fine Food

Perhaps the most astonishing factor about the mushroom is its double standard in terms of the relative merits derived from its eating. Although it is highly praised as a gourmet's dish and nutritionists and scientists claim for it rich nutritional benefits in the way of vitamins (especially the B vitamins) proteins and the germ-stopping properties of some of the chemicals found in it, the problem of the mushroom's potency as an allergen must be a strong consideration when including this food in your diet.

There are some 30-odd varieties of poisonous mushrooms which contain substances that can cause such symptoms as nausea, drowsiness, stupor, pains in the joints and even death in some instances. Avoiding such varieties is the means of protection in this case. Almost every person can remember childhood warnings about not picking and eating the wild mushrooms found in the forests and countryside. So, the problem of avoiding such dangerous species as the *Amanita verna* and *Gyromitra esculenta* seems to us a minor one, since very few people gather wild mushrooms for the table. Yet, there are always those few enthusiasts who can't resist the temptation to find their own and in doing so, rely on such folklore tests as a silver spoon's turning black to distinguish between the poisonous and nonpoisonous species. These tests are useless and misleading and in some cases, can result in mushroom poisoning. One such case is found in the *Lancet* for September 16, 1961.

A Case of Mushroom Poisoning

A 40-year-old farmer was admitted to the Cumberland Infirmary complaining of pain in the upper region of the abdomen and jaundice. The initial diagnosis was inflammation of the gall bladder. On the following day, the patient had a major epileptic fit and a reduction in the amount of urine excreted was noticed. After the fit, his mental condition fluctuated. "He became extremely irritable and swore at his medical attendants when disturbed. Spontaneous clonic twitching of the muscles of his limbs and face appeared." The initial diagnosis was changed to possible mushroom poisoning.

In questioning the family about the possibility of the patient's ingestion of poisonous mushrooms, it was confirmed that he had indeed picked and eaten a goodly amount of mushrooms. However, his wife and nephew had also eaten some of the same mushrooms, yet only the nephew experienced ill effects, complaining of vomiting as a result of the meal. On further investigation, it was discovered that the highly poisonous species, *Amanita phalloides,* could be found near the patient's farm. Treatment, employing such commonly used medical techniques as gastric lavage (the washing out of the stomach) and antidotes, covered a period of about 30 days, after which, the patient was discharged from the hospital feeling well and completely cured.

This case of near death from mushroom ingestion is, of course, an isolated case, a case, which, as we mentioned earlier, could easily have been avoided by observing the simple rule of not picking wild mushrooms. However, the case is interesting from another point of view, one which we think is really the crux of the matter concerning the possible hazards involved in eating mushrooms. This point is found in the following statement taken from the *Lancet* article. "Nothing strange was noticed by the patient about the mushrooms and a large stew had been eaten by the patient, his wife and his nephew on October 5, 1959. The wife suffered no ill effects, but the nephew vomited several times that evening and felt unwell for two or three days." Why didn't all the members of this family contract the poisoning, since they all ate from the same mushrooms? Why did the poison single out only one of them? The fact that the poison only affected one member of the family, certainly points up to the possibility that an exaggerated allergenic reaction could have been the culprit. Certainly the circumstances involved in this case compare favorably to those conditions which we define as allergy, food allergy to be specific. John P. McGovern, M.D., and Joseph I. Zuckerman, M.D., in their article "Nutrition in Pediatric Allergy," found in *Borden's Review of Nutrition Research,* Vol. XVII, No. 3, give this definition of food allergy. They say, "Food allergy may be defined as a condition of unusual or exaggerated specific response to those foods to which the patient is sensitive, and when ingested in similar amounts by the majority of individuals, are harmless." Isn't this what happened in the *Lancet* case described above? The patient was extremely sensitive to a food which the other members of his family could tolerate.

Allergy to Mushrooms

This implication that mushrooms are an allergenic food, we think, is the most important single factor in deciding on whether or not to include mushrooms in your diet. To be sure, it is of greater importance to most of us than the danger of outright poisoning from mushrooms. One can avoid the poisonous species by buying only commercially grown varieties.

However, what of the consumer who relies on the growers' integrity and know-how in the business of growing mushrooms and still finds that he becomes ill after eating these commercial brands? Should he assume that the grower has produced an inedible species? We think not, for there are over 700 edible kinds of mushrooms, certainly a wide enough range for mushroom growers to choose from. With this choice at their command, they need not turn to the growing of undesirable species. Reed Millard, in the June, 1956, issue of *Coronet* magazine, says this about the reliability of eating commercially grown mushrooms: "Only an expert can be trusted to tell them apart and even experts have made mistakes. This is true, of course, only of the wild mushroom. One need not question the edibility of commercially grown strains."

No, the real problem in such a case is an individual one—one in which the individual himself must bear the blame, for it is his bodily system which cannot tolerate the mushroom. We believe the explanation for this strange phenomenon can be traced back to what we have said earlier about the mushroom being a peculiar foodstuff. Remember, we said that the mushroom provides an amazing source of protein to the human body—the composition of some varieties being as high as 65 per cent protein. Yet, the very fact that the mushroom is high in protein may be the real essence of the problem many people face when they eat mushrooms. Their bodies simply cannot tolerate the type of protein found in a particular species of mushroom. An allergenic reaction is set up if the mushroom's protein does not combine favorably with the proteins already in the blood stream. Symptoms such as headaches, giddiness and colic are the result. A similar type of reaction is found in the sensitivity many people exhibit to milk proteins. Certainly, this is a strange turn of events—milk, a food rich in valuable nutrients turns against the body and causes such unfavorable reactions that death may be the end result in a few cases.

Nutritional Value of Mushrooms

Although there exists a similarity between mushrooms and milk, in so far as both can be classified as allergenic foods, the similarity ceases when we begin to think in terms of the nutritional value of both foods. Certainly, milk has many assets as far as health value is concerned, but the many hazards associated with its daily intake make us take a dim view of its worth to the body. On the other hand, mushrooms have as much and more to offer in the way of health-giving benefits and their faults are minor in proportion. Remember, avoid the wild mushroom—stick to eating mushrooms sold in today's markets, for they are grown carefully.

And the knowledge that mushrooms can create allergenic reactions in certain individuals should be caution enough while still enabling most of us to enjoy the rich nutritional treasures which can be found in the mushroom. Bear in mind that almost every food, even meat, carries with it the possibility of creating an allergenic reaction in certain people. "Allergy to the meat and organic tissues of mammalian animals occurs, but less frequently than to milk, eggs, cereal, grains, fish and certain other foods." (*Borden's Review of Nutrition Research,* Vol. XVII, No. 3.)

We cannot exclude mushrooms from the diet because of their allergenic properties, or we would have to do so with almost every other food known to man. Mushrooms are rich in folic acid, the yellow vitamin which, along with vitamin B_{12}, is the most potent weapon ever discovered against pernicious anemia. Mushrooms are also fairly good sources of other B vitamins as well, three-fourths of a cup containing about as much thiamin as a bran muffin, as much riboflavin as an orange and as much niacin as a serving of halibut. Also, surprisingly enough, we are told that mushrooms grown in the light, instead of the conventional dark cellars, are rich in vitamin D, which does not occur in any other food from non-animal sources. And perhaps the most amazing thing about the mushroom is its germicidal capabilities, as shown by the experiments of Dr. William J. Robbins and co-workers at the New York Botanical Gardens. These researchers found that certain chemicals in mushrooms exhibit definite germ-killing activity. One of these substances, pleurotin by name, showed an amazingly strong reaction against staphylococcus germs.

Now, do you see why we say mushrooms are such a valuable addition to your diet? Their fine record of nutritional benefits speaks for itself!

Non-Stick Frying Pans

The Story on Non-Stick Frying Pans

We have a letter from the president of the T-Fal Corporation on the subject of the new "non-stick" frying pans, which, he tells us, "have been widely accepted in both Europe and the United States. In the years 1959 and 1960, more T-Fal frying pans were sold in France than all other types of frying pans combined, from all competitors, including plain aluminum, stainless, cast iron, copper, etc. We have sold almost 3 million pans in the last 5 years and as yet, we have received no complaints from our customers of a harmful nature. Instead, these pans have been widely received as a health aid, since they are especially beneficial to those on low-calorie, non-grease diets."

Some of the Facts

Many people have written us asking for our opinion on these pans which are now being widely advertised, often with the notice that they have been okayed by the Food and Drug Administration. Let us review some of the facts:

1. Why do you want a frying pan? Cooking at the high heat implied in the word "fry" is quite destructive of many valuable elements in food. Foods—all foods—should be cooked at low heat to preserve these precious vitamins, enzymes and minerals. Roasting or broiling meats and baking vegetables or cooking them for the shortest possible time in as little water as can be—these are the best cooking methods to use.

2. The inside of the pan is lined with a plastic substance called Teflon. Now, of course, we do not believe that plastic substances should be used in contact with food, especially hot food. But let us take a little closer look at this particular plastic.

The chemical name for it is *TFE-fluoro-carbon* resin. The du Pont publication, *Journal of Teflon,* for July, 1960, states: "Effective immediately, the Food and Drug Administration has cleared an additional number of teflon TFE-fluoro-carbon resins as safe for service in food processing and handling applications."

A copy of a letter from J. K. Kirk of the Food and Drug Administration to the Dupont Company was sent to us by the President of T-Fal Corporation referred to above. This official statement of the Food and Drug Administration will, the T-Fal president believes, allay our fears as to the possible unhealthfulness of using the non-stick pans. The letter says, in part, "It is the conclusion of the Food and Drug Administration that the uses of these Teflon resins as outlined, whereby they will come into contact with food during processing or cooking, do not present any problems under the Food Additives Amendment. The data demonstrates that, in some cases, there is no transfer of the fluoride to the food and that in others, the transfer would be so small that the amount involved would be generally recognized as safe." He then lists 8 different kinds of Teflon to which this statement would apply.

Now, let us consider the official statement of the Food and Drug Administration whose only duty, remember, is to guarantee the complete wholesomeness of all food and medicine. *"In some cases, there is no transfer of the fluoride to the food."* The wording of this sentence can only lead one to believe that *in most cases, there is a transfer of the fluoride to the food.* In the other cases (we presume this means all other cases), the amount of fluoride entering the food would be "so small that the amount involved *would be generally recognized as safe."* What kind of an official statement is this from the bureau sworn to protect the health of the American people? No mention of any toxicity tests done. No mention of the years of work necessary to try such toxic substances with laboratory animals, under many different kinds of conditions, to guarantee the absolute safety of the substance. Nothing of the kind! We are told, simply, that the Food and Drug Administration believes that the amount of the plastic that gets into the food "would be generally recognized as safe." By whom? A toxicologist? Obviously, animal tests could not have been done, since, according to the *Journal of Teflon,* the material was not given to the FDA to test until 1960. Animal tests require a number of years to complete. Yet, this letter was sent to us by the president of the company selling this frying pan to assure us that there could be no question as to its safety. The advertising piece that accompanies the pans when they are sold says, "These and other governmental agencies cleared pure Teflon as safe! Pure Teflon was proved inert in cooking."

The re-wording, you see, is what is important. The FDA statement says "in some cases, there is no transfer of the fluoride to the food," and the seller of the pans prints on his advertising brochure "Pure Teflon was proved inert in cooking." A peculiar interpretation of the FDA statement, we think. But anyone would, of course, believe it implicitly, unless he wrote to the FDA to inquire.

Only Wooden Utensils Should Be Used

3. With frying pans now being sold, you get a wooden spatula for turning and stirring food cooked in the pan. In *Product Information Service,* published by the du Pont Company, you get this added piece of information: "Wooden or rubber spatulas only are recommended for use in the pan—never metal utensils. Nothing should be cut up in the pan and only a moderate heat should be used with it.

It should not be overheated when empty. Scouring with steel wool would be harmful to the finish."

In most kitchens, obviously, the wooden spatula might not be handy most of the time; the fried eggs or steak *would* be cut apart in the pan with a sharp knife and undoubtedly, at one time or another, whoever washes the dishes would scour out the inside with steel wool, just from force of habit. The plastic lining is apparently very easily scratched. Removing chunks of it by scratching the

Nightingale, Florence

Florence Nightingale, English nurse, hospital reformer and founder of the modern nursing program, was born in Florence, Italy, May 12, 1820. Early in her life she began to show a keen 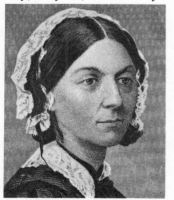 *interest in helping others, especially the sick and suffering. During a trip through Europe in 1837 and 1838, Miss Nightingale, witnessing the deplorable conditions existing in the hospitals, decided to devote the rest of her life to nursing, although at this time nursing was considered a highly degrading occupation. After receiving only three months of formal hospital training at Kaiserswerth, Germany, she became the head of a hospital for invalid women in 1853. One year later, she was sent to the aid of the wounded soldiers at a hospital in Scutari, near Istanbul. It was here that she became famous as "The Lady with the Lamp," for through her devotion to duty and improved sanitation and nursing methods, she was able to reduce the mortality rate in that hospital from 42 to 2.2 per cent. This remarkable feat earned for her world-wide attention and thanks. Yet, among the upper echelon of the Army, there was mixed emotion concerning her methods. Overcoming these difficulties, Miss Nightingale went on to reorganize the British Army Medical Service causing the needed reforms in hospital care to become a reality, most notable among them being her theory that "the maintenance of health by preventive measures is as important as the restoration of health by corrective measures." Before her death in 1910, she founded a school for nursing at Liverpool in 1910, helped set up others and was awarded the British Order of Merit in 1907.*

surface will obviously soon invalidate the purpose of the pan, for the aluminum surface will be exposed and the ungreased food will stick to this surface just as easily as it sticks to any aluminum surface. Of course, if you are stirring the food in the pan with a sharp instrument, the Teflon that is scratched off would almost have to become lodged in the food, now, wouldn't it?

4. "It should not be overheated when empty." Here is the most important aspect of the use of non-stick fry pans. Overheating the empty pans can be fatal. Literally. You put the pan on a lighted burner and someone calls you away. Let's say it's an emergency, you're gone for a long time and you have turned the burner to high. Under such circumstances, any ordinary pan will burn badly, even melt into an unrecognizable heap of metal. There will be unpleasant fumes from the overheated metal. But if the pan is lined with Teflon, the fumes can kill you.

Perhaps some people in your family aren't so forgetful, but perhaps others are. We know someone who forgetfully went to bed leaving a pan with water heating in it on a very hot burner. The water boiled away, the pan melted and at 4 A.M., our friend woke to find the house full of fumes. If this had been a Teflon pan, he might never have awakened.

Heat Causes Formation of Highly Toxic Gases

A mechanical engineer became concerned about the possible dangers of Teflon. He sent us a copy of instructions sent out to factories where Teflon is used. Here are some notes from the sheets (in every case, the comments in parentheses are ours):

"Investigation shows that a toxic gas, *perfluoroisobutene,* develops from thermal (that is, by heat) decomposition of Teflon. This gas is about 10 times as toxic as phosgene (poison gas, used in warfare). However, tests have indicated that the toxic decomposition does not develop below 400 degrees Fahrenheit (easily obtained in a hot oven or over a stove burner turned on high) and no ill effects have been reported by individuals exposed to Teflon heated below this temperature . . . Firefighting personnel can easily be exposed to the hazard, unless adequate respiratory protection is provided and maintenance personnel repairing such equipment after a fire, may be subject to exposure. . . .

"Because of the extremely toxic nature of the decomposition products of Teflon, disposition of waste Teflon parts becomes a special problem. These parts should not be disposed of in the usual manner of waste disposal, but should be buried in the ground. The reason for this extreme precaution is that minute quantities of decomposition products of Teflon can cause serious illness and even death. (Note: *minute quantities.*) A case in point is: An employee laid a lighted cigarette on the edge of a sheet of Teflon and later picked it up and continued smoking. The cigarette had become contaminated with enough Teflon to cause this employee to become violently ill and later to die from edema of the lungs caused by the decompositioned Teflon. . . .

The Fumes Can Be Lethal

"When a flash fire has occurred, the area in the immediate vicinity should be evacuated immediately. Employees should be instructed not to re-enter the area until sufficient time has elapsed to permit thorough ventilation of the area. Also, employees engaged in the repairs of equipment after a flash, should be extremely cautious in removing parts, so as to avoid contact even with the minutest quantities of the decomposition products of Teflon. (Note: *minutest quantities.*)

"All persons handling the Teflon parts must wash hands thoroughly with soap and water as soon as possible to avoid contamination of the mouth and digestive system, due to any Teflon residue on hands.

SPECIAL NOTE

"The hazards and procedures outlined herein should be discussed with all people concerned with the handling of Teflon parts."

If, after reading this information, you believe, as the Food and Drug Administration apparently does, that Teflon-lined pans are just as safe as can be to have around for use every day in the average kitchen, where the average housewife, doped with tranquilizers, cigarettes, alcohol, pep pills and aspirin, does her cooking with much of her attention elsewhere, then we can hardly keep you from buying one. They present one advantage, so far as we can see, over other kinds of pans. You may save yourself possibly a minute and a half a week that you would otherwise have to devote to scouring an ordinary pan. This adds up, of course, to 78 minutes a year. If you feel that such a saving is worth the risks, then there's really nothing we can say to dissuade you. But do be careful not to lay your cigarette down on one.

Novocaine

What Is the Truth About H₃?

During 1959, persistent reports crossed the Atlantic of a "youth serum" discovered by a Rumanian physician—a miracle drug that would reverse the process of aging, restore color to white hair and movement to limbs long crippled by arthritis. Hardening of the arteries would also yield to this new treatment, according to the reports. Minds clouded and confused because of aging blood vessels would return to clarity and serenity. Middle-aged individuals, wishing to postpone old age, could do so with some shots of the new drug.

The treatment is a series of injections of a substance called H_3 by the doctor who made it famous. H_3 is a certain form of a drug, well known in our country—procaine or novocaine—which is generally used for local anesthesia in dentists' offices.

Interest Aroused

Our file of clippings and reports grew, as did the volume of letters from people asking that we give them information about this new "miracle drug." It seemed to us, for a long time, that this was nothing relating to our program, which is concerned with promoting good health and preventing illness through a diet and way of life that will bring about such results. For about a year, we continued to collect reports, read and digest them.

The Rumanian doctor, meanwhile, was visiting other European countries. Dr. Anna Aslan, of the C. I. Parhon Institute of Geriatrics at Bucharest, was wined and dined in England and a group of 400 British specialists listened to her lecture on her H_3 treatment. The *British Medical Journal* for November 28, 1959, reviewing the lecture, stated that there was great difficulty in getting at the facts about results, as the slides of "before and after" pictures did not present patients in such a way that comparisons could be made. Unfortunately, too, tests made by giving one group of patients the H_3 treatment and withholding it from another group of patients, were not conducted scientifically, since they were not "blind" tests—everyone involved knew which patients were getting the treatment and which were not.

An editorial in the same issue of the *Journal* reviewed the history of novocaine, or procaine, as a drug, stating that it has been tried by many other investigators to improve circulation in various diseases of blood vessels. "It has been found useful in many allergic states and in anuria (suppression of the urine) and to relieve muscle spasm," the *Journal* article continues. "Perhaps one of its most valuable uses, overshadowed in the last 10 years by that of corticotropin and the corticosteroids, was in the treatment of rheumatoid arthritis, in which, somewhat mysteriously, relief often outlasted any possible local anesthetic effect. . . ."

Even in large doses, the drug is eliminated completely from the blood stream in 20 minutes. Overdosage can bring a feeling of dizziness, pins and needles, twitching, convulsions and, finally, loss of consciousness. A deficiency in vitamin C adds to the possibility of harm from overdosage.

Rejected by British Medicine

As a rejuvenating drug, the *Journal* says that "there is no real evidence that it is any good at all, and the extensive publicity given to it in the press will have the unfortunate effect of raising the hopes of many that, at long last, the elixir of life has been discovered."

We do not think that the unequivocal rejection of H_3 by British medicine necessarily means that it is no good. Orthodox opinion has been wrong before and will be wrong again. Only time will tell, we believe, whether or not the novocaine treatment will finally have a permanent place in medicine.

Vitamin B and Novocaine

Our interest in the story stems from the fact that novocaine, or H_3, breaks down into a B vitamin in the blood—the vitamin called para-amino-benzoic acid or PABA. The next question that naturally occurs is, if such excellent results can be obtained with the novocaine treatment because it breaks down into a B vitamin, why not obtain the same good results, or even better ones, by giving the B vitamin itself? Dr. Aslan says that she has tried this without success. Her explanation is that the drug keeps on breaking down into the B vitamin—thus providing a continuous supply of the vitamin. But surely, a continuous supply of the vitamin could be given in some other way.

If, as Dr. Aslan believes, the good results have been directly caused by the B vitamin, this, it seems to us, should open up new avenues of research among scientists especially interested in the B vitamins. Perhaps PABA is an extremely important one, far more important in large quantities than anyone has imagined up to now. Perhaps something in our modern environment is especially destructive of this particular vitamin, so that we all are deficient in it without knowing it. Perhaps something in the make-up of only certain people invites this kind of deficiency, and that is the reason why some people age so much more rapidly than others. Perhaps our bodies lose this vitamin as we grow older, due to some as yet not understood relationship with some other vitamin or mineral. Perhaps this is the reason why the novocaine treatment appears to hold off old age—it may supply this needed vitamin at just the right moment and in just the right amount.

B Vitamins in the Diet

All these are speculations, of course. We hope that the interest roused in Dr. Aslan's novocaine treatment will have sufficient impact on researchers to set some of them off on a quest for the significance of the part the B vitamin plays in this treatment. Meanwhile, make doubly certain you are getting enough vitamin B in your daily meals. PABA is one of the large complex of B vitamins—it comes right along with the others in food. These are the foods that are especially rich in the entire B complex: wheat germ, brewer's yeast, liver (fresh and desiccated), meat, nuts, fresh fruits and vegetables.

We understand that some doctors in America are giving the novocaine treatment. We do not know who they are or what results they are getting. Apparently, it does no harm, if one is not allergic to novocaine. We understand that the novocaine formula used in the Rumanian treatment is a little different from that commonly used for local anesthesia.

Nutmeg

Nutmeg Is a Poisonous Spice

The flavor of even a few flakes of nutmeg can be discerned in a very large recipe. It is a very pungent spice and most cooks use it sparingly. It was, therefore, with great surprise and interest that we read a rather lengthy report by Dr. Robert C. Green, Jr., in the *Journal of the American Medical Association* (November 7, 1959), describing the poisonous properties of nutmeg.

According to Dr. Green, nutmeg has been used for centuries in medicine as an aromatic stimulant, a narcotic and a laxative. In England and India, it has been widely used by the women there to induce abortion and initiate menstrual flow. Records from as early as 1576 tell of nutmeg poisoning and cases crop up periodically in medical literature.

An Actual Case

Dr. Green came upon such a case in his own experience and describes it in detail. The alarming aspect of nutmeg poisoning is the rather small amount necessary to bring about serious poisoning. In this case, 18.3 grams—about ½ ounce—did the job. A 28-year-old woman took the finely ground nutmeg at 10 P.M. one night to induce menstrual flow which had been delayed two days. She slept soundly until 5:30 A.M. the next day, when she was awakened by a burning sensation in the lower abdomen and an overwhelming feeling of impending death. She vomited, her legs felt as though they were asleep and she complained of feeling "funny all over." Then came a period of confusion in which the woman would scream wildly, and thrash her arms and legs about purposelessly. For the 4 hours before she saw a physician, this disorientation continued, interrupted by 3 short periods of lucidity.

The patient was admitted to a hospital and the condition persisted, with little change in the symptoms, except for increasing periods of lucidity, for 7 days. The data from this case and others in medical literature make it apparent that nutmeg taken in moderate quantities (5 grams or more) may produce a serious toxic state, and possibly death.

Experimental investigation revealed that the toxic factor is myristicin, a constituent of the volatile oil of nutmeg. It causes a marked depressive action on the central nervous system, as well as a less prominent stimulating effect. A toxic effect on the liver and/or the kidneys is also a likely result in nutmeg poisoning.

If a half-ounce of nutmeg can cause such serious consequences, smaller amounts must also be damaging to some degree. We believe that one should avoid the frequent use of this spice, even in small amounts or, if possible, discontinue using it at all.

Nutrition

Nutrition and Your Character

The cliché of modern nutrition is the slogan: "You are what you eat." It is true, of course, but we usually take the phrase to mean our physical make-up—the heart, the skin, the liver, the eyes, etc. We should remember that our temperament and character depends upon what we eat, too. Research has illustrated the brain's response to proper diet and nutrients. Editor Rodale has frequently written about the effect of the poor diet most teen-agers eat on their behavior. It was the basis for his off-Broadway play, *The Goose,* and he is convinced that the root of juvenile delinquency lies in the lack of nutritious food.

Apropos of this theorizing, we came across an interesting book entitled *Food and Character* by Louis Berman, M.D. An interesting aspect of the book is that it was published in 1932 and yet, the material and thinking in it are amazingly accurate, in the light of today's facts. Though the book is now out of print (your local library might have a copy), we would like to discuss some of Dr. Berman's points. They might be the key you need to get ahead, to make other people like you better, to make you like yourself better.

A fascinating project of Berman's was speculation on the eating habits of leaders in world affairs or in the arts. What makes a leader?

The author contends that, if one could canvass several of them for specific details of food and drink over a period of time, some sort of pattern would develop. It would also explain the calm passivity of Ghandi, the peppery wisdom of George Bernard Shaw or the iron-fisted militarism of Bismarck.

Oysters for Caesar

Dr. Berman tells us that Julius Caesar was a careful eater. He drank barley water in preference to wine and is said to have spurned a banquet prepared for him by Cleopatra for a dozen oysters. So, all militarists eat sparingly? No. The aforementioned Bismarck was called, by one biographer, a glutton. He indulged in enormous meals until the end of his life. At the age of 68, the Iron Chancellor, as he was called, weighed 247 pounds! "There are those," says Berman, "who would correlate these prodigious indulgences in food with the coarse brutality and the 'blood and iron' policy of the Chancellor." Certainly, humanity and compassion were not his strong points.

A contemporary of Bismarck, the English Prime Minister for Queen Victoria, Gladstone, was equally influential in his time, but of a completely different character. He was beloved by his countrymen and had none of the warlike tendencies of Bismarck. His eating habits were simple, and he was a disciple of the Fletcher school, so popular 50 years ago, which decreed that one must chew a mouthful of food 32 times before swallowing. "How much," asks the author, "were Gladstone's liberalism and abstemiousness connected."

Gandhi's Diet for a Quiet Man

Gandhi was one of the world's great men, who absolutely insisted that it was necessary to regulate what went into his stomach in order to control what entered his brain. He ate only goat's milk and dried fruit, such as dates. For the kind of life Gandhi led, Dr. Berman thinks his diet was perfect. It makes for a state of restfulness, not restlessness. "For one who seeks a life of meditation rather than of energy and action, such a diet is ideal."

Dr. Berman explains the varieties of diets these leaders ate in this way: "There are as many types of leaders as there are kinds of causes which they lead. But the kind of cause they lead is correlated with the constitution of their ductless glands, and so, with what they feed themselves. To this must be added the consideration of the climate of the times in which they live. Could any great man have been great if he had lived out of his time? Would Napoleon, in 1960, have been a great general, would Lincoln have been a great president or would Washington have been "first in the hearts of his countrymen"?

How do the ductless glands affect the whole man to the extent that a man who can literally change the world, owes his personality and character to the way they operate? The ductless, or endocrine, glands are those which manufacture the body's natural supply of hormones. The hormones act as catalysts, or promoters of chemical reactions, the causes of slowing down or speeding up body processes. To make hormones of the right types, in the right amount, at the right time, the endocrine glands must be supplied with the necessary raw materials—vitamins. The relationship between the hormones and the vitamins, shows that, apparently, one way to control the function of the glands is to control the variety and quantity of the vitamin intake.

Dr. Berman States It

"In conditions of character and personality defect or abnormality, where the status of one or the other of the endocrine glands has to be investigated, the nature of the food supply should be considered most seriously. It may be a possible factor in the production of the disturbance of the glands of internal secretion. And in the treatment of such a condition, the prescription of a diet calculated to affect the endocrine gland in question becomes a therapeutic necessity." This is Dr. Berman speaking and one can see the modern thinking behind his words. He continues: "That there is a definite relation between the vitamins and the nervous system, is proved by the occurrence of disturbances of the nervous system in such vitamin deficiencies as beriberi, scurvy, pellagra and rickets. These effects are of two kinds. First, there is a direct effect of the vitamins involved upon the functioning of the brain, as expressed in character and personality. And then there is an influence of the vitamins upon the endocrine glands, an indirect relation of vitamin deficiencies to deviations of character and peculiarities of personality. These conceptions have been found most useful in clinical situations presenting problems of the intellectual or emotional life of patients. The correction of dietary defects, especially in the vitamin content, has been of invaluable assistance in such instances. A host of researches, experimental observations in animals and studies of human beings now demonstrate that whatever affects the endocrine glands, deleteriously or favorably, affects the character and personality."

A Storage Organ

Dr. Berman then discusses each gland and its relation to vitamin supply. The thymus is a small endocrine gland close to the heart, which is characterized as a storage organ, "affording a certain amount of protection against the deleterious effects of a lack of food." Another author calls it "a barometer of nutrition and a very delicate one." Exhaustion, malnutrition and infection may have an adverse effect on it. The specific vitamin believed to be involved with the thymus is the B complex.

The adrenal glands, about the size of a man's thumb, are found atop each of the kidneys. They release hormones designed to mobilize all the body's assets in muscle and blood when struggle or stress are present. Emotions may also call this hormone into play. These secretions control brain growth, the development of sex glands, and the acidity of the body. Vitamin C is considered to be the most important nutrient in maintaining the glands' health.

"Gland of Glands"

The thyroid is called by Dr. Berman the "gland of glands because its activity makes life worthwhile." It controls vitality and growth and protects against poisons and injuries. It acts as an energizer and lubricator for an adult and helps in growth and development of tissues for a child. The thyroid is located in the neck near the larynx. This gland must have a constant supply of iodine in order to maintain the proper supply of thyroxine in the tissues.

The parathyroids are 4 little organs very close to the thyroid. They regulate the body's supply of calcium and vitamin D. A parathyroid deficiency is accompanied by a great sensitivity of the nervous system. A person suffering in this way presents temperamental characteristics quite peculiar to him, which tend to make him antisocial. Calcium and vitamin D are essential to a healthy parathyroid.

The gonads are the sex glands—in the male, the testes; in the female, the ovaries. Not only are these glands essential in the appreciation of sexual excitement and the natural results of it, but a degeneration in their function synchronizes the gradual breakdown of the tissues which leads to senility. The glands are also directly related to the personality. Protein is essential to the well-being of the gonads, as are vitamins A, B and C. But in 1943, Dr. Berman was able to say, ". . . the food substance which has been shown to be peculiarly related to the sex glands and the reproductive apparatus, especially the uterus, is vitamin E." Strangely enough, this important vitamin is given little credit today for its value in maintaining the health of the reproductive system.

The pituitary gland controls growth in childhood and adolescence and is very important in the development of sexual characteristics and metabolism. It has to do with blood pressure, the water balance of the body and the tone of the intestinal tract, as well as the pigment of the skin. Vitamin B is essential for the health of the pituitary and so, it is thought, is vitamin E.

The pancreas is the controller of the body's insulin output. It is, in effect, the body's insurance against diabetes. Without a proper output of insulin, the body's ability to use sugar is impaired. Without the proper use of sugar, the body's ability to do good work over a stretch of time is impaired.

A Summary

So let us summarize the effects of foods on the endocrine glands and of the endocrine glands on our emotions: thyroid (iodine)—excitability (mental agility and speed); parathyroids (vitamin D and calcium)—sensitivity (irritability); adrenals (vitamins A, B and C, tyrosine, cholesterol, magnesium)— driving power (resistance to fatigue); thymus (vitamin B)—immaturity (perversions); pituitaries (manganese, vitamin B, water, chloride, histidine)— maturity (intellectual control) and emotionality (emotional control); pancreas (sulfur, cystine, glutamic acid, glucose, nickel)—endurance; gonads (vitamins A, B, C and E, tryptophane, lysine, iron, linoleic acid)—sexuality.

It is clear from the above that the workings of these glands do have a decided effect on leadership, personality and character traits. It is clear, too, that each of them is concerned with the body's intake of specific nutrients. Dr. Berman reinforced his arguments by showing parallel effects of nutrients on the brain, sugar on the personality, fats and acidosis on the phlegmatic character, etc.

Dr. Berman was a man whose thinking was far ahead of his time. Even today, doctors with little vision refuse to investigate the value of his theories and, as a consequence, the accepted treatment for diseases of character and personality is tranquilizers instead of nutrition. Tranquilizers are not a cure, nutrition is.

Nutrition Is a Basic World Need

Most people think that, if they eat enough food each day to keep from feeling hungry, they have adequate nutrition. Of course, this impression is not necessarily true. The fellow who eats a hot dog, a soda and a candy bar for lunch can feel as satisfied as the fellow who lunches on an equal amount of roast beef with lettuce and tomato and a piece of fruit. The difference between the nutrition represented by these two meals is tremendous. The one is practically worthless, nutritionally, and will even rob the body of some of the nutrients it might have stored. The other abounds in protein, vitamins and minerals and will add to the protective store of these elements we all need.

The point of this contrast is that one cannot depend upon appetite, and the satisfying of it, as an indication of proper nutrition. As Dr. W. A. Odendaal says, in the *South African Medical Journal* (June 6, 1959), food has been so transformed by modern processing techniques, that "appetite has lost its path as a guide to good health." The doctor had occasion to say this in a paper on public health in which he stressed the need for proper direction of the public in choice of foods as a means of preventive medicine. He discusses several broad areas of public health, with recommendations intended to combat some common misconceptions. These recommendations prove to be as applicable to our own problems in America as they are in Africa.

Misinformation on Pregnancy Is Common

The doctor discusses the nutritional misinformation connected with pregnancy. How often do we hear, even today, the statement that the nutrition of the mother-to-be will not affect the child she carries. Yet, it seems that with each new day more evidence comes to show how sensitive the fetus is to the mother's nutrition. It has been found that some vitamins form essential constituents of some enzyme systems in the fetus. A nutritional deficiency, then, could be responsible for some congenital abnormality in the enzymatic system which is vital for normal development.

Sometimes, even though the mother-to-be is careful of what she eats, all of this is forgotten once the baby is born. If the new mother is nursing her baby, her nutrition is as important as before. Not only will what she eats affect the quality of her milk, but the large quantity is a drain on her tissues and this nutrition-rich liquid must be replaced. It is surprising to learn just how much liquid the mother loses to her baby in a nursing day. The average is a little less than a quart a day in infants, and about a quart and a half per day from 4 months on. A shortage of the proper food for the mother at this time may diminish the supply by a quarter, or even a third. Obviously, the nursing mother needs every bit of nutrition she can get.

The Answer to Dental Decay

Another of the common questions of public health, dental decay, is discussed by Dr. Odendaal. He notes that 95 out of 100 persons are plagued by this problem. Again, his opinion is that the beginning of sound, healthy teeth is the pre- and post-natal nutrition of the mother and child. The continuance of decay-free teeth is dependent on the elimination of refined foods from the diet and avoidance of sticky sweets.

Habits of the Aged

The nutrition of the older folks requires special attention, too. These people are most likely to suffer from malnutrition for a variety of reasons. Many of them have very little money and they try to skim by on cheap and filling foods, such as macaroni and cold cereals, which have little, if any, nutritive value. Some of these folks have problems in chewing because dentures are ill-fitting or nonexistent. The variety of their diet is limited and, again, they end up with foods lacking in nutritive value.

Loneliness is, among older people, a basic reason for not eating well. They have no one to eat with or cook for; there is no one to talk with while they eat. So they don't bother with a whole meal. They take a few crackers with jelly, or cookies, perhaps a piece of toast and a cup of coffee, or a soda. One's good health cannot long endure with such skimpy nourishment.

The physiological problems of the elderly cause difficulties in eating, too. In many cases, the sensation of taste or smell may be gone. Food loses its appeal under such conditions and special supplementary foods and drinks should be included in the day's schedule. Not enough secretion of digestive juices, dehydration of tissue and increase of body fat are other problems often found in this age group, and in each case, special dietary care is necessary to insure good health.

Not only should public health officials make every effort to awaken these older people to their particular needs, but provision should be made to assist them financially in acquiring the proper foods necessary to their good health. In Germany, persons over 65 are allotted an extra .2 grams of protein per kilogram of body weight. The *South African Journal* says calories should be restricted, but a good supply of protein, calcium, iron, vitamin A and the B vitamins is especially important. It has been found that a good protein supply in the elderly can arrest osteoporosis (brittleness of the bones) and promote recalcification. It is believed that protein may promote proper absorption of calcium. Of course, we know that vitamins are important, too. Vitamins A, D and C, especially so.

Mental Health

Increasing attention is being paid to the number of psychotic patients who show signs and symptoms of nutritional deficiencies. Dietary deficiencies are believed to affect both willingness and capacity for work and to alter the personality. Many believe that discoveries being made in the field of nutrition and mental health will revolutionize medicine as radically as antibiotics have.

Dr. Odendaal ends with a plea for more thorough grounding in nutrition for children in the grades and students in colleges and medical schools. We can add only a hearty amen.

The problems in public health are essentially the same all over the world: a lack of education, a lack of understanding and a lack of interest where nutrition is concerned. All the vaccines, the antibiotics and slum clearances and insect sprays will not erase the basic need all people have in common—if health is to be permanent—good nutrition. This is as true in the United States as it is in South Africa. We think this is the field in which the Public Health Service should concentrate much more than it has up to now.

What Vitamins Can Do

Every so often, the athletes get desperate enough to try nutrition and the success they experience is astounding. A clipping from the *Register* (February 12, 1961), a newspaper presumably published in the coal regions of eastern Pennsylvania, came to us. It told of the decision of Coach Bob McGrane of King's College, Wilkes-Barre, Pennsylvania, to "do something drastic" to pull his team and its ace scorer out of a slump. The ace, Mike Kwak, made only 38 per cent of his field goals. The team physician examined Mike and found that he had a vitamin deficiency. Vitamin injections before the next game were recommended. Kwak followed the doctor's advice.

The team, which had suffered 4 consecutive losses at the start of the season, suddenly reversed the trend to make the record in the next weeks read victory in 5 out of 6 games. Kwak, after beginning to take the vitamin supplement, upped his field goal average from 38 per cent to 53 per cent accuracy. He was selected to the Eastern College Athletic Conference Small Colleges All East Team for 3 weeks in a row (at the time of the clipping). He was leading all Pennsylvania players in scoring and his rebounding put him among the national leaders.

That a vitamin supplement could have such an effect, does not surprise us. What is especially interesting about this is the fact that a basketball star, described in the news article as a "muscular athlete" should be suffering from a vitamin deficiency. He is one of the specimens of our youth to whom we point with pride when the good health of American youngsters is questioned. Do you imagine that Mike Kwak's diet is any worse than that of most high school and college kids? We don't think so.

Too bad all youngsters aren't tossing baskets so that their efficiency would be important enough to merit investigation into their nutritional needs. Nobody checks diet when a boy or girl flunks a math test or hands in a poor English theme. Nutrition could be as responsible for this as it can be for poor basket accuracy. We believe that all youngsters, as well as adults, should be taking food supplements daily to prevent just such a lack.

Argument for Adequate Nutritional Testing

If scientific authorities and medical men would get together on what the facts are, we could devote our time exclusively to reporting on preventive medicine and diet. However, we keep reading about the harmlessness of insecticides on one side and see proof of their deadly effects on another; one group says atomic explosions are safe, another says they are killing us minute by minute. Why shouldn't we play it safe with these things by avoiding them if possible? The

same type of disagreement goes on and on about food supplements—
do we need them or not? We read that we are the healthiest nation
in the world and then we read that half of our young men are
physically unfit for military service. If this is true, we need something.

The talk of our nutritional superiority is so full of authority that
few persons question it, yet, judging from what Arthur N. Snider,
science writer for the *Chicago Daily News* says, in his column of
April 13, 1960, nobody knows what the status of our nutrition really
is. He says ". . . present techniques of establishing nutritional status
are crude and totally unsatisfactory. . . . Current methods largely use
height and weight tables (editor's note: These have been proven
totally unreliable and are completely useless for such a determination) and an inquiry into an individual's dietary habits." You can
imagine how much help this last is. Most people wouldn't even think
to mention the things which are worst for them nutritionally. Some
doctors are of the opinion that nutritionally bad foods—macaroni,
candy, cola drinks, etc.—are quite all right.

Biochemical Tests

At a meeting of the Federation of American Societies for
Experimental Biology, it was urged that biochemical tests for an
appraisal of a patient's nutritional condition be simplified and become
a common tool of physical examination.

Snider says, "The nutritional status of patients is taking on
importance because of the growing awareness that many diseases
can be traced back to long time dietary habits." These habits, of
course, deny the body some needed nutrient, a nutrient which can
easily be supplied by corrected diet and supplementation. How does
one reconcile such an attitude with the blistering articles which have
been appearing in papers all over the country, condemning those
who suggest that diet and diseases are often connected, and that
proper nutritional supplementation can lead to a cure in many cases?

We are firmly convinced that, unless a laboratory test of the
blood proves the patient is completely and adequately nourished, he
must supplement even a careful diet with vitamins and minerals. As
for the doctors who insist that we are well-nourished and need no
such analysis, ask them to fight it out with S. M. Garn of Fels
Research Institute of Antioch, Ohio. He warns that, while physicians
can spot the grossly overnourished or undernourished, they are on
unsure ground—they just don't know—when confronted with the
borderline individual. That individual could be you.

Which Nutrition Writer Do You Believe?

Have you just heard, for the hundredth time, that we are the
best fed country in the world and don't need health foods? Has your

doctor told you that? Or Frederick Stare's nutrition column? Or Dr. Crane? Or Dr. Alvarez? They all have about the same view, and it is often published beside a story such as the one which recently appeared in a Minnesota paper. This story told of a 10-year study conducted by 30 state universities, which concluded, according to Dr. Henry T. Scott of the University of Wisconsin, that the American teen-age girl has "deplorable eating habits, to say the least."

Dr. Scott went on to say that, "Girls between 13 and 19 years, as a whole, are on what you call a snack binge." These girls "take on a load of soft drinks, candy and fried potatoes after school," and when the family's dinner is served, they're not hungry. Such eating habits have marked the American teen-age girl with nervous instability, says Dr. Scott.

He takes it from there: "She is a good candidate for all sorts of illnesses. Calcium and some of the B vitamins are missing. She is loaded with starch. Her glandular system has not been built up to produce the hormones for all bodily functions, including reproduction." The trouble really begins when the girl becomes a mother, says Dr. Scott. That's the time the girl's physical health starts going downhill. "Her eventual destiny is some tax-supported institution."

The Real Truth

So these are the healthy citizens we're raising. This is the way the weak, young mothers who "can't stand" their children ate in high school. They're nervous, they're sick, they have menstrual troubles, miscarriages, difficult pregnancies. Their husbands don't understand them and bark irritably when their wives complain. No wonder— the husbands ate this way in high school, too!

If the 30 universities are wrong in their surveys, and this seems hardly likely, then our entire educational system is in jeopardy, since we depend upon such universities to teach our students and point the way to newer, more efficient methods of scientific investigation. If Dr. Stare and those who agree with him disbelieve these findings, they should challenge them and insist on undeniable proof. If they accept the conclusions, then they should modify their pronouncements, which are in direct contradiction to these findings.

The truth is that Americans are not healthy and each generation is even less so. All the oceans of advertisements for ready-mix cakes and nut-sprinkled candy bars will not change that truth. Sunday supplement nutrition writers' articles appear across the page from ads for cake icing you can squeeze from a tube and colas that mix with ice cream. Do you honestly expect them to write that people who indulge in such foods are getting poor nourishment?

Nuts

Have You Eaten Pistachio Nuts Lately?

Pistachio nuts have been decorating the tables of the human race since the earliest days of man. *Genesis,* the first book of the Old Testament, which deals with the creation of the world and the story of the Garden of Eden, mentions their use as a delicacy. In the United States, their fame rests mainly on their use as a flavoring for a rather exotic ice cream. We hope they will one day become a national favorite, as peanuts have.

An Anti-Cholesterol Food

The ancients thought pistachio nuts were useful as an antidote for liver ailments and as a kind of love potion. Today, Arabs consider them useful as a digestive aid. Whatever the legend or fact that surrounds them, we are always kindly disposed to the eating of nuts of any kind. We have stressed many times the values to be found in these foods. They are excellent sources of protein. They are rich in unsaturated fatty acids, the oils which help to combat the accumulation of cholesterol deposits in the blood stream and which are vital to the efficient operation of the body's most important organs. Nuts also have an appreciable content of valuable minerals and vitamins. They are a rich source of life-giving nutrients. After all, it is nuts that provide the nucleus of energy and growth that gives us our great, strong trees. The pistachio, of course, has all these desirable qualities.

The natural habitat of the pistachio tree is the warm, dry climate of the Near Eastern countries of Asia that border on the shores of the Mediterranean Sea. However, it has been found that the Southwest of the United States and the Gulf States can provide a suitable growth area for this tree. The trees grow slowly and only when fully grown, (about 6 feet high after 10 years) do they produce fruit. The nuts appear in bunches of 4 or 5 pounds all over the tree. The nut-bearing pistachio is one of those trees which require fertilization by a male tree; therefore, male and female must both be planted in the same area in order that the female bear fruit. The suggested ratio is one male (stamen-bearing) tree to about 10 female (pistil-bearing) trees.

What Does the Pistachio Offer?

An important consideration in discussing foods from a nutrition standpoint is, what does this food offer compared with others of a similar type? As far as protein content is concerned, the pistachio nut is hard to beat. The percentage of protein in pistachio nuts is greater than a similar portion of round steak, hard-boiled eggs, beans or raisins. Peanuts and black walnuts are the only two nuts, commonly eaten in America, that have more protein. Its carbohydrate content is quite low in comparison to most other nuts we eat. Its fat content is average, or perhaps a bit below average. Unfortunately, the calorie count is high—one of the highest of all nuts, so that those who are counting calories must be careful not to be carried away with their nibbling.

The idea of nibbling brings us to a very important point where nuts are concerned. We are strongly in favor of creating the habit, especially in children, of reaching for nuts, carrot sticks, raisins or fruit when in search of a snack, rather than something less healthful and actually less tasty. Kids dip into the potato chips, which have been fried in deep fat or the cookie jar, full of sugar or into the freezer for ice cream, loaded with sugar, artificial coloring and flavorings, emulsifiers, etc., not because they crave these things, particularly, but because they are around. Stock up on several kinds of nuts, fruits that are in season, celery stalks and fruit juices, instead, and you'll see that they are every bit as acceptable to nibblers. And if you're worried about calories, remember, that even the richest nuts won't do the damage to your figure that a plate of ice cream or a pretzel binge can do.

Your Family Will Enjoy Pistachios

We say try pistachio nuts on your family. If they haven't had them before, they will enjoy the distinctive flavor of pistachios. If they have, they'll welcome back an old friend, and you'll see them eat this healthful snack in a way that will gratify you.

As with just about every other food, commercial interests have led to the near ruination of pistachio nuts as they appear in most stores. They are dyed green or red or bleached white, depending upon the desired effect. Thy are heavily salted, too. Any advantages to be gained to your health from eating pistachio nuts can be lost in the dangerous effects of dyes and salt. Eat natural pistachio nuts, just as they come from the tree. These are the ones we recommend.

Old Age

What Happens as We Grow Older?

"Progress in medicine, discovery and development of new drugs, better personal hygiene and more adequate dieting, remove more and more obstacles to longer life. Yet we really do not know why people grow old. Why do some retain their youth long while others age early? Many theories have been advanced. One theory postulates the existence of 'A Primary Aging Factor,' undiscovered as yet.

This aging factor automatically limits human life to about 100 years. Another theory maintains that there is no such factor and that senility is due to the amount of stress endured during life."

So says Louis E. Graubard of the Galesburg, Illinois, State Research Hospital, writing in the *Illinois Medical Journal* for May, 1956. Dr. Graubard goes on to remind us that life has been described, not unjustly, as a gradual dying. We begin to age, of course, as soon as we are conceived. Some organs of our body age very rapidly. Milk teeth or baby teeth, for instance, are lost during early childhood—surely a sign of aging. The thymus gland, apparently important for infants and children, begins to atrophy or wither away during adolescence.

So, aging is a relative thing entirely. To the child, 20 appears to be a very great age. To a man of 80 being 40 is to be young again. Since aging is common to every living thing, it is only natural that we should all be intensely interested in just what it is, just how it affects us and, most of all, just what we can do to postpone its more unpleasant effects or perhaps avoid them entirely.

Here are a few facts we have gathered about what actually happens in one's body as one "grows old"—and we are using this term to refer to those over the age of 50, for, whereas some body processes begin to age early in life, as we have pointed out, most of us become aware of "growing old" around the forties and fifties, when we begin to slow down and changes in our health and appearance indicate that we have reached middle age.

Decrease in Minerals

According to *Science News Letter* for November 19, 1960, the older heart shows a very definite decrease in certain minerals, compared with the younger heart. Researchers at the University of Montreal found that, with the exception of phosphorus, all minerals had decreased in the older. Especially, there was a striking decrease in the amount of magnesium in the aorta or heart artery.

William Hobson, M.D., writing in the *Practitioner,* for May, 1955, states that the increase in blood pressure with advancing age is well known, but it is difficult to say when this becomes dangerous. Many older people live perfectly healthfully with raised blood pressure, he says. He reminds us that, as we grow older, cells tend to show fatty deposits. Today's research indicates that such deposits must be related to hardening of the arteries and hence, to heart and blood vessel disorders.

An article in *Newsweek* for October 2, 1950, quotes Dr. Nathan W. Shock, of the Public Health Service as saying that the notion that the older heart pumps less blood than the younger one is a theory that has failed to hold up. His report goes on to say that disorders of heart disease, hardening of the arteries and so forth, get their start in the thirties and forties. If we could prevent them then, perhaps we would not have to suffer from them later in life.

At a meeting of the American Medical Association in Miami, Florida, in 1954, a group of 4 doctors from New York Medical College stated that, starting at age 60 and going to 75, there is a reverse biochemical and physical process which can then enable a person to survive to 100. They obtained their information from a study of 1,000 old persons between the ages of 80 and 100. They found that, after the age of 75, cholesterol and other fatty substances in the blood went down instead of up. Between the ages of 60 to 75, they discovered, "the percentage of increase of aortic calcification over the preceding decade also reversed itself."

In assessing these findings, one of the doctors, Eiber, said: "In other words, during the age period 60 to 75, which we refer to as the 'threshold age,' certain biochemical and physical processes reverse and, instead of continuing their upward trend, actually reverse and go down. What the mechanism of this threshold period is, has not been fully worked out, as yet. It is some invisible, not clearly understood barrier.

"Most of us die before reaching that barrier or while going through it. But once we get through, our chances of living to be 100 years old are good."

It would seem, therefore, that a vigorous pursuit of health measures during this 15-year period would be an investment which could bring a handsome return in the form of additional years of life after age 75.

Lungs and Respiratory System

Dr. Graubard tells us that respiratory infections in old age are marked by a slow and imperfect return to good health and freedom from congestion. Dr. Shock, quoted in a *Newsweek* article for February 8, 1954, states that breathing becomes progressively more difficult as one grows older. From the age of 30 to 90, he says, the volume of the lungs diminishes about 30 per cent. The ribs grow more rigid and cut down on the amount of breathing a person can do under stress.

Digestive Tract

Dr. Hobson tells us that a decrease in the amount of hydrochloric acid in the stomach is common among about 35 per cent of everyone over the age of 60. Hydrochloric acid is one of the necessary digestive juices. Other digestive juices are decreased as well. Dyspepsia and constipation are common.

An article by John Esben Kirk, M.D., in the *International Record of Medicine*, for July, 1954, indicates that there are modifications in the intestinal flora as we grow older. These are the beneficial bacteria which occur in the intestinal tract. They are responsible for manufacturing many vitamins which we need and also for the proper absorption of food. So, along with losing the value of food because of too little digestive juice, as we grow older, we may also lose valuable nutriment because our intestines simply don't absorb it as they should. Many modern drugs, like the sulfa drugs and the antibiotics, incidentally, are extremely hard on these beneficial bacteria, so that one is quite likely to suffer from a serious lack, if one has been taking such drugs.

On the other hand, Dr. Shock has found that older people, in general, absorb their food as well as young people. "By giving doses of vitamin A, we found the older person got as much value from it as the younger one," he says. "This raises a serious doubt that old people are vitamin-deficient. *If they eat right, they will get all the vitamins they need.* And their digestion doesn't seem to fall off much later."

Throughout all the research we did on this subject, the above is the ever recurring refrain—almost every article stressed it. All the available evidence shows clearly that, if people do not eat properly, they will suffer for it—whether they are young or old. Old people have a tendency to develop bad food habits, partly due to circumstances, partly because they have not been taught the great importance of choosing food wisely. How can the digestive tract of anyone absorb vitamins, if he is not getting any to speak of in his food?

Health of the Skin

Dr. Graubard tells us that the skin becomes dry as we grow older and the most exposed parts (hands and face) begin to wither. Fluid is lost from tissues, which accounts for loss of weight. Hair whitens and falls out. There is an increase in facial hair among older women, due undoubtedly to the fact that the sex hormones which control such growth are decreasing in the older person. But lack of hair is apparent in other parts of the body. The *Lancet* for January 20, 1951, reveals that, in examinations of 100 women over 60, it was found that underarm hair was completely lacking in 40 and greatly reduced in the rest.

Bones and Skeleton

Dr. Hobson points out that changes in our body structure have a great deal to do with changing our way of life, even though they present no very serious health hazards.

Rheumatoid arthritis greatly limits the work that can be done by the hands. Osteoarthritis may be a crippling deformity for a man accustomed to earning his living by physical labor. Fear of falling becomes a terrible threat to older people whose bones show loss of calcium. Dr. Graubard tells us that some older people are so afraid of falling that they refuse to walk at all and either stay in bed or welcome confinement in wheel chairs. The certain inactivity that results leads to atrophy and finally, to immobility—they cannot move about any longer, simply because they have not moved about for so long.

A wonderfully helpful article which appeared in (of all places!) *Today's Health* for November, 1950, dwells on the absolute necessity of plenty of calcium in the diet for older people.

Says this author, "By the time we are 60, many of us are deficient in calcium, iron, proteins and vitamins A and B." He relates the story of an older man whose leg was broken in a fall. The doctor, setting the leg, berated him thus, "Why are your bones brittle? Because the ordinary American diet is calcium-poor, and a deficiency is built up over years. The blood needs and takes calcium. If you don't supply it by mouth, the blood appropriates what it needs from the bones, until, once resilient, they become brittle as toothpicks."

We were surprised to read this in a publication of the American Medical Association, whose official position these days seems to be that the American diet is perfect and no one needs to worry at all about deficiencies. Here we have confirmation, from their own magazine, that we "food faddists" are correct in saying that we need to pay strict attention to the calcium content of our diets, for we will not get enough if we don't. We recommend bone meal, to old and young alike, as the best possible source of calcium and all other minerals.

The article ends with the story of experiments at Cornell University, in which it was clearly demonstrated that rats who were given a diet *low* in carbohydrates (starches and sugars) lived until the age of 100 to 150, in terms of human age. They were seldom diseased and were more energetic in every way than their brothers who were fed "in the good old American hot-biscuits-and-cream tradition." Protein (meat, eggs, fish, nuts and seeds) should have top priority in your diet.

Aging and the Senses

Dr. Shock reports that after 50, nearly everyone suffers eye changes which interfere with good vision. At 60, there is a definite drop in color discrimination. Deafness increases from one per cent at the age of 20 to 5.9 per cent at 60. After 50, people lose the ability to hear tones of higher frequencies. This makes it difficult for older people to follow conversations where several people are speaking.

Dr. Hobson points out that the lens of the eye is a very sensitive index to age. It seems that, among otherwise healthy people, the ability of the eye lens to "accommodate" falls steadily with age until the age of 50, when it remains stationary. "We can say," he goes on, "with a fair degree of accuracy, that in the great majority of people, physiological senescence in the human lens is reached at the age of 50, but it begins at quite an early age—even before puberty."

In other words, the ability of the eye to see at long distances or to adjust itself immediately to seeing things that are quite close is actually at its lowest ebb at the age of 50 or thereabouts. It doesn't get much worse from then on. The inability of the lens of the eye to adjust to close work is, of course, the reason why most of us wear reading glasses or bifocals after middle age. It is interesting to know that this degeneration of the eye lens begins during adolescence and progresses quite steadily until the age of 50—and apparently does not get much worse from then on. So, if you have managed to do without reading glasses up to the age of 50, perhaps you will be able to do without them completely!

Dr. Hobson tells us that both visual accuracy and how quickly you see things are affected by age. The amount of light you need becomes increasingly important, too. These changes can be detected by the age of 20!

Deafness is more common in older men than women—could it be because they may be subjected to more noise, especially at jobs in heavy industry? Women, on the contrary, suffer more from vertigo or dizziness, as they grow older. He believes this may be due to hardening of the arteries in the delicate inner section of the ear—a good indication that a diet high in B vitamins and the right kind of fats and low in the unhealthful fats and carbohydrates, might be a solution to this problem.

Mentality and the Nervous System

Perhaps more important than any other disability in the consideration of older people is mental disability—the apparent degeneration of the mind which results in changes in personality. Coping with other problems of ill health seems easy, indeed, beside the problems that are ever present in caring for someone whose "mind is gone," as we are accustomed to speak of it. Senility or senile dementia are terms used by doctors.

Dr. Hobson tells us of tests given to people of various ages to note the difference in results among older people. "The ability to learn depends largely upon the intelligence," he says, "so that memory function, ability to learn new tasks and tasks involving the relinquishing of old habits are found to be more difficult for old people." Testing the ability to do logical thinking showed that older people tended not to draw logical conclusions based strictly on the statements given, but often confined themselves to general remarks upon the statements. On tests like vocabulary tests and general information, older adults do as well as youngsters. No degeneration here.

Even quite old people who have had university educations appear to have certain intellectual skills which never desert them. A special intelligence test, given at the time of college entrance and again, 30 years later, showed that, in general, the score was higher at the later time. Dr. Shock has found that old people with high intelligence actually grow more intelligent with advanced age, while "the dumb ones just get dumber."

However, there are some changes that seem to take place in all of us as we approach old age. We tend to forget recent events, but to have clear memories for old times. Apathy and depression are quite common among older folks. Dr. Shock tells us that the speed of nerve impulses diminishes rapidly after the age of 40. There is at least a 20 per cent reduction between the ages of 20 and 90. This reduction limits the aging person's activity when a quick reaction is required.

Earl Ubell, Science Editor of the *New York Herald Tribune,* tells us, in the February 26, 1957 issue, that perhaps the apparent loss of intelligence in an older person may reflect merely his slowed responses. If the older person is allowed to "set his own pace," perhaps this disability would disappear. He reminds us, too, that hardening of the arteries in the brain deprives nerves of food, resulting in poor memory, incoherent speech, lack of ability to recognize familiar things or places, difficulty in concentrating and so forth.

Dr. Graubard tells us that from 10 to 15 per cent of admissions to mental hospitals are cases of senile dementia. There is narrowing of interests, forgetfulness, dulling of emotional reactions, faulty attention. Gaps in memory may be filled with meaningless talk, patients may become lost on the street, may identify strangers as members of their families and in their confused state, may easily become the dupes of swindlers.

Dr. James E. Birren, who worked with Dr. Shock in his experiments testing mentality, declares that the aging process itself does not slow down the mental process, although poor eyesight may make the individual seem slower mentally. However, he does believe that aging, combined with brain damage caused by degenerative diseases, sharply reduces mental ability.

This brings us back again to hardening of the arteries and other conditions which affect the brain, just as they affect other parts of the body. If you would prevent degeneration of the mind in old age, it seems that the best precaution is to maintain a high degree of health and to avoid, especially, the disorders of the blood vessels which are so commonplace in modern times. We are convinced that attention to diet, especially fats and the B vitamins, is the key to the situation.

One researcher at Duke University has tested the Intelligence Quotients of many people over 60 and has found that, if you have an IQ of 116 or more—about one person in 7 does—your mental ability drops off very slightly as you get older. If you have an IQ between 86 and 116—about 7 out of 10 Americans fall in this group—there is a gradual but moderate decline. If your IQ falls below 85—about 15 per cent of adult Americans—there is a marked drop in mental ability as you become older.

Other Changes as One Grows Older

Among miscellaneous changes that take place as one grows older are some surprising ones. For instance, there is considerably more sensitivity to changes in temperature. The feeling that you don't enjoy the first few brisk days of winter as much as you used to probably represents a very real change that has taken place— the cold will be more uncomfortable as you grow older.

The body's regulatory apparatus shows less efficiency in coping with changes in blood sugar, so that insulin may not produce its usual effects in older diabetics. Symptoms and signs of disorder are less conspicuous than in a younger person and minor deviations from normal may be more important. Repair of tissues is slower and there is a narrower margin of safety. So anemia, for instance, would present a greater hazard to an older person whose blood supply may already be lessened by hardening of the arteries.

Older people use less oxygen than younger people and the older man cannot take in the extra oxygen during exercise, as the younger man does.

Sensitivity to pain is decreased as one grows older, two Canadian researchers tell us in the *Canadian Medical Association Journal* for October 29, 1960. "Pain sensitivity decreased with age," they say, "as manifested by increased average values of the pain threshold in the older group. This finding was constant in 3 racial groups studied."

Dr. Shock found that the one organ most frequently damaged or inadequate in the older person is the kidney. "The kidneys do not work so well in the older person," he says. "You can tank up these people on water, give them various substances and learn that the old kidneys do not respond as fast" as those of younger people. The 80-year-old kidney is only half as efficient as the 30-year-old one. Undoubtedly, one reason for this must be the increased load on the kidneys to excrete all the many poisons to which modern human beings are exposed. Avoiding as many as possible is the wise course.

There is general agreement that the glands must be closely involved with aging. The thyroid gland, for instance, which regulates many things that go on inside one's body, declines in activity as one grows older. Perhaps the pituitary gland (the master gland of the body) is the one which controls aging. Dr. Shock says that this gland acts as a trigger on the kidneys. However, he goes on, there is no one thing which causes aging. He believes it is a combination of gland action, diet and a "third item which I call the ability to keep an active interest in what's going on."

Dr. Shock lists the following criteria, if you are interested in knowing whether or not you are growing old:

1. Do you have a loss of immediate recall—memory for events that have occurred in the past 24 hours?

2. Does it take you longer to perform physical and mental tasks?

3. Do you tend to resist new ideas?

4. Do you have fewer goals to strive for than in the past?

5. Do you spend an increasing amount of time dwelling on the past?

However, there is no rule. And, as Dr. Graubard says, "We have seen, and still see some, who, according to normal standards, ought to be in wheel chairs, slobbering, trembling, mumbling and edentulous, effectively ruling the destinies of countries. Sophocles wrote Oedipus, still the model of the classical tragedy, when he was 90. Titian painted masterpieces at 85. Oliver Wendell Holmes was 85 when he wrote his famous essay, *Over the Tea Cups*. Verdi composed Otello when he was 80. And in our times, Bernard Baruch, Winston Churchill and Helen Keller are dramatic examples of real achievement in old age."

Olives

Olives and Olive Oil for Ulcers

In the better restaurants, the customer is often presented with a dish of olives as a "nibbler," or relish, before the main dish is served. Many Americans follow this custom in their homes—on special occasions. It is not usual, however, to find a family who uses olives regularly. It is also uncommon to find a family who is used to cooking with olive oil. The exceptions to this general rule are, of course, those families whose roots are in the Mediterranean countries. First and second generation Italian, Spanish and Greek cooks would be hard put to make a meal without using olive oil. They use it the way American cooks use salt and French cooks use wine—a pinch of it, a drop of it, a cup of it, will make anything taste better to them.

There are hints in medical literature, now, that olive oil might be more than merely a tasty addition to a dish. It might explain the mysterious fact that, while the Latins are highly emotional, hard-working people who eat highly seasoned foods as a rule, peptic ulcers and hardening of the arteries have a much lower incidence in Latin countries than they have in Britain and the United States.

A Coating for the Digestive Tract

No less an authority than Dr. Paul Dudley White (noted heart specialist) is mentioned in the Indian medical magazine, *Hamdard Medical Digest* (May-June, 1961), as attributing the low incidence of heart disease and hardening of the arteries, in part, to the Latins' consumption of more olive oil and fewer animal fats than other countries.

The Latins' fondness for olive oil goes back a long time. In 3,000 B.C., olive oil was used for cooking. It has been used ever since, both internally and externally. Aside from its value in cooking, it was long used as a dressing for wounds and a softening agent for the skin.

We have recently seen a good bit of information on olive oil as both a preventive and a cure for stomach ulcers. Olive oil is known to be soothing and protective to the mucous membrane which lines the stomach. Dr. J. Dewitt Fox, writing in the *Hamdard Medical Digest,* suggests that the ulcer patient use olive oil, instead of the cream usually advised as part of the ulcer diet by most doctors. He prescribes: "Two tablespoonfuls of olive oil with, or chased by, 6 ounces of milk will do the same, or even a better, soothing or healing job than the cream. It will also reduce stomach acid and because the oil is unsaturated, will not raise the blood cholesterol." We say skip the milk, too.

Dr. Fox went on to tell of a young Mexican doctor friend who took him out to dine at a Mexican restaurant. Dr. Fox was amazed at the amount of hot sauces his friend ate, with never a sign of digestive discomfort. When asked how he managed this, the Mexican friend replied: "First, I take a little olive oil. It protects my stomach."

Editor Rodale tells of a young relative who has, for several years, been troubled with a rather severe ulcer condition. Recently, the young man discovered the use of olive oil before meals lessens the discomfort he suffers after eating. Since then, he has made it a habit to start every meal with a teaspoonful of olive oil and the results have been marvelous for him.

Once inside the body, olive oil, aside from protecting the intestinal tract, causes vigorous contractions of the gall bladder and favors complete emptying, a good gall bladder tonic. While olive oil cannot dissolve gallstones once they are present in the gall bladder, it is helpful in throwing off accumulated cholesterol crystals.

Dr. Fox says that constipation can be combated by taking two teaspoonfuls of olive oil before retiring. The emptying of the gall bladder mentioned above brings out a copious amount of bile during the night and bile salts is one of the most effective laxatives known.

Does Olive Oil Reduce Cholesterol?

Dr. Fox's statements on the anticholesterol value of olive oil are amplified in the *Journal of the American Medical Association* (May 20, 1961). In the Questions and Answers section, Ogden C. Johnson, Ph.D., said that olive oil is, of course, an unsaturated fat. He went on to say that, in experiments, olive oil did not reduce the cholesterol level. However, he did state that olive oil, as a neutral, did not add to the level. Therefore, it is reasonable to assume that, if one were to adopt a continual diet of olive oil in place of saturated fats, the cholesterol excess already present would be used and eliminated, while the olive oil would not cause any future increase in the cholesterol level. Obviously, olive oil is a desirable substitute for saturated fats.

The French periodical, *La Vie Claire* (June, 1959), had something to say in favor of olives as a healthful food, that is, black olives. The short piece dismissed green olives as an incomplete fruit, not conducive to a happy digestive tract. But the ripe olive is hailed as a fruit that is precious to the irritated intestines and liver when they have been damaged by an excess of food or of alcoholic intake. Olives are advertised in the article as being rich in calcium and phosphorus as well as vitamin D, which aids in the assimilation of these elements into the cartilages, the bones and the teeth. One should make use of olives, says the article, especially when suffering from tooth decay which might be due to poor metabolism or lack of proper care of the mouth.

The Differences in Olives and Olive Oil

As might be expected, there are olives and there are olives— the quality varies. According to an article in the *New York Herald Tribune* (June 19, 1961), olives from the Greek isle of Crete are not "preserved" as are Spanish olives. The Crete olives are used on the island soon after harvest or they are pressed into oil for export. The oil is of two general qualities, depending upon how the olives have been harvested. Some growers cover the ground with a cloth, shake the branches and quickly collect the crop. Olives collected in this manner produce a finer oil than when the fruit is left to ripen on the tree and drop in its own good time. The fully ripened fruit is heavier in oil, but it is not so fine a quality.

The olive oil of Greece is not pasteurized. It is sent to the United States in the raw state. Unfortunately, or fortunately, federal laws insist that olive oil sold in the United States be pasteurized, so this process is carried out when the raw oil reaches these shores. Doubtless, some of the food value is lost in the process.

Hard to Recognize Difference in Olive Oils

A distinction made by olive oil experts which confuses the casual user of olive oil, is the difference between virgin oil and pure oil. Virgin oil is that which comes from a single pressed olive crop. Pure oil is a mixture of several virgin oils. Actually, the difference is one of flavor and is important only to the connoisseur of olive oils. For most of us, any olive oil has a unique taste when compared with other vegetable oils, such as corn oil, peanut oil, cottonseed oil, etc., but we are not able to distinguish one olive oil from another.

Most of the olive oil imported into this country is of the sweet variety, golden or pale straw-yellow in color and delicate in flavor. The other type is darker and has a more emphatic taste. Pure olive oil, as opposed to virgin oil, is a blend just as coffee is. Any one brand may be compounded of oils from Spain, Italy, Greece and perhaps North Africa. What olive packers try to do is to achieve a standard product that always tastes the same and has the same color.

Watch for Processing

It seems to us that the virgin oils bearing the specific country of origin on their label stand the best chance of avoiding excessive processing. These may be more expensive, but the value is there. The gallon-size container costs less per tablespoonful of oil than the smaller size bottles of two, four, six and eight ounces. Larger amounts of olive oil may be kept without refrigeration for a considerable time, since it does not spoil easily. This also eliminates the need for preservatives.

We are inclined to believe that other vegetable oils might have much the same effect as olive oil has on the intestines, in acting as a coating for the mucous membranes and acting to prevent and to cure ulcer. We do know that other oils have a definite capacity for actually reducing the cholesterol level of the blood. Safflower oil heads the list in this department.

Use Liquid Vegetable Oils

The evidence for the use of unsaturated fats is abundant. We are strongly in favor of the use of liquid vegetable oils in whatever way possible. Use them in salads, in cooking, over vegetables or by the tablespoonful if you wish. They are infinitely preferable to butter or margarine. Olive oil has a pleasant flavor that makes it appealing to many, and if you enjoy it, use it whenever possible. If you'd rather use corn oil, safflower oil, peanut oil or one of the others, go to it. Your health will benefit and you will have an excellent substitute for the dangerous hydrogenated fats used so frequently in American homes.

A word about whole olives. Most commercially packaged varieties are highly chemicalized with preservatives, plasticizers, colorings, etc., and the green ones are highly salted. We suggest, therefore, that you get your olives directly from an importer. Many Italian, Spanish and Greek grocers sell them directly from the barrel in which they were shipped from Europe. Even this is no guarantee of an unprocessed product, but chances that no adulterants were used are much better.

Organic Food

Why Organic Food Is Good

By Robert Rodale

As close as I can figure, there are 5 reasons why organic food is better than ordinary food.

REASON 1: There are no chemical residues in or on the food.

The lack of chemical residues ranks as the number one reason why organic foods are good. It is the advantage that convinces most people to start eating organic food. Specifically, what are these chemical residues? There are so many of them today that you can truthfully say that there is a book filled with their names—a book put out by the government saying how much of each chemical is permissible in different foods. And not only are there a lot of different chemicals being used, but they are being used for many different things.

Only a few years ago we did not have to worry about weed-killer residues in food, because no one used weed killers. Only a few years ago, you could eat a ham without wondering what was used to cure it. Now, you know that your ham probably contains calgon, the same water-softening chemical you use in your laundry. There is a chemical to make ice cream hold its shape as it melts. There are hundreds of different chemicals to kill insects and to cure plant diseases, some of them so poisonous that only one drop on your skin is enough to cause serious illness and possibly death.

The average person knows something about the chemicals in

his food and would choose not to eat them if he had an alternative. The steady growth of interest in organic gardening and farming is traceable to the desire of more people for pure food.

REASON 2: Organic food has superior nutritional quality as the result of growth on fertile soil.

The expanded use of chemicals on food has perhaps caused some people to overlook the fact that the original reason for growing foods organically was to get more nutritional value. The birth of the organic idea is traced to very near the time of Sir Albert Howard's experiment with the diets of two groups of children at a boys' boarding school in England. One group was fed ordinary food and the other was given organically grown food—the actual menus of each group being the same. The organic group showed dramatically better health experience than the normal group. They had fewer colds, better teeth and greater resistance to infectious diseases. It was that experiment which attracted J. I. Rodale's interest to the organic method and inspired him to found ORGANIC GARDENING AND FARMING magazine.

Humus-rich soil improves the food value of plants by providing them with all the nutrients they need in the proper balance. Balance is the key word to remember. When artificial fertilizers are used, the plants' roots are often saturated with an abundance of one nutrient, making it difficult for them to pick up other food that they need just as much. Since artificial fertilizers present their food in soluble form, the plant can't be selective and you can almost say it is forced to use the foods that are given to it.

To back up my claim that soil imbalance can cause serious defects, allow me to quote from the article, "Factors that Affect the Nutrients in Plants" from *Food,* Yearbook of Agriculture, 1959: "Raising the level of one mineral in the soil may depress the uptake or movement within the plant of another. The following are examples of some antagonisms that have been observed: nitrogen depresses phosphorous and calcium; magnesium depresses calcium; manganese, copper, zinc and cobalt depress iron." There is an unimpeachable source saying that the *balance* of food in the soil is of vital importance to the balance of the food that we eat. And humus is the one and only substance that always acts to balance out the nutrient components of the soil.

There are certain scientists, though, who still claim that the soil has no effect on the nutrient value of plants. They say that no matter how poor or how fertile a soil is, the crops grown on it contain the same balance of nutrients. Most of the scientists holding that view are the ones most closely allied with commercial farming. They want to believe that it is not their responsibility to provide proper food balance in plants—just high yields. Fortunately, it is not difficult to refute that outlook. The very same article that I quoted from before (from the yearbook, *Food*) tells how corn produces much higher protein content when grown on properly fertilized soil than on poor, neglected soil. The fertilizers used, over a 25-year period, were manure, lime and rock phosphate.

REASON 3: Organic food is not debased by overprocessing.

You can't call a loaf of white bread organic even if it is made from organically grown wheat. Having taken the life from the grain, you have taken its right to bear the label "organic." Fortunately, most growers and suppliers of organic foods appreciate that users want a product that is natural in all respects and they strive to treat their food naturally. And when you grow your own organic food you have control over it every step of the way. Most important, the average organic gardener doesn't have the knowledge or the means to overprocess food. It takes a lot of skill and expensive equipment to make whole wheat flour into white flour.

The effect of processing on food is not fully appreciated by most people. Again I am going to quote from the *Food* Yearbook of the United States Department of Agriculture. I hope you will forgive me for leaning so heavily on that book, but I am fascinated by the little nuggets it contains. The statement that I am now going to quote, was included by the author for the purpose of strengthening people's acceptance of food processing. I am giving it to you to show you that processing does more to food than you had suspected. Here it is: "A deficiency of trace elements is seldom a problem in human nutrition. One reason is that transportation and refrigeration enable most people in industrial countries to include foods from different areas in their diets. Furthermore, *procedures used to prepare and package foods for market often contribute several of these minerals to foods. Copper, iron and zinc, for example, may be added by processing machinery and cans and by cooking utensils in the home.*"

REASON 4: Better varieties of plants are used to grow organic food than are used by commercial farmers.

When you buy tomatoes in the store, you are getting the fruit of a plant that meets the farmer's requirements and not necessarily your requirements. The same could be said of almost every type of fruit, vegetable or grain. When a farmer grows tomatoes, for example, he wants plants that will ripen their fruit all at once, be easy to pick, stand up under shipment and yield the maximum number of bushels or tons per acre. Your wishes as a consumer are observed only so long as they don't conflict with his production problems. But when you grow tomatoes in your own garden, you can pick the variety that meets your needs 100 per cent. If you want high vitamin C content, you can grow Doublerich or High-C tomatoes. If you want an orange tomato with plenty of vitamin A, you can select Caro-Red. The day may come when super markets will handle superior varieties of plants because their customers demand them, but it hasn't arrived yet.

REASON 5: Growing food organically saves the land.

Any reckoning of the reasons why organic food is good must include consideration of the state of our soil. For it is from the soil that the true strength of America springs.

Commercial farmers today are too much concerned with events of today, and are making excuses for the failures they are breeding for tomorrow. They know that organic matter is essential to the health of the soil and they know that their farming methods are draining away that organic matter little by little each year. But they have to pay off loans on their big, new automatic machines, so they use methods to get highest yields that they know are really not sound. Tomorrow is time enough to put back the humus, they figure.

Even though the farmer is the custodian of the soil, you can't blame him entirely for slowly wearing it out. In our modern agricultural establishment, there are hordes of people who are helping him with that job. The chemical companies are spending millions of dollars to get new pesticides cleared for farm use, but they spend practically nothing to find out what those pesticide residues are doing to the soil where they accumulate. About a third of all the research done by the state experiment stations is financed by companies with some product to sell to the farmer. Many new farm scientists graduating each year have had their educations paid for by chemical company scholarships and grants. So you see, we have a lot of minds to change and people to educate to get across the organic idea.

Organic Food Proves Itself in Laboratory Experiments

In 1949, the Soil and Health Foundation published a bulletin describing a feeding experiment with mice which was conducted by Dr. Ehrenfried Pfeiffer at Threefold Farms, Spring Valley, New York. The experiment was undertaken in order to find out whether the treatment of soil with organic materials or with chemical fertilizers would show a difference in the feeding and health values of products grown under such farming methods. In this experiment, various groups of mice were fed food raised by different methods.

Results of the Test

It was found that the death rate from fighting was distinctly higher in the group fed food grown with chemical fertilizers. There were, in addition, more irritable and nervous mice in the chemical fertilizer group.

The mice were kept 6 in a box and each box was divided into two rooms, one for sleeping and one for eating. There was a tiny door in the partition—wide enough to permit one mouse at a time to walk through with comfort. Lifting the lids of the cages to let in the light produced panic and flight among the chemically fed rats who tried desperately to crowd through their tiny doorway by twos and threes. The organically fed mice reacted quite calmly, showing no panic.

Of the causes of death, stomach disorders were prevalent in the group fed chemically fertilized food to an extent of about 16 per cent. But they were present in only about 3 per cent of the organic group. The results of the experiment showed that the survival rate of the organic group was markedly higher than that of the chemical fertilizer group—32.63 per cent as against 21.38 per cent in the first generation. In another strain of mice, the survival rate was 64.41 per cent in the organic group as against 35.39 per cent in the chemical group. Larger litters were born to the organically fed mice.

Some time later, an interesting experiment was performed. It is a known fact certain chemicals, when rubbed into the skin, produce cancer. One of these cancer-causing chemicals was applied to the skin of all the mice. Among the mice fed with food that had been grown with chemicals, cancer of the skin reached as high as 71 per cent incidence, but in the organically fed group, only 45 per cent contracted cancer.

So it is apparent that laboratory experiments, conducted widely and fairly, would show, beyond a doubt, the superiority of organically grown food.

Osteopathy

Osteopathy

By Dr. A. Stoddard, M.B., B.S., D.O., M.R.O., Phys. Med.

This article is reprinted from the Cambridge University Medical Society magazine, Michaelmas, 1960 issue, by permission of the editors.

There are a great many misconceptions about osteopathy and it is the purpose of this article to clarify the position and state the case for and against osteopathy, as I see it, having myself had the advantage of an osteopathic and a medical training.

The misconceptions about this subject do not merely stem from the ignorance of medical men about present-day views of responsible osteopaths, but rather from the historical background of osteopathy and from the fact that proponents of the methods have in the main been practitioners outside the medical profession. This latter fact alone has been enough for most medical men to disregard all the claims of these unorthodox practitioners. In spite of official skepticism and outright criticism, the osteopathic profession continues to flourish and osteopaths do treat and do relieve a sizable proportion of the public in all walks of life from the heads of state down to impecunious old age pensioners.

A scathing criticism of osteopathy is to be found in a book called *What is Osteopathy?* by Drs. Hill and Clegg (1937), but when analyzed, we find that most of the criticisms were based on writings of the founder of osteopathy, Dr. A. T. Still. These criticisms might have been valid in the light of modern knowledge, but the autobiography was written in 1875. It would be easy to criticize medical methods in 1875 in the light of present-day medicine. We must remember that Dr. A. T. Still practiced in the early days of American history when the European settlers were pushing their way across the continent of North America, when fighting the Red Indian was commonplace and in fact, Dr. Still himself took part in some of this fighting. There were no definite medical schools then. The doctor was apprenticed and Dr. Still grew up in this type of training. He was a devout man and had an unshakable faith in divine law, so that when he lost 3 of his children with meningitis, it brought him up with a jolt and it is no wonder he started asking himself questions about the validity of the then existing methods of medical treatment. Was he not right to query the efficacy of drastic purgation, bloodletting and the drugs of those days? I see, on page 11 in the *British Medical Journal* of January 2, 1875, that diabetes was treated with mineral acids, bark and opium. In the same issue, Dr. Conrad says that vinegar had some power of modifying the eruption of smallpox; cancer of the skin was treated with arsenical paste; enuresis was treated with strychnine. In the light of modern therapeutics, these were foolish and dangerous practices.

Critics Should Examine Current Pronouncements

If criticisms are to be made about osteopathy, let the critics examine the pronouncements of osteopaths of the present day. The most reasonable account of the basis and scope of osteopathy can be found in the *Osteopathic Blue Book,* published by the General Council and Register of Osteopaths in 1958.

Even accepting the fact that many of Dr. Still's statements were false and exaggerated, there was at least a germ of truth in his claims, even if they were couched in rhetorical and Biblical phraseology. He drew attention to the effects of disordered mechanics upon the body in health and disease—an aspect of medicine still not receiving the attention it deserves, even though the present "disc" era has focused attention on abnormal mechanics in the spine.

Dr. Still had a mechanical turn of mind and he made several inventions for use in farming and his emerging ideas revolved round the conception of the human body being a machine. He also thought that, if the goodness of God was not to be questioned, surely the body should have within itself the capacity to combat disease. His theme was that, given a structurally sound body, then it should function healthily. Any disturbance of structure could account for the proneness of the body to disease.

Stopped Using Drugs and Patients Got Better

Basing his treatment upon this idea, he treated everything from typhoid to croup, from dislocated hips to "bloody flux" by manipulation of the spine and peripheral joints. He stopped using drugs. His patients got better—not really because he manipulated their spines, but because he inspired confidence and he stopped using the arsenic and mercury and leeches, as prescribed by his medical colleagues. The patients recovered because of their natural immunity unhindered by the deleterious effects of blood-letting, etc. It is clear that Dr. Still misinterpreted the reason for his patients' recovery and attributed it to his manipulation of the spinal lesion. So grew up the excessive claims of the early osteopaths that osteopathy was a complete system of medicine in its own right.

Osteopaths Slow to Relinquish Claims

Over the past 80 years, osteopaths have been slow to relinquish these claims, but the majority have now got the thing into reasonable perspective and the scope of osteopathy, the range of its efficacy, is more clearly defined and the role of the osteopathic spinal lesion better understood.

The American osteopaths defined the osteopathic lesion as any structural perversion which leads to functional disturbance. I prefer to define the lesion as a condition of impaired mobility in an intervertebral joint, in which there may or may not be altered positional relations of adjacent vertebrae. When altered position is present, it is always within the normal range of movement in that joint.

Most osteopathic spinal lesions are traumatically produced either by one single trauma or by a series of stresses of a mechanical nature. It is the state of the joint after the initial injury and prior to any subsequent pathological change in that joint. The moment when irreversible pathological changes take place in the joint, it ceases to be a purely osteopathic lesion. Similarly, when the altered position is such that the articular facets are not in apposition, it is no longer an osteopathic lesion. It is dislocation and this is outside the meaning of the term.

Lesions Easily Diagnosed by Thorough Examination

These lesions are easily diagnosed by those who are prepared to take the trouble to examine individual joints in the spine with sufficient care and attention to detail. The features of the lesion are restricted mobility, sometimes altered position and tenderness and muscle tension around the joint. There may be altered skin sensations and sudomotor changes locally around the joint. Detailed mobility tests are used and some practice is necessary in acquiring a proper assessment of the ranges in individual joints. It is not quite so simple as assessing the range of movement of a peripheral joint, like the knee joint. Rather, it is similar to assessing the range of movement in the carpal or tarsal joints.

These spinal lesions are undoubtedly the cause of local pain and referred pain. They do, also, sometimes cause a disturbance of autonomic reflexes in the area. There can be a disturbed somatico-visceral reflex just as there can be a disturbed viscero-somatic reflex. "The sharp distinction which is customarily drawn between the autonomic and somatic nervous systems, though useful for purposes of description, is to a considerable extent misleading. Afferent impulses from somatic structures may reflexly affect viscera." From *Applied Physiology,* p. 765, Samson Wright (1952).

One has frequently noted a disturbance of vaso-motion in the legs in cases of disc prolapse. Why should there not also be a disturbance of viscero-motion due to mechanical lesion, therefore? If the sympathetic nerves to a limb can be influenced by a purely mechanical disc lesion, why cannot those to a viscus be influenced and thereby alter the visceral function?

This is the basis for the osteopathic claim that spinal lesions can give rise to visceral disfunction and they claim, in due course, that this disfunction leads to disease. If this is so, then it is legitimate to treat disease by manipulating the spine.

Two Serious Objections to This Disease Theory

There are two serious objections to this theory of disease. The first is that the vegetative nervous system has an enormous capacity to balance itself in spite of considerable adverse influences. The vaso-motion upset by disc lesions is, in most cases, a purely temporary phenomenon—often so temporary that the patient fails to mention it and therefore, rarely is it elicited in the history of these cases. But if such patients are questioned, most of them admit to temporary coldness and blueness of the affected limb. By analogy, it is reasonable to suppose that any visceral disturbance from mechanical influence would have but a temporary effect. This does in fact tally with my own clinical observations.

Whatever the compensatory mechanism is, in the autonomic

nervous system, it certainly operates. Witness the return of vaso-motor tone in a limb which has, by all intents and purposes, been stripped of all its sympathetic nerves during the operation of sympathectomy.

The second serious objection to the view that structural disturbances cause visceral disease is that those patients presenting with the most serious and gross of mechanical defects (for example, structural scoliosis and kyphoses, gross spondylosis and osteoarthrosis, severe disc lesions and even fracture dislocations), are more often than not quite healthy subjects otherwise.

If the mechanical or structural fault does cause disturbance of the visceral reflex arc, then they do not tally clinically. Otherwise, the worse the structural fault, the worse would be the visceral disturbance. No, some compensatory mechanism is evoked on the part of the body and such visceral disturbance as does occur (and I am convinced that it does), is quite soon rectified by the spontaneous powers of recovery of the body.

However, ought we to ignore this even temporary disturbance of health by mechanical faults? I think not, for I have seen permanent vaso-motor changes from a disc prolapse and I have seen lasting visceral disturbance cleared up by manipulation of the spine.

Osteopath's Role Is That of Human Mechanic

The role of the osteopath is, in my view, that of a human mechanic, one who adjusts mechanical faults in any part of the loco-motion system. This is the field in which he can excel. He can also help in those disturbances which are labeled "functional" in nature. The term "functional" is oftentimes used with a disparaging implication by medical men whose only interest is in patients who have frank disease.

When a patient presents himself with indigestion and all the tests prove that there is no organic basis for the symptoms, the patient is labeled "functional" and very often little is done for him. He goes away disgruntled because he is told that there is nothing wrong with him and yet, his symptoms persist. Very often, the osteopath could help here. There may well be a structural fault in the mid-thoracic spine which is giving rise to dyspepsia.

When frank disease is established, then there is little point in treating the condition osteopathically. If the patient has a gastric ulcer, treatment to his thoracic spine may do some good, but it is not as effective as putting the patient on a diet or performing a gastrectomy. If the patient has pneumonia, it may do good to loosen his paravertebral muscles and ribs, but it is quicker and more effective to treat with antibiotics.

Osteopathic Work also of Psychological Value

Apart from purely local mechanical faults and functional disorders, there is still another role in which the osteopath can and does do a lot of good. This is in the realm of neurosis. Large numbers of patients have minor symptoms aggravated by anxiety. They are unhappy and uneasy about their health and very often refuse psychological help, believing their symptoms are of a physical nature. Such patients respond much better if a reasoned physical explanation is offered and a physical treatment employed. Certainly, this type of case tends to gravitate to the osteopath and, what is more, they respond and recover. If they recover, does the explanation offered to the patient matter all that much? Doctors are constantly employing this method of suggestion by using the bottle of medicine as a cure.

Much more could be said in detail about the use of osteopathic methods and lists of disorders effectively treated, but suffice it here to say that there is undoubted value in the method and osteopathy warrants closer attention and investigation by responsible medical men.

Overweight

What Do We Mean by Overweight?

How do you know what your correct weight should be? If you can no longer wear the size you wore several years ago, does this mean you are overweight, or should your weight go up as you become older? Or can you judge what is actually too much weight for you by the number of people who call you "Tubby"?

Overweight, today, is one of the most prevalent and serious of all "civilized" diseases, for it is a disease. Here are some facts and figures on overweight that should scare us into doing some constructive thinking about our condition if we number ourselves among the great army of overweight people.

Life insurance companies tell us that, among overweight clients, deaths from the following conditions are far more common than they are among those whose weight is average or below average: organic heart disease, diseases of the coronary arteries, angina pectoris, cerebral hemorrhage, chronic nephritis, cancer of the liver and gall bladder, diabetes, cirrhosis of the liver, appendicitis, hernia, gallstones, stomach ulcers, to name but a few. Asthma and bronchitis carry higher mortality risks when the patient is overweight. Too much weight complicates recovery in heart disease and arthritis. It has been suspected that obesity favors hardening of the arteries.

No one knows exactly how many Americans are overweight, but the figure has been set as high as 20,000,000.

USDA Issues Table of "Desirable Weights"

In *Food,* Yearbook of Agriculture, 1959, p. 103, appears a table of "desirable weights" for heights, as follows:

Height in Inches	Weight in Pounds	
	Women	*Men*
58	112 ± 11	125 ± 13
60	116 ± 12	130 ± 13
62	121 ± 12	135 ± 14
64	128 ± 13	142 ± 14
66	135 ± 14	150 ± 15
68	142 ± 14	158 ± 16
70	150 ± 15	167 ± 17
72	158 ± 16	178 ± 18

Katherine H. Fisher and Raymond W. Swift, both of the Pennsylvania State University, who wrote this chapter, tell us, in addition, that overweight means an excess of 10 to 20 per cent in body weight. When the excess weight represents more than 20 per cent of the desirable weight, we refer to the condition as obesity.

They tell us, too, that, "It has been suggested that one's desirable weight at age 25 should be maintained throughout life. We estimate, however, that one out of every 5 adults in the United States is overweight."

Most sensible of all, we believe, are the ideas of Dr. Charles F. Wilkinson, Jr., of New York University Post-Graduate Hospital, who believes that, at the age of 50 and thereafter, you should weigh about 14 per cent less than you weighed at 35. From 35 to 50, he says, body muscle will probably decrease, since physical activity lessens. As muscle content 'of the body decreases, it is replaced by fat. So the total body weight may stay the same, but the percentage of fat will be steadily rising.

How Can You Tell You're Overweight?

How do you know whether you are overweight? Here, we present some new tables on weight-height relationships which we think should give you the answer. These are not the old tables based on life insurance company figures with which we have all been familiar for years. And it seems there are very good reasons why those old tables should be discarded. Jean Mayer of Harvard School of Public Health explains in the August, 1955, issue of *Harper's* magazine how those old tables were compiled.

The figures represent not any ideal weight, remember. They tell us just what actual average weight was. In 1912, when the figures were compiled, height was taken with shoes on, weight was recorded with street clothes on. Apparently, many of the weights were estimated, not measured. Considering the amount of street clothing worn, especially by women in those times, it is not surprising to find that, even though you consider yourself rather heavy, you never seem to be overweight according to these ancient standard tables.

Furthermore, Dr. Mayer points out, the practice of buying life insurance in those days was confined largely to a relatively small group of prosperous individuals. "When you are using the 'normal' weight table and comforting yourself with the thought that your weight is 'normal for your height and age,' remember that you are pitting yourself against bankers, brokers, lawyers and physicians of the gay nineties, complete with handlebar mustaches, vests, striped pants, morning coats, spats, watch chains and carnations," says Dr. Mayer.

The weights for men were predicted on their standard weights at age 30, on the theory that any increase from then on would be pure fatty tissue. So it is quite possible that these figures represent the already almost middle-age spread of a nearly sedentary group of individuals.

An article in the *Canadian Medical Association Journal* for January 1, 1955, gives tables for the average weights for height and age of Canadians in 1953 (Table 8), compiled by the Department of National Health and Welfare of Canada. This is with ordinary indoor clothing, but no shoes.

Specific Gravity and Weight Calculations

An interesting angle in weight consideration is specific gravity. It is a system by which one measures the weight of objects or elements in relation to water. For example, the specific gravity of water equals one, so that anything weighing twice the weight of an equal amount of water has the specific gravity of two. The higher the specific gravity of an object, the more compact or dense is its structure. Consider the difference between a nail and a wooden peg of the same size. The nail is not porous as is the peg; it will not float, but the peg will. The specific gravity of the nail is higher than that of the peg. It is stronger. There is more substance packed into the nail than the peg, though their size is exactly the same.

In the human body, specific gravity is an important factor in considering who is overweight and who is not. A football player

Table 8: CANADIAN CHART FOR AVERAGE WEIGHTS BY YEARS

WOMEN: AGE IN YEARS

Height Feet	Inches	15	16-17	18-19	20-24	25-29	30-34	35-44	45-54	55-64	65 and Over
4	8	96	105	100	106	110	115	126	130	134	120
	9	99	107	103	108	112	117	127	132	137	124
	10	101	110	107	111	114	119	128	134	139	128
	11	104	112	110	113	117	122	130	137	141	132
5	0	107	115	114	116	119	124	131	139	144	136
	1	109	117	118	118	122	126	133	142	146	140
	2	112	120	121	121	124	129	134	144	148	144
	3	115	122	125	123	127	131	135	146	151	148
	4	117	125	129	126	129	133	137	149	152	152
	5	120	127	132	128	132	136	138	151	155	157
	6	123	130	136	131	134	138	140	153	158	161
	7	126	132	140	133	137	140	141	156	160	165
	8	128	135	143	136	139	143	143	158	162	169
	9	131	137	147	138	141	145	144	160	165	173
	10	134	140	151	141	144	147	145	163	167	177
	11	136	142	154	143	146	150	147	165	169	181

MEN: AGE IN YEARS

Height Feet	Inches	15	16-17	18-19	20-24	25-29	30-34	35-44	45-54	55-64	65 and Over
4	11	92	99	116	121	128	134	135	127	138	126
5	0	97	103	119	124	132	138	139	132	141	130
	1	102	108	122	127	135	141	142	136	144	135
	2	106	113	125	131	139	145	146	141	148	140
	3	111	118	128	134	142	148	150	146	151	144
	4	116	122	131	138	146	152	153	150	154	149
	5	121	127	134	142	149	156	157	155	157	154
	6	125	132	138	145	153	159	161	160	160	158
	7	130	136	141	149	156	163	164	165	163	163
	8	135	141	144	152	160	166	168	169	166	167
	9	139	146	147	156	163	170	172	174	169	172
	10	144	151	150	159	167	173	175	179	172	177
	11	148	155	153	163	170	177	179	183	176	181
6	0	153	160	156	166	174	181	183	188	179	186
	1	158	165	160	170	177	184	186	193	182	191
	2	163	169	163	173	181	188	190	197	185	195
	3	167	174	166	177	184	191	194	202	188	200

who weighs 220 pounds might not be overweight, while an office worker, of the same height, who weighs that much, definitely is. The difference lies in the specific gravity of each. The football player will be muscular, the office worker will probably be flabby. The athlete's specific gravity will be higher than that of the office worker because muscle has a higher specific gravity than fat. To go back to the steel nail and the wooden peg—the nail has more efficiency, or strength, than the peg, even though both have exactly the same outward appearance; the athlete has more efficiency, or strength, than the office worker even though both are the same height and weight.

This factor should be considered in using the tables provided here. You can fit the age and height descriptions for proper weight in every way and still be unhealthfully overweight as an individual. Certainly, your own experience has taught you that, of two women, each of whom is 5 feet 3 inches in height and weighs 120 pounds, one can be very different from the other in appearance and in the way she carries her weight. You might say one is too fat and the other just right.

You can increase your specific gravity by reducing the fat on your body and replacing it with muscle, through exercise. Also, you can concentrate on high specific gravity foods. Most fresh vegetables have a high specific gravity: green peppers, 1.12 to 1.15; beets the same; broccoli, 1.12 to 1.14; tomatoes, 1.14 to 1.20; a starchy vegetable, the potato, has only 1.06 to 1.07. Good eggs have a high specific gravity of 1.10, but poorer quality eggs, only 1.085. Fatty foods have a lower specific gravity and should be used sparingly: butter .86, lard .92 and milk 1.03.

Decreasing Weights

Table 9 is that developed by Dr. Wilkinson showing the rate of decrease recommended for each age over 35.

By comparing your own statistics with the charts, you can see the good sense in Dr. Wilkinson's ideas. Just because the weight of Americans and Canadians goes steadily upward as age increases, is no reason to suppose that this is the ideal situation, any more than one could suppose, for instance, that diabetes is a perfectly natural and ideal phenomenon since so many of us suffer from it. Certainly, with life insurance figures clearly showing the relation of overweight in later life to the incidence of degenerative disease, one could do no better than to follow the suggestions above and consider oneself overweight if one's weight figures are higher than those in Dr. Wilkinson's chart.

What then does overweight mean? Making some slight allowances for body build, we can say that overweight is weighing more than the desirable weight for one's age and height according to these revised and very sensible tables.

Table 9: RECOMMENDED WEIGHTS BY HEIGHT AND AGE

WOMEN (WITH 1½ INCH HEELS): AGE IN YEARS

Height Feet	Inches	15-19	20-24	25-29	30-35	35-40	40-45	45-50
4	10	107	111	114	117	111	105	100
	11	108	113	116	119	113	107	102
5	0	110	115	118	121	115	109	104
	1	112	117	120	123	117	111	105
	2	115	120	122	125	119	113	107
	3	118	123	125	128	122	116	110
	4	121	126	129	132	126	120	114
	5	124	129	132	136	129	123	117
	6	129	133	136	140	133	126	120
	7	133	137	140	144	137	130	123
	8	137	141	144	148	141	134	127
	9	140	145	148	152	145	138	131
	10	144	149	152	155	147	140	133
	11	149	153	155	158	150	143	136
6	0	153	157	159	162	154	146	139

MEN: AGE IN YEARS

Height Feet	Inches	15-19	20-24	25-29	30-35	35-40	40-45	45-50
5	0	113	119	124	127	121	115	109
	1	115	121	126	129	123	117	111
	2	118	124	128	131	124	118	112
	3	121	127	131	134	127	121	115
	4	124	131	134	137	130	124	118
	5	128	135	138	141	134	127	121
	6	132	139	142	145	138	131	125
	7	136	142	146	149	142	135	128
	8	140	146	150	154	146	139	132
	9	144	150	154	158	150	143	136
	10	148	154	158	163	155	147	140
	11	153	158	163	168	160	152	145
6	0	158	163	169	174	166	158	150
	1	163	168	175	180	171	162	154
	2	168	173	181	186	177	168	160

Your Weight and Your Emotions

Are you fat because of your emotions? There seems to be a large amount of evidence which points to the problem of overweight as having its root in psychological problems. We are not sure that mental attitude is the main reason for obesity, but many authorities are, so we think that this viewpoint should be presented in these pages.

That there is some definite psychological pattern involved in overweight is pretty well demonstrated by the work of Dr. Benjamin Kotkov, Clinical Psychologist at the Boston Dispensary in the New England Medical Center, in company with Dr. Stanley S. Kanter, psychiatrist, and Dr. Joseph Rosenthal, internist. (*Newsweek,* November 17, 1952.) From 300 obese women, some of whom weighed as much as 300 pounds, 131 were selected to be included in the tests. As controls for these, 80 normal-weight women were recruited.

The researcher worked with 6 women at a time, giving them the well-known Rorschach Ink Blot Test. This test is one of psychology's most successful tools for testing personality. One by one, 10 cards bearing strange ink patterns—or blots—were shown to the group. As each card was held up, the subjects were asked to write down what each design suggested to them. The things each person "sees" in these blots demonstrates, to the trained observer, the patient's turn of mind, his attitude about the life around him, in short, his personality. Dr. Kotkov concluded that the fat women's personalities were not nearly so well-adjusted as those of the normal-weight subjects.

The 6 traits common to the obese women were: repression of true feelings; lack of initiative; tenseness and suppressed anger that led to depression; they were self-centered and oblivious of the reactions of others, easily and deeply hurt at any real or imagined rejection; not disposed to seek out new friendships, because the risk of failure seemed too great; did not enjoy social relations or social occasions which they considered "painful experiences"; and they showed lack of interest in clothing since they did not feel at ease even in nice clothes.

It was recorded by Dr. Kotkov that this personality pattern was evident whether the woman was 15 per cent or 50 per cent overweight. Education and intelligence were not factors in determining the amount of extra poundage the women were willing to carry.

Fat People Are Bad Risks

If people are willing to be heavy and risk being unattractive and if their personalities, lacking though they might be, let them get by, why are we so interested in getting these people to slim down? The answer is, of course, that overweight is dangerous to good health. The *Bulletin of the New York Academy of Medicine* (May-June, 1960) tells us that obese persons have a mortality rate that is 20 per cent above the average. In cardiovascular disease, the rate is much higher for fat people than for others—150 per cent for men and 175 per cent for women. Diabetic deaths are 4 times more frequent in overweight people than in normal-sized ones; where gall bladder disease, cirrhosis of the liver and appendicitis are concerned, the rate among overweight people is double that of others.

One ray of hope that should encourage all overweight persons is that almost anyone can lose weight, and when fat people do reduce, their mortality rates return to normal. We will try to give one answer here as to why one hears this so often from overweight persons: "I've tried, but I simply can't cut down. I guess I'm just naturally heavy, and there's no use fighting it."

No One Is Naturally Heavy

No one is "naturally heavy." No one inherits a tendency to be overweight. What one does acquire from one's parents is a pattern of food selection. It is not surprising that, if one's parents have always started the day with buns and pancakes and have gone on through the day with snacks of candy and pretzels, pie and cake, the child will follow suit. Anyone who eats this way will probably put on weight; it's not due to any physical inheritance, but to the inheritance of bad habits in eating. It is extremely rare for a child to be born destined to be overweight due to some congenital imperfection. But a child's parents can easily teach him to eat in such a way as to make overweight inevitable. In this sense, obesity "runs" in certain families. When both parents are stout, more than 70 per cent of the offspring can be expected to be overweight. When the parents are of normal weight, less than 10 per cent of the children will be classed as obese.

Two solid indications that heredity is not responsible are: (1) fat people with obese parents do respond to weight reduction treatment just as anyone else does; (2) the weight of identical twins (those with the same inherited characteristics) varies greatly from time to time, while their coloring, height and general build remain the same. If the twins' weight were inherited, there should be no appreciable difference in weight between the two.

Is It Hunger or Appetite?

Dr. Max Millman, in *Today's Health* (August, 1950), wrote of an important distinction in the use of food: We must, he says, remember that there is a difference between hunger and appetite. Hunger is an instinct and all of us are born with it, an unpleasant sensation in the pit of the stomach, an awareness that we must have food to sustain our bodies. Appetite is an emotion which we acquire as we mature. It is a desire to repeat some pleasant sensation. When you feel hungry for some particular thing, and nothing else, that's appetite. When you're really hungry, anything will do.

Normally, appetite is an excellent regulator, as it was meant to be. It makes us want to eat the foods we need in some variety. That way we don't eat fruit exclusively, because we get hungry for meat sometimes, and that assures us of needed protein. We have an appetite for something sweet, at times, because our bodies need the natural sugar for energy. When we have had enough, our appetite tells us so. It regulates our food intake, and, if we are eating unprocessed, fresh foods, we can usually depend upon it to direct us properly.

Now, if the appetite becomes unreasonable in the demands it makes on us, the emotion which controls it has somehow gone haywire. The plump person who says he overeats because he's hungry really means that his appetite is out of control. The very thought of a dish of ice cream or a piece of cake awakens such desire in him that the desire is almost impossible for him to resist. It can be compared to the emotion that makes sportsmen play golf or go fishing at every possible opportunity. Just the thought of the pleasure it gives them to indulge in these sports, makes their eyes light up and the yearning is almost visible. However, they must control the emotion. They have responsibilities that won't allow them to spend every day at play. Anyone who refuses to be guided by his responsibilities and simply golfs or fishes all day, every day, without regard for the welfare of his family or his job, is considered to be abnormal, ill really. He doesn't control his appetite for fun and he should. The "overeater" is ill, too. He doesn't control his appetite for food and he should.

Just as some persons drown their anxieties in alcohol, others turn to food. Worry, fear and fatigue may rob one person of an appetite for food, while the next will react by overeating. Think of yourself and your friends. When faced with an emotionally upsetting situation, do you and they eat more or less? A large majority of several hundred fat people who were asked that question said they ate more. When worried or nervous, they said they just couldn't stop nibbling and chewing.

Defense against Responsibility

In many obese people, the weight they carry serves as a defense against assuming certain responsibilities which they fear they are inadequate to discharge properly. These might be anything from marriage to unpleasant jobs to difficult social contacts. Dr. Millman cites the case of a 16-year-old boy who was afraid to play football, baseball or any other athletic game, due to his parents' overprotection during childhood. He feared injury and yet was ashamed to admit his fears. He soon discovered that obesity was a perfect excuse for nonparticipation. He could make himself too fat to play. He overate whenever possible.

A young lady of 26 was anxious to avoid matrimony and the responsibilities that are involved with it. Rather than admit this to herself and simply refuse to consider marriage, with the healthy realization that it was not for her, she became fat to make herself less attractive to men. If she were never asked, she would never have to admit to herself or anyone else, her reason for not wanting to marry.

There are almost as many psychological reasons for overeating as there are people who overeat. For some people, food means security, so that whenever they feel insecure, they overeat. Boredom leads others to gluttony—"Whenever I have nothing else to do, I can always eat." Some people who feel wronged overeat as a gesture of self-pity. Then there are those who have a false sense of economy —they overeat because they can't bring themselves to throw leftovers into the garbage can. The list of reasons is endless.

Sugar in the Blood?

Most of the cases above are in need of some professional help. But one wonders why the psychological frustrations these people experience make themselves felt by this weight-gaining device. Not every insecure, bored, afraid or unrealistic person becomes overweight. Why does it happen to these people? One theoretical answer to that question appeared in *Science News Letter* (April 7, 1956). Drs. Albert Stunkard and Harold G. Wolff reported to the American Psychosomatic Society that the answer might lie in the rate at which some bodies remove sugar from the blood.

Emotional stress makes some people eat more because it upsets the body mechanism for handling sugars and starches. Apparently, sugar is removed from the blood too fast after eating and this lessens the feeling of having enough to eat, which in turn leads to overeating.

The two doctors reported that they had injected a measured amount of sugar solution into the veins of obese persons and it disappeared from the blood at higher than normal rates. Further study of 4 very fat people over several months showed that, when they were under stress of an emotional sort, injected sugar was removed from their blood at abnormally fast rates. But when the stress was absent and relatively calm periods ensued, the injected sugar was removed at a normal rate.

It was interesting to find that hunger contractions in the stomachs of starving people could be stopped with the injection of sugar into the blood stream, and without the least bit of food actually being consumed by the starving person. From this and other experiments, the doctors concluded that hunger comes when the sugar and starch stores of the body are depleted and the feeling of having eaten enough comes when these stores are replenished.

This brings us to the truism that appetite is indeed bound up with emotion. If the emotional aspects of life are pleasant, the body is better able to conserve the sugar in the blood, which is the key to a desire for more food. In obese persons, this blood sugar is more liable to quick depletion.

Blood Sugar Levels

The thing to do, then, is to maintain a diet which will insure a steady blood sugar level. This means avoidance of foods which induce an artificially high blood sugar reading which cannot be sustained. Imagine your proper blood sugar level to be a tight rope strung between two poles. The rope is set at 50 feet. The tight ropewalker sensibly steps onto the rope at the 50-foot level and calmly walks across. He is trained to do this with ease. You are geared to operate with ease at a steady blood sugar level. Now suppose he were to step onto the 50-foot-high platform and, instead of simply walking on the wire to get to the other side, he were to jump on a spring board which would catapult him to a trapeze 30 feet above the wire. He would hold the trapeze until he got tired and had to let go. Down past the wire he would fall, only to hit another springboard which would catapult him up to another trapeze 80 feet high, but a bit closer to the other end of the rope. Again he would tire and let go and again he would hit the springboard and bounce to a trapeze still closer to the platform he was aiming for. He would arrive there eventually, exhausted, with sore legs from the springboards and sore hands from the trapeze.

This gives some idea of the stresses our bodies suffer when our blood sugar is suddenly elevated with a candy bar or a soda, then, after a few minutes, is plunged low when the candy wears off, and must be boosted again with another sweet. A careful diet of selected natural carbohydrates, plenty of protein and the proper fats, eaten at mealtime in sufficient quantity to satisfy the appetite, will sustain the proper blood sugar until the next meal. Even the person who uses more blood sugar under stress will have what is needed until the next meal is due. If something extra is required, the person's needs will be met with natural foods, such as fruit, a piece of cold meat or the like. No need for fattening foods, no need for bouncing blood sugar levels.

Eat Proper Foods

We believe stable blood sugar is the best answer for all obese persons. The plan for acquiring it does not require the counting of calories or the painful reduction of food intake. We may eat normal and adequate amounts of food, but eat proper foods, properly prepared or as close to raw as possible. Some persons are willing to go on a starvation diet which allows only a quart of liquid per day or 5 hard-boiled eggs and a half grapefruit per day and yet, they will not follow our diet suggestions because they feel they can't do it.

You lose weight by eating your choice of natural foods in reasonable variety and amounts, according to your own appetite, provided the foods you choose contain no refined sugar, no added salt and are not prepared in hot fat. You will find that you are satisfied with what you eat at meals, most times, but when hunger pangs hit at other times, there is no prohibition against a glass of unsweetened fruit or vegetable juice, a chicken leg (or any lean meat) or a banana (or any other fresh fruit) as a snack. If you are overweight, this diet will restore you to a healthy level, and will do so without creating any complexes or other psychological problems.

A Modest Proposal

Every time we think we have come to the final horror in the thoughtlessness of modern medical practice, we are shocked anew by a piece such as the one which appeared in the *Lancet* (July 23, 1960). A Danish correspondent to this magazine actually suggested, in apparent seriousness, that, where overweight is a problem, a removal of a part of the intestine from which energy-producing nutrients are absorbed, should be attempted.

A couple of problems present themselves here: for one, how much of this organ, the jejunum, should be removed?

If too little is taken away, there will be no effect on weight and, if too much is removed, progressive uncontrollable starvation may result. Now, suppose the magical amount were to be arrived at and the patient were to lose weight because less calories were being absorbed than were being used—how would one stop it before the patient shriveled into nothing? The author's alternative is to cause a by-pass of the jejunum by the food, which can later be redirected to the jejunum for absorption once more via more surgery.

Even this solution has a few drawbacks: ". . . pernicious anemia may follow; but this could easily be mastered by hematological (blood study) control and adequate treatment. If other difficulties, such as ileus or severe dyspepsia should develop as a sequel to such jejunal cul-de-sacs, one might, as an alternate operation, remove part of the jejunum from the intestinal canal without resection . . ." At this point, we stopped reading. The only conclusion we could reach, under the circumstances, is that the author of the communication was either pulling the reader's leg or was mentally incompetent.

This man is advocating a major operation which is almost bound to have serious debilitating effects and could lead to fatal starvation, through lack of absorption, for the purpose of losing weight. Imagine advocating such radical measures when diet, nothing more, could remedy the situation absolutely. We wonder that any doctor would make such an insane proposal. We wonder too that a journal of the *Lancet's* stature stooped to print it. Finally, we wonder how many readers seriously considered the possibility of trying it.

Steer Clear of Overweight Drivers

Maybe you don't drive as safely as you'd like to simply because you're fat! In *Consumer Bulletin* (June, 1960), this theory was offered by Dr. Rosario Robillard of Montreal, Canada. Statistically, the overweight driver is more accident-prone than the slim one and the tendency to crack up rises as the poundage does.

Dr. Robillard's position is that, when overweight is really pronounced, driving licenses should be restricted to private automobiles; and when obesity is extreme, even a private automobile license should be denied.

Well, Dr. Robillard may have a persuader for avid drivers who won't go on a diet. Maybe they will respond to such measures and do themselves and those on the road with them some good. We think this item is important because it points out, once more, that overweight lowers the body's efficiency no matter what one tries to do. We're not meant to be fat. We can't take it and when we are, we simply can't do the things we want to do as well as as we'd like.

A decrease in efficiency is not the only consequence of overweight. Inside, the heavy person is having trouble, too—the heart, kidneys, circulation and elimination are only a few of the bodily functions that tend to go bad in the presence of overweight. Regain your proper weight by eating unprocessed foods and avoiding refined sugar and salt; get plenty of protein and fresh fruits and vegetables.

Pectin

Pectin Assumes New Importance

As reported in the *Journal of the American Medical Association* (November 18, 1961), there is hope that pectin in the diet may turn out to offer valuable protection against the accumulation of strontium 90 in the body. Laboratory experiments made with rats in Russia and described in the Russian publication, *Labor Hygiene and Occupational Diseases,* are cited in the *Journal of the American Medical Association* as claiming to "prove that pectin reduces the absorption and deposition of the isotope in the skeleton."

Like American scientists, those in Russia have been seeking

prophylactic agents that will help the body to eliminate radioactive strontium rather than to let it accumulate in the bones, where, in amounts much larger than those we are presently receiving from fall-out, it could cause leukemia and bone cancer. The various compounds tested have generally been found to be "inadequately effective and not without harm to the body."

Pectin derived from sunflowers, however, is believed to be superior on both accounts. According to the Russian researchers, the addition of pectin from sunflowers to the diet of rats "binds radio-active strontium in the gastrointestinal tracts of rats (and) reduces the absorption and deposition of the isotope in the skeleton." At the same time, it was concluded that using this common ingredient of food for "enrichment of the usual mixed diet, would not interfere with nutrition, metabolism or other body functions."

Are Reports Confirmed?

Can we accept this Russian report as conclusive? Certainly not. We know too much about how science in the Soviet Union is compelled to serve as the handmaiden of politics. There was certainly a need to allay the fears of Russian citizens over atmospheric bomb tests and this report might well have been developed for that purpose. Before we can accept it fully, we can only wait and see whether our own scientists can corroborate the Russian results.

However, we see good reason to hope and expect that it will turn out to be true. For one thing, Aleksei Golub, a Soviet scientist who defected to the West in Amsterdam, was reported by *United Press International* to have made the same claim after he was safely away from the Soviet Union and its pressures. For another, what we already know about pectin and its action in the body confirms that it may very well serve as claimed.

What Pectin Is

Pectin is a substance found in and between the walls of the cells of plants. In unripe plants, it is found as part of the protopectins, carbohydrate complexes that are not soluble. As the plant matures, according to Edna Brown Southmayd, Ph.D., of the research department of Sunkist Growers (*Nutrition Research*, December, 1961), enzyme action within the plant releases soluble and consequently, digestible pectin substances. Pectin has a strong water-binding property, which helps plants to retain their water and makes it useful in making jellies. Interestingly, it is the pectin of green fruit, which is indigestible, that has this jellying property. The pectin of mature fruit, which we do digest, for that very reason of its solubility, is not good for jelly making. This is probably one of the important factors entering into the established fact that ripe fruits and vegetables are more fully digested than the green ones.

The Russian reports did not state, apparently, whether the pectin used in their experiments was from mature or unripe sunflower seeds. Neither did they state whether they considered the aid to elimination of strontium 90 a characteristic of all pectin or just of sunflower pectin. We have long believed that, in addition to their known superb nutritive value, there are in sunflower seeds many as yet undiscovered or unconfirmed properties. In this case, however, we think it probable, because of already known attributes of all pectin, that it will turn out to be the pectin rather than the sunflower that is significant.

Pectin Prevents Lead Poisoning

It has been known for more than a hundred years that the ingestion of pectin would prevent lead poisoning. This, according to

---

Pasteur, Louis

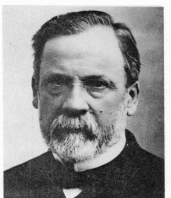

Perhaps one of the most important and influential men among the pioneers in the field of medicine and science was Louis Pasteur. One need only consider the many valuable contributions which he gave to the world as proof of this assertion. Pasteur's life in science began at the Royal College of Besancon and the Ecole Normale of Paris, from which he graduated in 1847. From this point on until his death in 1895, the list of Pasteur's accomplishments began to unfold. Early in his career Pasteur turned his attention to the study of the fermentation process, especially as it pertained to the beer and wine industries. He demonstrated that fermentation was due to the presence and growth of certain microörganisms. Removal of these organisms would halt the fermentation process and thus prevent unnecessary spoilage. From this principle evolved the famous Pasteurization process, which is based on the use of heat to kill these organisms in milk. Other achievements which earned for Pasteur the title of Founder of the Science of Bacteriology were his studies on the silkworm disease, yielding a method of eliminating this plague, and the development of the inoculation for rabies. Pasteur received many distinctions for his valuable work, greatest among them being his election to the Academy of Science of the United States.

Dr. Glenn H. Joseph, writing in *Nutrition Research* for September, 1955, is because pectin, in the digestive process, is transformed into galacturonic acid, which has the property of combining with certain heavy metals into insoluble metallic salts. These salts cannot be absorbed into the system and so they are excreted. Galacturonic acid from pectin combines in the same way with calcium, causing its excretion and, since we know that calcium and strontium 90 are molecular twins (the reason that strontium 90 lodges in the bones through ion exchange), we might speculate even without any evidence that pectin might be expected to combine, as galacturonic acid, with strontium 90 and prevent it from being absorbed into the system, so that it will be excreted instead.

This, as we have already pointed out, is still a matter of speculation. Only time and further experimentation can prove or disprove it.

Meanwhile, however, there is no need to wait for proof so far as our diets are concerned. The consumption of foods containing pectin will not do any harm and has strong nutritional benefits that make it important in every diet.

Nutritional Values of Pectin

Professor Ancel Keys, Director of the Laboratory of Physical Hygiene of the University of Minnesota and a noted research scientist, has been pointing out in recent years that pectin has a beneficial effect on the blood cholesterol level. In an address to the American Heart Association in November, 1960, he reported that experiments had proven that the addition of 15 grams (about ½ ounce) of pectin to the daily diet of middle-aged men caused the blood cholesterol to decrease by an average of about 5 per cent. Professor Keys also pointed out that eating pectin, by itself, is not as valuable an aid in blood cholesterol reduction as eliminating saturated fats and using unsaturated vegetable oils. But pectin is of definite value in this respect and Dr. Keys speculates that the high consumption of fruits, including apples, by some populations (like the Italian) helps to explain the low blood cholesterol levels in those populations.

Pectin nourishes the intestinal flora, helping them to carry on their vital work of combating and controlling the numbers of disease bacteria. The pectin, in its turn, is converted by these benign bacteria into fatty acids which arrest the development of the bacteria responsible for bacillary dysentery, infantile diarrhea and other intestinal disorders. Some of the pectin entering the intestine combines with calcium to form calcium gels, which aid healthy elimination by providing bulk.

According to Edwin F. Bryant, Ph.D., pectin removes toxic wastes from the body by combining with them into chemical forms that permit their elimination.

It also corrects constipation by its water binding properties, moistening and softening the waste to be eliminated.

All in all, it can be seen that pectin is a valuable element in any diet. For preventive purposes, one can get quite enough from a diet containing substantial quantities of apples, crab apples, sunflower seeds, currants, grapes, plums and cranberries. For such purposes as reduction of blood cholesterol, doctors use capsules of pure pectin, containing much larger amounts. Dr. Keys, in his experiments, used 15 grams a day, an amount derived from two pounds of apples.

Eat Sunflower Seeds

Of course, for reduction of blood cholesterol, pectin alone is not nearly as important as the unsaturated fatty acids, in which certain of the vegetable oils are particularly rich. We have long held that such valuable food substances are best taken, not as extracts, but in the natural combinations in which they occur in nature's foods. For this reason, we have long advocated the eating of large quantities of sunflower seeds as a health measure, even more important than the very valuable use of corn, safflower or soybean oil in salads and in cooking. We have maintained that there are special and potent virtues in organically grown, whole sunflower seeds that are only beginning to be understood.

Now that these new studies have demonstrated the value of pectin from sunflower seeds, as well as the oil and the rich vitamin content, our belief is reinforced that the sunflower seed, easily grown in your own back yard, is one of the most valuable and concentrated nutritive foods known to man. In Russia, where sunflowers are grown everywhere and the seeds are a staple of diet, millions have lived through famines eating practically nothing but sunflower seeds, while maintaining excellent health. We do not, of course, recommend such a restricted diet. But we do recommend that you eat some sunflower seeds every day. Whether or not they turn out, after further investigation, to serve any worthwhile purpose in eliminating strontium 90, they cannot help being beneficial in terms of general good nutrition.

Physical Fitness

Youth Fitness in Today's America

What follows is a report whose extremely serious nature should awaken all Americans to the dangers to health that accompany our modern way of life in this country. This press release originated with the American Association for Health, Physical Education and Recreation, a Department of the National Education Association. We are appalled, as were the authors of this report, at the physical condition among American youth revealed here. We are even more disturbed that the report does not mention diet as a contributing factor to the physical fitness or unfitness of youth. While we agree that lack of exercise and physical exertion are important reasons for the steady deterioration of the health of our young people, we are convinced that a much more important reason for this is their malnourished condition, resulting from diets low in most of the important food elements. Countless surveys have shown that this kind of diet is widespread, especially among American teen-agers. The next time someone tells you everyone in this country is getting all he needs for nourishment out of his daily meals, show him this report.

One of the scientists who gave tests to both British and American children which produced similar results stated, "Our poor showing is due mostly to the lack of physical training in the United States compared with that in Britain and the fact that our kids are more obese than theirs. Malnutrition isn't always undernourishment—the greatest malnutrition in America is overnourishment."

Can the United States be any stronger than the people who compose it? Is the state of physical fitness of American youth a real cause for national alarm? Are Americans blind or indifferent to forces which are causing erosion and decay of our most vital asset, our human resources—our people? What is the effect of today's living mode in the United States on health and fitness? Are we more concerned with exploring outer space than providing space for recreation and family activity here at home—space for living, space for leisure, as well as for work? These are real and valid questions being raised by thinking citizens in many places. They are the natural outcome of our population explosion, our rapidly increasing automation and its resultant lack of former activity and exercise.

The alert was sounded some 4 years ago with the exposure of comparisons between European and American children as a result of physical fitness tests using the Kraus-Weber Test. The comparisons at that time were anything but flattering to the American ego. Regardless of the hue and cry that the Kraus-Weber tests might lack sufficient validity and reliability as an index to fitness levels, the fact remains that we showed glaring physical deterioration.

Now, 4 years later, comes further proof from the American Association for Health, Physical Education and Recreation at the National Education Association Center in Washington, D.C., that America MUST take steps to compensate for recent fitness deficiencies which result from complacent and "fat" living. Fitness test results just released by AAHPER headquarters of OPERATION FITNESS—USA involve a research project in Japan conducted by competent Japanese fitness experts in collaboration with OPERATION FITNESS—USA and some American test leaders. Some 20,000

Japanese children were given the AAHPER National Fitness Test battery and the results are interesting and arresting to say the least.

Japanese children excelled American children in almost every basic component of physical fitness—in many cases by alarming margins. This is not a conjecture or a hunch. The team of research leaders carefully followed the American plan of fitness testing in minute detail. Children were selected on a sampling basis in all parts of Japan, in rural back country, in the cities, on remote islands, and in the exact fashion as was done in the United States when the Research Council of AAHPER developed national fitness norms for the AAHPER National Fitness Test. Each test item was carefully administered with American techniques.

The nation which was almost a shambles following World War II has surely and constructively built a program to conserve and strengthen its youth, and has accomplished this tremendous task with large amounts of American assistance.

Japanese leaders proudly point to the unusual results that have been obtained with required physical education instruction for all children at all age levels, beginning with grade one, for at least 3 times per week. They declare that, if the present rate of emulating and adopting American ways of living continues unabated, they will soon lose this superiority and lapse into a state of unfitness similar to that in America.

The tests in Japan revealed that Japanese children excelled Americans by wide margins in items involving arm strength. This was true for both boys and girls. Greatest deviation between the two races occurred when children in the lower quartile of results were compared. Here the Japanese girls excelled ours at various age levels from 18 per cent to 47 per cent. The only American solace in tests of arm strength was that the best American girls did exceed the best Japanese girls by a small margin. In tests of speed and agility, the agile Japanese make us look bad. This is partly due to basic anthropometrical differences between the races. Only at the 17-year-old level for boys do Americans approach achievement levels of the Japanese.

In tests involving leg power, the Japanese are clearly superior at all age levels. Japanese girls, as was expected, excel by larger margins than do the boys. At no age level did American boys equal Japanese test results. In tests involving sheer speed, Japanese girls excel at every age level, with the boys showing marked superiority at every level except from age 15 upward. In tests involving arm power, we see the first opportunity for consolation with equal test results. Younger American girls show slight advantage over their Japanese counterparts, but this edge is lost as Japanese girls mature. American boys are slightly ahead of Japanese boys at some age levels.

In tests which identify the degree of endurance for sustained activity, Americans again show up poorly in comparison. At no single age level for either boys or girls do we exceed Japanese test results. And finally, Americans emerged with superior test marks in items involving abdominal endurance over the Japanese. Both boys and girls showed superiority ranging from 1 per cent to 18 per cent. Structural differences again cause some of the differences which were noted in speed and agility tests, only this time the differences mitigated in favor of American youth.

Some doubters in this nation continue to raise the question to confuse the issue—"Fitness for what?" Other minority groups seek to deride the validity and use of all fitness test norms for one reason or another. But the great majority of professional leaders working in fitness-related areas have moved wholeheartedly behind the effort of OPERATION FITNESS—USA to sound the fitness alarm—to do something dynamic about our serious fitness problems in a push-button age. During the first 16 months of AAHPER's OPERATION FITNESS—USA, over 16 million American youth have been tested, and thousands have profited by several other projects in the program. Tests have been conducted in public, private and parochial schools, camps, recreation departments and youth-serving agencies and clubs.

The Japanese comparisons revealed above are all the more striking when it is realized that this nation has made significant progress in health and dental care, prevention and control of disease and the discovery and use of many wonderful drugs. It must be realized also that one cannot completely isolate the physical components of total fitness; that emotional, social and spiritual fitness are equally important. It is very doubtful whether real fitness levels of attainment in the emotional, social and spiritual can be made without rather sound and basic health and physical fitness status. It is obvious that substitutes must be found in America to keep this nation strong and vibrant in the face of increasing mobility, lack of leg and muscle use, disregard for balanced diet and growing apathy toward physical exertion. It is equally obvious that every step must be taken to bring the family unit together with the fitness motif and the recreational concept if American integrity is to be maintained.

President Kennedy's Statement on Physical Fitness

(As submitted to Good Housekeeping *for January, 1962.)*

Despite our unparalleled standard of living, despite our good food and our many playgrounds, despite our emphasis on athletics, American youths lag far behind Europeans in physical fitness.

"Softness on the part of the individual citizen can help to destroy the vitality of a nation. The physical vigor of our citizens is one of America's most precious resources.

"No matter how vigorous the leadership of the government, we can fully restore the physical soundness of our nation only if every American is willing to assume responsibility for his own fitness and the fitness of his children. We are, all of us, as free to direct the activities of our bodies as we are to pursue the objects of our thoughts. But if we are to retain this freedom, for ourselves and for generations to come, then we must be willing to work for the physical toughness on which the courage and intelligence of man so largely depend.

"All of us must consider our own responsibilities for the physical vigor of our children and of the young men and women of our community. We do not want our children to be a generation of spectators. Rather, we want each of them to be a participant in the vigorous life."

An Open Letter to President Kennedy

MR. PRESIDENT:

It is with enthusiasm and high hope that we welcome your efforts and your desire to "fully restore the physical soundness of our nation."

We have nothing but praise for your encouragement of the Council on Youth Fitness and your determination to improve the health and toughness of American youth. Such an improvement is not only necessary, it is imperative.

In 1947, of the young men appointed to West Point, 3 per cent failed the physical aptitude test. In 1960, 15 per cent failed.

In physical fitness tests given to freshmen at Yale University, 49 per cent failed in 1951. This was a distressing showing, and the situation has steadily been getting worse. In 1956, 57 per cent failed. And by 1960, the failures had increased to 62 per cent.

Even more significant was a comparison made last year in Japan by Japanese physical fitness experts in collaboration with the American Association for Health, Physical Education and Recreation. Some 20,000 Japanese children were chosen by the best statistical methods and given the AAHPER National Fitness Test. In tests for speed, agility, leg power, endurance, etc., in practically every case, the Japanese excelled American youth, who had been given the same tests here, by alarmingly wide margins.

When 10,000 British boys and girls were given the same tests, they also proved far superior to our own young people in physical fitness. In a comparison with European children made by a different series of tests, the Kraus-Weber test, American children were once again shown to be physically inferior.

These are facts that must be faced, and a frightening situation that must be changed.

Because you, Mr. President, have shown deep concern over the problem and a strong desire to find corrective measures, we ask you now to consider some facts about diet and nutrition that may not have been presented to you before. The Council on Youth Fitness seems to believe, and perhaps to have persuaded you, that a program of calisthenic and gymnastic exercise for children will solve the problem. We have nothing to say against exercise. We believe in it. We know its value and its necessity.

But—

Exercise alone cannot bring health to a malnourished child. That is obvious. And it is even more obvious that exercise and good nutrition both will not bring health to a child who is being slowly and systematically poisoned.

Virtually all authorities agree that, since 1946, when World War II ended, we have shown "glaring physical deterioration," in the words of an AAHPER statement. Yet we had no more planned and compulsory physical education before 1946 than we have now. We had no more gymnastics. We had no greater encouragement of exercise among the 97 per cent of students who are not team athletes. Yet the pre-1946 young people were in far better health and physical condition.

What happened in 1946 and since then to cause a glaring physical deterioration in our youth?

One thing that happened was the release, for public use, of a host of new chemical compounds that had been developed during the war. Poisonous insecticides, chemical fertilizers, hormones, antibiotics and food additives of a thousand kinds became standard ingredients of the American diet. The other significant happening, in our opinion, was the increase in prosperity which put more money into the hands of children and permitted them far more indulgence in sweets.

According to a recent county health survey in Hillsdale, Michigan, a typical school child's lunch consists of hot dogs, potato chips and a soft drink, followed, after school, by candy bars and more soda pop. Of 133 children surveyed in the fifth grade in a single school, only one ate anything resembling a nutritious lunch.

Let's take a closer look at such a typical school child's lunch. According to George Blumer, M.D., writing in *Annals of Western Medicine and Surgery,* some soft drinks contain harmful drugs, most of them have a chemical reaction strong enough to injure the teeth and other parts of the body and their constant use is almost bound to have a deleterious effect on other aspects of diet.

If the soft drink is a cola drink, 18 ounces of it contain as much caffeine as a cup of coffee. Most parents do not permit their young children to drink coffee, knowing that caffeine, a powerful stimulant, is dangerous to the heart and general health. But the parents do not even know that in drinking 3 Cokes or 1½ Pepsis, the child is getting the same caffeine as in the forbidden cup of coffee, *and forming a caffeine habit* that will make stimulants progressively more necessary.

To hold their sugar in suspension and prevent it from crystallizing, all soft drinks contain acid—usually orthophosphoric or citric—which eats away tooth enamel and can impair the appetite and digestive processes by creating an excessively acid condition in the stomach. Carbon dioxide—the bubbles of soft drinks—is suspected of contributing to eye weaknesses, according to Dr. Hunter H. Turner, writing in the *Pennsylvania Medical Journal.* The colors of soft drinks are frequently "certified" coal-tar colors, which means they are not instantaneously harmful so far as can be observed, but there is no guarantee of what their long-range effects may be. Many coal-tar derivatives have been proven causes of cancer.

And then your soft drinks contain large amounts of refined sugar, utterly stripped of all vitamins and minerals. The devastating effect of sugar in the mouth is so well known it requires no restating. But what you may not know is how sugar produces the characteristics of laziness and inactivity that have been found so dangerously prevalent in today's young people.

According to E. M. Abrahamson, M.D., and A. W. Pezet, in the book *Body, Mind and Sugar,* when sugar is eaten, it goes almost immediately to the blood, creating an abnormally high blood sugar content. This is the "quick pick-up" that sugar and candy manufacturers advertise. What they are careful not to advertise is that the pick-up is only momentary, after which the blood sugar level plunges far below normal. This creates abnormal tiredness, lethargy and a desire to eat more sugar to raise the blood sugar level once more.

As we are sure you know in your own household, Mr. President, it is impossible to keep a healthy, well-nourished youngster from being physically active. If our young people generally don't take enough exercise, doesn't it make sense to suppose their enormous consumption of soft drinks, candy bars and other sweets has a great deal to do with it? Isn't that why one of the American scientists who tested both British and American children stated: "Our poor showing is due mostly to the lack of physical training in the United States compared with that in Britain *and the fact that our kids are more obese than theirs.*" (Our italics.)

So much for the soft drinks. The candy bars consumed by the typical school child almost invariably contain some chocolate, which, unknown to parents, has a content of caffeine, of theobromine, another stimulant very similar to caffeine in its action and of oxalic acid, which robs the body of calcium, retarding growth and weakening bones.

The potato chips are deep fried, a cooking method that is one of the prime suspects in ulcers of the digestive tract. Is it any wonder that the *American Medical Association Journal of Diseases of Children* pointed out in 1960 that peptic ulcer in children is far from rare? In many others, of course, the ulcers that develop in adult life get their start in childhood.

The hot dogs, far worse, in all probability contain a variety of additives, including a dye to give them a bright red color, an anti-oxidant to slow down rancidity, a tenderizer and a "preservative" that prevents the meat from changing color when it is spoiled.

It is of such chemical additives, containing no nutritive value and added to foods only for commercial reasons, that Dr. W. C. Hueper, Environmental Cancer Chief of the National Cancer Institute in 1956 warned, at a symposium of the International Union Against Cancer: "The daily and life-long exposure to such agents would represent one of the most important of the various potential sources of contact with environmental carcinogens for the population at large."

Since then, new food and drug legislation has required the manufacturers and users of such additives to prove them harmless, but today, 4 years later, most of the more than 1500 additives in common use have not yet been proved harmless, yet continue to be used.

It is, in fact, generally accepted among scientists that acceptable proof of the effects of these additives will take generations to produce, because they may have long-range results that will only be determined with the passage of time.

Meanwhile, many of us have been guinea pigs subjected to these chemicals of unknown effect for 20 per cent, 30 per cent or half of our lives. *But our children have been fed these strange, unnatural substances all their lives.*

If we find the youth today in poorer health than their parents were at the same age, would you not say that the chemical diet of the past 15 years may well be responsible?

And let us not forget that the chlorinated hydrocarbons—DDT, Chlordane and other even more poisonous insecticides—first came into general use in 1946. These poisons are absorbed through the skins of animals, fruits and vegetables. There are residues of them in practically everything that is eaten. Not much is yet known of what their ultimate effects may be, but it is certain that they cause structural changes in the liver, that they drive Vitamin C out of the system and thus may cause partial or complete deficiency diseases and that they may well be the cause of our new or rapidly increasing virus diseases, such as serum hepatitis and Virus X.

The above evidence represents only a minute fraction of the

multitudinous ways our young people are subjected to malnutrition and poisoning of their systems. It is offered here to help you understand that, while we may be the best fed people in the world, we are by no means the best nourished. And if we are to find the way to improve the fitness level of our youth, the problem of nutrition cannot be ignored but must be given at least as much weight as exercise.

Throughout history, where nutrition has not been understood, abundant wealth has led to softness, ill health and shorter lives. We have abundant records from our own South of before the Civil War, where the plantation families got quite as much exercise as their slaves, but the slaves were still stronger, tougher and longer-lived, because they used molasses while their masters used refined white sugar, they ate coarser bread, green vegetables, wild fruits and berries, the unwanted organ meats and were denied the luxuries of coffee, tea and whiskey.

Today, we know how health, strength and energy can be built through proper diet. There is much still to be learned, however. One positive suggestion we can make is that the medical profession be urged and encouraged to expand its nutritional research, and to give up devoting all its attention to the search for magical cures for diseases that might not be much of a problem in the first place, in a country of healthy, resistant people.

We might also suggest that what is known about high-nutrition foods be more widely publicized and given greater official recognition. We refer to such facts as the way wheat germ oil, in training table diets, increases the strength and endurance of athletes. We refer to such readily available sources of excellent nutrition as rose hips, desiccated liver, halibut liver oil, wheat germ and other treasure troves of desperately needed vitamins and minerals.

You do not need to be told, Mr. President, how great is our national need for hardier, healthier young people. We hope and trust that you will develop the rounded program of fitness improvement that will preserve and enrich our greatest treasure—our children.

Yours respectfully,
THE EDITORS

Do You Break Training?

By Paul C. Kimball

In the fall of 1927, I went to Oxford University, England, and entered a university that is entirely different from anything that I know of in this country. It is a university of 6,000 students, nearly all of them men. Most of these students previously attended what are called public schools. We would call them private schools. There they are subjected to the severest kind of discipline. They have to be in bed at certain hours at night, specified hours are set for study and also for play and they are all watched very carefully that they do not smoke or drink. If they are found doing either, they are expelled from their school. They finish public school at about the age of 18; then they go to Oxford University, if they are fortunate in gaining admittance, and there they have no supervision whatever. You can imagine the condition that arises when approximately 3,000 young men are released from the supervision of public schools and are sent away to the university where they have no supervisor over them.

As a Result

The first thing they discover is that they don't have to go to class unless they want to—one of the delightful things, perhaps, about Oxford University. Also, there are no rolls called in the classes that are conducted. If a man wants to spend all his time reading novels, that is his prerogative. They don't have to take any examination at the end of each quarter. The only time they have to take an examination is at the end of 3 years, 4 years or 10 years, or such time as they feel they are ready to take the degree that they are after. As a result, a great many of these boys go in for smoking and drinking on a large scale; and I think a condition exists there that has not its equal in any of our American colleges.

When I arrived at Oxford, I found that everyone played some kind of game. I thought of playing English rugby, but soon found that it is entirely different from our game. In the first attempt I made to play it, I held the ball under my arm when I was tackled and went down as we do here. The rest of the players on the field crowded around me shouting, "Heel it! Heel it!" That's all I remember. I came to later and found that they had kicked at the ball and kicked my head instead, trying to get the ball away from me and then, after carrying me off the field, had gone on with the game. After this try, I decided to play some other game. So I started to practice rowing in the fall of 1927. In the spring, I rowed number 5 in one of the fastest college boats that has raced at Oxford—a boat that entered 6 races and won them all. When I returned to the Varsity the following autumn, a number of groups wanted me to coach for them. You see, at Oxford, there are no professional coaches, and a man who has rowed with a successful crew is usually asked to take on a coaching job the following year.

Rather Weak

One group of young men came to me and said, "We would like you to coach our crew for rowing. None of us has ever rowed before, but we think you can teach us the rudiments." Truthfully, I felt rather weak at that sort of an offer. I had never done any coaching.

However, I accepted their invitation, but said to them, "Now, if I am going to coach you, I am going to make you train according to my rules. I will not have a thing to do with you unless you will promise to obey them implicitly." The group said, "Well, that is all right with us. What are your rules?" I said, "First of all, you must stop smoking." They murmured at that and pointed out that they had just left school and apparently thought it would be "big" if they could smoke. I then said, "Secondly, you must refrain from the use of alcoholic drinks of all kinds." Having left their prep school and entered the Varsity, they believed it was their right to have their pint of beer for lunch. I said, "You must cut it out. You must also stop using tea."

More Like Mud

Finally I said, "You must also stop using coffee." But that did not hurt them so much because they said that English coffee was more like mud than anything else.

After the boys had agreed to my training rules (and it took them a week to make the decision), I took them in hand at about the middle of October. I worked with them every afternoon for 3 hours till February, when they competed against crews from all the other colleges of Oxford. There were approximately 50 crews in the races. My boys were competing against crews composed of men who had been rowing since they were tiny tots. This group that I had was made up of inexperienced boys. From October to February, those boys trained. Not one of them, so far as I know, used a cigarette during this period; not one of them had a cup of tea or coffee, or drank any alcoholic drink. Then came the day of the first race. No one thought they had the remotest chance of victory.

The race was on the Thames at Oxford, over a mile and quarter course. Two cannon were fired, starting the race. Every crew went as hard as it could. As coach, I had to run along the bank and shout words of encouragement to my crew through a megaphone. By the time I had gone about half the distance, I was so tired I could not run much farther. My particular crew had not gained anything, nor had they lost anything thus far during the race; they were just even with their competitors.

By Three Hundred Feet

I thought, "Well, that's a good thing; I will give them my last word of counsel and advice and sit down and rest." So I shouted through my megaphone, "Sprint!" They sprinted beautifully and within a minute, had stretched out a hundred feet between them and their nearest competitor. They won their race by 300 feet, with ease. Everybody said that the next day they would be beaten.

The next day, we tried the same tactics and won the race

handily. On all 6 days, a race being slated for each day, they won by large margins, but not because they were experts. They were not as finished a crew as most of the others, nor were they polished in their technique, but the best thing about them was they had stamina. They had some reserve, even after a hard race.

These boys won their races hands down. People came up to me after and said, "Mr. Kimball, how did you manage to get such success with that crew? They were just novices and yet, they made better crews look weak." I answered, "I made those boys live right. I made them cut out tobacco, alcohol, tea and coffee. When the sprint came, their lungs were clean, their systems were clean, their blood was clean, and their nerves were strong."

The *London Times*

The *London Times* gave a most creditable report on that particular crew, saying it was one of the fastest crews ever developed among the freshmen groups at Oxford. Their success was due to their hard work and clean living. I have seen this formula work so many times.

I took another group the next year. When races came, we had the same results as in 1929. I also had an opportunity to help coach the Oxford swimming team for two years. I coached two distance men who were victorious both years. I saw success come so many times from living the Word of Wisdom that nothing can change my belief in its value. It is not a teaching particularly limited to our Church. I saw the Kent school from Boston in the largest rowing regatta in the world at Henley on the Thames. There they defeated some of the best-known crews in the rowing world. Just a high-school crew from Boston, but they had trained as this group of boys that I taught to row trained.

In 1928, the University of California sent a crew to the Olympics, at Amsterdam. They raced against crews composed of picked men of wide and long experience, gathered from all parts of the world. They won their races because they had the stamina for a driving finish. They had lived the Word of Wisdom and really trained.

Another Incident

Another incident immensely strengthened my knowledge of the value of the Word of Wisdom. You know that Oxford is a university of tradition. According to historians, it was founded in 900 A.D. Among its traditions is that of the annual boat race against Cambridge on the Thames in London. They first raced in 1829 and have since rowed against each other 83 times.

Last year, the Oxford crew was reported by all of the newspapers to be the fastest crew that had ever been developed at either university. There were in this crew more men with experience than they had ever had previously.

The races stood 41 wins for Cambridge and 40 for Oxford. Everyone thought that this time, Oxford would win the race and even things up with 41 wins for each university.

A week before the race was to take place, another tradition was carried out. The Oxford crew went to Eastbourne on the coast of England for the week end. This crew had been in strict training since October, and it was, by then, the latter part of March. At Eastbourne that week end, they broke training, giving as their excuse the same argument so often made by young men who are in athletics: "Well, if I don't break training, I will be stale and I will not be able to put forth my best efforts when the race comes."

Fallacious Tradition

The whole crew broke training; they had their liquor; they smoked their cigarettes. Contrary to tradition, however, Cambridge did not break training. They maintained just as strict training, right up to the time of the race, as they had at any time during their training period.

The day of the race came. It is one of the largest sporting events in the world. Estimates are that over three-quarters of a million people watched that race over the four-and-a-quarter mile course. At the start of the race, the Oxford crew, as anticipated, went ahead with a spurt, and at the half-way mark, had established a time record for that part of the course. Had they been racing the fastest crew that had ever been on the Thames river, they would have been leading by 90 feet at that point. They were leading Cambridge by slightly more than that distance and were increasing their lead slightly. After they had rowed three-quarters of the course, Cambridge was even with them, and Cambridge won the boat race by 3 full lengths, better than 200 feet.

People wondered why Oxford had "cracked up." It was clear to me, and it was clear to a great many other people over there, they had broken their training. All of the reserve that they had built up over 5 months had been destroyed. Just once, they had broken their training habits, but it was that one incident that destroyed their victory. At the end of the race, the Cambridge crew was fresh enough to row their boat very smartly to the landing platform, get out, turn their "eight" over and dump the water out that it had shipped, and go in and change. It was 15 minutes before the Oxford crew had sufficiently recovered from the strain of the race even to row their craft over to the side of the river and get out; others had to lift the boat out of the water and put it on the saw-horses to dry.

Services Refuse Our Young Men

Would you say that the prime of a man's physical stamina and power occurs at the age of about 18 to 22? Well, the army thinks so, too. This is the best age for a man to serve his two years with the army—the easiest time to train him and the easiest time for him to take the training. It must come as a surprise to the armed forces of our country to find that almost half of the men examined for active duty, though they are largely in this most desirable age group, are unfit for service. Of those found unacceptable for service in 1959, about half were rejected because of poor mentality, the other half, but for a few refused due to criminal records, etc., were found to be physically incapable of soldiering. This report was published in the *Army Times* (January 21, 1960).

The story only begins with the rejections, according to Hanson Baldwin in the *New York Times* (December 12, 1959). He tells us that the average Marine recruit arrives at camp with 7.2 cavities in his teeth and this figure goes for the other services, too. Many of the recruits, despite prior examinations, are found, on arrival at camp, to be physically deficient, with cardiac trouble, orthopedic disorders, deafness and other conditions. Many others have psychological problems, being either immature, unstable or both.

At Great Lakes Naval Training Center in Illinois, the problems are similar. Almost 20 per cent of the incoming recruits between February and October of 1959 required specialized medical, dental, psychiatric or other services before qualifying for basic training.

Of those received by the Second Infantry Division between April and November, 1959, the average age was 20.2 years. Ten per cent of these were pronounced unfit for combat duty, and 15 per cent more were rated fit for only combat support, not actual fighting.

The concluding paragraphs of Mr. Baldwin's article are the most startling, however, for in them, the columnist says there is general agreement in the services that 1959's recruits are an improvement over the two preceding years! What could they have been like? If Americans are the best fed of all peoples, if most of us are eating a good diet, if we don't need food supplements, if our preserved and gimmicked foods are so wonderful, then why are so many of our young men, who should be bursting with vitality, in such bad shape?

We say raise your children on natural foods and supplements if you expect them to be able to hold their own with others, should they be called to the service. And if you want them to hold their health, whether they become soldiers or not, keep them away from a refined foods diet.

Plastic

Scrap Plastic in Water Pipes

The *Industrial Research Newsletter* (Vol. 9, No. 11) carried a statement by Walter B. Tiedeman, Executive Director of National Sanitation Foundation Testing Laboratory, which should set the record straight on plastic water pipes for once and for all. Mr. Tiedeman said that water pipe is often made of "scrap plastic," and that such material presents a hazard to public health. He added that the word plastic "covers a myriad of products, including many from which toxic substances are readily extractable by slightly aggressive potable waters." In other words, water that is fit for drinking might contain an acid or other substance which would react with the plastic, releasing some poisonous element.

Few of us as consumers are qualified to say which of the many plastic products offered for sale are made from "scrap plastic." The plastic container for juice might be scrap, the nursery bottles, now being promoted because they're unbreakable, could be scrap, too. Both of these are intended to contain liquids far more "aggressive" than water. What about the foods which come in plastic bags and are intended to be boiled with the food in them and the plastic dishes and cups? If these are made of "scrap plastic," there can hardly be a doubt that the toxic substances Mr. Tiedeman speaks of will be transferred to the user.

We have continually recommended against the use of all plastics in connection with foods or liquids to be drunk, because of the toxic substances used in their manufacture and the likelihood of their penetrating the foods coming in contact with them. Scrap plastics, or any other kind, carry a potential danger which is well worth avoiding and not too difficult to do.

Poison Ivy

Jewelweed for Poison Ivy

Poison ivy sufferers are members of that hearty breed who are so miserable with their affliction that they'll try anything for relief. They will take shots, eat poison, rub it on themselves and take any pill or slather on any lotion that offers a glimmer of relief. In the *Annals of Allergy* (September-October, 1958), there is suggested a different sort of therapy that just might work. At least it comes highly recommended by Dr. Roger A. Lipton.

Dr. Lipton uses a tincture of jewelweed, and mixes this with water, at about 4 parts of water to one tincture, then applies it topically to the affected area. Of 115 patients treated with jewelweed, 108 responded "most dramatically." It caused prompt disappearance of the dermatitis and relief of the symptoms within 2 to 3 days. Jewelweed is a succulent, tall weed, sometimes called "touch-me-not" which is found in many parts of the country. The botanical name is *Impatiens pallida.*

Caution: jewelweed taken internally acts as a cathartic, emetic and diuretic and is too dangerous to be used in this way.

Poisons

A Poison Bottle You Can't Mistake

Mistakes are made with bottles of poison every day by people who should be able to protect themselves by reading a label. Think of the number of children who cannot yet read a label, persons who cannot read English or older folks whose eyesight is not up to reading fine print. These are the individuals most likely to mistake a poison bottle for one containing aspirin or seltzer powder. The children are likely to be just as curious about the taste of one as they are of the other.

The *New York Times* (January 29, 1961) printed an idea endorsed by the Canadian Medical Council and other kindred organizations, which would, in our opinion, save many lives lost through accidental poisoning every year. It's simple, actually: make a standard shape and color for all bottles containing poison, which would be distinctive enough for anyone to recognize by sight or even touch without having to read the label at all. A 6-sided bottle of heavy blue glass has been proposed for this purpose. A problem presented by this choice, however, is the fact that only 3 manufacturers in all of North America make blue glass, and their formulas are secret.

There are so many dead ends to efforts at life saving—dead ends involving lack of knowledge, or inability to translate knowledge into a practical treatment—that it is hard to see such a simple way to save lives go unused, only because the material proposed is not available cheaply or easily. An idea of the potential of such a device is apparent in the fact that 600,000 persons in Ontario, Canada, alone have a limited ability for reading labels. That is only one province. Think of all those in the United States who could benefit.

Write to your Food and Drug Administration about this idea and demand that it be given serious consideration. If the blue glass really turns out to be an obstacle, what is wrong with another color in a distinctive shade—purple, green, black? It's a good idea; let's see it gets somewhere.

Pollution, Air

An Inch above the Water

By Jim Keefe

This article is reprinted from the Missouri Conservationist *for May, 1961.*

"Who would want to live in a world which is just not quite fatal?" This question was posed by Dr. Paul Shepard, Jr., at a resources conference in Kentucky not long ago. He was referring to the steady poisoning of our environment, a poisoning that he likened to yeast in a vat of cider, which manufactures alcohol in its environment until it kills itself off with its own wastes. And he asks if this is to be the way of mankind.

Two great conservation problems are before us now, he said: a population explosion and the poisoning of our environment. "Only the self-cleansing capacity of the air, water and soil has saved us from the fate of the yeast," he declared, "but our cities now wear a permanent grey cap of toxic gases." He pointed out that DDT, formerly heralded as the conqueror of the housefly, has now become suspect because of its menace to human health, while the flies still buzz merrily around us.

But other, more potent, chemical pesticides pour from our laboratories in a steady stream, each more deadly than the next. These, plus X-rays and atomic radiation add their bit to the poisoning of our air, water and soil. Their effects on humans have brought forth a little game of "figuring the maximum safe dosage," and the more we learn, the lower falls the limit of "safe dosage." "A safe dose of DDT yesterday may poison our lives tomorrow. Safe roentgens received by X-ray technicians earlier are now known to have increased their chances for defective offspring," Shepard declared.

This is wrong—the guessing game of "maximum safe dosage"—because the more we know, the more it is revised downward. But it is even more wrong in that "it idealizes life with only its head out of water, inches above the limits of toleration of the corruption of its own environment."

Dr. Shepard asks: "Why should we tolerate a diet of weak poisons, a home of insipid surroundings, the noise of motors with just enough relief to prevent insanity? Who would want to live in a world just not quite fatal?"

But Dr. Shepard poses an even deeper question: Maximum safe dosage for whom? What is the safe dose for bacteria that live in our soil? For swallows that feed on insects poisoned by insecticides? For the myriad plants and animals that, in a virtually unfathomable chain, form the base of all life on this planet? No one knows. And if we extend this to its end we must ultimately decide on "useful" and "useless" life forms, and who wants to sit in judgment on that?

Men of good will toward life have to find a middle ground, between the fanatic Jain wearing a face mask to keep from killing gnats and the technician-manipulator of environment envisioning the complete subjugation of nature.

Remember those two human dilemmas: population and poison. Unless we can solve them, the hubbub about the space race is academic. We'll only be trading one poisoned environment for a fresh new one to poison.

A Cure for Smog Poisoning

The smog fighters in California have gotten around to vitamin C, at long last. In the *Los Angeles Examiner* (February 7, 1959), the science editor reports that vitamin C counteracts ozone poisoning and might serve as a shield against the harmful effects of smog upon the nose, throat and lungs. Dr. Sidney Mittler of the Armour Foundation found that mice exposed to ruinous, even fatal, doses of ozone, could be protected from damage by giving the animals vitamin C by injection.

Ozone is recognized as one of the most harmful substances in smog. It leads to formation of peroxides, which are irritating to the body.

Now here is a chance for mass medication on the fluoridation scale, the difference being that everyone agrees that vitamin C can't hurt you and any excess is easily eliminated from the body. Why shouldn't Los Angeles County make free vitamin C tablets available to all residents who want them, as a public health measure? It's cheap and it's effective.

Pollution, Water

Insoluble Detergents and Water Pollution

The acute problem of unsanitary water supplies in the United States gets scant attention from the government and from most of the citizens. People worry more about another war and the price of meat than they do about safe drinking water. It should be remembered that we might avoid another war and one can exist on less meat or cheaper meat cuts if need be, but good water is essential to life and without it, we haven't a chance.

Perhaps the problem which concerns most of us directly is the contamination of our drinking water by detergents. Each day, new evidence of this pollution is reported in our newspapers. One such appeared in the *Minneapolis* (Minnesota) *Star* (August 2, 1960), which ran a series on the local water supply. They noted the phenomenon of foaming water from the kitchen faucet. They also told the story of Chanute, Kansas, which had a spectacular show when, during a drought, the city recirculated sewage into its water treatment plant for reuse. Detergents produced drifts of from 10 to 14 feet high atop the treatment basins. On a windy day, a "snowstorm" would come up when the foam was blown off.

Unscientific Remark

The article goes on to say that detergents are "harmless" and without their foaming, scientists would never know of their presence in waste water. It is difficult to imagine a less scientific remark. If detergents are harmless, then why have we read of several deaths of small children due to swallowing detergents from the boxes kept under the sink? And if "invisibility" means safety, then poison gases in the air from industrial plants and nuclear fall-out shouldn't occupy our thoughts for a second.

In the same newspaper article, there is talk of the problems in safe water created by new industrial wastes. Some chemical industries in the Minneapolis area have been "advised" to dilute their chemical wastes when tests showed that the wastes would kill fish. Such waste dumping goes on in cities all over America, on a greater or lesser scale. Most of the time, no one in the water department is even aware that the contamination exists. Even if more help is called in to determine the dangers faced by the citizenry, chances are that they'll okay whatever it is in the water because they probably won't know what they're looking at. The above-quoted *Minneapolis Star* tells us that even government investigators were unable to identify 143 parts out of 150 parts per million of soluble organics found in river water. The 7 parts that were identified were detergent components. The rest could have been anything dumped from any industry into the river—that includes paints from mills, dyes from textile manufacturers, acids and other corrosive materials from chemical factories, which, if they can kill fish, can kill us eventually, no matter how much they are diluted.

Poisoned Fish Offshore

This ties in well with an article in the New York *Mirror* on July 2, 1960. In place of his usual outdoors column, Jim Hurley printed a reader's letter. The letter told of the policy of the National Lead Company which allows the dumping of deadly sulfuric acid, iron sulfate and other wastes, into the fishing water off the New Jersey shore. While there are other means of manufacture which would result in a safe waste, the company, according to the letter, refused to change its methods, regardless of the damage to the fish, because it would be less economical. The danger of eating seafood taken from these waters was taken up with the Department of Health, Education and Welfare, and there it lies amidst a jumble of arguments about territorial waters, contiguous waters and international law. Meanwhile, the National Lead Company continues to dump its dangerous waste into the waters, and we continue to buy and eat fish caught there. If the fish are poisoned just a little, we will be poisoned just a little. If it makes us ill or kills us, it is supremely unlikely that the National Lead Company will be concerned, or even know of it, because we won't know ourselves exactly what the cause was.

Finding a Solution

These difficulties do have a solution—they must! For example, the detergents in England have been altered, in experiments, so that they do decompose in the same way that soaps do. The *Lancet* (April 30, 1960) reported on this. Detergent manufacturers agreed to supply two urban areas with detergents based on an alternative alkyl benzene sulfonate. Though not all of the substance was decomposed (due, in part, to ill-equipped treatment plant), the results were good enough to cause the Standard Technical Committee on Synthetic Detergents to remark that: ". . . the replacement of the old material (detergents) by the new throughout the country would substantially diminish the troubles which have been caused by the increased use of synthetic detergents, but it is, as yet, uncertain whether it will provide as complete an answer as we could have wished."

Of course, this statement doesn't say that they have the perfect answer to the detergent problem, but in England they're trying! They know something must be done and they are experimenting to find a solution. We don't even admit to the public that detergents are a problem and conceivably, this attitude will result in a wall-to-wall carpet of detergent residue from the Atlantic to the Pacific. The manufacturers have a responsibility here, and the government should make every effort to see that they face up to it.

It is also up to the government to protect us from such hazards as those described in the column on the National Lead Company. Who else can? If other companies can and have found safe methods for accomplishing the same operation, National Lead should be constrained to do so as well.

Your voice in these things is your representative in Congress. Let him know how you feel about water pollution. Ask him to introduce, or vote for, legislation which will prevent the abuse of our water system and curb the manufacture of harmful detergents. Don't wait! Write and ask what has been done and is being done now.

Is Our Water Becoming a "Fountain of Death"?

The latest facts on the water you're drinking may be hard to swallow. Nevertheless, it's important that you know what's happening —and start doing something about it. As Senator Robert Kerr of Oklahoma said at the 1960 National Conference on Water Pollution, "If most of you got an analysis of the water you drink, you would be shocked and uneasy. The results might drive you to drink—but not water."

Exaggerated? Let's look at the record: The incidence of infectious hepatitis, a debilitating and sometimes fatal disease of the liver, which can be transmitted by polluted water, is soaring more than 71 per cent over 1959 figures. A typhoid outbreak in Keene, New Hampshire, two years ago was traced directly to contaminated water; it killed one person, struck down 18 others. Widespread outbreaks of water-borne diseases are on the rise. An epidemic of infectious hepatitis in Rhinebeck, New York—where the municipal water supply is chlorinated, as it is in thousands of other communities across the land—is just one instance of several jaundice epidemics traced to their water. Within a month, 70 cases were reported and in all, 83 people were stricken, many of them requiring hospitalization.

In the first 3 months of 1961, the United States Public Health Service reported 77 additional cases of hepatitis in Mississippi and Alabama, caused by seafood from the heavily contaminated Pascagoula River. The service also reported an outbreak of typhoid fever in Chicago and 6 cases of diphtheria in Pennsylvania—all attributed to supposedly pure water. Nationally read columnist Drew Pearson, on February 13, 1960, stressed: "The Public Health Service is collecting water pollution reports that read like horror stories. Government doctors have traced *paralytic polio* in Camden, New Jersey, *typhoid fever* in Milwaukee, Wisconsin, *dysentery* in Cincinnati, Ohio, and *yellow jaundice* in Utah, all to polluted water!"

Representative John D. Dingell of Michigan has collected over 200 articles and editorials on pollution, labeled them "Poison in Your Water," and had them printed in the Appendix of the *Congressional Record*. Among them are scores giving specific evidence relating polluted water to illness. One, for example, is an editorial from the Salt Lake City *Desert News and Telegram* listing 3 Utah rivers as health hazards and linking them to "an alarming increase in the incidence of infectious hepatitis." Another is an article in an Arkansas newspaper in which a physician pointed out that all but one of 34 Arkansans stricken with paralytic polio resided in areas of the state that have no sewers.

Polio, Worms and Dirty Water

From the Robert A. Taft Sanitary Engineering Center in Cincinnati, Ohio, the nation's foremost water research station, Doctors

Norman A. Clark and Shih Lu Chanz report that an "explosive outbreak of poliomyelitis" in Edmonton, Alberta, Canada, was "reasonably correlated" with sewage pollution, and that a similar outbreak in Nebraska was probably traceable to the same sources of infection.

At Rensselaer, New York—which, along with other upstate cities, depends on the filth-ridden Hudson for its water—residents were ordered to boil their drinking water during a 1958 crisis. The head of the county board of health there warned that "city water in Rensselaer is so polluted, it is dangerous for human consumption. . . . A disastrously widespread epidemic (of infectious hepatitis) . . . is greatly to be feared."

Perhaps one of the most disturbing bits of news regarding the sad state of our water is another contaminant—this one a disease-bearing worm. A lengthy Public Health Service survey revealed that drinking water in 13 out of 14 rivers sampled, contained microscopic worms called nematodes. Their potential threat is frightful. Tests have shown that those which breed in sewage plants can ingest disease-causing bacteria and viruses. Furthermore, these nematodes are indestructible by chlorination and *completely protect the germs they carry*. If 13 of the 14 municipal water sources investigated now have such worms in them, how do you feel about your own water?

Pesticides Most Toxic

And if sewage is a dangerous problem, chemical wastes—particularly pesticide residues—represent an even greater threat. Along with solvents and detergents, these insect and plant killers are classed as petrochemical compounds. At the Taft Sanitary Engineering Center, scientists have identified approximately 100 of them as actual water pollutants. Dr. Bernard B. Berger of the research center emphasizes: "We have no idea how many petrochemicals are in our streams. But we believe that for every one we've found, we have missed hundreds of others. *Our ability to protect water quality has not kept pace with the development of these compounds.*" Reporting on the Taft Center's findings, *Time* magazine (September 20, 1960) commented significantly: "The new contaminants are difficult to spot and control; *they cannot be removed from the water by current treatment methods.*"

How treacherous are such compounds? Dr. Clarence Cottam, a highly respected wildlife expert, summarized the situation pointedly at the 1960 National Conference on Water Pollution, indicating that Americans now invest more than two billion dollars a year attempting to protect their crops from pests—and *run the risk of poisoning their drinking water in the process.* "Some of these poisons are not very toxic to man," said Dr. Cottam, "while others are among the most toxic materials known. . . . *It is too dangerous to ignore the effects of even small quantities of pesticides in the water supplies.*"

Effect on Wildlife

As for what's been happening to wildlife, the reports have been plentiful—and certainly should be a stern warning to man, industry and agriculture. The nation's fish and other aquatic life have been finding our waters increasingly unbearable. Just a short time ago, 10,000 canvasback and redhead ducks were destroyed on the Detroit River by the release of poisonous wastes. Insecticides thrown into a stream wiped out 300,000 salmon, trout and togue in New Brunswick. Dead fish by the thousands completely littered the shores along Columbus' (Ohio) polluted Sciota River, while small dead fish have been reported popping right out of the water faucets in Chicago.

In California, Governor Brown's special committee to investigate agricultural chemicals heard testimony from the State's Department of Fish, Game and Wildlife, stating that birds were known to have died after as long as 3 years as a result of eating fish and plankton from waters polluted by air-borne chemical dusts and sprays. Tons of dead fish have turned up in the Passaic River, from which many northern New Jersey communities had been taking their drinking water. Fish kills in lakes, streams and rivers throughout the entire continent have curbed sports and recreation. Fish can no longer survive in parts of New Hampshire's Merrimack, once famed for its fishing. Deer, along with fish, are being killed by pesticide pollution in Maine. Up at Bangor, the pool of the Penobscot once held more salmon than any other on the Atlantic seaboard and its first fish of the spring was traditionally sent to the White House. Today, the pulp mills and chemical wastes "have deadened it as thoroughly as if they had used hand grenades," according to an *Atlantic Monthly* writer.

Even the Great Lakes, the world's largest source of fresh water, are suffering. Industrial wastes, farm poisons and sewage are defiling them faster than they or overburdened sanitation men can cope with them. Experts now predict that these tremendous bodies of once-pure water are becoming rapidly doomed, that they are "aging" faster than they would naturally. "They can eventually die," said University of Michigan oceanographer John C. Ayers.

And that is by no means all. "A sudden and mysterious outbreak of cancer among Rocky Mountain rainbow trout is forcing health officials to destroy all rainbow trout in Idaho and Montana government and private hatcheries." So wrote Drew Pearson on August 17, 1960, adding that the National Cancer Institute and government officials "warned that the sudden cancer epidemic in trout illustrates how insect sprays, the dumping of industrial waste in rivers, food additives and radioactive fall-out can cause cancer." It's surely not enough to shrug our shoulders and say "poor fish" when such conditions are not only a positive threat to human health, but are worsening every day.

Other experts, medical doctors among them, testified before the California investigating committee that DDT and other chlorinated hydrocarbons and organic phosphate pesticides were "delayed reaction poisons," which are known to be accumulative in human tissues and to "trigger" cancer, sometimes years after the original exposure. "The Columbia River," continued Pearson, "is so contaminated in some areas that *mere motorboat spray can cause disease.* In Washington, D. C., residents have been warned against eating fish caught in the Potomac, and swimming in the Potomac (as in hundreds of other rivers and lakes) is now almost nonexistent."

Some Statistics

Some cut-and-dried, yet almost unbelievable statistics may help reveal the shocking condition of our water supply.

"Two-thirds of the nation's people get their drinking water from sources into which are discharged disease-carrying bacteria, viruses and toxic material." (*Los Angeles Times,* February 24, 1960.)

"Where two million people got their drinking water from streams in 1900 and 24 million dumped sewage into them, today, 100 million depend on the same streams for their water and 120 million are dumping sewage into them." (*Los Angeles Mirror-News,* March 25, 1960.)

"More than 70 million Americans out of 117 million having public water supplies, now drink water that had been through a sewage or industrial plant at least once." (*New Republic,* June 6, 1960.)

Figures reported by *United Press International* indicate that sewage pollution has increased 600 per cent in the last 60 years and that industrial and pesticide pollution has skyrocketed more than 1000 per cent in an even shorter period.

Detergents Pose a Bubbling Dilemma

Still another troublemaker seeping more and more into our water is the residue of household and factory detergents. In Milwaukee, for example, foam from detergents recently appeared in the city's drinking water at the filtration plant. It came from an intake more than a mile out in the lake and 55 feet below the surface. Numerous other cities have started experiencing episodes of detergent-caused bubbling coming from their water faucets, making glasses look like beer steins. Lakes and streams receiving these far-from-clean detergent residues have been frothing 15 feet or more up into the air, resembling grotesque outdoor bubble baths and creating sudsy "snowstorms" on windy days.

The important question, as asked by national health authorities at the pollution conference, is "What will happen to people if they drink detergent-contaminated water for 25 or 30 years?" Said former United States Surgeon General LeRoy Burney about detergents: "They're not killing us or making us critically ill. But how does the human body react to steady doses of diluted chemicals? What happens if the concentration increases, either suddenly or gradually? We cannot say we know the answers." Sanitation scientists see detergents as a cue to much wider hazards of the many petrochemical by-products now gushing into water supplies. "What if poisonous by-products, reacting like detergents, cannot be detected in waste water?" the sanitation men ask.

Poisons Beget More Poisons

Also presenting some pretty disconcerting evidence at the pollution conference were many other leading engineers, medical researchers and chemical scientists. One after another at the December, 1960, Washington conference emphasized how little was known about the poisonous flood of present-day water contaminants.

"Man has always adventured far beyond his knowledge or even his awareness of his ignorance and has always expected to be rescued miraculously from the consequences of his foolhardiness," said Dr. Robert A. Kehoe, Director of the Kettering Laboratory at the University of Cincinnati. Metallic stuff (inorganic matter present in pesticides, industrial wastes, detergents, etc.) is immune to the natural process by which water can dispose of plant and animal debris through bacterial action if it contains enough oxygen, the conference noted. Such chemical compounds resist the attack of purifying bacteria. Kehoe described as "stupid," the somewhat general notion that water pollution can be handled by applying good sanitary engineering principles. "Let us be honest with ourselves," he said. "Specifications for human health and welfare, in relation to the common contaminants of many of our sources of water, do not exist and we shall not be able to deal effectively with their problem of public health until they can be formulated on sound physiological facts." (That is, their effects on bodily functions.)

The difficulty of setting tolerance limits for the multitude of contaminants was outlined by Dr. Kehoe. He said it had taken 30 years of "somewhat pedestrian efforts" to arrive at a basis for fixing permissible concentrations of lead in water, food and air. Dr. Chauncy D. Leake, Dean of Ohio State University Medical School, commented that compounds of lead so widely used and dissipated in water, air and food, accumulated in the body and that this "should suggest to an alert physician that there may be a possibility of chronic lead poisoning whenever a diagnosis is difficult to establish in an obscure ailment." Much the same thing has been said about pesticides by a Mayo Clinic specialist, who reasoned that some persons can take less than others.

Rolph Eliassen, Sanitary Engineering Professor at the Massachusetts Institute of Technology, suggested that the chemical industry devote efforts to producing substitutes for detergents and other synthetic chemicals which contribute to pollution problems. The "public of the future," he noted, might reject products which could not be broken down so that they would not add to water contamination.

The chairman of the medical science division of the National Research Council, Dr. R. Keith Cannan, observed candidly: "The engineers—chemical, mechanical and electrical—are now so busy modifying man's natural environment out of all recognition, that they have little time to consider the effects of their enterprises on man's essential well-being. They leave to the sanitary engineers and medical guardians of the public health the task of tidying up after them."

Concluded the expressive Dr. Kehoe: "A discerning eye cannot fail to perceive the overwhelming artificiality of the future human environment. Out of this will come, inevitably, an enormous growth of the problems of waste disposal. How can we fail to appreciate the urgency of developing methods whereby the facts may be learned, and of establishing the facts as they are needed for our guidance in matters of human health and safety?"

Pesticide Industry Sidetracks Public Interest

As for the poisons most responsible for fouling our water, agricultural sprays and dusts, along with manufacturing wastes, must be accorded a notorious first place. The United States Public Health Service reported *Tampa Tribune* (October 26, 1961) that these two wiped out over 6 million fish of the 6.3 million killed by pollution in 1960.

In his report on pesticides and water pollution, presented at the Washington conference, Dr. Cottam put a telling finger on the reason for this mounting danger. "The pesticide industry," he wrote, "is growing by leaps and bounds and entomologists predict, and chemical manufacturers hope for, a fourfold expansion in use of pesticides during the next 10 to 15 years. Today, well over 12,500 brand name formulations and more than 200 basic control compounds are on the market. Most of the currently used pesticides were unknown even 10 years ago. Furthermore, and contrary to the public interest, most new pesticides are decidedly more toxic, generally more stable and less specific in effect than those of but a few years back."

Dr. Cottam went on to cite the fact that "at least 3 billion pounds of these chemicals were sprayed over more than 60 million acres of our crops and timberland last year. . . . There also is considerable evidence of serious side effects that are generally overlooked because of the delayed action when highly toxic, stable and broad spectrum poisons are used in quantity. . . . There is much evidence that some of these chemical poisons are getting into our water systems."

And as another speaker at the pollution conference stated: "We are running an unnecessary risk when we just blithely go ahead and use these things because we have not died yet." If there is any doubt at all about your own water supply (including the detrimental addition of fluorides, incidentally), it's a healthy idea to use bottled spring water.

While we rely on the fact that science has conquered the great water-borne diseases, in reality, the source of the diseases—pollution —has not been stopped. Consider that it was 60 years after scientists had discovered the link between cholera and polluted drinking water before methods for purification began to bring typhoid, endemic diarrhea and dysentery under control. Are we dashing madly backward now?

Pure water cannot be taken for granted. If sickness and disaster are to run from our faucets, it's time to check the whole plumbing system on a national scale. Neglect won't solve the problem. Neither will burying our heads in the foul mud of our river banks, nor bickering over the costs involved. Health cannot be measured in money. If the abuse of our natural resources, the short-sighted greed of our economic system, industry and over-chemicalized agriculture have jeopardized our water supply and brought the very real danger of a "fountain of death," as Senator Kerr termed it—then it is time to act. It is time for all of us to be roused, to demand and work for better, safer methods and uncontaminated water. The time is now— before our chance goes down the polluted drain.

A Conference on Water Pollution

We are plagued in the United States with water problems. We don't have enough for growing our food or watering our lawns. We barely have enough for drinking purposes and, of that, very little is truly safe for drinking. The dangerous pollution of the water we are expected to drink resulted in a Conference on Physiological Aspects of Water Quality, held in Washington, D.C., September 8 and 9, 1960. The purpose of this gathering of outstanding scientists was to evaluate present knowledge of the physiological effects of consuming, over long periods of time, water that contains either minute amounts of potentially toxic chemicals or excessive amounts of common minerals. What are the effects of insecticides in drinking water, for example?

As can be imagined, the subject is a vast one. The report pointed out that "many of the constituents of water, both natural and man-made, have never been identified." The scientists are faced immediately with this basic decision: is it better to investigate fully the substances we already know or should we try to discover unknown substances in the water which could be even more dangerous? We say there is plenty to be done in the areas that are already familiar to our scientists. The speculation on new dangers is important, but it can wait until we take care of the problems we know about now.

Insecticides a Major Problem

Major consideration should be given to the insecticides which wash from the forests and fields, upon which they have been sprayed, into nearby waterways which serve as drinking water. Depending upon the length of time between spraying and the rain, the local community can get quite a dose of the poisons in its tap water. Then, too, there is the problem of insecticides sprayed directly on the water to kill mosquitoes, etc. Much of this sprayed water works its way into municipal water supplies, and the insecticides are left in it to do their damage. There is no known way to remove them.

Industrial wastes are another type of pollutant. These are usually chemicals which are conveniently dumped into rivers and lakes, or even the ocean. Oftentimes they are so diluted that the residue left in the water you drink is minute, perhaps one part per million or less. It is undetectable and tasteless. But we all know that this is no guarantee that the water is safe. Minute amounts of poison can kill; if not at once, they can be accumulated in the body and, when they get sufficient strength, kill in a year or 5 years or 20 years.

We are all facing the problem of radioactive particles which shower down on our water supplies. Some areas have very high readings. In some places marine life is contaminated or destroyed by radioactive fall-out, just as it is by industrial wastes. No one can be sure just how much poison one is eating with the flounder dinner one orders in a restaurant or the lobster one broils at home. The waters in which these creatures live influence the healthfulness of their flesh, which we eat. The spring of 1961 saw a great furor in New York City over the fact that hepatitis germs were being carried by oysters gathered in nearby waters, waters polluted with hepatitis organisms.

Don't Forget Detergents

We have spoken, before, of the threat of detergents in our drinking water. Detergents are poisonous beyond a doubt. Bad enough that they are used in washing dishes so that the family is bound to consume some of the residue when it eats or drinks from the dishes and glasses. Now, however, detergents are used so commonly that they bubble up in the reservoirs that hold community water supplies, and come right out of the tap into your water glass! Detergents do not disintegrate, hence they are passed through sewage systems into the streams intact; nor are they caught by municipal filtering systems, so they turn up in the water supply of the houses downstream, and they kill or contaminate marine life on their way.

We have not yet mentioned the poisons we deliberately introduce into our water systems. Chlorine, for example, is a deadly poison put into our water to act as a disinfectant. The choice is a difficult one for us to make. Without the chlorine, serious disease could be carried into our home through infectious organisms; however, the chlorine itself is a threat to our good health since it is a poison. Certainly, scientists could figure out a better, safer means of protection. Water pasteurization is a good, healthful way to purify water. Waterworks officials tell us it is "too expensive."

The addition of fluorides to many municipal water systems is another man-made water hazard. No one really can tell what the added fluorides will do to the systems of the people who ingest them. What we do know is that the commercially manufactured fluorides being added are poisons of the most deadly type, and that they are cumulative. There is no way of predicting when they will damage our systems or which persons will be first to be hurt. We know only this: the human body is not compatible with these fluorides and ill effects are certain to occur. There is no proof that the fluoridation scheme works at all and there is much evidence that it is totally impractical. Where chlorine is in our water to protect us from the definite danger of infection which is inherent in the water, and that can be met in no other feasible way at present, fluoridation is intended to reduce tooth decay, which has no relation whatsoever to water, and can be fought effectively by good diet and careful mouth hygiene.

These are just a few of the known dangers our scientists could tackle before exploring the unknown. Let us dip into the *Proceedings of the Conference on Water Quality* we mentioned above and see how our scientists are thinking on some of these points.

Peppermint to Sweeten Our Water

When fluoridation comes up for consideration in the various communities, those of us who oppose it point out that the addition of fluorides to prevent tooth decay could lead to other additions: aspirin to prevent headache, perhaps, digitalis for heart disease, sugar for energy, etc. This argument is usually dismissed as hysterical stone-throwing by the lunatic fringe. In the *Proceedings,* J. E. McKee, Professor of Engineering and Environmental Health at California Institute of Technology, writes: "Fluoride and, formerly, iodide, are but the first of many elements that might be added to water. It is not difficult to envision traces of cobalt or copper that might improve bone structure or skin. Perhaps 0.5 milligrams per liter of boron could be added to make grass grow better on watered lawns. Indeed the day may not be distant when odor-masking or deodorant compounds are added to improve the taste of water. Certainly a slight peppermint taste would be preferable to that of dilute hydrocarbons. Truly the role of trace substances represents a new frontier of American life, and the water supply may be chosen to deliver some of these substances to every household." . . . Even to households which don't care to have them, we are sure.

One is so staggered by the fact that a man, bright enough to be teaching in a university, would even consider such an insane proposal that comment comes hard. Imagine, boron in your drinking water so that your lawn will grow! And peppermint flavoring in the water you use in making soups, coffee, tea or stew—we know people who become positively ill at the thought of peppermint flavoring, not to mention the dangerous synthetics that would be used to get the mint flavoring! And what chemical poisons do you suppose would be used to mask unfortunate tastes and odors in the water? Might they be harmful to humans? It is likely, judging from past performances, that no one would know or really care.

A Note of Sanity

A very sane attitude was added to the *Proceedings* when W. C. Hueper, Chief, Environmental Cancer Section, National Cancer Institute, Bethesda, Maryland, spoke on the subject: "Cancer Hazards from Natural and Artificial Water Pollutants." He stressed the relationship between cancer and water supply by citing the work of two Dutch scientists, Diels and Tramp, which showed that municipalities receiving their drinking water from rivers had a higher death rate (606 per 100,000) than those who obtained their water from bodies of water in leaths (595), dunes (585) or wells (568).

Dr. Hueper talked, then, of the carcinogenic (cancer-causing) possibilities of radioactive fall-out in water, industrial wastes, arsenicals in water, detergent residues—in fact, all of the dangers we mentioned before, but he labeled them all as possible causes of cancer.

In an open discussion following his statement, Dr. Hueper was asked to comment on the rash of cancerous fish which have been occurring in the rivers, streams and hatcheries throughout the country. Rainbow trout appear to be the most frequent victims of cancer of the liver and it occurs in the fish of almost all hatcheries. Dr. Hueper stated that this condition had been reported in 1955, but that the report "had escaped attention." The cause of the cancer is not known, but tests are being run to find out. As Dr. Hueper pointed out, there is a federal law which forbids the shipment of meat from a diseased animal across state lines. Therefore, the hatcheries must either cut their shipments drastically, or break the law. Hatcheries can't stay in business if they can't sell their fish. Because there is money involved, perhaps the answer will soon be found and we will be safe from cancerous fish, at least from those raised in hatcheries.

No One Eats the Liver Anyway

It was then asked of Dr. Hueper if, since the condition affects only the liver of fish and no one eats the liver anyway, it is safe to eat trout from streams and lakes.

DR. HUEPER: Let me ask you this question: After you have seen fish having cancers illustrated in the picture I have shown, would you eat the meat?

DR. GAUFIN: Well, I have seen some fish in which there is just a mild infection. It doesn't seem to extend to the rest of the fish. In such cases, is there danger of transmission of cancer?

DR. HUEPER: We don't know . . . I will cite the experience in my own laboratory. I brought back the affected fish and posted (dissected) them in my own laboratory. That day, 3 assistants, who are very fond of fish, were present. After they had seen the tumors, I offered them one big 10-pound trout which was normal. Their emphatic answer was, "Oh, no, Doctor."

Asked his guess as to the possibility of arsenic in the food or water being responsible for the cancers, Dr. Hueper said he doubted that to be the cause. "In my opinion, one ingredient in ordinary food which isn't suspected at all must be responsible." (The ingredient was, of course, unknown to Dr. Hueper at this time.) What could it be? Who knows, we all might be eating it daily!

In a summation of the Conference's findings on insecticides and their effects on fish and other aquatic organisms, Dr. Gaufin remarked that, in the United States, production of insecticides had reached a level of 560 million pounds in 1956. These include some 90,000 different insecticide formulas, which are sprayed on 30 million acres of crop lands and 6 million acres of forests *every year!* With such vast usage of insecticides, "many of them are likely to get into water resources and cause rather severe kills of aquatic organisms."

A Shocking Illustration

To illustrate the severe losses that are possible, we are told that, in the Yellowstone River during 1955, about 95 per cent of the aquatic insects were wiped out by the use of DDT. Some 3 months later, there was a fish kill. There was speculation as to what caused the vast number of fish to die. When it was suggested that their food —the water bugs—had been killed, and hence, they died of starvation, the idea was discounted, because an expert noted that in 3 or 4 months, the remaining insects had repopulated the river to its former level. What the fish ate in the 3 or 4 intervening months is not explained. Our guess is that they ate the DDT-ridden bugs and died as a result of the poison they took in.

Dr. Gaufin stated that, "the effects of these insecticides upon fish are quite different than upon other animals; in fact, many fish actually store rather vast amounts of these insecticides. What the long-term effect of this may be no one knows. We eat the fish, so we eat the insecticides. Who knows how many of these Yellowstone River fish were caught and eaten in the 3 months before the kill? Who knows what eating those diseased fish did to the people who ate them?

"What the long-term effect of this may be, no one knows." That sentence should be carved on the tombstone of our age. We don't know what the food additives will do to us. The same goes for pesticides, fluorides, drugs, radiation. We don't know what any of these things will do to us, but we use them with the enthusiasm of a miser let loose in a mint. Why don't we wait till someone *does* know what the long-term effects will be, instead of continuing to use these things and adopting the use of more and more new ones? We can't do anything but wish we'd waited, if we once discover that using insecticides, additives and all the rest, has doomed our people to early annihilation from cancer and other diseases. The time to stop and consider that danger is now! It may not be too late. As long as there is even the possibility of ill effects from the sprays, drugs, etc., we use, their use should be severely limited. We are children playing with dynamite! When someone warns us that it could blow us to kingdom come, we shrug and say that none of us has been blown up yet and we keep on playing. Children have an excuse for this sort of behavior, but it's hard to see how we adults do.

Posture

Take Your Rest with Your Feet High!

There seems to be little doubt that man suffers a serious disadvantage in comparison with other animals because he walks erect. The 4-footed beasts, with their internal organs swung neatly, hammock-like, between 4 staunch supports, never experience many of the uncomfortable and mysterious disorders that plague two-legged man. Varicose veins, for instance, or phlebitis of the legs and Buerger's disease. One can't help feeling certain that much of the difficulty stems from the fact that man's feet are so far from his heart and head, and the job of pumping blood all the way down and back again, against the strong force of gravity, is a tough one.

Then, too, we human beings abuse our feet and legs fearfully. Aside from encasing our feet in shoes which cramp, disable and deform them, we stand on them for long painful hours, we walk on hard floors and sidewalks, putting a frightful strain on the delicate, curved arches of our feet, we never exercise them properly, we allow bad posture to twist the way we use them.

Stand on a corner of a busy street some day and watch the passers-by. Count the number of women you see over the age of 25 who do *not* have varicose veins. The men suffer only slightly less than the women, but of course, their disability is concealed by their trouser legs. One cannot continue to abuse any part of the body and expect it to remain in good health. Feet and legs are no exception.

Varicose Veins and Rest

In talking about varicose veins, as well as health in general, we always recommend that, when you are resting, you make certain to keep your feet as high as possible. Obviously, you can't sit with your feet on the desktop during lunch hour at the office or prop them on a neighboring chair in a restaurant. But any time you are at home, you can certainly rest your feet on something so that they will be on a higher level. The relief you can get from this simple change is amazing. The lasting benefits that may ensue from a daily habit of resting or even sleeping with one's feet higher than one's head are something we sincerely wish scientists would devote some time to investigating. It is probably too simple and easy a thing for anyone to bother with.

Slant Boards Recommended

Slant boards have come into prominence recently and have been recommended by many writers on health. A slant board is simply a well-polished piece of wood built on a slant so that you can rest on it with feet higher than head. Gayelord Hauser, in his book *Look Younger, Live Longer,* has this to say about the benefits to be attained from spending some time each day on a slant board: "The spine straightens out and the back flattens itself. Muscles which ordinarily are somewhat tense, even in easy standing or sitting, are relaxed and at ease. The feet and legs, freed from their customary burden and the force of gravity, have a chance to release accumulated congestions in the blood stream and tissues, and thereby reduce the possibility of swollen limbs and strained blood vessels. Sagging abdominal muscles get a lift and the blood flows more freely to the muscles of the chin, throat and cheeks, helping to maintain their firmness. The complexion, hair and scalp benefit from this increased blood circulation and the brain also is rested and cleared."

He does not quote a medical authority, but we assume that he has had considerable experience himself and has heard from readers of his books about their experiences with a slant board. You can make your own board using any suitable board (like a large ironing board) propped up on something firm so that, as you lie on it, your feet would be a foot or so higher than your head.

Important for Prevention of Varicose Veins

Varicose Veins by W. A. Black and I. O. Justinius illustrates exercises that can be performed while lying on the slant board. It is interesting that these authors also mention the importance of avoiding constipation, as they feel certain the pressure exerted by an overloaded colon affects the legs just as will tight garters, crossing the legs constantly or standing too long. Of course, the most common cause of varicose veins among women is pregnancy, when supposedly the heavy weight of the pregnant uterus exerts pressure on the blood vessels of the legs.

What about the various reclining chairs which claim for their users considerable health improvements? We think anything in the nature of a reclining chair is a fine idea. We are especially interested in those which maintain excellent posture while they raise the feet and legs high. By excellent posture, we mean, simply, that they do not encourage one to slump. Sitting with chest caved in and knees high, as most low modern chairs encourage one to do, can mean only harm, for when your chest is sunk and shoulders slumped, efficient breathing is interfered with and lack of oxygen can bring harmful results.

Besides, encouraging bad posture while you are sitting means

FIGURE 1: *How to Sit in an Easy Chair*

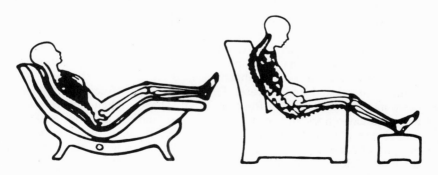

Correct Posture   Wrong Posture

that it's so much more difficult to coax your hip, stomach and shoulder muscles to maintain good posture when you are not at rest. So the idea of a "lounge," wherein you sink low and sit on the end of your spine, with your back curved into a semicircle, is not a happy development in modern furniture. Figure 1 shows what we mean.

The Correct Sitting Posture

To sit correctly, one should rest firmly on the buttocks, one's back should be at right angles to the thighs and one's stomach should be pulled firmly in so that the small of the back rests against the back of the chair. Figure 2 shows the sense and also the attractiveness of this way of sitting. It is admittedly hard, in such a position, to lift one's feet and place them on a hassock or another chair, with any degree of comfort.

FIGURE 2: *How to Sit in a Straight Chair*

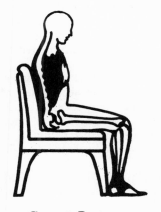
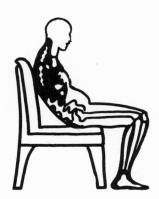

Correct Posture   Wrong Posture

A reclining chair, which maintains the body in this right-angle position, but tilts it back so that the feet can be high is ideal, we believe—for rest. One cannot very well carry on a stimulating dinner conversation in this position, or shell peas for dinner. It is surprising however, how many restful activities lend themselves to this position —reading, listening to music, watching television and, of course, napping.

It always seemed to us that such a chair should provide extra comfort for someone with poor circulation, especially an elderly person. Surely, sluggish circulation is stimulated when the feet are raised in this position. Since the rest of the body is perfectly supported, as well, there is no chance for a napping head to slide down on a shoulder or fall forward on one's chin. Dr. James F. Toole, a neurology teacher at the University of Pennsylvania, at a convention of the American College of Physicians, advised that napping in a chair was not advisable for elderly people who were suffering from some types of heart trouble or arthritis of the neck. The tendency was for the head to drop to one side, thus obstructing the blood flow. He stated that a turning or twisting of the head could vary the blood flow to the brain.

We have always approved highly of the design of the Contour Chair—a rather expensive, but quite attractive piece of furniture. We were interested, therefore, to learn that the Contour Chair folks made a laboratory test of the pulse rate of individuals resting on one of their chairs compared with that of the same people sitting in an ordinary arm chair.

No Significant Difference Noted

Eleven young subjects participated in the test, which was conducted completely scientifically. After preliminary adjustments to remove any chance that something else in the environment might influence the results, each subject was asked to exercise for 60 seconds, then sit in one chair or the other. His heart activity was being tested thoroughly.

It was found that the heart rate of the subjects relaxing in the Contour Chair was 7.25 per cent lower than their heart rates when they were sitting in an ordinary arm chair. This may seem like a small difference, perhaps, but considered over a period of days, months and years, one could surely say that resting in this reclining chair might make a difference to one's heart, especially if one is a heart patient.

An added advantage for a bedridden patient is that he need no longer be bedridden. Such a chair, in the middle of the living room, puts him in the center of family life, without any strain and without the nuisance of propping pillows to hold him up.

Get your feet up off the floor whenever you can for good health: Put them on chairs, hassocks, stools, beds or any other piece of furniture that is near at hand. Rest during the day with your feet high—on a slant board, in a reclining chair or simply flat on your back with your feet propped up on a chair, a cushion or the wall. If you suffer from any kind of vascular trouble, especially varicose veins, we think these recommendations are even more important.

Pregnancy

Make Sure Your Expected Baby Is Healthy

A baby has the right to be as healthy as it is possible for him to be. If he is anything less than that, his future must be clouded with nervousness and susceptibility to disease, poor mentality or with inefficient working of vital organs. That is, of course, if obvious deformities, which deprive the child of a normal limb or good hearing and eyesight, or which force him to speak poorly, are not present, instead.

Women Take Chances on Normal Births

Each year, many thousands of pregnant women are, in effect, deciding on whether to chance a normal birth, or to do their best to insure it. If they continue to smoke, snack on sweets, drink alcoholic beverages and make no effort to supplement their diets with fresh foods and vitamins, it will take plenty of luck and native good health to bring forth a perfect baby. And even with both of these latter attributes, one can't be sure. Will a baby, whose heart has not quite developed during gestation, show it at birth? Possibly not: he might become a heart case at 23 or have a fatal stroke at 38. Suppose the baby's nervous system falls just a little bit short of perfection. It might not show up for years. He may fret a bit as a child, be jumpy or excitable in his 20's and have a nervous breakdown at 32, when the first emotional crisis hits. The possibilities are endless. Who is to say whether or not a diabetic of 40 has become a diabetic because of improper nutrition in his mother's womb when the pancreas was being formed? Can one be sure that deafness at 60 would have occurred if the victim had been well nourished in the womb when the hearing apparatus was being formed?

Weaknesses May Not Appear for Many Years

The point we are trying to make here is that, in each of these cases it would be difficult, or impossible, to forecast the occurrence of such difficulties upon the birth of a healthy-looking baby who seemed quite well. Any of the weaknesses we've mentioned, while present, might actually not show up for years and years. Then rare would be the mother who would relate it to a binge of chocolate eclairs or smoking two packs of cigarettes a day for her nerves during pregnancy. She would have to be even rarer to recall the time of such excesses in her pregnancy and link it up with the fetal development going on just then. Scientists, however, can do just that. They know the proper schedule of a baby's development, just as well as a train dispatcher knows where a train will be at a given moment. They know what organ is being made on the 27th day of gestation, what bone is formed on the 86th day, which day fingernails develop, how far up in the gums the teeth are supposed to be moving at a given date.

All of this information has been used in experiments of various kinds to see what effects changes in environment can cause in the development of the fetus. If it is known, say, that the palate is formed in the 11th week of pregnancy or that the kidney is formed on the 28th day, studies can be made of mothers lacking this or that nutrient at that time in their pregnancy and the effect can be noted when the child is born.

Animal Experiments Significant

Of course, from a practical point of view, animals are much more suited to such observations than humans, since their eating habits can be absolutely controlled and, since most of them have a shorter gestation period, which makes for quicker observable results, than man. The results, while not exactly the same as in man, are strongly parallel, and many scientists are convinced that the reactions of a pregnant mouse or guinea pig to dietary changes can be assumed to be the reactions of a human, with allowances for size and gestation period.

We are convinced that one should pay close attention to the findings in animal and human experiments concerning pregnancy. We say: do everything you can to insure a healthy baby. In 9 months, the creature that will be your baby changes from a single-cell organism to a 200 billion-cell human being. The process is a complex one. It cannot be thwarted in any way if it is to be properly accomplished. It is up to the mother to provide the raw materials for the job through diet and a proper environment, by maintaining good health and even disposition. Medical literature is full of reports on prenatal observations concerning diet and other factors. We would like to present a few which will give some idea of the complicated process that pregnancy is and the factors that can affect it.

Vitamins Are Necessary to All Human Life

Vitamins are necessary to all human life and the fetus is no exception. It is interesting to note that some vitamins are used faster by the developing child than by the mother. In the *Journal of the American Medical Association* (January 30, 1960), we read of a series of tests in which the serum (blood) vitamin B_{12} concentrations were compared between mother and fetus in 25 cases. In each case, the fetal content was higher. The observers also found that, even when vitamin B_{12} was injected directly into the veins of pregnant women about to deliver, it was passed to the baby so quickly that, in 6 hours, the fetal reading for vitamin B_{12} content was higher than the maternal reading.

Here is a perfect illustration of what we've been saying. It is obvious the fetus needs a large supply of this vitamin, else why would nature provide for an amount in the fetus even greater than the mother's supply? Why would there be such a speedy transfer provided for, if the vitamin weren't absolutely essential? But suppose the mother weren't getting enough vitamin B_{12} in her diet. Suppose even the swiftest transfer to the fetus would not yield enough to help in the proper formation of nerves and organs? Development of the fetus would not stop or hesitate. The day's work would go on in building a human—but some part would be missing. It might show at birth, or in a year, or in 40 years, but the defect would be there and, at the first sign of severe stress, it would reveal itself. The material must be available to a growing fetus when needed; if not, the flaw is knitted right into the pattern.

In a previous issue of the *Journal* (December 15, 1958), the values of several other vitamins which are passed on to the fetus from the mother were catalogued. Vitamin A taken by the mother is passed to the fetus at the rate of 50 per cent to 62.5 per cent; of vitamin E, 88 per cent to 100 per cent is passed on; vitamin D is also believed to be 100 per cent.

In *Scope* (November 6, 1957), the status of proper diet in the proper development of a fetus was defined by Dr. Albert Hogan, Professor Emeritus of Animal Nutrition at the University of Missouri. He said that inadequate nutrition in some form is one of 3 causes of abnormalities in the newborn. The other two factors are genetic defects and positive injury. Now, remember, these are the only 3 things that can cause abnormalities. The genetic factor has long ago been discounted as the sole cause of malformations. Dr. Douw G. Steyn, writing in the *South African Medical Journal* (January, 1954), among others, has emphasized that stress, through emotional problems and through harmful drugs and their side effects, etc., and dietary lacks are far more prevalent causes of malformations than actual hereditary tendencies.

Each Nutrient Catalogued

But Scientific literature is more specific. Each nutrient has been catalogued as to the job it is intended to do during gestation. Here, according to the experts, is what can happen to the fetus when a nutrient is lacking in the mother during pregnancy.

If vitamin A is in short supply in pregnant experimental animals, such as a pig, a rabbit or a rat, it is likely that litters born to these animals will have defective eyes, urogenital systems and diaphragmatic hernia. In the *Sight-Saving Review* (Summer, 1954), Dr. Josef Warkany of the University of Cincinnati corroborates this, adding that the young of female rats with vitamin A deficiencies also developed heart malformations. About 75 per cent were so affected, though the majority appeared perfectly normal until they were dissected. Human babies are, of course, not subjected to dissection, so the record on such malformations at human birth cannot be complete. We have no real way of knowing if such defects as tendencies to heart, eye and urogenital weakness are present at birth or not.

In the *Journal of Nutrition* (June, 1944), Dr. Warkany told of the results on pigs of vitamin A-deficient diets in the mothers. One sow produced a litter with some limbs completely missing. In another case, the pigs were born without eyeballs. To other sows on vitamin A-deficient diets, piglets arrived with harelip, cleft palate, accessory ears and misplaced kidneys.

B Vitamins also Important

The B vitamins are equally important in fetal development. A shortage of these can result in abnormal brain development, defects of the heart, eyes, urogenital system, as well as the skeleton.

An oft-quoted example of the value of B vitamins in fetal development is the observation of 612 pregnant women in Norfolk, Virginia, who cöoperated in an experiment to discover the effect of vitamin supplementation on the intelligence of their expected children. Some were given vitamins and others, a harmless, useless pill, but neither group was aware of which they were getting. A follow-up on the children, for a period of 4 years, showed that those whose mothers received supplements had a significantly higher rate of intelligence. Benefits were most apparent in mothers who had received higher concentrations of thiamin, riboflavin, niacin and iron. The report of this experiment, which appeared in *Drug Trade News* (October 22, 1956), stressed the fact that the brain and the rest of the central nervous system, continue to develop through the first two years of life, and optimum growth results from improved nutrition through infancy.

The Importance of Riboflavin

In animal experiments, riboflavin has shown itself vital. For example, the eggs of a hen on a low riboflavin diet will have a low fertility, and chicks hatched of such eggs are likely to be poorly developed and short-limbed. They tend toward abnormal livers and anemia. In rats, riboflavin deficiency is likely to show up in short limbs, fusion of fingers and toes and cleft palate. In the *Journal of the American Dental Association* (August, 1955), we read of facial deformities in rats whose mothers were short of riboflavin. Teeth and supporting bones are said to be definitely influenced by such deformities.

In the *South African Medical Journal* (August 29, 1953), we are told that the need for riboflavin is considerably increased during pregnancy. Borderline deficiencies of riboflavin are the situations which result in congenital malformations. The *Journal of Nutrition* (June, 1944) explained that such cases have enough of the vitamin to continue gestation, but not enough for differentiation. If the level were a bit higher, a normal baby would result; if a bit lower, the fetus would die. Imagine anyone's taking the chance that an expected baby would be born malformed or dead for the want of a little extra riboflavin intake!

Pantothenic Acid Necessary

When the B vitamin, pantothenic acid, is missing in pregnancy, it has been found that, in some cases, the covering of the brain—that is, the skull and scalp—are not developed and the brain of the offspring is completely exposed. Failure of eyeballs to appear is another predictable consequence of a lack of pantothenic acid.

When the expectant mother's supply of folic acid, another B vitamin, is short, cleft palate and heart trouble have been found to be frequent results. The *New York Times* (November 27, 1954) carried a short article in which it was asserted that mother rats deprived of folic acid during critical periods of their pregnancy (2 or 3 days), produced "astonishing numbers" of defective offspring. They suffered most commonly from defects of the heart and blood vessels, but also from deformed skeletons, bad eyes, lungs and kidneys.

The very survival of the fetus is responsible in a large measure to vitamin E, say Woollam and Miller in the *British Medical Journal* (June 2, 1956). They also note that a wave of muscular disorders in newborn lambs appeared to be the result of an insufficient supply of vitamin E. At the Ohio State Medical Convention, as reported in the Toledo (Ohio) *Blade* for January 16, 1958, Dr. Ben H. Landing, Professor of Pediatrics at Cincinnati University, attributed the major portion of congenital damage to the failure of the infant brain to get enough oxygen before and after birth. Vitamin E is known to preserve a higher oxygen content in the blood, and it is certain that this oxygen would be passed to the fetus if the mother were to take advantage of the power of vitamin E as a dietary supplement.

Diseases Affect Pregnancy

A lack of sufficient vitamin C in the pregnant woman may show up in her child as sores in the mouth and hemorrhages under the skin. But of even more importance, vitamin C can help to prevent infections which cause diseases actually known to have harmful effects on the expected infant. German measles, or rubella, is the best known example of a disease in the mother which can seriously affect an unborn child. In the *Journal of the American Medical Association* (August 21, 1954), it is estimated that the risk of malformations (cataracts, deafness, mental retardation, heart disease) resulting from rubella in the mother range from 10 per cent to 90 per cent. Another authority offers the more tangible figure of 30 per cent risk.

The flu, which has been with us in epidemic waves during the last few years, is another danger in the occurrence of congenital malformations. The *Lancet* (November 28, 1959) reports on a survey taken in Dublin, Ireland, among 66 pregnant women after the flu epidemic there in 1957-58. Of those who had flu, the incidence of congenital malformations in the children they bore was 240 per cent greater than that of the control group. The abnormalities were almost entirely of the central nervous system. The risk was found to be greatest if infection took place within the first 3 months of pregnancy, tapering off thereafter.

First 3 Months Most Critical

Many people are puzzled at the fact that the first 3 months of pregnancy are so critical as compared with the rest of the gestation period. In the *British Medical Association Journal* article, Woollam and Miller say, ". . . the effect of a vitamin shortage during the first stage (corresponding to the first 3 months of pregnancy in the human) will be to interfere with the development of vital organs, such as the heart and brain, which are then in a critical stage of development."

Douw G. Steyn agrees when he writes that the younger the embryo, the more active is the development of the tissues, and the more active the development when nutrients are lacking, the more extensive will be the resultant abnormality. So the most important time to prepare for a baby, nutritionally, is the moment the mother becomes aware of her pregnancy. Actually, women of child-bearing age should be extremely careful of their nutrition, lest pregnancy begin several weeks before they are aware of it. These weeks are crucial.

Medications and the Fetus

The medications given to a pregnant woman can also have serious effects on the child she carries. William R. Thompson of Wesleyan University is given, in *Science News Letter* (April 27, 1957), as the source of the information that hormones like ACTH, cortisone and adrenalin given to the expectant mother may have drastic effects on the newborn. Douw G. Steyn says that cortisone may not only prevent proper tissue development, but destroy tissue already developed. *Nutrition Reviews* (October, 1957) blames a high incidence of cleft palate on the fact that the mothers of the animals observed had been given cortisone after the 11th day of gestation.

The problem of a diabetic mother-to-be can really be a serious one if the assumption made in the *British Medical Journal* (October 30, 1954) is accurate. In writing of a mentally defective child born to a schizophrenic woman who had been receiving insulin from the second month of pregnancy, the writer suggested that it was possible that the insulin was the cause of the child's mental loss. It is possible, he went on, that insulin is harmful only when given before the 11th week. This is an unusual viewpoint, one which we have seen nowhere else and one which should certainly be further researched.

We are, in general, wary of the use of any drugs unless there is no other choice to save a life. They might combat disease, but they do not add anything to the well-being of the baby. The side effects are often seriously dangerous. If this is true in all persons, how much more so in the delicate condition of pregnancy? The body then cannot spare any of its resources to deal with side effects from drugs and, if it does, the fetus might well suffer.

What About Stress?

Stress in pregnancy is difficult to avoid, because women, at this time, are even more likely to be susceptible to stressful situations than at any other time. The factor of stress was discussed by D. H. Stott in the *Lancet* (May 18, 1957), and he concluded that stress in pregnancy can be the cause of congenital defects. This was the result of interviews with 102 mothers of mentally retarded children and 450 mothers of normal children. Of the 102, all had had some form of illness during pregnancy (toxemia, rheumatic fever, ulcers or cardiac disease), while of the 450, only 30 per cent had been ill. Of the 102 mothers of abnormal children, there were 38 instances of emotional stress or harassment, including matrimonial trouble, eviction threats and quarrels with relatives. It was also noted that the incidence of ill health among the infants shortly after birth was 3 times greater among the abnormal groups.

And if stress should plague you during pregnancy, do not seek to drown it in narcotics. The *New York Times* (July 14, 1957) reported on the problem faced by the babies of women addicted to narcotics—the babies were addicted, too! One reads of the dreadful withdrawal symptoms of narcotics addicts and it has now been established that babies born of such women, deprived of their narcotics supply from the mother's blood, suffer as intensely in their bassinets as their elders do in the wards of the federal hospital for addicts in Lexington, Kentucky.

Smoking Creates More Stress Than It Relieves

Another way to meet stress is smoking, say many men and women. Of course, it has been shown that much more stress is created by smoking than is ever relieved by it. Whether a woman believes the evidence against smoking or not, whether she cares for her own health or not—smoking during pregnancy and while nursing, entails serious risks for the baby's health. How can the pleasure of a cigarette be worth such a chance?

In January, 1958, Ann Usher, in an article for *Better Homes and Gardens,* marshaled a number of startling facts which should have some influence on mothers-to-be. Body poisons (toxemia) which sometimes develop in pregnancy are more frequent in smokers. Thyroid disorders are 7 times more frequent in smokers. Even exposure to tobacco has an effect on the reproductive capacities of women. Those who work in tobacco factories have fewer pregnancies than is average in other fields. They have more miscarriages when they do conceive; those who do carry their babies to birth face a greater death rate for their infants in the first 3 years of life than do other mothers. A study in Brazil showed miscarriages and stillbirths among these women to be more than double that of other women.

Nicotine In Breast Milk

When mothers smoke as they nurse, it is known that the breast milk they give contains the deadly poison, nicotine. How much can an infant take? No one knows. How much depends upon the number of cigarettes smoked? What effect does the nicotine have on a baby? One can only guess, bearing in mind that an amount of nicotine equal in volume to what is present in a week's smoking, can kill a man.

An important fact uncovered by Miss Usher is that the rate of premature births among smoking women exceeds that of non-smokers by an appreciable margin. Premature babies are at a serious disadvantage in terms of good health. They are usually much lighter in weight than full termers. The *British Medical Journal* (December 8, 1956) tells us that very light birth weights in babies (less than 3¼ pounds) indicate a 10 per cent likelihood that the child will be backward or defective (a proven aid in avoiding premature births is vitamin E).

At Baltimore City Hospital, 2,736 women were observed to discover how smoking would affect the time of their delivery. In one group of 48 women who smoked more than a pack of cigarettes a day during pregnancy, the prematurity rate was 22.9 per cent, as against 11.1 per cent among 1,547 women who did not smoke at all. Among 1,019 women who smoked half a pack to more than a full pack a day, the rate was 18.4 per cent. There were 154 women who had been smokers, but stopped by the second month of pregnancy; their prematurity rate was 11 per cent. The national prematurity rate in 1958 was 12.9 per cent. The non-smokers in this group were below the average; the smokers, considerably above it.

Dr. George H. Davis of the Baltimore Health Department suggested that the nicotine, which acts to narrow the blood passages, could cause a reduction of the blood supply to the placenta. Also, mothers might substitute smoking for nourishing food. Dr. Davis then said he would advise his private patients to discontinue or cut down on smoking.

If the mother-to-be refuses to recognize her responsibility to stop smoking, it is urgent that she supplement her diet with vitamin E. This vitamin will at least assure her of the best efficiency of the blood that does pass into the placenta, if the supply should be curtailed by the action of nicotine.

The information here only scratches the surface of what has been written to prove the value of food supplementation in pregnancy. Space does not permit more than an indication of the proof that is to be seen.

Unwise to Risk Tragic Outcome

Can we say that a deformed child will surely be born to any mother who does not eat healthfully and supplement her diet with vitamins and minerals? Obviously, we cannot. You might be lucky and have a perfectly normal baby, even though you eat nothing but your regular, not-too-commendable diet. But, then, you could be unlucky, too. Could you bear to think that such a little bit of dietary care might have spared you and your child the unpromising future open to an abnormal child?

Women who have one deformed child have a 25 per cent chance of having a second. In the Oakland (California) *Tribune* (November 4, 1957), writer Jack Ryan told of Dr. Beverly Douglas of Vanderbilt University Medical School, who has been putting pregnant women who have already borne a deformed child, on diets rich in vitamins, but especially in riboflavin. "No mother in this group delivered a second deformed child when fed this diet during pregnancy."

If Dr. Douglas had been in charge of these women from the beginning, they would probably never have had a defective child. No one, barring injury or heredity, need ever have a defective child.

Protein

Protein in Your Diet

A book on proteins has been published by the National Research Council, which is the official group for making decisions on things nutritional.

We thought many readers would be particularly interested in that part of the book which deals with protein deficiency and which parts of the body are chiefly affected by it. Experimenting with animals, researchers are able, by carefully controlling the diet, to produce protein deficiency—or, if they wish, deficiency in one or another of the amino acids, or forms of protein.

Here are some of the symptoms of protein deficiency in animals. Bones are affected. We usually think of bones as being made of minerals, but there is considerable protein in them, as well as in the cartilage which links bones together. Growth of young animals is slowed or stops entirely when they are deprived of protein. Their bones become rarefied or porous. There is also disturbance of the structure of the teeth and the gums. In animals depleted of protein, there is a delay in the healing of wounds, because the cells which produce collagen (connective tissue) have no raw material to work with.

Reproductive organs may atrophy or waste away. Glands are affected, too. The hypophysis, the thyroid, the thymus, the adrenals, the spleen are all affected. There may be some thinning or even loss of hair and the skin may become atrophied or shrunken. The lens and the cornea of the eye are dependent upon an ample supply of protein for their health. They may suffer in protein deficiency. Cataract has been observed in animals depleted of protein or of just one of the important amino acids. The pancreas and the kidneys suffer. Muscles in the heart and skeleton may shrink.

There is a decrease in the production of hemoglobin—the red coloring matter in the blood—hence, a decrease in the number of red blood cells, leading to anemia. The liver—that most important organ of all—suffers perhaps more than any other part of the body. Many of its functions are dependent upon a constant supply of protein.

Most interesting is the revelation that reaction to infectious disease is controlled partly by the protein in the diet. The antibodies in the blood which fight germs are made of protein and any deficiency in the supply of protein is reflected in a decrease in their number; hence, a decrease in protection against disease.

The Importance of Protein

Proteins are made up of building blocks called amino acids. Of these, there are about 20 which it is essential for us to obtain in food, since the body cannot manufacture them. Deficiencies in these are not the kind of thing we see in human beings, usually, for considerable care must be taken to devise a diet in which only one or several amino acids would be deficient. However, when this is accomplished in a laboratory, we find such things as these to be the resulting symptoms in laboratory animals: loss of hair or graying of hair, death of muscle cells, accumulations of fat in the liver, convulsions.

The book goes on to say that protein deficiency is not common in our country and is confined chiefly to people suffering from serious diseases or, possibly, from those which involve loss of protein or poor absorption of protein. Alcoholism is a disease in which the poor diet eaten may contribute to liver disease, which is caused chiefly by lack of protein.

Protein Requirements

It has been suggested that adults should have a minimum of 70 to 80 grams of protein a day for good health. Teen-agers need from 75 to 100; children 40 to 70 grams. Note that this does not mean getting 70 to 80 grams of meat or eggs or fish. Not all of a high-protein food is actual protein, of course. They contain also water, carbohydrates, minerals and so fourth.

In general, meats, fish and eggs contain 10 to 20 per cent protein. One serving (100 grams) of each would equal about 1/7 to 1/4 the amount an adult might require daily. This suggests that many of us may not be getting nearly enough protein every day to keep us in good health. Surely, if we depend on cereal products and sweets to fill up on, we will be short on protein.

Government agencies have done some surveys on the protein consumption of Americans. They find, they say, that enough protein foods are consumed in families with higher incomes, but that, in lower income groups, there may be serious deficiencies. Protein foods are, in general, more expensive than starchy foods.

They say, too, that "there is evidence that, in spite of generous protein supplies in the nation's households, family members do not share in these supplies in accordance with their nutritional needs. Whether because of food preferences, notions about food needs or other reasons, diets of many individuals provide less than recommended amounts of protein. . . . Women, for example, are found more often than men to have poor diets compared with dietary recommendations. Older people with decreasing food intakes are likely to have diets lower in protein and other nutrients than young adults. In a study of one-day diets of over 1,000 Iowa women, the proportion of diets furnishing less than 50 grams (of protein) increased from 26 per cent for the 30 to 39 decade to 64 per cent for those 70 years and over. . . . Usually, the diets of younger children are relatively better than those of older children and, in general, boys do better than girls. Diets of adolescent girls especially are likely to be low in protein and other nutrients compared with recommendations." We cannot fail to note that the one-day survey disclosed a frightening percentage of protein deficiency in the diets of the women observed. Twenty-six per cent of the 30 to 39 year olds were not getting nearly enough protein for good health. And 64 per cent of those over 70 were not getting enough! Doesn't this explain a lot about the many chronic illnesses that begin to afflict one around middle age and continue to worsen as one grows older?

This suggests, certainly, that any housewife, charged with feeding a family, should concentrate on the groups mentioned above to make certain they are getting enough protein. Chances are the baby and any young children will be eating meals so closely supervised that there is little danger they will be short on protein. The grown men of the family will probably get enough protein from animal sources for their needs, since they are less likely to depend on make-shift meals. But teen-agers (especially girls) and older folks are in danger of neglecting protein at mealtime. We suspect the girls are afraid of gaining weight. Older members of society frequently do not get enough protein, because it is easier to prepare and eat soft, starchy, sweet foods. And, of course, they are less expensive.

Meat Substitutes

What about "meat substitutes"? There aren't any, really. You can substitute eggs and fish and poultry for meat, but that's about all. Substituting a cereal dish like macaroni or noodles for a meat dish will not provide enough protein of good quality, for the quality of protein as well as the quantity is important.

Amino acids must be considered. Cereal or vegetable foods tend to be lacking in one or another of these. So take foods of vege-table origin along with meats and eggs, so that the amino acids supplement one another and you get most benefit from all the differ-ent kinds. Don't get all your protein at one meal, dinner, let's say, and eat whatever happens to be around for lunch and breakfast. Protein meals should be distributed throughout the day—about a third of the day's quota at each meal, if you want to be sure of getting enough protein and also getting the most economical use of the protein in all your meals.

We think the book on amino acids would be useful for nutri-tionists and others who work with food professionally. It is a bit difficult for the average layman who does not have reference books at hand. The title is *Evaluation of Protein Nutrition,* publication number 711 of the National Research Council. It is available from the National Research Council, Washington, D. C.

Proteins for Posture

The posture of your child is a good index to the type of nourish-ment he is receiving. In *Nutrition and Health,* a du Pont publication (November, 1958), Dr. Genevieve Stearns of the University Hospital at the University of Iowa is quoted as saying that, "Some children never get enough protein to develop the normal amount of muscle. . . . These children tire easily and have little excess energy. They are always nutritionally below par."

This tiredness referred to by Dr. Stearns results in what she calls "fatigue posture," characterized by hollow chest and protruding stomach. The muscles needed to keep the chest out and the stomach in simply aren't strong enough to do the job. This is due to lack of muscle-building protein.

"Unless the child is fed enough protein so that his muscles can develop normally, he just does the best he can with what he gets." How is the protein supply in your children? Is their bad posture due to the lack of the stuff muscles are made of? Be sure to include plenty of meat, nuts, eggs and fish in their diet to help their bodies to develop properly.

Radiation

A Look at the Problem of Radiation

We can't escape the problems presented by the radioactive elements being released into the earth's atmosphere by nuclear explosions. We know radiation is actually harmful to the human body, but the idea is kind of fuzzy for those of us who have no detailed scientific background. *California's Health* (January 15, 1961), a publication of the California Public Health Department, carried the most understandable explanation of this very important phenomenon that we have seen up to now. It was written by Simon Kinsman, Ph.D., who is a Radiological Health Consultant for the United States Public Health Service. We would like to give some of the highlights of Dr. Kinsman's article, for the information is valuable and deeply concerned with good health.

Radiation occurs in a variety of forms—light and heat are two types we can perceive with our senses; X-rays and ultraviolet rays are two types which we neither see nor feel. Now, radiation from radioactive material (the material used to make nuclear bombs and in nuclear power plants) is a stream of very fast flying particles or waves which we neither see nor feel coming from tiny units of matter called atoms.

In the past 65 years, we have learned much about radiation. Man-made radiation in the form of X-rays was discovered in Germany in 1895. Then came uranium and radium. Invisible rays from radium were soon found to be of 3 kinds: heavy particles which travel only an inch or so in air, lighter particles which travel a few feet and, finally, waves similar to light waves, but too short to be seen by the human eye, which penetrate considerable distances, even through several inches of lead. These 3 types of invisible radiation are called, respectively, alpha, beta and gamma rays. (There are also cosmic rays which come from outside the earth's atmosphere, which are largely intercepted by the earth's atmosphere. They are not man-made nor controllable by man, so we are not especially concerned with those in space.)

Natural radioactive substances are everywhere—the water we drink, air we breathe, food we eat, soil we cultivate, etc. Along with cosmic rays from space, these tiny sources have been sending out radioactive signals for millions of years. This is what we call background radiation. Man has lived with this type of radiation since time began. The variation of this type of radiation from one locality to another is slight. Rain or snow do have some effect upon it.

Danger Varies with Exposure

Danger from radiation depends upon degree of exposure. (Degree here means the type and amount of radioactive material and one's distance from it.) Any exposure is undesirable. But taking radioactive materials inside the body is considered dangerous, even when it is part of a treatment. Dr. Kinsman says that one should "avoid inhaling radioactive substances or getting them into your food or drink, just as you avoid taking arsenic, lead or other poisonous substances." We wish we had as much control over radioactive substances as we do over arsenic and lead. How can we avoid ingesting radioactive substances when every substance in the world is being constantly bombarded by the very radiation we are discussing, due to the fall-out from bomb tests by ours and other countries? These explosions must be outlawed before they lead to their logical end: our own extermination.

Radioactive materials differ widely in the rate at which they lose radioactivity. The length of time they are kept in the body varies also. Radium and plutonium remain active for thousands of years and may be retained for long periods in the body, while others, such as radioactive sodium will be quickly eliminated and will decay in a few days. Naturally, one must be especially careful to avoid the ingestion of even small amounts of the more deadly materials into the mouth or lungs. That is why even eating or smoking is forbidden in some radioactive areas.

Exposure Limited in 3 Ways

Exposure to radiation may be limited in 3 ways: in time, by distance and by shielding. If you must be exposed to some source of radiation, get away from it as soon as possible. Stay as far away from any radioactive source as you can, if for some reason you must be in the vicinity of one. Use every safeguard you can get in the form of shields—gamma rays are stopped by substantial amounts of lead or concrete. Insist on lead shields—especially over the lower torso—when being X-rayed, unless, of course, the lower torso is the area to be investigated. Shielding of the spleen and appendix has been found effective in protecting experimental animals from leukemia after exposure to radiation.

Actual contact between an individual and a source of radiation is even more of a problem than exposure to rays. If, by accident, one gets a small quantity of radioactive material on one's hands or feet or clothes, it might find its way inside the body through a piece of food touched and eaten or through a cut. Any chance that contamination has occurred should be carefully checked and clothes changed and hands washed. Of course, we are still faced with the everyday contamination which we encounter in food that was grown

---

Reed, Walter

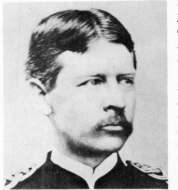

Walter Reed, famed as the army surgeon who stamped out yellow fever among the United States troops in Cuba, was born at Belroi, Virginia, September 13, 1851. In 1869, approaching the age of 18, Reed earned the first of two medical degrees, receiving his second in 1870 from Bellevue Hospital Medical College, New York. For some time thereafter he engaged in private medical practice, working at the same time for the boards of health of the cities of New York and Brooklyn. Giving up his practice, he entered the army medical corps in 1874 and was assigned as attending surgeon and recruit examiner in Baltimore. After his promotion to major, he was sent to the newly organized Army Medical School in Washington, D. C., where he did research work in bacteriology. In 1900 Reed got the chance to evaluate his bacteriological studies when he, together with Dr. James Carroll, was sent to Cuba to investigate the yellow fever epidemic. Working on the theory that yellow fever could only be transmitted from person to person by mosquitoes, Reed and his commission proceeded to submit 8 volunteers to the sting of mosquitoes which had bitten yellow fever victims. Through experiments such as this, Reed definitely established that the Aëdes Aegypti mosquito was the carrier of the dread yellow fever. This truly outstanding discovery earned for Walter Reed world-wide attention, for, with this knowledge, yellow fever could be controlled, better yet—eliminated entirely.

under a layer of fall-out, water supplies that are showered with it and milk high in strontium 90, due to the contamination of the cows' fodder. There is no way we know of that will eliminate these sources of contact, especially if nuclear testing continues.

Dangers We Face

Just what type of danger do we face from radiation in the nuclear world we inhabit? Are there risks? Have there actually been physical changes in our world, in ourselves, in our children? Are we being protected? Do we need protection? Let us take a sampling of the material in our files on this subject and see how the situation looks.

The pronouncements on the actual dangers we face today as a result of nuclear explosions and the fall-out they produce, are monumental in their contradictions. The New York *Herald Tribune* (August 19, 1960) carried two articles reporting the findings of a Columbia University research team, which concluded that, in the words of one headline, "Fall-Out Peril Exaggerated." The scientists guessed that, away from the central location of the explosion, "the strontium 90 level in the diet and bones of noncombatants would probably rise an amount equal to the radiation now hitting man from natural sources, such as cosmic rays. This would double man's present exposure . . . Thus, long-term survival of large populations, even in countries under attack, would appear to be feasible. . . ."

The *New York Times* (August 21, 1960) got on the bandwagon to report this optimistic view, too. The same paper reported, on the previous April 18, the opinion of Dr. Ralph E. Lapp, a Washington physicist, that those who said regions of heavy radioactive contamination would not be habitable for 40 years or more were wrong. The land could probably be inhabited and cultivated in a few months after attack. Obviously, no need, then, to be concerned about fall-out. Another *Times* (July 19, 1960) story tells us that fall-out in the Southern Hemisphere is less than that of the Northern. For those who live in the Southern Hemisphere, that must be good news. It must be good news, too, for those living on the low-lying plains to hear that fall-out there is less dangerous than at the foothills of mountains and areas of very high altitude. The New York *Herald Tribune* (July 21, 1960) shrugged off any danger to food from strontium 90, in an *Associated Press* report from the United States Public Health Service. The report concerned studies which showed that Americans "are not getting enough strontium 90 in their foods to add up to a health menace that should be regulated."

Officially, then, our government agencies are not concerned over our being seriously affected by fall-out in the atmosphere. One can readily understand their reluctance to express concern about a dangerous situation, which they are, in fact, sponsoring. What can they do, as they plan another explosion, but pat us comfortingly on the shoulder and assure us that there is nothing to fear? The contradiction in all of this lies in the fact that, while we are being told there is no danger, the maximum allowable dosage of radiation set by government agencies, is being changed frequently because newly discovered dangers in exposure are being recognized.

Until early 1960, apparently, the government's assurances of safety were based upon the investigations of a skeleton crew of scientists. In *Scope* (January 27, 1960), we read of an expansion of the government's program to control effects of environmental radiation on human health that was to start March 1, 1960. The then Secretary of Health, Education and Welfare, Arthur S. Flemming, promised the publication of both evaluated and unevaluated data on the extent of radiation in air, food and water in the United States.

Though the government says it believes that the danger of fallout is exaggerated, we see, in the *New York Times* (February 23, 1960), that the National Committee on Radiation Protection and Measurement, an arm of the United States Bureau of Standards, recommended a lowering of the maximum possible radiation exposure level for the public. The recommendation calls for a reduction to one-fifth of the doses previously allowed by that group, and about 70 per cent lower than those agreed upon in the previous November by another group, the International Committee on Radiation. The National Committee, in setting the new tolerances, said that the maximum permissible dose of man-made radiation for the general population should be approximately the same as the average national background level. That is, the level which occurs naturally in our atmosphere—about one-tenth of a roentgen (standard unit of radiation) a year. By contrast, the old allowance was half a roentgen a year, or 5 times the newly recommended amount.

Radiation in Food

The National Committee also made recommendations regarding the radiation levels permissible in foods. A drop to 40 per cent of the previous allowance was concluded to be best. *Food Field Reporter's* article (March 14, 1960) went on to say that the permissible strontium 90 level was cut from 80 to 33 micromicrocuries. "Strontium 90, like radium, settles in the bones and, in sufficient quantities, can create bone cancer and leukemia . . . Some foods have already shown concentrations of radioactivity above the new permissible limits."

The *New York Times* (September 7, 1960) carried the announcement of the Atomic Energy Commission, that workers in atomic industry, normally allowed a greater limit of radiation exposure than the rest of the population, would have a sharp reduction of their permissible lifetime accumulation of radiation. The new regulations served to limit the accumulated dose to one-third of the previous limits (15 roentgens a year to 5 roentgens a year). The regulation also sets up new standards for those not connected with atomic energy. They are restricted to an exposure that is 10 per cent of that permitted as a maximum for radiation workers.

The government is saying, in effect, that it realizes that it was mistaken in its previous estimates of the dangers of radiation. They were too low. We are now told that atomic workers were allowed 3 times too much radiation up to now; the general public has been permitted 5 times the safe limit of radiation, due to the 1957 recommendation of the Atomic Energy Commission. Is it possible that, in 1964, the level which is now recommended will be judged 3 times or 5 times more than we can handle? The most learned scientist will admit that the levels set are only a guess. We've seen plenty of wrong guesses in this area in the last 15 years. Who is to say that there isn't another mistake in the making?

Whatever happens in the future, the important thing now is to make Americans realize that radiation is a serious danger. If it is not, then why are the estimates of our ability to withstand its effects constantly being revised downward? If it is dangerous, then how can we, or any other nation, even contemplate the release of still more deadly radiation into the atmosphere? If we must flex our muscles before the world, let us do it in some other way, one that won't result in our own destruction, perhaps before we even have occasion to use such a weapon in war. Don't be misled by statements on the lack of danger in strontium 90. It's dangerous and it's increasing in our atmosphere—the atmosphere in which we breathe and grow our food and have our children.

The Sky Is Falling

An article in the *National Guardian* (February 1, 1960) summed up the current fall-out situation quite well. The data, all documented, give cause for alarm. One of the most interesting aspects of the problem lies in the fact that scientists seem to have misjudged the speed with which the radioactive debris is falling. They at first assumed that it might take 100 years to fall and, if it would, 92 per cent of the radioactive material would decay before that time had passed. However, recent observation has led to the conclusion that all of the fall-out will possibly have landed within about 10 years and, if this is the case, only 22 per cent of the radioactivity will have time to disappear before it falls. That means we are likely to be hit with about 70 per cent more radioactive fall-out than was anticipated.

A good deal of this debris is finding its way into one of the nation's staples—milk. In March, 1959, *Consumer Reports* concluded: "There is incontrovertible evidence that the strontium 90 content of milk has been increasing since 1954." The government announced an expansion of its testing of milk for this harmful substance. *Consumer Reports* commented: "As welcome as the increase will be, it still represents a good deal less than what may be necessary."

Science News Letter (July 2, 1960) described a series of 53 experiments with 44 cows, in which the radioactive products were artificially introduced into the diet of the animals and their milk was then checked for radioactivity. Three weeks after contamination of the land on which the cows grazed, strontium 90 levels in their milk were 5 times as great as on the first day. The test was one of many which proved the same point: cows and other animals whose milk we use and which graze on land which has been contaminated by fall-out (as has all land by now), transfer the deadly radioactive substances to their milk—the milk we drink!—in high concentration.

Roentgen, Wilhelm Konrad

Wilhelm Konrad Roentgen, German physicist and discoverer of the X-ray, was born in Lennep, Prussia, March 27, 1845. He earned his Ph. D. from the University of Zurich, after which he 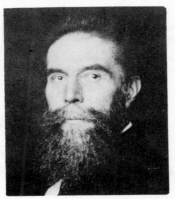 *spent 16 years as a professor of mathematics and physics. His enthusiasm for study and research in his technical field next brought him to the Physical Institute of the University of Wurzburg. It was here that Roentgen discovered the X-ray. While carrying out some routine research with a glass tube known as a Crookes tube, he observed that the passing of an electric current through the tube caused the illumination of a barium, platino-cyanide coated piece of paper which was placed near the tube. This phenomenon incited Roentgen to do further research on this tube, which resulted in his discovery of a new kind of ray which could pass through many kinds of light materials. Roentgen named this unfamiliar ray the X-ray. Although it at times has been called the Roentgen ray, the more familiar X-ray has been kept as the name of one of the greatest contributions to the science of medicine.*

Removing Strontium 90

One way out of this dilemma is suggested in the removal of strontium 90 from milk. *Food Field Reporter* (February 15, 1960) gave out the news of a method that would remove 80 per cent of this dangerous element from milk. The operation would be cheap and simple—just pass the milk through a column of bone meal. The calcium in the meal will attract and hold the strontium 90. The bone meal, according to Dr. Leon Singer of the University of Minnesota, could even be used again and again. But now comes a surprising statement: Dr. Singer stressed his opinion that the strontium levels in milk are not yet high enough to necessitate commercial treatment, but the treatment will be useful if it should ever become necessary.

But how could Dr. Singer be so sure that the levels are safe? *Consumer Bulletin* (July, 1960), in discussing the problem of fallout and strontium 90, stated that a primary problem is establishment of the minimum amount of strontium 90 which can be ingested daily without accumulation of significant amounts in the body. "Experiments on animals may establish such balances, but we do not know anything about them for human beings with their long life span. One cannot kill human beings that have been subjected to constant observation and tests under controlled conditions to make the necessary measurements. . . ." How long are we to wait before we begin to protect ourselves! When levels of strontium 90 become higher, we'll be in real trouble. We're in real trouble now! Why not begin using this bone meal filter to protect ourselves from just *one* hazard?

The *Science News Letter* article of July 2, 1960, quotes Dr. Gilbert B. Forbes, writing in *Pediatrics* magazine: "The peaceful use of atomic energy will, in time, provide fully as great a potential hazard as the bomb-testing program. . . ." If this is true, and indications are certainly compatible with this conclusion, we should be using every tool and investigating every suggestion to control the damaging effects we are warned to expect.

The government's official opinion having been stated, many intelligent, well-qualified persons in public life and in the scientific fields still show a healthy respect for the problems of the nuclear age. The *National Guardian* (February, 1960) quotes a federal judge of the United States Court of Appeals who was dealing with a suit to halt nuclear tests, as conceding that: "There is no question in anybody's mind that more damage from nuclear tests is possible than a human mind can comprehend."

Some Risk in the Smallest Dose

The *Ad Hoc* Committee (an objective scientific group) of the National Committee on Radiation Protection and Measurements concluded that, "Even the smallest dose is associated with some risk, and exposure of the general population to any increase in radiation should not occur unless benefits are expected." What benefits can be expected, we wonder, that will outweigh the cancer, congenital malformations, cataracts, etc., that we know can and will be brought on by excess radiation?

The *Lancet* (January 23, 1960) carried the opinion of T. C. Carter and other writers, that effort was made at first to set a safe limit of exposure beyond which bodily damage in radiation workers would occur, but ". . . we now believe that there is no dose threshold for the induction of genetic (hereditary) damage, and that there may be no threshold for the induction of some types of somatic (body) damage." In other words, there is no level of radiation, no matter how low, which can actually be considered safe.

With the above statement in mind, is it not staggering to contemplate the possible consequences of this news in *International Medical Digest* (March, 1960): "Radioisotopes alone are saving United States industry millions of dollars annually through improving processes. Also, 3 atomic reactor plants in different parts of the United States are already furnishing heat and electricity for homes and industry. More than 300 industrial reactor plants are planned for the immediate future. . . . The great increase in its (atomic energy) use and the increasing number of persons exposed to ionizing radiations may result in an increased incidence of radiodermatitis, either acute or chronic, and other radiation injuries. Without doubt, the greatest danger attending the use of atomic energy in industry is the danger of internal absorption of radioactive substances, because, once lodged in the body, they irradiate it from within, 24 hours a day. . . . It (the atomic industrial revolution) offers untold opportunities in research and development which will benefit all mankind—but with these benefits, goes a serious health problem."

May we mention here that the arbitrary raising of the radiation dosage permitted for the personnel in nuclear plants is a constant source of surprise to us. The Atomic Energy Commission tells us that atomic workers are safe at 10 times the exposure permitted to the general public. What logic is there in such an announcement? Is there some way of making atomic workers more able to withstand radiation than the rest of the population? If so, then we should all be able to avail ourselves of this defense. Perhaps atomic workers are chosen from some special breed of humans? Otherwise, we warn our readers very strongly against taking any type of job which brings them into close contact with radioactive substances. No salary could justify the risk involved to the life and health of the worker as well as that of his family and the children yet to be born.

Would You Risk This?

Perhaps you may have seen the article carried in *Look* magazine (April 12, 1960) which told the story of Jackson E. McVey of Houston, Texas. This case illustrates the potential tragedy faced by those working in atomic plants. Mr. McVey and co-worker Harold E. Northway were exposed in a laboratory to radioactive particles from decomposed pellets of iridium in 1957. The invisible particles drifted onto their skin and clothes. The two men unsuspectingly carried the particles to their homes, which then became contaminated, too. Of course, the families living in the homes were also affected.

As a result, the men and their families have become social and economic outcasts. Former friends and acquaintances are afraid that contact with either family will result in the spread of the horrible effects to their own houses. Businessmen have the same fear for their business places. Northway has developed cancer. McVey balances on the verge of leukemia, says his doctor. Both men have developed cataracts due to exposure, so has Mrs. McVey. An 18-year-old son, Eddie, is also suspected of having cataracts. Of course, the question of Eddie's future as a family man is still a problem. He is not even sure that he can father children. No one knows if the radiation to which he was exposed through his father's bad luck will affect the normalcy of any children he might have, but scientific findings seem to indicate that it will. Eddie, at the time of *Look's* article, was going steady with Diane who was willing to take that chance. Said Eddie, "My children—even if they are mutations—I'll love 'em just as much." Could a statement like this 18-year-old boy's, be the first of many similar ones to come from the better world promised by the Age of the Atom? The McVeys are in the process of continuing a suit against the company at which the accident occurred. One court has already ruled against them.

Another suit on radiation damage was reported in the Allentown, Pennsylvania, *Evening Chronicle* (April 24, 1960). Preston Mitchell, a rancher of Belle Fourche, South Dakota, ran into trouble in 1959. Many of his sheep became sick and died. Others staggered drunkenly around the rolling hills of the ranch. In all, 127 of the animals died of a mysterious malady and the Mitchells sold 327 others. Then Mitchell, his wife and their 6 children, also were afflicted with a strange illness. Their hair fell out. They became violently ill, apparently without cause. It is their contention that negligent handling of radioactive material by Atomic Energy Commission personnel caused a radioactive fall-out on the Mitchell ranch on April 17, 1959. They say the fall-out contaminated water and vegetation on the ranch. There are no atomic testing facilities in the area. It will be difficult for Mr. Mitchell to prove that fall-out is responsible; it would be harder to show that it is not. Unfortunately, the burden of proof is on Mitchell. The Atomic Energy Commission is presumed innocent unless he can prove otherwise.

Mentality and Radiation

The physical dangers of radiation are catalogued in more detail in other publications. In *Science News Letter* (September 17, 1960), there is the warning that mental retardation and loss of memory may result from long-term exposure to radioactive fall-out or other exposures to low dose levels of radiation. Soviet radiologists have found that dogs, after such exposure to radiation, do not learn as readily as before and may forget recent experiences. Both Soviet and United States scientists agree that the nervous system is afflicted by radiation. They differ only on the extent of the damage that can be done.

In *Drug Trade News* (September 19, 1960), the question of radiation damage to the nervous system (hence the brain) was discussed by Dr. Paul S. Henshaw of the United States Atomic Energy Commission. Dr. Henshaw is quoted as saying, "Although the information now available is limited and fragmentary, it is sufficient, nevertheless, to show that radiation can and does have late as well as acute effects on the nervous system and, thereby, on residual capabilities of the individual and group minds."

The article went on to state that the nervous system of human adults, because of its advanced development, may be more easily affected by radiation than the nervous systems of other animals. "If this impression be regarded as having merit," Dr. Henshaw went on, "we would scarcely be justified in concluding at this time that levels even a few times background (radiation) are inconsequential, particularly if we attempt to take into account the still more complex intellectual powers of population groups."

Dr. Henshaw discussed what happens to irradiated cells when the dosage is less than the 2,000 roentgens known to cause death in two or three weeks. Sometimes, there is recovery stemming from irradiated cells that survived. However, the surviving tissues do not perform as well in later life as do similar tissues which did not receive radiation. Also, it should be remembered that the cells which regenerate from the damaged ones are likely to be modified in some way and make their abnormal influence felt somehow at a later time. It may take one year or ten, or perhaps a generation, for the undesirable influence to show itself.

Radiation exposure of embryos in the uterus, even in doses of a few hundred roentgens, have adverse effects on learning ability, emotionality and locomotor coördination. Dr. Henshaw added that doses of 5 to 25 roentgens produced brain abnormalities in mice embryos, and foreign investigators have said that impairment of intelligence in these mice occurred after exposure to even one roentgen or less. In monkeys placed in an area of radiation when testing was done in Nevada, it was observed that a decrease in ability to see, while not shown after one year, emerged 3 years after radiation exposure.

Coloring may have something to do with the effect of radiation on one's body. In a study of 530 women given radiation treatments after surgery for genital cancer, it was found that fair-haired patients developed more severe radiation illness than women with brown hair. Symptoms included gastrointestinal disorders, increased blood pressure and redness of the skin. (*International Record of Medicine,* December, 1960.)

Protecting Ourselves

The problem we face today is not the intended radiation we are likely to get from X-ray. Nor is the danger of a job in atomic energy the difficulty for most of us. Instead, we are caught in an atmosphere of radioactivity over which we have no control, and one in which we increase our exposure merely by doing the everyday things we must do to stay alive. We must eat fruit, eat vegetables, drink liquids, touch metals, etc. As you will see, each of these holds the threat of more radiation.

Radioactive Waste in Bodies of Water

In *Science* (129, 94-5, 1959) two researchers stated that trace amounts of radioactive zinc (Zn^{65}) were being dumped into the Columbia River. The later use of this same water for irrigation permits the concentration of this radioisotope in farm produce and its eventual deposit in man. The researchers concluded that, "It is apparent that food organisms of man could accumulate hazardous levels of certain radioisotopes from water which contained concentrations of the contaminants that were well within the permissible limits for drinking water." (Second United Nations Geneva Conference.) This means that, if a level of safety is set for water that is to be consumed in its liquid state, there is no guarantee that this same water, used to irrigate crops is safe. The ingredients of the water are concentrated as they are absorbed by the plants and thus, the danger of any radioactive substances present in the water is greatly multiplied in the plant.

Consumer Bulletin (August, 1960) noted a report that radioactive fall-out is concentrated in the leaves of plants, more than in fruits, seeds, grains and edible roots. Beans and radishes were found to be higher in strontium 90 content than carrots and barley. Think of the leafy foods we eat: spinach, rhubarb, kale, cabbage, lettuce, etc.

Do you wear a watch with a luminous dial? A German journal, *Strahlen therapie* (110, 606-621, 1959), described observations which showed that wrist watches, travel alarm clocks and other clocks with luminous dials give off undesirable radiation. The dosage is mild—negligible, say the authors—but what standards do they have for making such an assertion? The radiation levels we had been told not to worry about for 10 years after the explosions in Japan, have since become something to worry about. Will someone find, in 20 years, that we should have worried more about luminous dials?

A *United Press International* dispatch on August 30, 1960, told of the Atomic Energy Commission report which said that small amounts of radioactive metals have found their way into alloys used by jewelry makers in rings, ring settings and mountings. The metal, ruthenium 106, probably made radioactive due to atomic testing, was said to present no health hazard as it occurred in the rings, but jewelry makers were ordered not to make any more rings using it. If it's so harmless, why the order to stop using it? Another unsuspected radiation source that you might have on your finger as you read this.

A Means of Preserving Foods?

Food Field Reporter (February 13, 1961) detailed with relish the answer to the fish industry's market problems—radiation. The fresh fish market would be tremendously expanded, it said, if the shelf life of fish could be extended through radiation processing. The added cost of one cent per pound for processing was considered acceptable, but the cost of an appropriate educational program to overcome initial consumer resistance was considered a major disadvantage. There appears to be no doubt that consumer resistance would be overcome if enough money were spent to do it. Advertising can convince Americans that anything is safe.

The whole question of the radiation of food as a means of extending its shelf life has been discussed and experimented with for more than 10 years now. The Army has been the chief proponent of the plan. The thought is, of course, to find a cheap way of preserving food as it is transported to soldiers in battle. Unfortunately, irradiated food has what has been described as a "wet-dog taste," and many foods change appearance as well as flavor to a degree that makes them so unappetizing as to be objectionable.

From a health standpoint, the taste and looks of irradiated foods are the least important aspects of the process. In order to forestall spoilage, the enzyme activity in a food must be slowed or halted. Refrigeration suspends this activity and, upon thawing, the enzymes resume their activity. Radiation simply destroys enzymes, along with much of the vitamin value of the food. The steak that will stay 3 months on a shelf, unrefrigerated, without spoiling is devitalized, dead meat, with a great deal of its food value gone in the processing.

Then, there is the problem of the danger in such food from the standpoint of radioactivity. Those in favor of radiating food say that the rays pass through food just the way X-rays pass through the human body. The value of any such reassurance vanishes as we recall that X-rays do not simply pass through the body, but are likely to lodge there tor some time. Radiation accumulates in anything that has been treated with it. That means meat, corn, apples or tomatoes that are radiated to preserve them, have accumulated some of the radiation. If you eat any or all of them, you will acquire some of their radiation. If you eat irradiated foods daily, your accumulation of roentgens will increase in direct proportion.

Some Means of Protection

There are some rays of hope through avenues for avoiding radiation damage, or at least reducing it. *Science News Letter* (May 21, 1960) told of the experiment of Dr. James K. Ashikawa of the University of California, which showed that mice could survive lethal doses of X-rays through treatment with common vegetable oils. Dr. Ashikawa injected the oil—an amount equal to about 1/30 of the mouse's weight—directly into the abdominal cavity of irradiated animals. As many as 90 per cent of the treated animals survived a moderate X-ray dosage, compared with survival of only 45 per cent in untreated mice. And after much stronger irradiation, which killed all of the untreated animals, some 7 per cent of the treated mice survived.

No one has been able to explain the exact mechanism which allows fats to ward off radiation sickness, although it is suspected that the answer lies in some biochemcial action involving the cell membranes, which are known to be weakened by radiation exposure. (Vitamin C is involved in holding cells together.) The best reaction was achieved through the use of olive oil, high in saturated fat, stearate. Dr. Ashikawa supplemented the natural content by adding pure methyl stearate. Stearate is also expected to play a role in rallying the body's natural defenses against radiation sickness.

Tannic Acid Recommended

Time magazine (August 10, 1959) told of Dr. Teiji Ugai, who remembered that strontium chloride combines with tannic acid to form an insoluble compound. From this, he reasoned that, instead of being deposited in the bones to do serious long-term damage, strontium might be eliminated from the human body if there were enough tannic acid present to combine with it. Experiments, showing that mice stored 30 per cent less strontium in their bones when they also got tannic acid, seem to bear out his theory, at least where animals are concerned. Dr. Ugai favored a standard brew of green or black tea as a source of tannic acid.

Nutrition Reviews (July, 1960) takes a view to which we are attracted. The idea is that, if one can ingest large amounts of calcium, while the strontium 90 is being ingested, the two will combine rather than be absorbed into the bones. They will then be eliminated from the body through its natural processes, as is normal for any excess of calcium, before the strontium 90 has a chance to lodge in the bones. The article calls the reader's attention to milk as a rich source of calcium. We would like to suggest bone meal instead. It is as rich or richer in calcium, with none of milk's drawbacks as an allergen, a growth inducer, a penicillin carrier, etc.

Researchers Working on Anti-Radiation Drugs

From *Missiles and Rockets* (September 26, 1960), we learned that Walter Reed Army Institute of Research is working on drugs that "may radically reduce the horrors of radiation damage to living organisms." The Army is building its research around protein-binding elements found readily in nature. They are synthetically produced because the scientists say that man could not consume enough in his natural food to give the necessary protection. However, the synthetic compounds being used now are not well tolerated. Toxic effects include nausea, low blood pressure, nervous disorders, abnormal animation.

Perhaps a human could not consume enough of these protein-binding elements, either synthetically or in foods, all at once, even to protect himself, but if they are useful in large amounts, surely smaller doses of natural foods rich in these protein-binding elements would be of some help. A good natural diet, rich in protein, minerals (calcium in particular), vitamins (vitamin C in particular) and unsaturated fatty acid foods such as peanut, olive and safflower oils, would go a long way toward supplying some kind of insurance against the hazards of radiation. If the body's own defenses are our best weapon against radiation illness (and they seem to be), let's give them something to work with!

Foods and Fall-Out
By Robert Rodale

What foods you eat govern, to a large extent, the amount of radioactivity from fall-out that will accumulate in your bones. Also —and equally important—it has been found that building up your health through an adequate diet and the use of certain natural food supplements, is likely to provide protection against the effects of radiation build-up.

The role of food in both introducing radioactivity into your diet and protecting you against the effects of radioactivity assumes renewed importance in view of the large-scale Russian and American atom tests. During the moratorium on testing, the amount of strontium 90 in the atmosphere and in our food had begun to decrease, and there was a cautious feeling that the worst was over. Now that feeling of relief (however slight) is gone and we must gird for future bouts with strontium 90 and possibly other fission products—radioactive iodine and cesium.

Exactly how serious the fall-out problem will become in the future, no one can say with certainty. It should be kept in mind that the fall-out from these tests creates an entirely different problem than the fall-out that might result from an atomic war. Our concern at this time is primarily for the changes that slight increases in radioactivity might have on our persons and our environment over a long period of time. The Atomic Age has given man, for the first time, the ability to work a change over the entire atmosphere. The degree of that change is admittedly slight, but it will remain for many years.

Any immediate harm that might be done by atomic test fall-out would be to susceptible groups in the population who would either contact fall-out "hot spots" in our environment or who would encounter higher than average doses of strontium 90 through their own eating and living habits. While the government spokesmen are probably right in saying that the *average* person has nothing to fear from fall-out at this time, we are not all average in our habits or bodily health. For example, whole wheat is more susceptible to strontium 90 contamination than almost any other food, but the government has not seen fit to call attention to that fact, because only 3 per cent of our wheat is consumed in the whole grain form, while 97 per cent of wheat is consumed as white flour, from which much of the strontium is removed when the bran is separated from the rest of the kernel. However, there are some people who eat all their wheat in whole grain form. By so doing, they are subjecting themselves to amounts of strontium 90 in excess of that received by the average American, who eats nothing but white flour.

Perhaps even more important than knowing how to peer behind the averages, is to understand how your body reacts to strontium 90. We respond to this poison in a way that makes it difficult to know just how much of it is being retained in our systems. Much of the strontium 90 we consume passes right through us, so it is with the portion that is retained in our flesh and bones that we are most concerned. Strontium is a very close relative to calcium and the two are usually found together. But animals and human beings have a very important safety mechanism built into their systems that enables them to select calcium for absorption in preference to strontium. For that reason, we are most concerned to find out the proportion of calcium to strontium 90 in a food. The mere knowledge of how much strontium 90 alone is present is meaningless, for that knowledge gives little or no clues as to what damage that strontium 90 might do. For example, milk contributes roughly 40 per cent of all the strontium 90 that is *consumed* by Americans. But because milk is relatively rich in calcium, we *retain* only 1/5 to 1/20 as much strontium 90 from milk as we do from vegetables, cereals and other items of the diet. (*Nutrition Reviews,* July, 1960, p. 199.)

The Strontium Unit

To simplify the problem of understanding strontium 90 contamination, the scientific world wisely developed the figure known as the "strontium unit" which expresses the number of micromicrocuries of strontium 90 *per gram of calcium* in a food. So if you know the strontium unit value of a food, you know not the total amount of strontium 90 in that food, but the amount that your system is likely to retain—which is vastly more important.

The foods with the highest strontium unit value are vegetables, cereals and fruits. The reason is that these foods are most exposed to air-borne fall-out. Corn has about 28 strontium units, cauliflower has 22 units, okra 18 units and Brussels sprouts 12 units. Husks and shells protect some foods to a certain extent. Lima beans, for example, rate at about 8.5 units. Evidently, the fact that their husks are discarded reduces their strontium content. Wheat averages about 25 units, although values of from 10 to 300 units have been reported for isolated samples. White flour has 12 strontium units, according to a report of bread sold in New York City made by the Atomic Energy Commission. Fruits have a slightly lower strontium 90 unit value than vegetables and cereals.

Foods produced by animals—meat, milk and eggs—generally have about one-third the strontium unit value of vegetables, cereals and fruits. An average strontium unit figure for these foods would be about 6, with variations according to the diet of the animals and their geographical location. Meat, milk and eggs afford more protection against strontium 90 contamination because the bodies of the animals have acted as filters, taking in larger proportions of calcium than strontium. When we consume the animals, we get the benefit of the selecting that they have done. The ability of cattle to prefer calcium over strontium is illustrated very well by reports of the condition of a herd of Hereford cattle that has grazed for two years at the Nevada Proving Grounds of the Atomic Energy Commission. Over 100 atomic explosions have taken place at this 600 square mile area. Yet, when these cattle were slaughtered, they showed only normal amounts of strontium 90 in their meat and bones. So it is apparent that by using meat as an important part of the diet, we are protecting ourselves to a degree against strontium 90.

Fall-Out in Foods and Environment

The lowest strontium unit value of any food is found in ocean fish. There are two reasons. First, the ocean provides tremendous dilution for fall-out. Unlike the soil, the ocean has no solid surface on which strontium 90 can accumulate. Second, ocean water contains liberal amounts of calcium. Fish living in the ocean always have a liberal supply of calcium and can, therefore, select it for absorption in preference to strontium 90. Tests of ocean fish made by a commercial laboratory show a rating of roughly one-quarter of a strontium unit for fish meal. By comparison, that is about 1/100th of the amount of strontium 90 in wheat. The value of the ocean as a fall-out-free source of food is recognized by the government, for the research director of one of the large fish processing companies told us that, in the event of nuclear war, plans would be put into action to attempt to feed the United States population from the ocean.

While we are primarily concerned here with fall-out in foods, it should also be mentioned that the air and the water we drink are carriers of strontium 90. However, the amounts we receive from those sources are much smaller than the amounts we receive from our food. There is one exception that I am aware of, and that is water from cisterns. It has been reported that cistern water, collected from roofs of dwellings, is considerably higher in strontium 90 than well water. If a cistern is your only source of drinking water, it might be advisable for you to attempt to obtain bottled well water or spring water.

Fall-out risks, such as the drinking of cistern water, should also be weighed in terms of the susceptibility of the people in the household. Children are depositing much more calcium in their bones than are adults and, therefore, strontium 90 contamination is a matter of more concern to them. The average child today has retained several times more strontium 90 in his body than the average adult. And since it seems likely that the atomic age is here to stay, children will have to face the radioactivity problem for years to come.

Whether or not you should change your diet to attempt to take in less strontium 90 in your system is a difficult question to answer. The government advises that at this time, the hazard is not serious enough to warrant any changes in diet. However, no one knows what the future will bring and the ultimate effect of the amounts of strontium 90 we are now subjected to are not completely understood. The use of calcium supplements will help reduce that amount of strontium 90 that is retained by the body and is a practice whose worth can not be denied.

Reducing

Don't Count Calories, Count Nutrients

We are a people of fads. It shows in our buildings, our clothes, our cars and in our diets. Diet fads come and go rapidly and frequently, and anyone who has been reading newspapers and magazines for even a few years can tick off 4 or 5 diet crazes that Americans have undergone in that time. Remember the rice diet, the Rockefeller diet, the 900-calories-a-day meals, to name a few?

Each of these has the same basic fault: nobody can or will stay with them indefinitely. The fellow on the canned liquid meals is living for the day he can sit down to a roast beef dinner and the lady who has been suffering with bland rice can't wait for her first banana split. Of course, a return to the same foods that made one heavy before will make one heavy again. No reducing diet is realistic and practical unless it consists of normal food schedules that can be used indefinitely to maintain a safe and healthful body weight. If the diet you are eating to lose weight is not the type that you would be willing to maintain for the rest of your days, it is likely to be a waste of time.

With this general attitude in mind, we approached a best-selling book on diet, *Calories Don't Count,* by Herman Taller, M.D. In many ways, we were pleased to discover, the suggestions in the book do give the dieter the hope of losing weight by eating a diet he can hope to live with. Principally, Dr. Taller's theory on losing weight has, as the title of his book would infer, nothing at all to do with the number of calories one ingests in the course of a day's eating. Instead, the amount of carbohydrate in the diet is severely limited and the amount of fat is unlimited. It is interesting, first of all, to notice that both fats and carbohydrates are elements that are high in calories. So, in effect, Dr. Taller is saying, "Substitute this high-calorie food for that one."

Dr. Taller's Reasoning

The reasoning behind Dr. Taller's theory is simply this: the body burns fat much more efficiently than it burns carbohydrates. Dr. Taller says that a fat person eating a large amount of fat burns it up at 3 times the rate of a lean man eating fats. This stepped-up fat metabolism works not only on fats just taken in, but on the fat that has been around for a while—the fat that makes heavy thighs and bulging midriffs.

Eating carbohydrates has almost the opposite effect. True, they are converted, in part, into energy, but fat people always seem to eat more energy than they can use. The balance accumulates in the

691

system, in the form of pyruvic acid, and is itself ultimately converted into more fat.

It is only fair to remark here that there is plenty of argument about Dr. Taller's theory among medical men, but the fact is that, if positive proof of what goes on inside the body is demanded, his guess is as good as the next man's. A large body of medical science insists that the number of calories one eats will tell the story. It says that whether one consumes 5,000 calories in walnuts or whether one consumes them in the form of chocolate eclairs, the end result is the same: the body is saddled with 5,000 calories it must burn off, otherwise they will accumulate to form heavy arms, unwieldy buttocks or necks that won't allow a collar to be buttoned. Dr. Taller's view is that a great deal depends upon the kind of food that contains the calories. The body can handle some kinds of foods with ease, while it cannot handle others nearly as efficiently. Eat your calories in a food your body can process and worry no more; eat calorie-rich foods that present a problem to the body and the calories will accumulate.

Up to this point we go along with Dr. Taller's general reasoning. We believe, too, that it is the *kind* of food one eats, not how much, that counts. It is possible that the time of day at which calories are consumed can have an effect, because of our personal activities schedule.

We have often expressed dissatisfaction with the theory of calorie counting. We believe it is discouraging, annoying and likely to be unhealthful. Who would deny the discouragement a big eater can feel in surveying the meager dinner a 1,200 calorie diet affords? What dieter does not feel a strong temptation to throw it all over as he carefully measures out his calorie quota of baked potatoes and chopped beef? But most important, what calorie counter has not indulged himself in unhealthful foods at the expense of the kind of foods he should be eating?

Every Bite Must Count

When one is limping along on a minimum calorie intake, every piece of food one does eat has to count in the maintenance of bodily health. A candy bar doesn't help a bit; it actually takes away from the body's stores of important nutrients. A piece of liver, on the other hand, does the double duty of satisfying hunger and bolstering the body's nutritional store.

Many dieters, given 1,200 calories to spend in a day, tend to ignore the importance of *how* they spend them. They might feel like having a pecan roll for breakfast—so they eat the roll with a calorie-free cup of coffee as a substitute for the eggs and fruit their diet suggests. If similar substitutions occur throughout the day, then the successful dieter must expect, not slim good health, but skinny malnutrition.

We believe that *everyone,* weight watcher or not, should pursue a diet of natural unprocessed foods and with few exceptions, eat as much of them as he likes as often as he likes. Dr. Taller differs with our concept in that he says one *must* eat as much of the fatty foods as one can—hungry or not—one must scrupulously avoid all but a small percentage of the whole range of carbohydrate foods— natural or not.

Foods rich in unsaturated fats have always been high on our list of recommendations. We are in favor of all types of liquid vegetable oils to be used in salads and in cooking, at every opportunity. They stimulate production of hormones which release fats stored around the body. We think fat-rich avocados and soybeans are two excellent foods. We do not believe, however, that these fats should be compared for health value with vegetable fats used in frying and those contained in margarine. Dr. Taller recommends a deliberate attempt to include fried foods and margarine in the daily diet. Researchers have shown that fried foods present a variety of dangers to the body, even if it were true that the fats used to prepare them help one to lose weight. More to our liking is the book's recommendation that one eat fish or sea food each day for the valuable unsaturated fatty acids.

Dr. Taller advises against saturated fats (the solid shortenings that come in cans), yet he is in favor of margarine—50 per cent of which is saturated fat in the form of hydrogenated vegetable oil. He would have his dieters avoid animal fats, even to cutting visible fat from the meats they eat, then he specifies such fatty meats as pork, ham and bacon, over the leaner meats. We believe that fatty meats are to be avoided whenever possible and that animal fats, whether one can see them to cut them off or whether they occur in the fiber of the meat, present the body with just the same kind of problem. Dr. Taller includes butter in this list of animal fats to be avoided and suggests curtailment of one's milk intake. We, of course, agree.

Carbohydrates Do Not Have to Be Complex

The question of carbohydrates is a simple one from our viewpoint, while Dr. Taller raises it to a new high in complexity. Of course, the body needs some carbohydrate to function. It is the energy food. Generally, one does not go too far wrong if one classes sweets as carbohydrate foods—candies, ice creams, sodas, cakes, etc. These are rich in carbohydrate; sometimes, they are almost pure carbohydrate. They are also unnatural sweets. We are opposed to their use, less because they are carbohydrates than because they are artificial foods which the body is not prepared to handle. We see no reason, though, for eliminating such nutritious foods as apples, grapes, peaches, fresh pineapples, figs or raisins, merely because they contain more than 5 per cent carbohydrate. They have elements the body needs for its operation. The same holds true for carbohydrate-rich fresh vegetables.

Calories Don't Count is strong in condemning bread as a source of unwanted poundage. Aside from being high in carbohydrates, the grain products offered today are so processed that they have little left to offer in the way of nutrition. So they are useless by both Dr. Taller's yardstick and ours. Slim nutrition, allergies and constipation are 3 marks of modern breads. Bread is the most prominent cereal food, but macaroni, crackers, doughnuts, noodles, all American favorites, are also included in the ban. Dr. Taller favors only gluten bread (a bread free of most carbohydrate). We are against its use as well as other breads.

Salt and Cereal Foods

Salt is another of those common foods which hold on to extra weight in the body. Dr. Taller advises, and we agree, that one eat as little as possible, though Dr. Taller promotes such high-salt meats as bacon and ham. He makes the interesting point that cereal foods (bread, crackers, doughnuts, etc.) are responsible, in a large way, for the great amounts of salt many of us eat. Cereal foods contain considerable amounts of potassium, which, once in the body, lowers the amount of sodium there. This means the body craves more sodium —in the handy form of salt (sodium chloride). So, if one stays away from bread and other cereal foods, one can avoid undue use of salt with much less effort.

In one section of his book, Dr. Taller summarizes the dieter's do's and don't's. We must take exception to a few points. He encourages the eating of foods fried in vegetable oils (preferably safflower or corn oil or margarine). We oppose all food frying—with the possible exception of scrambled eggs ever so lightly fried in vegetable oil. We see no merit in margarine for spreading and frying. Dr. Taller forbids the use of high-carbohydrate dried foods. If they have been dried by natural means, we believe the nutritional value of foods preserved in this way is unquestionable. While he opposes the use of butter and heavy cream, Dr. Taller is in favor of all cheeses. Are they not rich in the type of fats he would disallow? We say avoid all milk products, including cheese. In the case of soft drinks, Dr. Taller's only objection is the use of the pure carbohydrate sugar in them and will allow soft drinks sweetened artificially. We frown on unnatural sweets of all kinds, as well as the artificial colorings and flavorings in today's soft drinks. There is no emphasis on exercise in the book. Editor Rodale believes this to be an important factor in any reducing plan. Walking is one of the best types of exercise.

We Agree on Essentials

We are in agreement with *Calories Don't Count* on many important points. Where we disagree, it is because Dr. Taller's main interest in dieting is to lose weight, while our main interest in diet is to maintain good health. In our program, establishing proper weight level is an effortless bonus. While Mr. Rodale does not condemn all carbohydrate foods (for many are rich in nutrients), those foods he does condemn turn out to be the highest in content of useless carbohydrates—the very ones Dr. Taller says will put on weight fastest. Mr. Rodale is in favor of foods rich in unsaturated fats for their health value; if they also burn off unwanted fat in the body, so much the better. Cereals are opposed by Editor Rodale and Dr. Taller for reasons of health and weight gain.

We are happy to see public acceptance of a diet such as Dr. Taller's. It is believable and possible for one to lose weight following it and to form good eating habits in doing so. Aside from the few objections we have already registered and the easy changes that suggest themselves in the light of these objections, we believe that Dr. Taller's can be a healthful, effective reducing diet.

What About the Liquid Reducing Diets?

"No fuss, no bother, just pour and serve!"

"Now it's convenient to take your diet with you!"

"Diet with a purpose!"

"Easy, simple way to reduce!"

"Weight control formula—now fresh, ready to drink!"

These are some of the enticing headlines over ads for America's latest craze—the liquid reducing diet that you carry with you and mix with water or pour from a carton—the less-than-a-thousand-calories-a-day, synthetic, lifeless, powdered concoction that bears as much resemblance to food as shredded cardboard does. Except that it's flavored, of course—with anything from vanilla through chocolate, butterscotch, coffee, orange, eggnog, banana or scotch and rum.

Competition and Quality of Formulas

The new craze started on a nation-wide scale in 1959 and *Advertising Age* for December 5, 1960, advised us that the market had gone from zero to nearly 100,000,000 dollars, while the amount spent on advertising was expected to be $20,000,000.

The actual content of the new concoctions is carefully designed to meet the official requirements for dietary need. One half pound a day, which is all the dieter has to eat, according to the directions, contains the proper amount (officially) of protein, fat, carbohydrate, all the vitamins for which official requirement levels have been set and several others which have not been so recognized officially, all the officially important minerals and several trace minerals. The "food" is composed of powdered milk, soybeans, sucrose, corn oil, brewer's yeast, coconut oil and lots and lots of synthetics—vitamins, flavorings, etc. As competition grows more intense and cut-rate products begin to appear, there is no doubt that the formula will get steadily less nourishing.

Different Types of Reducing Tests Made

Long before the first of these popular dieting foods, *Metrecal,* was released, it was tested by a Florida physician on 57 patients who were trying to reduce. Dr. H. J. Roberts reported on his experiences in the November-December, 1960, issue of the *American Journal of Clinical Nutrition.* Dr. Roberts worked out a number of different ways the preparation could be used—alone, as the sole food for a given period of time, alternating with carefully restricted diet of real food for certain days or as an addition to real food at certain meals. Of his group of patients, 21 per cent lost 20 pounds or more, 48 per cent lost from 10 to 19 pounds. He says that these results compare favorably with other suggested diet regimes.

Let's go a little further into some of the results. Dr. Roberts believes that constipation is a natural accompaniment to any reducing program and hence, he was not surprised that some of his patients complained of constipation. One of the original patients dropped out because of it. Three others developed diarrhea, 3 others believed they could not stand the cramps from constipation or the other digestive disorders they encountered. One woman could not stand the smell of the preparation, so she dropped out. The constipated folks were given a laxative; the nervous ones, who might go on food binges if they encountered some emotional stress, were given sedatives. Participants were allowed, nay, urged to drink non-fattening liquids —coffee, tea, clear bouillon, etc. to help combat the tendency to constipation. Lettuce, tomatoes, celery and other raw vegetables were added to the diet from time to time. "Other gastrointestinal symptoms, relating to abdominal cramps, gas and heartburn, were encountered in 10 patients," says Dr. Roberts. Most of these, however, already had a history of disorders of this kind. Several patients complained of a bad taste in the mouth or a coated tongue after taking the reducing diet.

Patient First Needs Dietary Education

Wasn't the diet terribly monotonous? Well, you could always use different flavors of *Metrecal,* drink lots of tea and coffee and eat raw vegetables.

We are glad to say that Dr. Roberts states that such a diet program should not be undertaken just as a short cut to weight reduction, without some effort being made to educate the patient as to what he should eat to maintain proper weight. He says, too, that "close medical supervision is highly important when any weight-reducing diet which contains less than 1,000 calories per day is undertaken." He reminds us that one would do well not to lose weight at all, rather than to lose large amounts periodically and then put it right back on again. We were astonished to read, too, this statement: "Patients beginning a long-term weight reducing program should be continually reminded that this is one of the most severely disciplining experiences with which a person in our society can be challenged."

What a shameful admission of the terrible states of modern eating habits and the condition of modern food! What must it sound like to starving peoples in other parts of the world—one of the most severe disciplines a modern American can be subjected to is cutting down on food!

We believe that all the so-called "calorie-metered" liquid reducing foods (there were at least 75 at last count) are harmful and to be avoided by any health-conscious person. The reasons are obvious. Overweight comes from eating the wrong kind of food and taking too little exercise. A "crash" diet, dramatized and made much of for a period of several weeks or months, may take off a few pounds after which the hungry reducer will go back to eating just what he ate before and in a short time, will be back where he started.

It's all very well for Dr. Roberts to point out to his physician readers the necessity for education as to proper diet that *must* accompany any successful use of these reducing preparations. Safe to say, no part of that 20,000,000 dollar advertising budget will be spent telling Americans anything about what they should be eating. We haven't a doubt that many overweight people will take one of the diet drinks *in addition* to the badly planned diet they are already eating and will merely increase their problems many times over.

Dr. Frederick Stare and other widely read columnists whose financial backing comes from the food companies, will continue to attack any writer who recommends a soundly nutritious diet, with diet supplements, thus leading our poor obese friends even farther from the path they should be following.

And finally, the craze will die, as other crazes have died, and no one will have learned anything about how to prevent overweight, no one will have established the good food and exercise habits that must be established if one wants to avoid overweight. The drug companies and the dairies will be many millions of dollars richer and once again, a discouraged John Public and his missus will have been the victims of another "easy-way" scheme to quick success—this time, success in losing weight.

Definition of a Fad

Perhaps most astonishing of all, is the fact that no one will call the manufacturers of the liquid reducer "faddists." Indeed, we have the word of the American Medical Association on the subject. Answering a question on "faddism" in the January, 1961, issue of *Today's Health,* the spokesman for the medical association says that anything which lasts for only a short period of time is a fad. So, says he, if the current craze for liquid reducing diets "settles down" and becomes an accepted thing, then it is no longer a fad, but sound nutritional practice.

We recommend eating sunflower seeds which men have been eating for centuries—a fine, well-balanced, high-protein food. This is characterized as food faddism, simply, we suppose, because the big food manufacturers do not sell sunflower seeds. We recommend eating fresh, raw fruits and vegetables, which mankind has done for thousands of years. "Food faddism" shout the "experts" who believe that fruits and vegetables should be thoroughly processed and almost ruined from the point of view of nutrition before they can be eaten. Refining sugar and flour is a fairly recent development in food technology—a "fad," by the definition given above. But let us recommend eating wheat germ rather than the worthless starch that white flour is, and the cry of "food faddist" goes up from the very same people who define a fad as something of recent origin which does not last!

Avoid Liquid Diets

We urge you to shun the liquid reducing diets for the following reasons:

1. Using them, even for a brief time, will postpone even further that happy day when you will have established a set of good eating and exercise habits, which will keep your weight at exactly the right level for the rest of your life.

2. A survey has shown that losing weight by a "crash" diet like this, then regaining, then reducing, then gaining again, is far more dangerous than simply being overweight and staying that way.

3. Quite apart from the monotony and inconvenience of the liquid diet, there is every possibility, as Dr. Roberts suggests, that you can do yourself serious harm by undertaking a syntheic diet low in calories, without doctors' supervision. Every individual is different. You may become badly deficient in some necessary food element by following such a diet.

4. Dr. T. L. Cleave, surgeon in the Royal Navy of Great Britain, has written at length on why we overeat. He tells us that the body has a perfect mechanism for regulating the appetite which can *always* be depended upon to work, *so long as you eat foods in their natural state.* If you are hungry for an apple, your body will guide

you in knowing how many apples you should eat. If, instead, you eat apple pie, the body has no "built-in" way of regulating your appetite for this food, so you are bound to eat too much. If you are hungry for something sweet and you eat a bunch of grapes, your own appetite will tell you when you have had enough, and you will not eat too many grapes. But if you eat a chocolate bar, the highly concentrated sugar in such a food is something not encountered in natural foods, your body has no mechanism for dealing with it, so you are bound to eat too much. If you are hungry for a potato, your body can tell you how many potatoes to eat, but if you French fry the potatoes, thus adding a large amount of unnatural fat to the food, your appetite regulating mechanism will not be able to tell you how much of such a food to eat. We think there is a great deal of merit to this point of view and we urge readers to try an all-natural, unprocessed diet if they wish to reduce.

5. Exercise is just as important as diet for keeping your weight at the proper level. If you cannot take regular outdoor exercise every single day, then make it a point to walk every day for as long as you can.

Eating Meat to Lose Weight

In reducing your weight, the kind of calories is far more important than how many of them you eat. This point of view receives fresh confirmation in a new book, *Strong Medicine* by Blake F. Donaldson, M.D. Based, like *Calories Don't Count,* on new scientific knowledge of the role of fats in promoting a proper fat metabolism, *Strong Medicine* contends a natural diet of fatty meat and water is all that man needs to achieve proper weight, health and vigor.

Dr. Donaldson's recommendation of the kind of fat to be eaten—meat fat—derives from primitive man. He stresses from the beginning that his recommendations are a definite departure from what most people think of as normal eating and normal dieting habits. His entire program is based upon the theory that good meat, fat left intact, regulated liquid intake and a schedule of morning walking is all one needs for losing excess weight. By that he means *all* one needs. After all, meat and water were primitive man's only food, says Donaldson, and he survived admirably. The meat intake at mealtimes is unlimited (though ½ pound is recommended). The rest (including the 30-minute walk each morning, the 6 glasses of water, and the ½ cup of coffee at meals) must be as carefully regulated as a train schedule.

We think the reasoning behind the meat intake is the most important part of the book. Dr. Donaldson began with the fact that primitive people eating primitive foods appear least likely to be overweight. He found this to be borne out in his observations of the Eskimos. Though they have the native characteristic of a round face and their heavy, loose-fitting clothes add to the bulky look, the impression they give of excessive body weight is quite mistaken. They are small and slim.

With the diet of Eskimos in mind, high in fatty meat, Dr. Donaldson set up an experimental reducing diet which called for a half pound of fresh, unsalted ground meat, preferably beef or lamb, at each meal—the meat to have about one part fat to three parts lean. In other words, eat the fat from the steak you cook, instead of removing it. The fat eaten 3 times a day is intended to stoke the systemic fires that burn off one's own excess fat.

Along with the meat, the diet allowed in some cases for an average portion of fruit of a baked or boiled potato (no salt) and one cup of black coffee or clear tea.

There was no allowance for any intake between meals, except for 6 glasses of water taken by 5 o'clock in the afternoon. (Dr. Donaldson believes that the time is important. Absence of water in the evening apparently helps the anti-fat forces to do their work, he says.) A 30-minute walk before breakfast was also part of the routine. The experimental diet was such a success that no basic changes in it have ever had to be made.

Dr. Donaldson makes a very interesting observation on the way eating carbohydrates prevents the breakdown of fat. Carbohydrates turn to sugar in the blood stream. The normal pancreas responds, when presented with sugar, by producing insulin to burn up the sugar. This hormone, insulin, is an enemy of the hormone from the pituitary gland and it will interfere with the intended action of the pituitary hormone, which is the burning of stored fat.

Dr. Donaldson's formula of ground lean meat and suet, mixed into a patty, plus coffee and the 30-minute walk, seems to be a panacea for many types of diseases. He tells of using these foods to treat ulcers, heart diseases, diabetes, arthritis, etc. We are inclined to think that it is not so much the food these patients *do* eat, but that which they eliminate that makes them well.

One Is Bound to Feel Better

What obese person suffering from arthritis or from a heart ailment would not improve if he eliminated all wheat products, all salt, all sugar products and most milk and cream products from his diet? These are the pies, cakes, breads and sauces which add weight and usually come with minimal nutritional reinforcement. Any person is much better off without them.

Once that is done, if the dieter turns to fresh, wholesome meat, with enough fat for lubrication of the intestines and energy, with some fruit or a vegetable later on, he is eating the body-building protein he needs and avoiding the unnecessary weight-adding foods. He *must* lose weight and he *must* feel better on such a regimen!

Editor Rodale is, of course, strongly in favor of Dr. Donaldson's recommendations for walking. Dr. Donaldson holds that, regardless of how much exercise one gets on the job, there is no substitute for the regular unbroken swing of a long walk. He insists on this activity with just about as much emphasis as the meat diet. He is reluctant to excuse a patient for the walk (exactly 30 minutes) in even the worst weather, and he starts the weakest of them on a walking schedule as early as possible. Many of them report a newly found feeling of well-being which they attribute in part to the regular, daily walk.

The Addiction to Bread

On the subject of bread, Dr. Donaldson writes, "Bread addiction is little different from that of alcohol or cocaine or heroin addiction and sometimes, it seems even more dangerous." In his chapter on allergies, the author puts wheat flour into a group with milk, cream, cream cheese, ice cream, eggs and chocolate. He is convinced that allergenic difficulties arise from the use of foods which were unnatural to primitive man; that is, foods which are cultivated and must be processed. Meat and fruits and certain vegetables were eaten by primitive man as they grew. There was no preparation involved for him—even meat was eaten raw.

Grains and cereal products do not fit into this primitive category—man had to *learn* to use grain products. The same is true of the milk of animals. Dr. Donaldson holds that human breast milk is the only milk that is not foreign to man and the only type, therefore, which does not introduce foreign protein (always a possible allergenic source) into his system. Dr. Donaldson defines allergy as "failure to get used to new things." His understanding of "new" is anything introduced to the human environment within the last 8,000 years. Perhaps one-third of us, he says, are so equipped by nature as to be freely adaptable to changes. The rest are likely to react in an unusual and frequently, unfortunate way. This is, of course, an allergenic manifestation.

We believe that the nutrients contained in fruits and vegetables are important as a means of reinforcing the food value of the protein and fat of meat. We are not convinced that one should choose to survive on a meat diet exclusively, even though it might be possible to do so. We believe one should take advantage of the appeal and nutrition of wholesome fruits and vegetables. Few of us have a nutritional store so rich that we can afford to ignore safe sources of vitamins and minerals.

However, if one is considering a special diet for weight loss, we would certainly prefer that one use Dr. Donaldson's suggestions rather than the liquid diets or the sheer starvation of unreasoned calorie-counting techniques that people seem to go for today. One quarrel we have with the Donaldson diet is its monotony. Though he insists that his patients do not get bored with meat, meat, meat, we believe we would. Is it not asking too much for a patient to stay on such a diet for months at a time? Of course, we are aware that the exclusive meat diet is augmented with other foods as time goes on, but we often say that good diet is one which one can maintain indefinitely without change and we doubt that one could do this with the Donaldson diet.

Dr. Donaldson's results are remarkable, as one can see by the case histories he includes in his very readable book. Following his suggestions might be just what you need to begin losing weight. Certainly, his opinions on cereal foods, dairy products and exercise will be valuable to anyone interested in maintaining good health, whether weight is a factor or not.

Religion and Diet

Some Religions Influence Diet

There are several religious groups which have in their tenets specific directions concerning the types of food and drink to be avoided by their members. It is gratifying to see that these rules usually add up to sound nutritional practices and result in better health for the people who follow them.

One of the best known of these groups are the Seventh Day Adventists. These people are exhorted by their religion to remember that their bodies are Temples of the Holy Spirit and, as such, must be carefully preserved out of respect for this function if for no other reason. To accomplish their greater bodily health, Seventh Day Adventists are directed toward vegetarianism, are advised against coffee, tea or other caffeine-containing beverages (that includes cola drinks, for they do contain caffeine). They are forbidden to smoke or to use alcoholic beverages.

That these few prohibitions have accomplished their purpose is obvious in a report given at the annual meeting of the American College of Cardiology, as described in *Food Field Reporter* (June 5, 1961) by Dr. Richard Walden, of the College of Medical Evangelists, Loma Linda, California. The report concerned 130 Seventh Day Adventists employed at the College. Their blood was checked for cholesterol levels, which were found to be 10 per cent to 30 per cent less than typical American levels. Further, it was discovered that the sharp increase in cholesterol levels usually experienced by

American males between their 20th and 40th years, was delayed 20 years in Adventists. In general, coronary disease occurs about 40 per cent less in Seventh Day Adventist males than in the general population. Aside from the obvious advantages of the non-smoking, non-drinking, non-caffeine rules, it was shown that Adventists eat 25 per cent of their calories as fats, of which more than a third are the desirable unsaturated fats. Other Americans consume an average of 42 per cent of their calories as fat, and only 15 per cent are the healthful unsaturated ones found chiefly in raw, unprocessed seed foods.

All Visible Fats Removed

The 130 subjects were divided into two groups. One was instructed to remove all visible fats from the diet—no butter, margarine, shortenings, dairy products and bakery products, except bread. They were allowed 4 eggs, 4 avocados, 40 olives a week, plus a limited quantity of raw almonds, cashews and peanuts. Carbohydrates and proteins were substituted for the lost fat calories.

The second group also cut all visible fats, but substituted liquid corn oil as shortening, a corn oil margarine, corn oil mayonnaise and baked goods made with corn oil.

Both new diets caused a drop in cholesterol levels—about 15 per cent lower than they had been at the start of the study. This new low level was characterized as about the level common to so-called primitive populations, who are very rarely troubled by heart disease. The conclusion was that either the elimination of many fats or the substitution of as many as possible with unsaturated fats will lower the average cholesterol level.

Of course, it goes without saying that the fats were not totally responsible for the values shown in this experiment. It means only that they are a factor. It shows that persons whose circulatory system is healthy can approximate the optimum cholesterol level in their blood with very little effort. Good habits make the healthy circulatory system 40 per cent more likely than if one eats, drinks and smokes indiscriminately.

Healthy Teeth, Too

The Seventh Day Adventists came out on top again in a test for healthy teeth, which was conducted in Maryland and reported in *Public Health Reports* (March, 1961). Dr. C. J. Donnelly made a study of 290 Adventist children with a control group of non-Adventist children in the same area. It was found that the Seventh Day Adventist children, between ages 10 and 13, had 40 per cent fewer decayed, missing and filled teeth than the control children. Two doctors, who conducted a similar test previously, were quoted as saying that "the lower rate (of decay) among the Adventists might result from their educational program which discourages the excessive use of sweets and snacking between meals."

In Colorado, another dental test was conducted in which Seventh Day Adventist children made a showing of 300 per cent less cavities than their contemporaries who came from families not health-conscious. The test was repeated, and again Seventh Day Adventist children were found to be superior. Why not? They avoid soda and sweets.

The Mormons have similar prohibitions concerning diet. They are forbidden to use tea, coffee, cocoa, soft drinks, alcohol and tobacco. As a consequence, their cancer rate is comfortingly low.

A Salvation Army Experiment

The Salvation Army does not have any dietary regulations for their members, so far as we have been able to discover. However, in 1949, the Army decided to try out a health diet at their children's home, The Haven, in London. They began gradually. The 30 children were to eat 3 substantial meals a day containing meat, cheese, fish, eggs, etc. Fifty per cent of the food was to be served raw, along with "hard" food (crusty bread, etc.). Raw fruits were substituted for desserts and plenty of raw vegetables were included in the menus. In telling of the experiment, A. B. Cunning, M.B., and F. R. Innes, M.B., in their book, *We Are What We Eat,* say: "What has astonished the authorities are the high spirits of the children and The Haven has been called The House of Merriment. Here, the children have glossy hair, their skins are clear, they get over colds or other little minor ailments quickly. Their teeth are good, not perfect, but much above the average school child."

Christian Science prohibits injections and the use of drugs. We believe this rule will save more lives than it will cost. Drugs and vaccines have serious side effects and are often used indiscriminately, without necessity. Careful diet will help the body in preparing to defend itself against invasion by infectious bacteria. The body is equipped to do this job very well if it is properly nourished. No drugs needed.

Religious dietary regulations sometimes offer a good means of comparing the effects on health that the absence of certain foods can have. The two experiments with Seventh Day Adventists definitely showed that heart disease and tooth decay are less likely to occur when smoking, alcohol, sweets and caffeine are kept to a minimum or completely avoided. One does not have to change religions to take advantage of this clue. Observant parents will use this information to protect themselves and their children from uncomfortable and very serious disabilities.

Reproduction

Help for the Childless Couple

For most people, conception of children presents little or no difficulty. In the United States, according to generally accepted and often quoted figures, 85 per cent of all married couples have children, and of the remaining 15 per cent, about half are childless by choice. That leaves only 7½ per cent actually unable to have children.

Yet, the desire for offspring is so basic, the failure to have them so bitter and emotionally disturbing, that reproduction has been considered through all history to be a major concern of medical practitioners. In ancient times, the chief hold of pagan goddesses, such as Ishtar, Isis and Aphrodite, on their worshippers was their supposed ability to confer fertility. The Book of Genesis records the lifelong struggle of Sarah to have a child. The "wise women" and witches of the Middle Ages, had a steady clientele of childless women. And our doctors today find ready subjects for their experiments with hormones in unhappy, childless couples.

The possible causes of infertility are so many, varied and complex, it would take a substantial book to examine them all in detail. But that is hardly necessary here, for what is most important is that modern researches are now tending to demonstrate that in most cases, infertility can be overcome without resorting to dangerous and unpredictable drugs, and certainly without surgical techniques of internal treatment. For this, our principal thanks are due the Wistar Institute of the University of Pennsylvania, where Dr. Edmond J. Farris pioneered a remarkable new technique for accurately timing ovulation.

The Rat Hyperemia Test

Known as the rat hyperemia test, the technique consists of taking a urine specimen every morning for a period of from 5 to 10 days following the end of the menstrual period. Each day, the urine is injected into a female of a special strain of white rats developed and bred for this purpose by the Wistar Institute. Two hours later, the rat is painlessly killed by illuminating gas and her ovaries examined. From the particular quality of redness (hyperemia), it is determined on which day ovulation has begun.

Repeated over 3 successive months, this test will accurately predict, within 6 to 12 hours, the time ovulation will begin.

This is remarkable in itself, but even more remarkable is the fact that women from all over the country, who have unsuccessfully been given estrogenic hormones and whose husbands have been dosed with testosterone in efforts to achieve conception, have finally managed to have children without any drugs when they found a doctor who would take the trouble to time their ovulation by the rat hyperemia test.

Writing in the *American Journal of Obstetrics and Gynecology* in 1952, Dr. Farris was able to report then that, in experiments with 148 women, all given up as infertile by their own doctors, he had helped them to achieve 150 conceptions.

Typical of what the actual problems turned out to be was the one of Mrs. Agnes Wolf, which she described in an article in *Cosmopolitan* (December, 1954). Mrs. Wolf had a very short—one day—ovulation period, and had a blockage in one of her Fallopian tubes. This meant that she was able to conceive on only 6 days in an entire year. By pinpointing the times of ovulation, she was able to have two children.

Few Causes of Barrenness

In terms of our theoretical understanding of the problem of childlessness, the success of the Wistar Institute experiments confirms what many of us have long believed. In the words of Dr. T. N. A. Jeffcoate in the *British Medical Journal* (July, 1951), "Fertility and infertility are relative rather than absolute states, comparatively few individuals being either completely sterile or fully fertile. "What this means to us is that there is practically no such thing as a naturally barren person. There are practically always causes for lack of offspring. In some cases, such as the closing of both Fallopian tubes due to an infection in the uterus, venereal disease, etc., there does not seem to be anything that can be done except to discover the hopelessness of the situation and make it known to the woman.

In most cases, however, the real problem is not barrenness but simply low fertility. In other words, it is not that conception is impossible, but just that it does not take place. Dr. Jeffcoate, who is Professor of Obstetrics and Gynecology at the University of Liverpool, says in the same *British Medical Journal* article, in discussing male infertility: ". . . it is by no means uncommon for men with extremely low sperm counts to be responsible for an occasional pregnancy. It should never be said that pregnancy is *impossible,* even if *no* spermatozoa can be found."

Treatment of the Male

Since reduced fertility of the husband is found in approximately half of all childless marriages, it is apparent that one broad avenue of help for the childless lies in increasing the fertility of the male partner. Doctors have experimented with a wide variety of techniques and substances to accomplish this end.

In a paper read to the Symposium on Infertility Problems at the 104th Annual Meeting of the American Medical Association (1955), Edward Tyler, M.D., and Heron Singher, Ph.D., made a comprehensive report in which they examined the results of various therapies. These included administration of thyroid extract testosterone, gonadotropins, liver and lipotropic substances, weight reduction and improvement of health habits and prostate massage. They concluded that none of these measures was spectacularly successful, but the most successful of them was the eating of therapeutic amounts of liver and lipotropic substances.

It seems most significant to us that combining the successful results obtained by liver therapy with the successes attributed to "general measures" for health improvement, we find that 26 per cent of the men participating in the experiment were helped by what was basically improved nutrition. This is a far higher figure than that for men supposed to be helped by any other means. It is almost 4 times the figure for men aided by prostatic massage and 3 times the figure for men who gained an increased sperm count through the use of testosterone.

Drs. Tyler and Singher made no mention of vitamin E therapy, which we can suppose was unfamiliar to them, even though, as early as 1952, Dr. Evan Shute of the Shute Clinic in London, Ontario, had reported, in the *Urologic and Cutaneous Review,* that he had personally achieved numerous improvements in spermatogenesis, in many cases bringing complete normalcy, with a dose of 10 milligrams a day of vitamin E (alpha tocopherol) for two weeks. Dr. Shute did not claim success in all cases. He did point out, however, that vitamin E is helpful in many cases and, where it is not going to help, it is possible to determine that fact within two weeks.

Dr. Shute's results showed that vitamin E therapy increased the sperm count in 48 per cent of the men treated, helped 67 per cent to generate only live sperms when they had previously had either all or a high proportion of their sperms dead and produced all normal forms in 56 per cent of the men that had morphologically abnormal sperms before treatment.

If we project a synthesis of Dr. Shute's results with vitamin E with the other nutritional measures reported on by Drs. Tyler and Singher, we find that we are justified in supposing that a clear majority—in fact, a very large proportion—of infertile men can achieve a marked increase in fertility through proper nutrition.

Among the facts cited, but not interpreted, by Tyler and Singher, we find that in the seminal fluid, the sperm are protected by ascorbic acid (vitamin C) and that the seminal fluid of infertile men shows abnormalities in its amino acid composition.

A Problem of Overall Health

This gives further reinforcement to our idea that fertility, like so many other supposedly medical problems, may turn out, in most cases, to be simply a problem of overall health. This is not true in all cases, of course. It is well known that mumps, gonorrhea and other diseases can result in sterility. Where there is such a cause, a medical check-up and analysis will reveal it.

But most failure to conceive has no such specific cause and there, we can be sure, overall health plays a major role. In fact, in view of the general low level of nutrition in our modern world, it seems to us miraculous and a testament to man's fantastic survival potential that 85 per cent of married couples *do* have children without any apparent difficulty.

It is also fantastic, in view of the failures, reported over and over, of hormones, prostate massage and X-ray therapy to alleviate infertility in any but a few isolated cases, that so many doctors turn to these measures first, without any consideration of general health factors. In the *British Medical Journal,* as far back as May, 1951, Drs. Margaret Moore White and Mary Barton pointed out that it was incorrect to suppose that hormone treatment was necessary for low-grade sperm. ". . . it is the first duty of the physician to eliminate nutritional and other adverse conditions affecting general health."

It is our firm belief that a large proportion of barren marriages can achieve children by improving the general health of both partners, with particular emphasis on certain elements:

1. Be sure the diet includes substantial amounts of high-grade protein. Eggs, liver and other organ meats and desiccated liver supplements should be especially helpful. The eggs, by preference, should be fertile.

2. Eliminate, or at least cut down on, smoking. Smoking drives vitamin C out of the system. This vitamin is essential to health and, as we have seen, it plays a special role in protecting and nourishing the sperm.

3. Eat plenty of wheat germ and sunflower seeds, both rich sources of vitamin E. Corn oil in salads will provide more. The unsaturated fatty acids in these foods are also thought by some investigators to have a beneficial effect on fertility.

4. Take a good supply of vitamin and mineral supplements derived from natural organic sources.

5. Do enough walking or other mild exercise to maintain good tone in your circulation. Get plenty of rest and, if it is at all possible, spend as much time as you can outdoors, breathing fresh country air.

Sexual Technique

In addition, there are certain elements of sexual technique that can help to achieve conception:

1. Each month, for 3 months (as recommended by Dr. Farris of the Wistar Institute), count the exact number of days from the end of one menstrual cycle to the beginning of the next. Add the 3

figures obtained and divide by 6. The resulting number (say 12, for example) will give you the number of days after the end of menstruation (12 in our example) until the midcycle day.

2. Starting two days before midcycle day, the 10th day after menstruation ends in our example, practice coitus once a day for 3 days. To achieve the greatest activity of the sperm, coitus should first be practiced 5 days sooner, and then abstained from for 5 days.

3. If fertilization is not achieved in 4 months, put the entire schedule back one day. If that doesn't work in 4 months, put the schedule ahead two days.

4. It is not necessary for the woman to have an orgasm. She should, however, experience enough vaginal stimulation, to have a good vaginal secretion of mucus.

If, after following this schedule with variations for a year, there still has been no conception, then medical examination of both partners is advisable. In such a case, the precise ovulation timing of the rat hyperemia test will very often help bring about the desired result, without resort to the dangers of hormones, X-ray and surgery.

Rh Factor

Understanding the Rh Factor

"Rh factor" is a common medical term these days. You hear it most from newlyweds or expectant mothers. These are the groups most aware of the Rh factor, due to premarital blood tests and to the problem the Rh negative finding presents during pregnancy. People talk about Rh factor, but most people don't have any idea of what it is and why it creates a problem.

Most People Possess the Rh Factor

Rh is a factor, or ingredient, in the blood. Most persons possess it and these are described as *Rh positive*. There are some individuals who do not have this Rh factor in their blood and they are designated as *Rh negative*. It is no more abnormal to be Rh negative than it is to have natural platinum blonde hair. It's just something out of the ordinary. The individual who is Rh negative is perfectly well and healthy. However, when Rh positive and Rh negative blood is mixed in the unborn child or as the result of careless transfusions, the situation must be viewed in a new light.

When Rh negative and Rh positive blood are mixed, the Rh negative blood fights against the stranger (the Rh factor) by manufacturing antibodies, just as it would any other invader, such as a virus or an infectious organism. The antibodies destroy the Rh positive cells. These broken-down blood cells are extremely poisonous.

Care Must Be Taken to Use Proper Type

Of course, such a mixture of the blood can only occur in blood transfusions or in pregnancy. In transfusions, care must be taken to use the proper blood type. If an Rh negative woman conceives an Rh positive child, the reaction caused by the possible mixture of the two blood types can lead to serious danger for the child. The child may develop a disease known as erythroblastosis, a blood disease of the newborn.

Erythroblastosis is the result of the interaction between the Rh negative blood of the mother and the Rh positive blood of the child. It is not uncommon for some of the infant's blood accidentally to leak into the blood stream of the mother, even though both blood streams are essentially independent. This causes antibodies to form in the mother's blood. These antibodies do not endanger the mother, but when they get back into the circulation of the infant, they begin to destroy its red blood cells. The result is erythroblastosis.

What Can Be Done

The disease itself varies in severity, depending upon the number of antibodies produced in the mother's blood stream. The case may be so mild that the infant will recover on his own or it can be so severe that the child will die, even in spite of prompt treatment. The treatment now commonly employed consists of exchange transfusions immediately after the baby is born. This procedure involves slowly removing from the circulation of the infant its partly destroyed poisonous blood, at the same time replacing it with fresh, healthy blood.

If a married couple finds that they have unlike Rh factors, there is bound to be concern about the chances of having children who are afflicted with erythroblastosis. An article which appeared in the *Journal of the Kentucky State Medical Association* (June, 1955) offers some reassurance. The author, Glenn W. Bryant, M.D., stated that the vast majority of Rh negative women do not produce antibodies. Even those who do usually have one or more normal children before any problem develops. Husbands who are Rh positive still father Rh negative children in 50 per cent of cases where the mother is Rh negative. These children are, of course, perfectly normal. Overall, there is only one case of erythroblastosis in 200 recorded births, and one case in 26 births resulting from incompatible Rh matings. Finally, the chance for complete normalcy in an afflicted infant is much better today, with the exchange transfusion technique.

Predicting Severity

An expectant mother who knows her blood is Rh negative should be checked frequently for the development of antibodies in her blood stream. There are laboratory tests which can determine the presence of antibodies and their rate of increase. If they increase rapidly in the last stages of pregnancy, erythroblastosis can be expected in the infant. Preparations can then be made in advance for the exchange transfusion.

Dr. Bryant mentions that there was, at one time, a tendency for some doctors to interrupt the pregnancy of an expectant mother whose blood showed a high level of antibodies, by means of Caesarean section. However, the infants delivered in this way fared badly and many developed severe disorders of the central nervous system.

Dr. Bryant says that the procedure has been abandoned, except in rare cases in which a patient has already had an erythroblastic stillborn baby, whose death in the womb can be placed at just a few days before term delivery. In such cases, Dr. Bryant believes labor should be induced before the full term of pregnancy has been completed. Otherwise, the baby afflicted with a conventional case of erythroblastosis seems to have some protection so long as he is in the uterus. It is only shortly after delivery that he develops jaundice and increased anemia. With these facts evident, it was realized that most pregnancies in Rh-sensitized patients should be allowed to continue to term and go into labor spontaneously.

Prevent Rather Than Cure

While most researchers were resigned to anticipating Rh trouble and preparing for it as best they could, Warren M. Jacobs, M.D., was researching a hunch he had concerning the transfer of positive Rh factors from the fetus to the blood stream of the Rh negative mother. In 1956, he reported on his preliminary investigations, using bioflavonoid compounds in connection with controlling the transfer of the Rh factor from child to mother.

He reasoned this way: "It is fairly well accepted that Rh positive cells enter the maternal circulation through a break in the placenta's capillary system. Investigators have shown that, even in normal pregnancies, varying degrees of placental capillary breaks occur with some bleeding and escape of blood cells from the developing infant into the mother's blood stream. If these "breaks" could be eliminated, thought Dr. Jacobs, the transfer of these dangerous cells would be reduced or stopped entirely. Because much has been written on the use of bioflavonoids to prevent capillary weakness, this seemed to be the logical thing to use in his experiments.

In these experiments, detailed in *Surgery, Gynecology and Obstetrics* (January, 1960), Dr. Jacobs used two sets of pregnant women who were Rh negative. One set received bioflavonoids in the amount of 400 to 600 milligrams each day, the other set did not. No other intentional difference existed in the treatment of either group.

Experiment Shows Bioflavonoids Helpful

The two sets of women were further divided into 3 groups according to their experience with the problem of Rh factor as presented in pregnancy. Group I consisted of mothers who had delivered one or more infants mildly or moderately afflicted with erythroblastosis, but who had survived, and of Rh negative mothers who had had no previous pregnancy. Thirty-two such patients in the non-bioflavonoid group were observed. One infant was stillborn, 9 had severe jaundice and anemia and died shortly after birth, in spite of attempts at exchange transfusions. Twenty-two were moderately affected, were given one or more exchange transfusions and survived. The survival rate was 22 out of 32 or 68.8 per cent.

Sixteen patients in the same group were given bioflavonoids. One infant born to this group died soon after birth. Fifteen were moderately affected and all survived after transfusion. The survival rate was 15 out of 16, or 93.7 per cent.

Group II consisted of mothers who had delivered one or more live-born babies who died shortly after birth in spite of therapy. Twenty-four such patients were in the non-bioflavonoid group. Seven of their infants were stillborn and the other 17 died within hours after birth. None survived in this group.

Six patients whose histories were the same as the above, were given the bioflavonoid supplement. One infant born to these was stillborn; two died in the immediate time after birth; 3 survived after one or more transfusions. The survival rate was 3 out of 6, or 50 per cent.

Group III consisted of mothers who had delivered one or more previous stillborn infants. Fifteen such patients made up the non-bioflavonoid group. All were delivered of stillborn infants. Ten such patients were in the group given bioflavonoids. Two of their infants were stillborn. Two died almost immediately after birth. Six infants survived after therapy. The survival rate was 6 out of 10 or 60 per cent.

Worth a Try

Dr. Jacobs was quick to note that he considered the bioflavonoid group too small for drawing definite conclusions about bioflavonoids and the Rh factor, and that more studies were being done. We hope to see the results very soon.

While Dr. Jacobs declines to label his findings as conclusive, we do believe that they are worth the attention of any gynecologist or obstetrician, as well as any mother-to-be who is concerned because of an Rh incompatibility with her husband. Bioflavonoids are nothing more than natural elements found largely in citrus fruits and green peppers—in the white membranes. What is the harm in trying Dr. Jacob's regimen, especially when a chance for serious damage to the child exists if you do or if you don't? The bioflavonoids are absolutely harmless, with no side effects; they are inexpensive and easy to take. Ask your doctor to read Dr. Jacob's report in the original, if he cares to send for it, but ask him to prescribe the bioflavonoids for you if you have an Rh factor problem.

Of course, even without Rh factor difficulties, bioflavonoids should make up a part of your diet, as they occur in fresh fruits and vegetables. People who bruise easily, who have nosebleeds or who have high blood pressure should pay special attention to bioflavonoids in the diet.

Rose Hips

Roses for Health
By Robert Rodale

It is a rare flower that doesn't have a story to tell. One of my favorite flower stories relates how the rose filled an important gap in a plan to produce natural vitamins.

The story begins in 1950, when Editor J. I. Rodale decided that the organic method should be applied just as strongly to the lives of men as we apply it to the lives of plants. Why should we load up our plants with compost and mulch, he reasoned, without giving our own bodies that extra measure of protection? After all, nature is just as good a guide for the feeding of men as it is for the feeding of plants. With that thought in mind, he founded PREVENTION, a health magazine that was intended to teach people how to remain healthy by following a natural regimen.

Keystone of the Prevention system is a diet of natural foods. But J. I. Rodale realized that many people could not obtain organic foods, and that even the good values of organic foods are often wasted in cooking and storage. And sometimes it just isn't practical to get all the vitamins and minerals we need through ordinary food. What was needed to round out the Prevention plan, J. I. Rodale realized, was a complete selection of vitamins and food supplements made from food sources. Prior to that time, almost all vitamin products were synthesized from coal tar substances or other artificial sources. Just like most farmers were using chemical fertilizers, most people were taking artificial vitamins.

The Search for Food Supplements

The PREVENTION editors soon had worked out a good list of food products that were so rich in various vitamins and minerals that they could be easily concentrated into food supplement form. There was bone meal for calcium and phosphorus, yeast and desiccated liver for the B vitamins, wheat germ oil and its concentrates for vitamin E and fish liver oil for vitamins A and D. But something was missing. Where was the vitamin C to come from? Synthetic vitamin C (ascorbic acid) was synthesized from corn and potato starch and could not really be called natural. Citrus fruits are fairly rich in vitamin C, but not rich enough to concentrate into food supplements. The PREVENTION editors searched everywhere for information about foods high in vitamin C without luck. They were about to give up, and were even considering accepting synthetic vitamin C as a desperation measure, when J. I. Rodale came across an article telling how the British and Scandinavian people used rose hips—the fruit of wild roses—as vitamin C supplements during World War II when the ships carrying South African oranges could not get through. Children scoured the countryside collecting the hips, which were used in soups, preserves and tea. It was worth noting that some sources reported the health of the people in those countries was better during the war than it had been before or has been since. Children suffered from less dental decay.

The search for a vitamin C supplement was over. Inquiries were made overseas and soon, vitamin manufacturers were receiving supplies of rose hips from Europe to be made into tablets. Solving the vitamin C problem was not the end of the rose hip story, though. It was really just the beginning. One day the editors of ORGANIC GARDENING AND FARMING magazine awoke to the fact that rose hips were a subject of prime horticultural interest. Which species of roses produced the largest and richest hips, we wondered? Could they be grown in American gardens? How would the rose hips be harvested, processed and prepared? Soon, a research project was under way. Studies were made of all the garden literature, and field tests of different varieties and species were conducted at the Organic Gardening Experimental Farm. We even had hopes of eventually fostering commercial rose hip production in the United States.

Discovery of *Rosa Rugosa*

Out of our studies, one species of rose emerged head and shoulders above all the rest—*Rosa rugosa*. Not only did it have largest usable fruits of any rose, but its hips were richest in vitamin C. Vitamin analyses showed that they had as much as 3,000 milligrams of vitamin C per hundred grams—60 times as much as orange juice. We found that it grew readily in our temperate climate, and its fruits had a pleasant flavor that would incorporate well into many recipes. Rugosa hips could even be eaten right off the bush when fully ripe. Just to compare the vitamin C potency of rugosa with that of some other species, *Rosa canina* has about 1,000 milligrams of vitamin C per hundred grams and *multiflora* only 250.

Several years ago, I began growing *Rosa rugosa* in my own

garden and only then did I begin to appreciate it fully. Up to that time, I had looked on it as a food plant and had not really paid much attention to its flowers or foliage. Now, I would grow it and like it, even if it didn't have any hips at all. Not only is the shape of the bush more pleasing than that of most roses, but its leaves are a deep, shiny green with a most interesting, wrinkled pattern. Rugosa flowers liberally, not just in spring, but a few in the summer and many in the fall. They're not tiny, wild-looking flowers like those of some shrub roses, but magnificent, large-petaled blooms. And at the risk of making rugosa sound like some sort of super-plant, I will say that its fragrance is unrivaled in the plant world. It is one of the few roses that even perfumes the air around it.

Rosa rugosa has only one pest that I have noticed—the Japanese beetle. But the main blooming period of the rose comes before the beetle season starts, and many parts of the country are free of Japanese beetle infestation. Nothing attacks the foliage and the plant seems to grow well under any sort of conditions, even in the salt air of the seashore.

Rugosa characteristics have been bred into many different kinds of roses, but I prefer the pure strain. There are several different pure rugosa varieties available—with different-sized bushes and different-colored flowers. They're all good.

Salad Greens

Health from Your Own Salad Garden

Home gardening is easy—and it's fun. If you've never grown so much as a reluctant dandelion, you'll quickly find the simple knack of growing things nature's way. More than that, too, you'll discover the double pleasure of a healthful pastime that puts really wholesome, tasty foods on your dinner table.

Let's begin with a handful of popular salad vegetables—lettuce and tomatoes, radishes, onions and peppers—all hardy plants, good producers and among the least difficult for the novice to grow.

Getting Started

If you've shied away from gardening until now because you felt that it was too much work, take heart. We have a plan that cuts down the work of gardening drastically—and has been proven successful in use by thousands of gardeners. Basically, the idea is to follow the "no-digging, year-round-mulch" system which has been made popular by Ruth Stout of West Redding, Connecticut.

Her method consists simply of keeping a thick, permanent layer of hay over every inch of her plot—a constant *mulch*. It's never removed or dug under, but merely added to as fast as it starts to decompose. Whenever she wants to put in some seeds or plants, Ruth just rakes enough mulch aside and plants. Later, when they've sprouted, the mulch is pulled close around the plants, thereby keeping the ground around them moist and outwitting the weeds. With her technique of a "constant surface cover"—literally a top-of-the-ground compost—Ruth Stout has grown peak-quality vegetables in abundance for 18 years with a minimum of work.

Uses a 6- to 8-Inch Mulch

Miss Stout uses "spoiled" hay—that is, hay intended for feeding animals, but which has been wet or slightly damaged by weather and time so that it's not suitable for livestock feeding. It *is* perfectly suitable for gardening, however, and there's plenty of it available. Farmers in every section of the country invariably have some spoiled hay, and most of them are glad to have gardeners help use it up. Combined materials are fine, too, especially if some are compact, others loose and bulky. How much mulch to use? Ruth Stout advises keeping a 6- to 8-inch mulch over the entire garden area.

The big, important thing is what a permanent mulch accomplishes. Ruth Stout's type of mulch eliminates plowing, tilling, weeding, cultivating, everyday stooping and squirming. It holds moisture and lessens the need for extra watering. Most important—mulch helps build topsoil; it's an endless source of decomposing material adding humus to the soil. Any soil can be made good if plenty of humus is put in it—*and good soil is the secret of easy gardening.*

These Steps Bring Garden Success

Here is how we recommend you begin this spring: (1) Prepare the spot you plan as a garden, using the few conventional practices outlined a little further on. (2) Start collecting and placing mulch, if at all possible, in advance of putting out plants or sowing seeds. (3) Locate a good source of *started* tomato plants, peppers and lettuce, onion sets and radish seed. Seeding plants should be stocky, firm and have a deep-green color. A few cents extra in price for well-started plants will more than repay itself in the long run.

For the first-year garden only, start by preparing the piece of ground. Clear it of debris and large stones; dig under light top growth or weeds if these are sparse—but pull most of them out, roots and all, if there are many. Cutting under the roots with a sharp-ended spade helps make quick work of this task.

Healthy Plants Resist Insects and Disease

Now ready the bed for sowing seed or transplanting started seedlings. Cultivate the top several inches as early in the spring as the soil can be worked—*but never when it's wet.* Besides being more difficult to work, a wet soil will puddle, bake and often form brick-like clods. Keep in mind that the purpose is to loosen and aerate the soil so plant roots can penetrate and develop, and so that water, air and fertilizer—all essential to strong, rapid growth—are easily available.

The final step in advance preparation is to rake the top two or three inches of soil fine and smooth for planting and sowing. Don't overdo it; the surface need not resemble a fitted sheet—in fact, it's better if there are shallow furrows to catch moisture and air currents.

Once your soil is in shape, the biggest factor for success is on your side. Sticking to organic methods means the major part of your work is done. Gradually, you'll discover that vigorous, natural plant growth resists insect pests and disease; that hardy, unpampered and well-nourished plants don't require an arsenal of costly and toxic compounds to insure proper growth and production.

Salad Vegetables

TOMATOES—By far the most popular home garden edible, tomatoes will bear in as few as 65 days. They can be planted—and are—in millions of gardens everywhere in the country. A 50-foot row will take care of more than a dozen unstaked plants or about 25 if supported. Staking will let more plants occupy the space you have. For each plant, drive a 5-foot stake into the ground alongside it. Tie the plant to this with soft yarn or strips of old cotton clothing; make the tie tight around the stake and loop it loosely around plant stems just below a leaf node.

Staked tomatoes contain more vitamin C than those which have been allowed to ramble on the ground. Apparently, the sun increases the vitamin C content of tomatoes, so it is best to harvest them as soon as possible after several days of bright sunlight. Tomatoes are also a good source of vitamin A and the B vitamins, phosphorus and calcium.

Set the started plants you buy out in the garden after all danger of frost is past, disturbing the roots as little as possible. Choose an open, sunny, well-drained location and have the soil porous, fairly light, containing a moderate amount of humus.

It is important to remember that the amount of vitamin A in a tomato varies with the type and also with the growing method, weather, soil, etc. "Doublerich" is a recently introduced variety which has twice the vitamin C content of ordinary varieties. "Caro-Red" is another newcomer with 10 times the usual amount of vitamin A contained in its orange-red flesh.

LETTUCE—A cool-weather plant, lettuce grows best in early spring or fall in the North and in fall, winter and spring in the South. The secret of raising fine plants is to keep them uncrowded and growing rapidly. Almost any fairly good garden soil that is well-drained and not excessively acid is suitable.

Set purchased transplants to stand about 15 inches apart in two-foot-wide rows. Get them into the garden as early as you can; light frost won't hurt. Young plants particularly appreciate mulching with a humusy material to keep down weeds and later supply extra plant nutrients. Be sure the moisture supply is kept constant; if rain is sparse, water generously during early growth period to keep plants developing rapidly. To halt damage by cutworms, surround the stem of the plant with a cardboard collar about two inches long. If hot weather arrives before plants head well, you can provide helpful partial shade by driving a few stakes along the sides of rows and stretching a canopy of double netting or cheesecloth across these.

Lettuce Rich in Vitamins A and C

Of 4 popular lettuce types, the loose-leaf or nonheading is easiest to grow and produces an abundance of mineral- and vitamin-rich green leaves, higher in food value than the white or balanced heading varieties. Leaves may be harvested by stripping, while the plant continues to grow. Newly picked lettuce should be eaten as soon as possible, as wilting means that valuable vitamins and minerals are being lost. Lettuce should never be soaked for this drains vital nutrients from the leaves into the water. While lettuce is not overly rich in all of the vitamins and minerals you need, it does contain an abundance of vitamin A, as well as some of the B vitamins and vitamin C. Phosphorus and iron are its two major mineral constituents.

RADISHES—Just about the easiest vegetable to grow, radishes will spark your salad appetite and contribute some vitamin C and minerals. A very quick-growing root crop, they are frequently used to mark rows in the garden.

The early or forcing radish requires cool spring or fall weather to develop best. They prefer a moist, loose, fertile soil. Early varieties mature in 20 to 30 days, so space your planting time to provide a succession of yield.

Four small radishes contain only 4 calories and provide 5 milligrams of vitamin C, 10 milligrams of vitamin A, 7 milligrams of calcium, some phosphorus and iron, and traces of the B vitamins: thiamin, riboflavin and niacin.

PEPPERS—Tasty suppliers of lots of vitamin C, fresh green peppers are a must for the salad fancier. Five or 6 plants will yield plenty of peppers for the average family. Because the pepper plant's requirements are so similar to those of the tomato, many gardeners substitute a pepper here and there in the tomato rows.

Peppers are not actually ripe until they are red, so that a red pepper has much more vitamin C than a green one. A ripe bell pepper may contain as much as 300 milligrams of vitamin C, while an average size orange contains only about 50 milligrams. When peppers turn red and feel firm, they can be harvested by cutting them within ½ inch of the stem. From the moment of harvest, the amount of vitamin C begins to dwindle; therefore they should be picked immediately before use or refrigerated as soon as possible. Cutting or shredding the vegetable further diminishes its vitamin C content. Vitamin A is plentiful in peppers. The B vitamins, calcium, phosphorus and iron are contained in peppers, too.

ONION—The onion is another easy-to-care-for plant which makes a tasty contribution to any salad. It is rich in essential minerals your body needs: calcium, magnesium, potassium, sodium, sulfur, and iron. It contains traces of silicon and iodine. Vitamins A, B and C are found in onions in appreciable quantities.

For the beginner, a good way to become familiar with onion growing is to start by using sets—small bulb seed onions. The best

Schwann, Theodor

Theodor Schwann, a German biologist and physiologist, is credited with the development of the animal cell theory. He was born at Neuss, Prussia, December 7, 1810, earned his col-

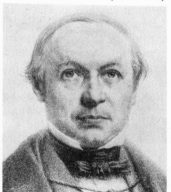

lege degree from the Jesuit College in Cologne and in 1834 graduated from the University of Berlin, having acquired a firm background in medicine and the related sciences. Utilizing his newly gained knowledge, Schwann in the same year made the first of his important contributions to medicine—the discovery of the enzyme pepsin. It was at this time also that he did some pioneer work on putrefaction and fermentation, which aided greatly the work of both Joseph Lister and Louis Pasteur. However, these two research projects assume only minor importance in comparison to the work for which Schwann is most famous—the explanation of the growth and development of plants and animals based on the cell theory. Schwann proved to the scientific world that plants and animals are composed of cells, that each cell has its own life and that the life of each individual cell is based on the life of the whole organism. This cell theory proved to be one of the most important aids in the advancement of medicine. Schwann died at Liege on January 11, 1882.

sets to plant are those no smaller than a dime. A pound of sets is enough for 50 feet of row.

Planted as early in the spring as possible, sets will grow rapidly, need only shallow cultivation while coming up and nothing but the protective cover of a labor-saving mulch once they're on the rise. By 5 weeks, young plants should make good growth and, if pulled at this stage, are known as scallions or early green bunching onions— fine for spring salads. For onions left to mature (about 100 days), draw extra mulch up close when plants are 10 to 12 inches tall to help preserve moisture needed while forming bulbs.

Benefits Are Many

There are more rewards to gardening than you might imagine. If your mental picture of a vegetable garden is limited to visions of struggling with weeds, insects and uncoöperative weather, you'll make some pleasantly surprising discoveries by looking into the organic idea a little more closely.

For one thing, treating the back yard's soil and plants organically is an ideal form of out-in-the-air recreation—both invigorating and relaxing, and one in which you can pace yourself. You don't need a degree in agricultural chemistry to get good results, nor do you need any expensive and dangerous sprays or commercial fertilizers. Furthermore, even with a postage stamp sized plot, you'll reap a tidy share of tastier, more healthful produce. And at the same time, you'll spare yourself the far less enjoyable market-counter search for "acceptable" (but not poison-free) salad ingredients.

To be sure, your greatest anticipation in planting a garden is the enjoyment of its harvest. Nevertheless, you'll soon realize there are multiple benefits—cheerful outdoor activity, healthful exercise and an indescribable feeling of well-being in working with the earth and growing plants. What's more, there's the delight of sinking your teeth into better-tasting, *better-for-you,* home-grown vegetables. If you've never had a garden before, you'll never be without one once you try this method.

Salt

Adding Salt Is Unhealthful

The occurrence of salt (sodium chloride) in processed foods is on the increase, and the consumption of these foods by Americans is increasing as well. It has come to the point at which a whole week's rations for a family frequently consists of nothing but processed foods. Of course, there are many undesirable elements in processed foods, but sodium added at the factory, added in the kitchen and added again at the table is a serious threat to good health and should be avoided whenever possible. The body does need some salt to operate, but this need is adequately filled by that which is contained in natural foods. When the body gets more than is necessary, trouble begins.

Heart trouble is one of the most common conditions attributable to an excess of salt. One of the scientific illustrations of this danger appeared in the *Archives of Pathology* (May, 1961). The project, reported by Robert Belliveau, M.D., and M. Elizabeth Marsh, Ph.D., was designed to discover just what influence sodium chloride would have on the development of atherosclerosis (hardening of the arteries) and myocardial (heart muscle) and renal (kidney) infarction (loss of blood supply due to a circulatory obstruction) in rats.

The procedure was this: 106 rats, 6 to 8 weeks of age, were used. Eighty-six of the rats were divided into 4 groups and fed a diet conducive to causing hardening of the arteries, plus either tap or saline (salt) water. Group II drank one per cent saline solution; Group IV increased to two per cent saline water. A fifth group of 20 rats on stock rations and tap water was used as controls.

Trouble from Saline

The rats on one per cent saline solution remained free of infarcts. But those 21 which were given a two per cent saline solution to drink, showed 10 cases of blood obstruction to the heart and 6 cases of blood obstruction to the kidneys in 11 of the rats. Of those 43 rats on plain tap water (and eating a diet conducive to hardening of the arteries), one heart problem and one liver problem developed. The 20 controls on plain water and regular rations showed no heart or kidney infarcts.

From this test it is obvious that salt added to the diet of normal animals does have an adverse effect on the kidneys. It was noted that the saline solution significantly increased the deposition of fat seen in the aortas (main artery) of all animals on the arteriosclerosis-inducing diet. This accumulation of fat did not show up in an increase in blood pressure. That means, of course, that one cannot depend upon a warning, such as high blood pressure, when circulatory disease is building.

In *Annals of Internal Medicine* (February, 1961), G. Douglas Talbott, M.D., and others, submitted an interesting report on the needs and the habits of man concerning salt. The articles noted that consumption of salt varies greatly throughout the world— ". . . whether or not more salt is added seems to be determined solely on the basis of palatability. Some investigators feel that palatability in turn depends chiefly upon habit, while others maintain that it is an inherent quality of the food itself."

More Salt with More Processing

A look at the history of man's salt consumption gives some indication of why our use of salt has come to be so universal. "History shows," says Talbott, "that the further a group's customs depart from the primitive, the greater is the desire for salt as a seasoning. Primitive man did not add salt to his food so long as he lived by the sea or ate his meat raw. Even when fire was first tamed for cooking, salt was not needed, because meat that had been roasted retained sufficient sodium chloride (salt) to satisfy the unsophisticated palate. . . . Sociologists have noted that, through the ages, the use of salt has consistently increased with each move inland, with each advance in cereal (grain) consumption and with each new wave of urbanization . . . it is said that many Eskimos add no salt at all to their food and that some African tribes use less than two grams per day."

If a departure from the primitive means an increase in salt, we can better understand why some of us use as much as 24 grams of salt per day and why the average American consumption is 10 grams of salt per day. We're "progressing" ourselves towards a salt intake that will leave little room in our diets for anything else! What could be further from nature than a totally synthetic orange drink that tastes "something like orange juice," or a maraschino cherry, or a cake mix with icing from a tube? Is it any wonder that Americans crave salt?

More Salt—More Heart Disease

Dr. Talbott and his colleagues noted that heart disease has increased directly in proportion to the amount of salt in our diet. Interestingly, this same relationship has existed in previous times in other civilizations. Since accumulated fatty deposits in the blood vessels are acknowledged to be largely responsible for heart ailments, it was decided to conduct an experiment to determine what interference if any, is presented to the body's proper use of fats when salt is ingested.

The subjects were 20 normal males, ranging in age from 18 to 39 years. They were placed in solitary confinement and given a carefully measured diet. During the first week, the diet contained an ordinary amount of salt (average, 4.126 grams per day). At the end of the week, blood samples were taken to ascertain the individual amounts of fat, among other things, in the blood of the subjects.

Fats Increased by Added Salt

After this, the blood fat of the men was raised artificially by an injection. The blood was measured immediately after the injection for its fat value, then again at 2, 4 and 24 hours thereafter. This showed the average speed with which the body normally deals with fats in the blood stream.

In the second week, the experiment was repeated exactly, except that each man was given 20 grams of salt a day in the form of a tablet to be swallowed and a drug to inhibit urinary excretion of the salt. After a week of this, blood values were again determined. Again, tests were done to see how long it took the blood to clear itself of unwanted fats.

The results showed that sodium chloride caused a significant increase in the triglycerides, strongly suspected as being the most active lipid factors in hardening of the arteries.

Semmelweis, Ignaz Philipp

Ignaz Philipp Semmelweis, a Hungarian physician and obstetrician, was born in Ofen on July 1, 1818. After receiving his M. D. from the University of Vienna in 1844, he took up the 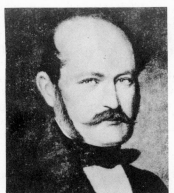 *specialty of obstetrics, and it is in this field that he gained his mention among the great men of medicine. Semmelweis, like Joseph Lister, became almost obsessed with the idea that cleanliness and sterility should be the foundation for all operating procedures, whether it be in the field of surgery or obstetrics. During his career as an obstetrician at the Vienna Hospital, Semmelweis searched for but could not find any explanation for the high incidence of childbed fever with its resultant death until one day he observed that students came directly into the maternity ward from the dissecting room with only a soap and water wash of their hands. Linking this procedure to the high death incidence of childbed fever, Semmelweis, in 1847, insisted that students and, in fact, all personnel coming into contact with maternity patients, wash their hands in a chlorinated lime-water solution. Through the introduction of this procedure, the death rate from childbed fever dropped to about 3 per cent and two years later fell to the low of 1.25 per cent. Due to this then unorthodox method, Semmelweis met with such heated opposition that he lost control of his mind and was placed in an asylum where he died on August 13, 1865. Ironically enough, his death was listed as due to a dissection-wound infection.*

When to Limit Salt Intake

One investigator in this field has suggested that, in his opinion, the most important time to apply restriction of salt intake is during youth. "This would suggest that limiting the ingestion of salt early in life might serve as a prophylactic (preventive) measure for those whose family history or individual constitution indicates a special tendency toward atherosclerosis."

Though Dr. Talbott is careful to admit that testing 20 men and their fat metabolism is not conclusive, he does say: ". . . the statistical significance of the fractional lipid variations noted in this experiment, may indicate the desirability of restricting excessive intake of sodium chloride as a means of controlling coronary heart disease."

Meniere's Disease Reacts to Salt

Meniere's disease, characterized by headache, dizziness, ringing in the ears, etc., has been known to respond to the variations in salt intake. Patients on a low-sodium diet had fewer attacks than when using their usual amount of salt. Yet, we were astounded to see, in the *Lancet* (July 8, 1961), that some doctors use a hormone to overcome the normal physiological processes involved with sodium intake! Imagine—they were ignoring any of the other complications salt *and* a hormone drug together might cause in any type of patient. They were using this combination on a person with Meniere's disease, a disease which usually hits older people whose circulatory and kidney systems are likely to be bad in the first place, instead of cutting salt intake.

It's Possible to Break the Salt Habit

The use of added salt is a habit that can be broken, just as other bad habits can be. We get used to salt's taste on certain things and continue to expect the same flavor. It isn't a nutritional need that makes us use salt at all. Taper off, if that's easier for you. Use only half as much salt as before, or salt only *some* of the foods you used to salt. You will find it only takes a small effort. Soon you'll be using still less salt, then none. You'll prove to yourself within a month that you can live without added salt and you won't mind doing it.

These 3 papers we've discussed are only a fragment of the vast amount of medical literature which notes the dangers in the use of salt for everyone. Lack of added salt can only be harmful to the body in rare, abnormal cases. Most of us get far more salt than we should, by eating the food just as it is set on the table, without picking up the salt shaker at all.

Sciatica

Surgery for Slipped Disc or Sciatica?

Sciatica is one of those common diseases which is well defined in the physiology books and in the medical journals. The main trouble is that no new treatments have been devised and the old ones appear to be either very radical or ineffective.

The disease itself is characterized by a strong discomfort—sometimes a deep ache and sometimes a sharp stabbing pain—that runs down the back of the buttock and thigh to below the mid-calf of the leg. One would assume that this pain is due to an irritation of the sciatic nerve itself, because of a bump or a strain of some kind. Experts believe this to be untrue, except in the rarest cases. They say that the pain is referred to this area from nerve roots which could have been damaged due to such widely diverse reasons as a slipped disc, tuberculosis of the bone, vascular injuries which affected the spinal cord, meningitis and syphilis. The degree of pain varies with the patient, but in the worst cases, the victim may be unable to stand or walk due to pain. Sneezing or coughing, or any sudden movements or jolting of the spine, can aggravate the irritation and cause searing pain. Sitting or lying can be as uncomfortable as standing, so it is not surprising that serious sciatica victims are ready to do anything for relief, including submitting to surgery.

The surgical treatment is intended to correct a misplacement of a vertebra due to a loss of support by the disc, which then causes the spinal column to list to one side. This results in the nerve's being pinched and the pain we sometimes call sciatica follows from that. One of two courses is usually followed in the surgery employed to alleviate this situation: the surgeon may place a support between the vertebrae to keep them the proper distance apart or he might "fuse" the spinal column so that it cannot bend to either side at that point, and needs no support to keep it from leaning and closing the gap between the vertebrae.

What It's Like

When a patient suffers from a so-called slipped disc, there is stiffness in his forward bending, but the sideways bending is effortless. X-rays show merely a narrowed disc space. There is a chronic low backache, usually worse after or during exercise, also there is a lump or protrusion as a result of the disc displacement.

Burns and Young, writing in the *Lancet* (February 3, 1951), stressed the need for reserving surgery as the last resort in treating sciatica. The authors estimate that only one in 40 cases of sciatica or low back pain needs surgery for a cure.

What else can one do? Some go to chiropractors and find the

results well worthwhile, with nothing more radical being done than a simple manipulation. Burns and Young say that, while manipulation sometimes leads to improvement, sometimes it makes things worse. Of course, this can be said of many treatments. The patient simply has to make his own decision.

Sciatica attacks are usually of short duration, if the problem has not progressed too far. The *Lancet* article says that, in an acute attack, the patient should be put to bed, for this is usually a comforting move and the attack may be shortened. If the patient refuses to go to bed, wearing a corset, which restricts movement of the lumbar spine (lower back), might help.

Apply Heat

Most other forms of treatment are considered by Burns and Young to be "ineffective." Physical therapy is characterized as not beneficial. Heat, as sometimes applied by a physical therapist, is said to temporarily diminish spasm, but a hot water bottle or a hot bath at home is cheaper and just as effective, say the authors. They also tell us that the condition tends to improve on its own. ". . . in a year, even the severest attack of sciatica is likely to subside either completely or, less often, into a chronic grumbling ache in the back or thigh. Recurrent attacks of lumbago and sciatica also tend to improve, becoming less frequent and less severe." There again is excellent reason for holding off on surgery until the condition is so severe as to allow for no other course.

If the patient is hospitalized and no immediate surgical activity is planned, there is an argument as to the best means of treating him. One school says that complete bed rest for a month or more is the only sure way to relief. They are opposed by another group which insists in early activity. A doctor, E. Schack Shaffeldt, writing in a Danish journal *Ugeskrift for Laeger* (February 25, 1960), reported on two sets of sciatic patients, one of which was treated with complete bed rest, the other required to attempt normal movement as early as possible. The 100 patients who rested stayed in the hospital an average of 50 days each, while those 100 who were active were released in an average of 30 days. This observation would seem to bear out our opinion that prolonged bed rest is not often an effective prescription.

The *Practitioner* (February, 1960) schedules treatment for a severe disc injury in this way: bed rest for 14 days, with a fracture board under the mattress; local heat should be applied to relieve pain; non-weight-bearing exercise on lower limbs (lifting legs and moving them from side to side) on the 10th day. Once the patient is considered recovered and is released, he should do no heavy work and he may have to wear a cast or corset for support.

There is very little literature to be found on the use of food supplements as a therapeutic agent in treating sciatica. *Vitamins in Medicine,* a book by Bicknell and Prescott, mentions that some researchers have claimed relief of sciatica through the use of thiamin, but that "these claims have never (up to 1953) been confirmed. . . ."

While no definite therapeutic effect was proven with thiamin, we believe that diets rich in the B vitamins to strengthen the nerves, protein to build firm tissues which will properly place the disc and reinforce it and bone meal to strengthen the bones of the spine and each vertebra in particular, can contribute much to the prevention of sciatica.

Shoes

What Are Good Shoes?

"If only children's shoes wouldn't last so long!" It's the nation's chiropodists talking. Shoes for kiddies are one of the very few of our modern commodities that outlast their usefulness. Unfortunately, parents are reluctant to part with shoes that still have plently of wear left in them, even though the child who wears the shoes has far outgrown them. The results can only be cramped toes and discomfort, leading to a bad walking gait and a life of tired, sore feet.

To start at the beginning, chiropodists think children should be kept out of shoes and stockings as long as possible. Even after they have begun to wear shoes, children should be encouraged to go barefooted indoors, on the beach, in the garden or any place else that presents a surface safe from the hazards of infection, broken glass, etc. (*Medical Press,* June 22, 1960). We know, of course, that when surfaces are resilient, in the way that wood and ground and sandy beaches are, the bare feet take hold of it and function naturally in the way that our outdoor-living ancestors used their feet.

Walking barefoot may even be physically beneficial, as well. We are reminded of the treatments of Father Kneipp, whose book, *My Water Cure,* brought him great fame in Europe. He recommended walking barefooted in the dewy grass of the morning as a preventive and a cure of many disorders. He told of a friend who was completely cured of chronic catarrh by a daily walk, barefoot, through the woods in the mornings during pleasant weather. Just why that system is effective, Father Kneipp does not say. Editor Rodale suggests that there might be great benefit in absorbing the electrical charges given off by the wet grass.

Too Good to Throw Away

On the whole, the experts agree that a wide range of sizes is available in children's shoes, but too often the best selection is on the expensive side. These shoes are far too expensive to be discarded as quickly as they should be, so parents either put off buying a new pair when they're needed or plan to hand them down to the younger children, even though the fit may not be a good one for them. The *Medical Press* article says that the shoes should be cheaper and less hard-wearing.

The best type of shoe for a child is a relatively lightweight one that will permit the sole to bend with some ease. This allows the child to walk with a natural springy gait, instead of ploddingly picking them up and laying them down, as though the shoes were soled with wood. A heavy shoe is not necessary for support. A firm lace-up shoe or one with an adjustable strap will usually do the job quite well. After all, the main function of a shoe is to protect the foot from cold and injury, and this requires only a reasonable covering and a fairly thick sole, not an impenetrable wall! In the summer, a toeless sandal will do admirably and in winter, a shoe that fits well around the heel, has plenty of room in the toe box and is waterproof, is all that is needed.

Fashionable Footwear

As the children become a little more mature, they become conscious of what is fashionable in footwear. Casual shoes are very popular at this age, and this term includes loafers, moccasins, ballerina shoes and a dozen others that have no laces or straps across the instep. Chiropodists find two things wrong with such shoes: to stay on the foot they must either be so short that the toes are cramped or, if they are large enough, the wearer must "hold" the shoe on by curling his toes; either way, such shoes mean that the toes are forced into unnatural positions and eventually, the foot becomes deformed. If you can't fasten a shoe to your foot, you shouldn't be wearing it.

Once the upper teens are reached, outrageous footwear is worn by most women. Among other abominations, sharply pointed toes and high heels are doubtless the worst. Such shoes are made and bought for and by the average teen-age girl, as well as her elders. No wonder. In the *Lancet* (March 12, 1960), P. Chapman put his finger on the main reason for their popularity: "So long as mothers wear deforming shoes, their daughters will crave to wear them also. Why women want to wear them is a matter for conjecture. Probably the explanation is their desire to appear as rich and leisured women, a motivation similar to that of Chinese ladies in past times who cultivated enormous fingernails." The Chinese ladies mentioned above couldn't use their hands effectively and our women, hobbling around, can hardly hope to use their feet to any comfortable degree.

The fashionable shoes of today have no relation in shape to the feet they have to cover. Only a deformed foot would come to a point in the center. The longest part of the foot is on the inside and that's where the longest part of the shoe should be. It is generally agreed, in design, that form should follow function; the shape of an object should be governed by the job the object is intended to do. It is not difficult to see how women's shoes shatter this rule.

Are Manufacturers to Blame

Manufacturers who make badly shaped shoes blame the fashion setters. It is not their fault if women insist on foot-mangling styles. A constructive suggestion for overcoming this situation came from A. W. Fowler in the *British Medical Journal* (April 2, 1960). He notes that sensible shoes for children have caused no financial impasse for shoe manufacturers. On the contrary, most parents demand them because they have been educated to the importance of well-fitted shoes on growing feet. Mr. Fowler suggests that shoe manufacturers get together and produce educational advertisements describing the principles of good footwear for adults and let them back up the campaign by producing sensible and smart shoes for all age groups. Such industry ads are common in many other groups of manufacturers, and they create much good will and dispense much worthwhile information.

Do you buy sensible shoes for yourself and your children? Does your favorite shoe manufacturer make shoes that will help your feet, not ruin them? Perhaps a letter from you asking for a good selection of properly shaped shoes will influence him to offer better, more healthful designs.

When the child is a toddler, the type of socks used are important, too. The newer type of stretch nylon socks tempt parents because they offer the promise of a good fit in spite of rapidly growing feet. However, *Medical News* says that such socks continually restrict movement of the toes because they grip so tightly and the toes have no chance to develop properly.

Skin Diseases

Unsaturated Fats for Skin Conditions

In laboratories where the complexities of nutrition are studied, animals on a fat-free diet develop a disease called fat-deficiency disease. Rats show arrested or retarded growth, changes in skin and hair, kidney disorders, impairment of reproductive function and a raised metabolic rate. This means that they burn up their food more rapidly.

The skin of these animals becomes dry and scaly and covered with dandruff. Cold weather accentuates the condition. Just adding fats—any kind of fats—to the diet of these animals does not improve the condition. But adding unsaturated fats, chiefly linoleic and linolenic acids, reverses the process and cures the skin conditions. It seems reasonable that similar conditions in human beings might indicate a shortage of these important fatty substances.

Eczema is, to a great extent, a disease of infants and children. *Medical Times,* June, 1958, relates the experience of one investigator, B. M. Kesten, who studied 2,000 cases of eczema. About 2/3 of the group were less than 6 years old, the largest concentration of patients being between 9 and 24 months.

It is noteworthy, we think, that human breast milk is rich in unsaturated fatty acids—far richer than cow's milk. Could it be that the widespread aversion to breast feeding which exists today among new mothers has something to do with the prevalence of eczema among infants and children? Certainly the fact that human breast milk is rich in unsaturated fatty acids indicates that these are essential for the new baby or they would not be provided by nature in such abundance. Where can children who are not breast fed obtain these valuable fats?

Treating Eczema

There is considerable evidence in medical literature that giving the unsaturated fats is beneficial in cases of infant eczema. Bicknell and Prescott, in their book *Vitamins in Medicine,* tell us of many cases where unsaturated fatty acids greatly improved eczema. In some instances, asthma also cleared up at the same time. The oils were given by the tablespoonful or used in cooking. In one case, corn oil was given, since it is high in the unsaturated fats. So are the sunflower seed, soybean and wheat germ oils. In fact, any oil from a vegetable or cereal source seems to contain, in general, more of the unsaturated fats than fats from animal sources.

An article in *Münchener Medizinische Wochenschrift (Munich Medical Weekly),* Vol. 26, p. 1308, 1961, discusses the work of Dr. Sigwald Bommer who used various unsaturated fats in treating eczema and other skin conditions—psoriasis, boils and certain kinds of ulcers. He tells us there is no disagreement about the importance of these fats in the diet. He says they have a direct effect on the function of blood vessels and circulation, although exactly how they figure in this respect is not understood. There is also general agreement, he feels, about the wrong proportions of fats people get today —too much of the saturated fats and too little of the unsaturated ones.

Dr. Bommer reports on 6 years of his own experience in giving oils rich in unsaturated fats to his patients. He used oils rich in vitamin E and the unsaturated fats. He says that an optimal supply of unsaturated fats does not appear to be present in our daily diets and "abnormal disturbances may result from an excess of fat, which consists predominantly of saturated fatty acids or of a mispropor- tion of these with the unsaturated ones. It is certain," he goes on, "and has been substantiated by observation, especially in children, that too great a restriction of the total supply of fat reacts definitely also on the skin and can produce pathological changes (impetigo, eczema, etc.). In connection with this, it is interesting to know that Norwegian breeders of furred animals feed linseed cakes to their silver foxes in order that these animals may grow an especially beau- tiful coat of fur."

To put it simply, it seems that the average diet today contains too little of the unsaturated fats which occur in seeds and unprocessed cereals, as well as vegetable and seed oils, and too much of the saturated ones—in general, those of animal origin like butter, milk, fat meat and so forth.

Worst offenders of all, we believe, are the fats which have been deliberately converted to saturated fats from the unsaturated state. These are the processed fats—margarine and the solid shortenings, as well as lard. The solid shortenings are made by forcing hydrogen through a liquid oil. The process is called hydrogenation. In the process, the unsaturated fats are largely changed to saturated fats. It is important to remember, we think, that merely avoiding margarine and the solid shortenings will not serve to improve your diet with respect to the unsaturated versus saturated fats. You should also make an effort to include in every day's meals some of the rich sources of unsaturated fats—seeds, nuts, wheat germ, vegetable or cereal oils. Avocados are another excellent source of these fats. And you should especially avoid processed foods, for you can be certain that fats used in their preparation were saturated ones.

Since the earliest investigation, in 1933, researchers have known that unsaturated fats can be used to treat eczema. Treating seborrhea, another skin disease, Dr. Bommer tells us he uses vitamin B_{12}, given twice weekly to the mother of a nursing child or to the child.

Vitamin E Added

Giving vitamin E, along with unsaturated fats, to a group of patients resulted in improvement and acceleration of the healing process in 60 per cent of the cases treated, although there were no complete cures. There were no unpleasant aftereffects, either. Of course, one would expect that there would not be, since these are foods, not drugs.

Believing that vitamin E would aid in the treatment, Dr. Bommer added a preparation of this and got no significant improvement. However, when he changed to vitamin E in wheat germ oil, there was an immediate difference. The question then arose as to whether the vitamin E or the unsaturated fats in the wheat germ brought about the improvement. It seems to us that the question is not important. The important thing is that the wheat germ oil got results.

Treatment for Other Disorders

Three other researchers have reported good results in treating boils with unsaturated fats, says Dr. Bommer. Linoleic and linolenic acids (both present in the various fats and oils we mentioned above) were the fats used. Dr. Bommer treats patients who have boils with a diet that completely avoids sugar and other sweets, canned fish and meat, including sausages. The diet is supplemented with vitamin C, and vitamin A. Adding unsaturated fats to this diet did not improve the results, he says.

It has been found that unsaturated fats are 25 to 50 per cent lower in the blood of psoriasis patients than in healthy persons. Dr. Bommer gave a wheat germ oil preparation to one patient who was completely cured within a few weeks of a stubborn case of psoriasis, which she had had for many years and which had resisted all treatment. Other patients did not find this complete relief. At present, Dr. Bommer gives folic acid (a B vitamin) for psoriasis.

He also uses vegetable oils for treating ulcers externally—leg ulcers specifically. This oil, he says, is far superior to other local preparations for ulcers. He still does not know, he says, whether it is the vitamin E or the unsaturated fats which do the work. And we still say, what does it matter? Using an unsaturated fat preparation, he obtained "surprisingly rapid granulation and regeneration of the skin, even where there were many ulcers and several of a considerable size. The ointment is also well tolerated by a sensitive skin."

Dr. Bommer recommends the unsaturated fats treatment both internally and externally for infantile eczema and the eczema that older children and adults may have which comes from some systemic cause, not from an allergy. We think psoriasis patients should try it, too, as well as persons suffering from boils and ulcers.

Our Recommendations

There seems to be little doubt that the good health of the skin is closely tied in with the fat content of the diet. Is there enough of the right kind of fat and not too much of the wrong kind? By "right" kind, we mean, first of all, unprocessed fats—those of vegetables, nuts and seeds, uncooked and untampered with. Wheat germ is another rich source of these fats—either the flakes, which also contain good protein and lots of B vitamins, or the wheat germ oil, which does not contain B vitamins (they are water-soluble) or protein, but does contain considerable amounts of vitamin E. Other vegetable and cereal oils are readily available in your grocery store—corn oil, peanut oil, soybean oil, sunflower seed oil and cottonseed oil. These have been processed, true. They have been refined and deodorized. Olive oil is the only vegetable fat, so far as we know, that reaches us in an unprocessed state. It has been pressed from the olives— that is all the processing that has been done.

How can you use such oils in your diet? You can, of course, take them in a spoon like medicine, but this seems most unnecessary, since they are food and very pleasant, agreeable food. We hope you eat salads. Over the salads should go salad dressing, using one of the oils mentioned above and a little vinegar or lemon juice, plus herbs, garlic or whatever else you like for seasoning. You should use liquid oils whenever you use oils in cooking, rather than butter, margarine or the solid shortenings.

And this brings us to the final recommendation: shun all fats that are solid at room temperature. These include margarine (any margarine) and the solid white shortening used for baking, as well as fatty meats and butter. Since saturated fats are almost universally used in the processing of foods, don't eat processed foods—crackers, fried TV dinners, rolls and muffin mixes, cake mixes, bakery products and so forth. Prepare your own food in your own kitchen.

Sleeping Pills

Why Permit Over-the-Counter Sale of Sleeping Pills?

"The only reason the Food and Drug Administration allows quiet pills to be sold without a prescription is that the amount of drugs in each dose is well below what would ordinarily be needed to produce untoward effects . . . The danger lies in the fact that persons who are not educated in pharmaceutics and who are disturbed may take double or triple doses and perhaps more often than recommended on the label. . . . For example, high doses of bromides taken over a long period of time can cause habituation, or bromide intoxication, the main symptom of which is mental disturbance."

The above statement appears in the American Medical Association *News Release* for September 22, 1961. It reinforces, once more, our view that so-called "harmless" medicines are not harmless at all. The person who takes too many aspirins or too much of a laxative is in trouble. The person who takes too many nonprescription sleeping pills or quiet pills is in trouble, too.

No effort is made by the druggist to discover whether or not the purchaser of quiet pills is "disturbed" or "educated in pharmaceutics." How many orders of pills would be sold if an education in pharmaceutics were a prerequisite? The whole system is unrealistic.

People who use such drugs seldom pay any attention to what is printed on the label. They have been sold on the idea that the pills can't hurt them, so the purchaser keeps taking as many as necessary to knock him into a state of tranquillity.

"Persons who buy such pills are deluding themselves into thinking that, for a dollar or two, they can avoid professional treatment . . . Actually, they stand the risk of aggravation of mental turmoil and worsening of their condition. When they finally do consult a physician, they may require more extensive treatment than if they had sought help in the first place."

Here we are, confronted with full recognition of the problem presented by nonprescription tranquilizing drugs and yet, there is no action by the government to legislate against the problem. Why should there not be a law which prohibits the purchase of any such products without a prescription? We are aware that a prescription does not lessen the danger these drugs carry, but at least the extra bother involved in acquiring a prescription, and the possible rejection of such a request by the physician, would lessen the number of victims.

Poisoning and Cataracts from Sleeping Pills

It is appalling to find that drugs which are being used every day by patients, at the prescription of their doctors, can cause serious illness and death. These drugs, in spite of their known danger, are not outlawed.

In the *British Medical Journal* (December 5, 1959), an article by Robert Crawford, M.D., tells of a 42-year-old man who complained of blurred and double vision for a week. Examination showed the formation of cataracts, with no apparent reason. It later developed that a sleeping pill, "carbital," which the man had been using for 5 years, was the cause. He stopped using the drug and his eyes cleared in several weeks. The author writes that these so-called "toxic cataracts" are not uncommon, and describes several drugs which cause such effects.

In 1933, 2, 4-dinitrophenol was first used in the United States as a slimming agent. By 1938, 150 cases of cataract of both eyes had been reported due to its use. During the First World War, 2, 4-dinitrophenol was used as an explosive, but caused 31 deaths from *poisoning* in France, England and the United States.

Another drug used in the treatment of obesity, 3, 5-dinitro-*o*-cresol, has caused several deaths and one known case of glaucoma and cataract. It is also widely used as an insecticide, fungicide and weed killer and has been found severely toxic.

Paradichlorobenzene, widely used as a clothes moth killer, is known to be toxic to humans and may cause "delayed" cataract. In one case, cataract occurred 14 months after the onset of regular toxic symptoms and 12 months after the patient had ceased contact with the chemical.

Can Cause Toxic Symptoms

Carbromal, another sleep inducer, has been found to cause toxic symptoms and death. Long-continued use may cause chronic poisoning. Two deaths are recorded from 20 to 50 tablets (10 and 25 grams). Among cases of acute poisoning admitted to the psychiatric division of the Copenhagen Municipal Hospital, 1943 to 1946, it was the third most common agent, with a mortality of 6 per cent. Chronic usage leads to loss of energy and ability and to depression. Several doctors have expressed concern over the difficulty in dealing with addicts (one case ending in death) and the unrestricted sale of carbromal. Dr. Crawford, in the same paragraph, writes that carbromal "has been regarded as a relatively safe hypnotic (sleep inducer)." What can we expect from the ones regarded as less safe? It would make one think twice when a doctor assures one that this or that medication or sleeping pill is safe.

The article ends with a list of 17 preparations containing carbromal which are available for use as sleeping pills or tranquilizers. Your doctor might prescribe them, not having read of their toxicity. Surely the drug companies selling them won't emphasize the danger in the literature they send to him. We are convinced that no drug should be used in any but emergency cases. Prolonged or habitual use of drugs is especially dangerous. Sleeping pills can and often do lead to addiction and poisoning. They should not be used without the most serious consideration.

Smoking

The Teen-Ager and Tobacco

Back in the days of rural America, it was the custom for a lad and his buddy to sneak a few matches and a bit of cornsilk, settle behind the barn or some other out-of-the-way place and try an excitingly daring thing: smoking a home-made cigarette. Punishment for engaging in this type of adventure sometimes came in the form of a whaling from dad or an upset stomach from mother nature.

Times change, of course, and today, we find, in practically every public place, vending machines which dispense countless brands of cigarettes to any child possessing a bit of cash and some mechanical know-how. It is a common sight to see young folks smoking cigarettes as they trudge along to junior or senior high school. Some schools have even set up smoking rooms to which pupils may retire for a noonday smoking break. Admission to such rooms may be open to all or limited to only those who have written parental permission.

As more and more parents smoke, they see no harm in granting such permission to their children. This does not mean that the much-publicized dangers of smoking to health have ceased to exist. The late Dr. Raymond Pearl, Johns Hopkins University, said that every cigarette you smoke shortens your life 25 minutes. Yet, teenagers and adults willingly submit themselves to this prospect.

Young, restless, eager to grow up, a teen-ager is not entirely to blame for becoming a cigarette, pipe or cigar smoker. Smoking, to many young folks, has become a symbol of maturity because adults, not children, smoke. Parents, teachers, that popular new movie or recording star, adult friends and acquaintances—all smoke. The teen-ager is an imitator of their actions. Obviously, as they can see no harm in smoking and they know so much about other things, why shouldn't they know if smoking were dangerous? Advertisements have a way, too, of surrounding cigarette smokers in an aura of glamour, adventure and success.

How Healthy Are Teen-Agers?

Why get all excited about smoking teen-agers? After all, they are young and healthy, strong enough to overcome any possible dangers which smoking may present. Teen-agers are bursting with glowing health, full of limitless energy, exuberance and pep. Are they?

By the teen-agers' own admissions, they are not. A nation-wide survey conducted by the University Opinion Panel and reported in *Pageant,* June, 1961, reveals that more than half of the thousands of teen-agers interviewed were worried about their health. One out of 5 teen-agers fears that his hearing is defective, 40 per cent of them complained that they had no pep, more than one-third claimed frequent headaches and colds, eye difficulties and upset stomachs, 25 per cent suffered from poor appetite. Are these the fine specimens of perfect health which can so easily throw off tobacco's poisons?

When one considers the diet on which most of America's teenagers exist, it is possible to see why so many of them have reason to worry about their health. Dr. Henry T. Scott, University of Wisconsin, says that the American teen-age girl has "deplorable eating habits, to say the least." She is forever going on crash diets or indulging in diet fads. She stuffs herself on soft drinks, candy and French fries at the local lunchroom after school and then, comes suppertime, she just isn't hungry. She isn't getting enough calcium and some of the B vitamins.

The girl marries and becomes a mother and her real troubles begin. How can her malnourished body provide for the added burden of a baby? Warns Dr. Scott, "Her eventual destiny is some tax-supported institution." An isolated opinion, you may scoff, but Dr. Scott has based his comments on a 10-year study conducted by 30 state universities.

The diet of the teen-age boy differs little from that of the girl, except that he probably consumes greater quantities of the stuff. The diets are identical in their content of worthless foods. Such foods are displacing nutritious foods full of vitamins, minerals, protein and other nutrients needed by the growing body. A deficiency of some degree must result. A teen-ager on this type of diet who smokes cigarettes, is in for trouble.

Vitamins B and C Depleted

Amblyopia is a condition of dimness of vision or its loss due to tobacco poisoning. A British publication, the *Lancet* (August 9, 1958), points out that one symptom of this disease seems to be evidence of a deficiency of vitamin B_{12}. Our investigators have discovered that recovery from amblyopia is practically assured when this vitamin is administered. Previously, in order to effect the cure, the patient had to give up smoking, but with vitamin therapy, this is not necessary. From this, it would seem that B vitamins are used up when a person smokes.

Vitamin C, our protection against poisons, is also used up in the process of smoking. The smoker destroys his own defense against colds and infections, especially those of the nose and throat membranes. At the same time, he irritates them with tars and nicotine. Smokers suffer from 65 per cent more colds, 167 per cent more throat and nose irritations and have a 300 per cent higher incidence of coughs than non-smokers, according to an insurance handbook put out by the National Underwriters Company.

We see a vicious cycle. Smoking robs the body of its essential vitamins and creates a deficiency. Cigarettes are substituted for nourishing foods and then the smoker becomes more deficient. A semistarvation diet, like that eaten by too many of our teen-agers, may produce this type of craving for tobacco.

Roger William Riis wrote an article on the effects of smoking on throat membranes, lungs, stomach, etc., for *Reader's Digest* in January, 1951. "When I began research for this article, I was smoking 40 cigarettes a day. As I got into the subject, I found that number dropping. As I finish the article, I am smoking 10 a day. I'd like to smoke more, but my investigation of the subject has convinced me that smoking is dangerous and worse—stupid." What did Mr. Riis find so convincing in his research?

He found that nicotine is a deadly poison, 400 milligrams of which would kill you as quickly as a bullet. This is the amount of nicotine taken in during the course of a week by the pack-a-day smoker. The only reason it does not kill you immediately when you smoke is the fact that you do not inhale all the nicotine a cigarette contains; your body eliminates as much of the poison as possible between puffs to keep a lethal dose from building up and the body builds up a tolerance toward the expected dosage.

A beginning smoker often experiences acute nicotine poisoning because his body has not yet developed a tolerance to nicotine. Nausea, vomiting, cramps, diarrhea, blurred vision and clammy perspiration are symptoms of this type of poisoning. As the body adjusts itself to the poison introduced into its system, nicotine poisoning occurs less frequently and less violently.

Mr. Riis found that tobacco tar, that greasy accumulation left on your ashtray, fingers or cigarette holder, is an irritant to delicate membranes and is as deadly as nicotine to heavy smokers. He found a whole series of diseases which could be traced to cigarettes, cigar or pipe smoking.

Many Diseases Traced to Tobacco

Lung cancer is probably the most widely known disease associated with smoking. Studies by Dr. Ernest L. Wynder and other doctors indicate that the longer a person smokes and the more he smokes, the greater are his chances of developing cancer of this type.

The dangers of smoking to the heart patient are also emphasized. Smoking, the *Journal of the American Medical Association*, March, 1955, notes, can have a damaging effect on the myocardium (muscular wall of the heart). An increased pulse is one result of smoking a single cigarette. Inhaling smoke every 20 seconds steadily decreases the flow of blood through the hand during the smoking period, according to the *British Medical Journal* (Vol. 2, p. 1007, 1951).

Buerger's disease is a circulatory disease which seems to confine itself almost exclusively to male smokers. This disease involves the constricting of blood vessels; the smaller the vessel, the more tightly it is constricted. The hands and feet become numb and tingle as though they were asleep. Unnourished tissues die and if gangrene sets in, amputation must be attempted.

Ulcers have been related to smoking. Dr. Arnold S. Jackson, President of the National College of Surgeons, has discovered that chain smokers comprise 90 per cent of his ulcer patients.

Poor muscular control, nervous conditions, impaired senses of smell and taste are a few of the afflictions of the smoker. Temporary night blindness is still another condition created by cigarette smoking. A Mayo Clinic doctor, Dr. C. Shard, notes, "Smoking two cigarettes will cause a 15 to 30 minute delay in the time the eyes require to adjust themselves to see in dim light."

Sterility is a major problem the smoker faces. There is at least one case on record where the husband's smoking resulted in his producing well-formed but dead sperm. Soon after he stopped smoking, his wife conceived. He resumed smoking and again his sperm were found to be dead. Tests with rats have revealed that dosing them with nicotine produces fewer litters and more infertile pairs. Descendants of pairs continually dosed with the poison were less fertile than control pairs. Dr. Alton Ochsner of the Ochsner Clinic, New Orleans, says, "The decrease in sexual activity of men in their 30's can very often be traced to excessive smoking." This was reported by Ben Solomon in the *Youth Leader Digest,* May, 1960, Vol. 22, No. 8.

Smokers Less Masculine, More Shy and Inhibited

A Study of Harvard Alumni also was reported by Mr. Solomon. It was begun in 1938 with Harvard sophomores. It yielded this discovery: "Smokers are physically less masculine, lower in physical fitness or hard muscular work, frequently shy, have more inhibitions and are more self-conscious than non-smokers.

Teen-agers who smoke, Mr. Solomon finds, are reluctant to join in work, games and studies and if they do, are generally less successful at it. The degree of their reluctance and success are in direct proportion to the amount of smoking they do.

This may all be true, admits the smoker, but I get a "lift" from smoking that I enjoy. That "lift" or feeling of well-being the smoker gets from one cigarette occurs because the nicotine has caused an immediate rise in blood sugar. The nicotine is powerful enough to keep the blood sugar level from returning to normal for about 30 minutes. The nicotine, animal experiments have shown, has stimulated the adrenals to release blood sugar, which produces that relaxed, good-all-over feeling. Because you feel good does not mean that the nicotine has been good for you.

The type of reaction which releases sugar into the blood is a protective one used by the body for sudden demands in times of stress. Infectious diseases, the administration of morphine, cocaine or similar drugs, fear, anger and pain—all stimulate the pouring of additional sugar into the blood. The chain smoker is constantly forcing his body to use up blood sugar from the adrenals and from storage places in the liver. As a consequence, his nerves, glands and secretions are wearing themselves out to promote a temporary feeling of well-being. In times of real stress, will the smoker's body be too exhausted to provide the necessary protection?

The wise teen-ager, and the wise adult, too, will realize that smoking can do his health no good. If he doesn't smoke now, he will refrain from taking up the habit. If he is already a smoker, he will try to stop.

How to Break the Tobacco Habit

Reading books on smoking may help strengthen his resolve to shake off the smoking habit. Gloria Swanson bet one of her friends 10,000 dollars that she would not begin smoking again. And she won the bet. Perhaps the temptation to smoke can be overcome for you by the thought of the loss of money.

Dr. Geolo McHugh, psychologist of Duke University, suggests, in the *New York Times,* March 13, 1952, that a person trying to give up the habit not give up abruptly, because, if he fails, giving it up again will be harder. He advises against limiting the number of cigarettes smoked per day, as this plan leads to too much concentration on smoking. He would advise setting aside a certain period each day when one will not smoke; for example, two or three hours in the morning. The rest of the day, smoking is unrestricted. Research over a period of 5 years dealing with 600 people indicates that smoking the rest of the day will not increase. As the body adjusts itself to living without nicotine, a complete break can be made more easily later on.

Adopting a substitute habit may help. Some people smoke as a result of frustration, irritation or boredom. Writing down an analysis of what has happened prior to the time the desire to smoke presented itself, may reveal the reason for smoking and a solution to the problem of giving up tobacco.

Another way, and perhaps the best way, to stop smoking is to keep the blood sugar level high for several weeks to see if this has some effect on smoking. Eat meals high in protein and cut down on all starches and sugars, eliminating especially all white sugars and flours. A high-protein breakfast will help you start the day right. A couple of nuts, sunflower seeds or hard-boiled eggs can be nibbled on as a substitute for smoking. Meanwhile, make certain that your body gets plenty of all the B vitamins and sufficient amounts of vitamin C each day to protect you from the poisonous nicotine.

Parents of teen-agers who smoke can try to provide high amounts of protein in attractive meals and in prepared nutritious snacks at home. Be certain, parents, that you are first setting a non-smoking example for your young adults to follow.

Remember, as Mr. Solomon points out, "Tobacco is a loaded lethal weapon and time pulls the trigger."

Dangers of Smoking Need Emphasis

At least one jury decided, on the basis of evidence presented, that lung cancer can be caused by smoking cigarettes. It would seem that those who are conscious of the danger to health presented by smoking should seize upon the advantage of such a decision to start a strong campaign against starting the habit. The Public Health Service and the FDA should be releasing articles in newspapers and magazines, acquainting the people with the unfavorable percentages for acquiring serious disease they face if they smoke. After all, such a campaign is periodic with these agencies in warning against quacks and food faddists. It has been said that, if evidence equal to the amount on smoking as a cause of cancer were presented to show that a bridge were unsafe, the bridge would surely go unused and petitions would flood the authorities to have it torn down. Why do our government agencies hold back on what is obviously their responsibility to inform the people of a serious peril? Can it be that they are too much influenced by powerful tobacco lobbies?

Doctors also seem to take the matter much too lightly. They light up a cigarette while they're telling the patient that smoking is dangerous to health. How dangerous? Well, not enough to cause the doctor to break the habit.

Somewhat more concern was shown by a correspondent to the *New England Journal of Medicine* (June 16, 1960). He repeats the indisputable fact that lung cancer is 10 times more frequent in smokers than non-smokers, regardless of sex, locality or occupation. He notes that 157 in 100,000 heavy smokers die of lung cancer as compared to 3.4 in 100,000 of those who never smoked.

The tobacco companies argue that we live longer and hence, more lung cancers get a chance to develop; that improved techniques in diagnosis show up more cancers than before. They forget, or want to forget, that non-smokers live longer, too and that they also benefit from improved diagnosis.

The author gives 3 facts on smoking that can't be denied: some association exists between smoking and lung cancer; smoking certainly does not improve health, but rather impairs it; and smoking is habit-forming. He calls for regulations that would force a change in advertising methods by which the tobacco industry makes smoking appear to be a desirable social grace. Doctors and teachers who do not smoke should emphasize the dangers involved and point out that living a full life has absolutely no dependence on smoking. These are all worthwhile steps that should be taken.

How Smoking Affects the Unborn Child

Women who smoke are ever so relieved if they get a doctor who does not forbid their smoking during pregnancy. They are quick to defend his opinion against that of the so-called fuddy-duddy who says smoking is dangerous to the unborn child. Admittedly, proof to support the latter opinion has been hard to come by, but a recent study published in the *British Medical Journal* (October 10, 1959) should convince everyone of the connection.

Dr. C. R. Lowe surveyed the histories of 2,042 pregnant women delivered in the summer of 1958. Of these, 1,155 were classed as non-smokers and 668, as smokers.

It was statistically concluded that smoking during pregnancy reduces the birth weight of the infant, and "the reduction of weight is by no means trivial." Since the period of gestation was apparently not affected by smoking, a direct retardation of growth in the fetus is considered to be caused by smoking. It could happen in several ways: the tobacco might have a direct drugging effect on the fetus, since the fetal heartbeat is known to increase with the mother's smoking; or smoking may reduce the circulation in the placenta, retarding the growth of the fetus by reducing its blood supply and, thereby, its nutrition.

While researchers are puzzled as to which of these effects, or others, cause this serious change in the normal development of the fetus, there can be no doubt that an undesirable change does occur as the result of the mother's smoking. As we see it, a mother who wishes to be certain that her unborn child has every opportunity to be born healthy and fully developed, has no choice but to discontinue smoking as soon as she is aware of pregnancy or, preferably, as long as there is any chance that pregnancy might occur.

Smokers Should Ask Permission

The *British Medical Journal* (May 14, 1960) had a most interesting letter in its correspondence section, and it might explain a phenomenon that has puzzled all of us. Why do doctors treat the problem of smoking so lightly? Why, indeed, do so many of them smoke? Says Dr. John Dancy, "The truth, surely, is that doctors who smoke become laymen for this purpose and have a blind spot for their own addiction. Tobacco has become indispensable to them and so, it must be at least harmless for everyone else. Tobacco sensitivity, if it exists at all, is the plea of the crank or the social misfit."

The letter goes on to tell of a London doctor who complained that one of his women patients had stopped keeping her appointments because the doctor chain-smoked while examining her. This, in spite of a conspicuous sign on the wall forbidding smoking in that area of the building.

The question of smoking in public is a serious one. Almost no one regards "No Smoking" signs with any responsibility these days; even fewer are the authorities who would try to enforce such rules. There was a time when politeness required that the permission of all in the room be obtained before one lit a cigarette. Such refinement is no longer in vogue. It is not any more impolite to ask a person not to smoke in your presence, than it is for him to have lit up without asking your permission. The fumes from a cigarette are dangerous, too. Don't be afraid to demand your rights.

Soap

Soap and Skin Infections

Those who are frequently pestered with boils and infections of the pores where hair follicles emerge might profit from the words of Dr. F. Ray Bettley, a physician for diseases of the skin at Middlesex Hospital in London, England. He says that much of this trouble can be traced to the use of soap. Studies show, says Dr. Bettley, in the *British Medical Journal* (June 4, 1960), that the use of soap increases the permeability of the skin and allows alkali to reach and irritate cells below the surface of the skin. This acidity which soap usually destroys is actually the skin's means of self-sterilization, so it is no surprise that the germs which cause boils, etc., have easy entry in frequently soaped areas. Dr. Bettley says that the avoidance of shaving soap is often enough to cure folliculitis, a common disease of the hair glands. (Certainly anyone with serious skin problems from shaving should try using an electric razor and save himself the unnecessary discomfort the use of shaving soap can cause.)

For most of us, use of soap should be curtailed or completely eliminated. We lather ourselves in the bath or shower out of force of habit, rather than the need to get rid of grime. Perspiration and the little smudges of modern living wash off easily without soap, so why expose the skin to it. Soap can cause serious skin problems.

Soft Drinks

Cola Drinks for Burping Baby?

Dr. Joseph Molner writes a syndicated newspaper column on medical questions, as do several other doctors and psychologists and nutritionists. It is true that we frequently disagree with what these writers have to say, because they often parrot the misconceptions about health and merely repeat advertising slogans put out by drug houses and food manufacturers. In at least one instance, however, we found cause to cheer a column by Dr. Molner which appeared in the *Milwaukee Sentinel* (November 8, 1960). The good doctor wrote an answer to a letter which asked about the efficacy of cola drinks for babies. They were suggested by a doctor from the child's second week instead of milk or juices, because "it makes a child burp and is good for children." The letter went on to tell of a little boy who drinks 3 bottles of cola drink every day at this same doctor's orders.

Doctor Molner wrote, first, that he could hardly believe that a doctor would suggest cola for a baby. We are inclined to question Dr. Molner's experience or association with other medical men if this is his true feeling. We have heard this advice dozens of times, as you probably have, and frequently meet mothers who use colas regularly to relieve their children's upset stomachs—often at their doctor's suggestion. Anyway, Dr. Molner calls the idea "idiotic," and we certainly must agree with him there.

He goes on to discuss what is in cola drinks—water, bubbles and sugar, plus flavoring and some caffeine. We add to the list carbonic acid, artificial coloring and phosphoric acid. Certainly there is nothing here that baby needs and can't get from milk, says the writer. But there also are some things he doesn't get—no protein in colas, no vitamins, none of the natural sugars he should be getting from natural foods.

Will the cola make him burp? Probably. But the only reason for burping a baby is to help him get rid of the excess air he swallowed with his food. If a baby is drinking cola instead of food so that he can burp, he is only burping the air he swallowed with the cola!

"Ridiculous . . . Harmful"

Says Dr. Molner: "It is ridiculous to feed such stuff to a baby. A ridiculous deprivation of the food a baby should be getting, and besides, it's probably downright harmful. The harmful part, for a child, is the caffeine. It is a stimulant, just as the caffeine in tea or coffee is a stimulant. Babies don't need stimulants. Excess stimulation can lead to lack of sleep and nervousness . . . large amounts of caffeine can make an adult nervous and jittery. Do that to a baby? What a disgraceful thing to do!"

Of course, infants should never be exposed to colas or any soft drinks, but neither should anyone else, especially children. Think of the nervous and jittery young children and teen-agers we keep trying to diagnose through psychology, psychiatry, medicine, etc. What about nutritional diagnosis? How many of these drink colas?

Soil

Soil—Key to Proper Mineral Nutrition

By Robert Rodale

Does good soil produce good plants and, in turn, healthy people? That is one of the most challenging questions facing anyone studying human health. It is a question that is pregnant with immense benefit and is, likewise, immensely complicated to answer. There can be little doubt that health starts with the soil, which is the source of most of our food, but so many other factors can create health or take it away that it is difficult to maintain a sharp focus on the direct effect of soil on health. Clever investigators, though, have developed ways to trace our strength or weakness directly to the soil beneath our feet, and it is to these studies that we can look for guidance.

Mineral nutrition is influenced by different soils and that is the area we want to probe most deeply. The soil is the agent that transports minerals and mineral salts from their source, which is the rocks that make up the crust of the earth, to plants and animals and ourselves. These minerals are divided into two categories—macronutrients and micronutrients. The macronutrients are those that are used in relatively large quantities and the micronutrients are the trace elements, usually needed in only very minute amounts. It is simpler to present information about these nutrients to you in chart form, so please refer to table 10.

In addition to the minerals, we should at least take note of the "energy elements"—carbon, oxygen, hydrogen and nitrogen. These elements do not originate in the crust of the earth like the minerals, but are largely obtained from the atmosphere and from water. Ninety-five per cent of the structure of mammals and green plants is made up of these energy elements. Except under desert conditions, plants are seldom short of carbon, oxygen or hydrogen. The nitrogen supply, of course, can be a problem in certain soils and a shortage of nitrogen can make difficult the production of foods with high protein content.

Because minerals make up only 5 per cent of the plant and animal structure, we should not feel that they are unimportant. They exert an influence all out of proportion to their quantity. Plants and animals can't live on protein, carbohydrates, fats and water alone. They need minerals, too. I don't have the room in these pages to review the general function of minerals, but I did want to point out to you the difference between the energy elements, which originate in the atmosphere, and the structural elements (minerals) whose source is the crust of the earth.

Forces of nature are constantly at work to break up the rocks that compose the earth's crust and wash the particles into the oceans.

Table 10: THE MINERALS ESSENTIAL TO LIFE			
The Macronutrients (*Needed in large amounts*)		The Micronutrients (*Needed in trace amounts*)	
PHOSPHORUS CALCIUM MAGNESIUM POTASSIUM SULFUR CHLORINE	} *Essential to plants and animals*	IRON COPPER ZINC MANGANESE	} *Essential to both plants and animals*
SODIUM	} *Essential only to animals*	COBALT IODINE FLUORINE (possibly)	} *Essential to animals, but not to plants*
		BORON MOLYBDENUM SILICON GALLIUM VANADIUM } (possibly)	} *Essential to plants, but not to animals*
		ALUMINUM	} *Found in plants and animals; no demonstrable value*

The soil is no more than a temporary resting place for these mineral particles on their trip from rock to the sea. Because of that constant washing process, soil is a very changeable commodity. On one farm, you may find several different kinds of soil, each with a different make-up of minerals. The plant, the middleman between us and those minerals in the soil, can not move around from one type of soil to another to select its diet of minerals. It is locked in position by its roots and must forage for whatever minerals it can get from the spot where its seeds happened to sprout. If a plant is growing in a spot that is lacking in a particular mineral, it can react in two ways: (1) by failing to grow to full size, thereby reducing crop yield or (2) by failing to incorporate normal amounts of that mineral in its leaves, stalk or seed. It is that second reaction that we are concerned about, because a plant whose edible part is lacking in proper mineral balance will not provide a healthful diet for man or beast.

There is abundant proof that the mineral balance of plants is varied by the mineral balance of the soil on which it is grown. The lack of iodine in the soils of certain areas of the Midwest is the cause of the "goiter belt." Plants growing on those low-iodine soils don't pick up enough of that vital element to provide proper thyroid gland health to people living in that area. Another proof of plant-soil mineral relationship is the fast-expanding use of plants as guides to prospecting for useful ores. Modern prospectors collect samples of plants from likely looking mineral sites and have them analyzed for such elements as copper, zinc, manganese and molybdenum. If the plants check out unusually high, workmen will return to the site and make test drills to find out what underground rock or ore is causing the imbalance in the plants above. The Russians have advanced far in the science of plant-mineral prospecting, because it is the fastest way to survey their vast land areas for underground mineral wealth. There has also been much work done relating animal health to soil conditions. Phosphorus deficiency in livestock has been reported from at least 20 states. Calcium deficiency problems are also widespread. Few self-respecting farmers today would consider doing without mineral supplements in animal feed, often presented in the form of mineralized salt.

Minerals Affect Health

Now, let's dig into the subject of the effect of mineral imbalances in plants on our health. Orthodox medical science takes the position that goiter is the only disease that can be caused by a deficient soil. There is a certain amount of real truth in that position, since goiter seems to be the one disease whose primary cause is food grown on a soil deficient in a trace element. But it is not correct to say that soil deficiency can not be a *contributing* cause of other diseases. Minerals are so vital to our health that the continual eating of food with wrong mineral balance can have a weakening effect that leaves us prey to one or more of a variety of ailments.

In England, there has been much study of the possible relationship of soil quality to stomach cancer. In the small English villages, families produce a sizable amount of their own food in their gardens and the habit of the English of living many years in the same place, allows scientists to make valid studies of the quality of garden plot soils on people's health. C. D. Legan reported, in the *British Medical Journal* (September 27, 1952), that people living on the peat soils of northern Scotland showed a higher incidence of stomach cancer than people living on more mineralized soils. He speculated that a lack of trace elements was the cause.

Soil and Tooth Decay

Cancer, though, is perhaps not the most meaningful disease to use to search for soil-health effects. The incidence of cancer is so limited that researchers find themselves working with only a small group of the total population. If we are going to determine the effect of good or bad soil on a whole population, we should check the incidence of a disease that meets at least these 4 goals: (1) it occurs among a large segment of the population; (2) it is a condition that reflects general bodily health; (3) it can be easily and quickly observed without complicated diagnosis; and (4) it should be a disease that has been related to soil deficiency by theoretical studies.

Tooth decay (caries) meets those 4 requirements. It is a degenerative disease whose incidence has been linked by some studies to soil conditions. Although diet and other health habits also play an important part in tooth health, I think that researchers are on firm ground in using it to attempt to find out how soil is related to human health.

New Zealand is the place where some of the best studies on tooth decay and soil conditions have been carried out. That country has had a high incidence of tooth decay and the fact that there are wide differences in soil conditions in New Zealand and a racially uniform population, makes such studies meaningful. New Zealanders also are in the habit of consuming locally grown produce, so the influence of eating food from different areas is minimized. But, strangely enough, it was an earthquake that created the most ideal conditions for a soil-health survey in New Zealand. On February 3, 1931, near the village of Napier, an earthquake raised a land mass 60 miles long and 10 miles wide out of a seacoast lagoon. Soil that had been collecting silt under water for many years suddenly raised 9 feet in the area and, after 13 years, came into use for growing food and truck crops. The city of Napier found itself with a source of food grown on "new" and highly mineralized soil.

Not far from Napier is the town of Hastings, similar in all respects, except that its food is grown on "older" and leached soils. The New Zealand Medical Research Council saw the opportunity to make a study of the dental health of Napier and Hastings, and received coöperation on the project from the United States Navy Dental Corps, the Soil Bureau of New Zealand and even the United States Public Health Service. The project began in 1954, about 10 years after the town of Napier began receiving a large amount of food from the land that had been raised from the lagoon. Soil analyses were made, and it was found that the primary differences in the Napier and Hastings soils were in soil acidity and the micronutrient content. Not only did the Napier soils have higher concentrations of trace elements, but the plants grown on those soils revealed, after analysis, that they had more of certain trace elements, also.

When checks of dental health in the two towns were first made in 1954, it was found that the Napier children had much less decay than Hastings children. The picture began to be complicated somewhat, though, by the fact that Hastings instituted fluoridation in 1954, recognizing the poor dental health of its children. Hoping to keep their survey free from the influence of fluoridation, the researchers brought into the experiment the nearby town of Palmerston North, which was similar to Hastings in all respects, but whose water was not fluoridated. The final results of the experiment, published in the December, 1961, issue of *Soil Science* magazine, show that Napier children continue to have better dental health than those of Palmerston North and even better than the children of Hastings, which has fluoridated water. The authors of the report conclude that minerals in the soil, especially trace minerals, have a definite effect on dental health. They feel that the higher amounts of molybdenum in the Napier soil is possibly the chief factor, but are continuing their investigations to see if other trace element differences could also be significant.

Studies in the United States

Some useful studies of the relation of soil to dental health have also been carried out in the United States. Chief sources of information have been reports of the condition of teeth of draftees. During World War II, the Navy checked the number of cavities in the teeth of 70,000 draftees in order to find out how many dentists it would need to get them in shape. Dr. William A. Albrecht, Chairman of the Soils Department of the University of Missouri, related the findings of these dental checks to soil conditions in the draftees' home areas. Here is what he found: Men from the East, where farm soils are "oldest" and most leached, had an average of 17.55 filled and unfilled cavities. Those from the midsection of our country, where soils are richest, had between 12 and 13 cavities. West Coast men averaged over 15 cavities. Dr. Albrecht feels that the soil of the western states cannot match the balanced richness of the midsection soils, so he claims that these results show a definite relationship between dental health and soil conditions in the United States.

As you may know or suspect, however, the position of United States government agencies and official medical bodies is that soil quality is not reflected in better health. Their view is that any deficiency in macro- or micronutrients in food from one area will be balanced out by food from another area, since most people eat food grown in different parts of the country. The only trouble with that viewpoint, though, is that the people who hold it can't prove that they are right. There is so much tooth decay and so much degenerative disease of all kinds in the United States that the good health of the American people can't be used as evidence by the people who claim that soil quality doesn't make any difference and that the different geographical origins of our food wipe out any deficiencies that may exist.

Some Questions

Instead of trying to ignore the question of soil and health, our research organizations should be seeking ways to find valid answers. Enough evidence has already been produced right here and in other countries to convince even the skeptics that there is *some* relation between soil and health and that more studies should be made. There are so many more questions waiting for answers. Here are just a few:

Are rural people more susceptible than city people to soil-health relationships, because of their tendency to eat more locally produced food?

Can the eating of more ocean fish, with their rich complement of trace elements, help to prevent mineral deficiencies caused by food grown on exhausted soil?

Is excessive fertilization of soils with concentrated major nutrient fertilizers causing trace element problems?

Can we develop ways to detect if plants or animals suffer from "hidden hunger"—that invisible poverty of trace elements?

Most important, we should begin to think of the soil as a source of quality nutrients, not just bulk to fill our stomachs. If that attitude could penetrate through all layers of our food-producing industry, our health would surely benefit.

Soya Milk

Soybean Milk Safe and Valuable

A short time ago the papers picked up a story of allergy in a child to soybean milk. Much was made of the faddists who insist on using soybean milk on infants who have allergenic family histories and even on those who don't. Since we advocate the use of soybean milk in preference to cow's milk, we were, naturally, the recipients of many letters calling our attention to this situation and demanding that we explain our position on this point more fully. The *New England Journal of Medicine* (March 30, 1961) did that for us when it printed a letter from a Hawaiian doctor who said that "condemnation of soybean milk is as unwarranted as would be a condemnation of breast feeding, because extreme sensitivity has been reported to human breast milk." Dr. Moore goes on to say that the use of soybean milk in infants who show strong allergy to cow's milk has been a boon to physicians. "In these infants, the risk of soybean sensitivity is far less than a risk of a reaction to cow's milk, even in populations where soybean products are in daily use."

Soybeans are a natural food, though they are not as familiar to our diet as other foods, and a perfectly healthful one, rich in protein. Their protein does not seem nearly so hostile to the human blood stream as cow's milk does in many cases and so, soybean milk serves as an excellent substitute for cow's milk in infants who have a sensitive or allergenic background.

Of course, there may be a child here and there who is sensitive to soybean milk, but the incidence is much lower than for cow's milk. No food is absolutely acceptable to every human. Some individuals are allergic to strawberries, eggs, carrots, celery, etc. In this context, an occasional allergy to soybean milk can be understood. It is much less likely than an allergy to cow's milk.

Spleen

The Spleen, Scavenger of the Blood

For many years, it has been customary for physiologists to consider the spleen a largely vestigial organ. Knowledge of its function in the body was (and still is) incomplete. Although certain protective activities, such as blood purification and regeneration, have long been known to be performed by the spleen, medical authorities have generally believed that all such functions are performed, and performed better, by other organs as well.

This is probably the chief reason that the spleen remains a mysterious organ about which little is known, and even less is known absolutely beyond dispute. Medical researchers, like most other people, like to concentrate their efforts on what they consider important.

Now, however, it has been shown that the spleen plays a vital role in helping the body to recover after exposure to radiation.

In a recent article in *International Forum* (Vol. 3, No. 9), Professor Maxwell M. Wintrobe, head of the Department of Medicine of the University of Utah and Director of the Laboratory for Study of Hereditary and Metabolic Disorders, points out that, "it has been shown that recovery of hematopoietic (blood-making) tissues following whole body irradiation is significantly hastened by lead shielding of the marsupialized spleen. It was found that the dose required to produce death in 50 per cent of spleen-shielded mice was 1100 roentgens, whereas only half this amount produced the same number of deaths in unshielded animals."

In non-technical language, what Professor Wintrobe is pointing out is that, after exposure to radiation, a healthy spleen is the most important single element in regeneration of the blood. It not only plays its own role in cleansing the blood stream, but seems to be necessary to the proper functioning of all the other organs that participate in the manufacture of new, good blood.

This, of course, is one more demonstration of the truth of what Editor Rodale has often pointed out: there is no such thing as an unnecessary part of the human body. Whether it be spleen, tonsils or vermiform appendix, if it seems unnecessary, that is only because we don't understand enough about it. Every cell we possess has a purpose and is necessary to full, healthy functioning. Surgical removals may sometimes be necessary, but they should never be done casually or without evidence that they are inescapably called for.

In another study cited by Professor Wintrobe, animals that had had their spleens removed developed anemia when injected with radioactive strontium, but those that still had their spleens did not develop anemia.

Nobody, as yet, seems to have made a sufficient study of the role of the human spleen in fighting radiation to have published results. It is surely a justifiable supposition, however, that these days our spleens are active every minute, defending us against damage from the radioactive fall-out in the air we breathe, our food and our drink. It's a good time to learn as much as we can about our spleens, and to take the best possible care of them.

What Is the Spleen?

The spleen is an abdominal organ located on the left side of the body, just under the diaphragm. It is made of both muscle fiber and glandular tissue suspended in a membranous sac. In appearance, it is like a large lymph gland. Its normal weight is about 200 grams, and at that weight, it cannot be felt by palpation (hand pressure). If it enlarges as much as 25 per cent however, to a weight of 250 grams, it becomes palpable.

A direct supply of arterial blood is received by the spleen, and is then fed right into a major vein for immediate return to the heart and the circulatory system.

In the prenatal embryo, the spleen participates in formation of the blood. After the child is born, this function seems to be suspended, but the organ seems to be ready to resume it at such time as it may be necessary, as for instance, when radioactivity destroys the red cells of the blood at a rapid rate.

Ordinarily, the spleen's relation to the red cells is more that of a scavenger. As the red cells are used up, they are reduced to dust-like particles which the spleen removes from the blood stream. The organ will also remove whole red corpuscles that are badly formed as part of its work of keeping the blood in the healthiest and purest possible state.

The spleen seems also to play an important role in regulating the number of leucocytes (white cells) in the blood. These are produced principally in the bone marrow, but the rate at which they are produced or inhibited seems to be controlled by secretions of the spleen. Lymphocytes, one type of white blood cell that appears with miraculous speed at a source of infection, are apparently stored in the spleen and released at the first sign of foreign matter entering the blood, dispatched right to the heart through the portal vein and from there, sped on their way to combat the infection.

Disorders of the Spleen

One of the serious disorders that can happen to the spleen—lymphoid hypoplasia—is caused by a deficiency of vitamin A. When this occurs, the glandular tissue of the spleen shrinks and ceases to function.

The other disorders to which the spleen is subject, while not directly traceable to vitamin deficiency, are equally well averted, for the most part, by a devotion to the principles of proper diet. These are all disorders of overwork of the spleen. If called upon continually to correct improper composition of the blood, the spleen may become enlarged and overactive, and continue so, even when there is no longer any need for it. Hypersplenism can be a cause of congenital hemolytic jaundice, anemia and various other disorders of the blood. But hypersplenism seems to occur only when there is originally a blood disorder that causes the spleen to work over-time in the effort to correct it.

The maintenance of a pure, healthy condition of the blood that will not overwork the spleen, of course, is largely a matter of good diet. There are also definite bacterial infections, such as malaria, that are known to have a pathological effect on the spleen. But it is our belief that the diseases we may get—even the contagious or infectious diseases—can be greatly reduced by building our resistance with good nutrition.

Since it has now been shown to be a vital element in our ability to withstand and survive radioactive fall-out, guarding the health of the spleen has become more important than ever before.

Sugar and Sweets

You Don't Need Refined Sweets for Energy

Every commercial for candy, sodas or other sweets makes a point of the energy your child or you, yourself, will get from eating the advertised products. "Contains pure sugar," the announcer says, "for quick energy." Gradually, the attitude we are accepting is that a diet lacking in "pure sugar" is a diet which will leave us without any energy at all. This is the reason mothers give for allowing their children's high consumption of sweets at the expense of their appetites for nutritional foods.

Can anyone really believe that eating candy, or any of its relatives, is the only way a boy can get the pep to play ball or a girl to jump rope? What did the Greeks do for energy when the original Olympic Games were held in ancient times—chew on a piece of peanut brittle and wash it down with a swig of cola? Of course not; they got energy from the natural sugars that appear in most fruits and vegetables. And with the natural sugars, came the vitamins and minerals which bodies can translate into healthy muscles and vital organs.

Many Types of Natural Sugars

When we think of sugar, we think in terms of the small bowl of white grains or wrapped cubes always to be found on a restaurant table or the counter in a diner. Actually, there are many types of natural sugars which we eat every day and which can satisfy our need for energy safely and fully.

Glucose, sometimes called dextrose, is what we refer to as blood sugar. It occurs in the blood and in almost all fruits and vegetables. In grapes, for example, and in honey, more than half of the solid matter is glucose.

Fructose, as is implied by the name, is found in most fruits and vegetables.

Lactose is a sugar we hear of frequently. It occurs only in milk. It is quickly and easily digested and in the process, is changed into glucose and galactose. Lactose is especially prized as food for the friendly intestinal bacteria we need to prevent infections.

Maltose is a natural sugar we find in malt-germinated grains.

Cellulose is a sugar, too, but is indigestible to humans. It consists of such things as the skins and cores of vegetables and the husks of grains. These elements are valuable for their bulk, however, which is important for good digestion and avoidance of constipation.

Inulin is another of the sugars that we humans are not able to digest efficiently. It occurs in onions, garlic and Jerusalem artichokes.

Sucrose, which we find in fruits and vegetables, is the chemical name for the white sugar Americans sprinkle on their cereal and stir into their coffee. It makes up about half the solid matter of a carrot. Of course, when we eat sucrose in the form of a sugar cube, we eat the product left by the manufacturers after they have managed to scrape away all of the vitamins and minerals offered by the carrot or the sugar cane or sugar beet. The sucrose, or white sugar, we know is pure carbohydrate; that is, combined carbon, hydrogen and oxygen.

Refined Sugar Is Not a Food

This sucrose is no more a food than a teaspoon of iron filings would be if it were edible. However, refined white sugar doesn't pass through the body without affecting it. For example, when the body calls for energy needed to do some special job, the refined sugar, instead of fat which is the body's legitimate store of energy, is burned to provide that energy. That is the reason sweets tend to make people put on weight—the body never gets a chance to burn the fat which it has been accumulating for use in an emergency and the accumulation just continues.

Another of the problems refined sugar brings to the body is the processing it requires. It demands all sorts of special attention upon entering the body. Enzymes must rush to it to help the sugar get ready for the intestines. Once there, all sorts of involved mechanisms are called into play to handle the sugar. Vitamins, especially the B vitamins, are stolen from the job of repairing frayed nerves or rebuilding liver cells and are transferred to the sugar project. The calcium-phosphorus balance is upset. The added complexities of handling sugar are infinite and largely unknown. But, while these things are going on, other jobs are left undone, due to lack of material, and these unfinished projects throughout the body can result in the chronic illnesses and weaknesses so many of us complain about.

Why We Prefer Natural Sugars

When sugars are taken in their natural state, as they occur in vegetables, fruit and milk, they are not the unexpected, undesirable guest in the body that refined sugar is. They are not to be pampered and waited on, they come ready to pitch in and do their part in keeping the body on its feet. They bring not only enough vitamins, minerals and enzymes to take care of their own processing in the body, but more besides. Naturally occurring sugars add to bodily health; they do not make demands on the body that will tear it down. Furthermore, the body is geared to take care of these sugars easily and efficiently, if they are eaten in reasonable amounts, and to make use of them.

Will there be enough sugar in the food you eat daily to take care of your energy needs even though you lead an active life? Well, just think of the number of sweet-tasting foods you can eat every day without using a pinch of sugar. All fresh fruits taste sweet and all are rich in carbohydrates (the collective name for all sugars and starches, which are converted to sugar by the body). Many foods, which do not taste sweet at all, are full of carbohydrates. Here are the amounts of sugar, or carbohydrates, you get with some commonly used, readily available, fresh or dried, fruit, as shown in *Nutritional Data,* published by H. J. Heinz Company:

BLACKBERRIES	12.5%	DRIED FIGS	68.4%
RED RASPBERRIES	13.8%	GRAPES	15.5%
ORANGES	11.2%	PEACHES	12.0%
APPLES	14.9%	PEARS	15.8%
APRICOTS	12.9%	PLUMS	12.9%
BANANAS	23.0%	PRUNES	71.0%
CHERRIES	14.8%	RAISINS (DRY)	71.2%
DRIED DATES	75.4%		

The readings on the carbohydrate content of some of our vegetables are interesting, too:

BOILED SWEET POTATOES	27.9%	CARROTS (RAW)	9.3%
BAKED WHITE POTATOES	22.5%	ONIONS (RAW)	10.3%
KIDNEY BEANS (COOKED)	16.4%	LIMA BEANS (COOKED)	18.3%
SWEET CORN (COOKED)	20.2%	PEAS (COOKED)	12.1%

Nuts offer plenty in the way of carbohydrates. You will be surprised at how much sugar you can get in a nut without making any additions whatsoever.

ALMONDS	19.6%	PEANUTS (ROASTED)	23.6%
CASHEWS (ROASTED)	27.1%	PECANS	13.0%

Cereals and Bread

If you or your children eat processed breakfast foods (of which we disapprove), your carbohydrate intake skyrockets:

CORN FLAKES	85.0%	BRAN FLAKES	78.8%
PUFFED RICE	87.7%	WHEAT FLAKES	80.2%

This means that, if you put a cup of cereal in your bowl and eat it all, even without sugaring it, your body will get between ¾ and 9/10 of a cup of sugar from that part of your breakfast alone. Cereals of this type are almost as useless to the body as white sugar, but they serve to illustrate our point that artificial sweets, added to the average diet for energy, are certainly unnecessary.

We have not yet mentioned the bread most people eat each day. White bread is 51.8 per cent carbohydrate; rye, 52 per cent; wholewheat, 49.0 per cent. Then there's macaroni at 76.5 per cent and spaghetti at 30.2 per cent carbohydrate.

We Eat More Than Two Cups Daily

Most of these and other high-carbohydrate—hence, "high-energy"—foods appear on American tables several times a day. We eat well over two cups of sugar a day, even in a completely natural diet, before adding any sweetener to our food. Champion athletes break records without sucking candy squares or drinking pop, why should American children need a "burst of energy" for playing with dolls or climbing trees? A healthful, natural schedule of food and rest is the best way to retain sufficient energy. There is no need for any refined sweets. If extra energy is somehow needed, an apple or fig or prune will supply all that is needed and do so healthfully. Remember, the announcer who tries to convince you that energy comes only in candy bars is not nearly so interested in your health as he is in the money you can spend on his product.

We are convinced that most people have too much carbohydrate in their diets. Americans, especially, seem to have a taste for artificial foods that are rich in carbohydrates. We say, make an effort to avoid overindulgence in all carbohydrate foods. If you're hungry, eat some protein in preference to carbohydrate. If you insist on high carbohydrate foods, stick to natural ones.

We're Using More Sugar

Some time ago, there appeared a story in a food trade paper in which the head of the Sugar Research Foundation said that canners should prepare their fruits with 60 per cent more sugar than they use now (in canned peaches, it is 35 per cent) to gain maximum consumer acceptance. He said that best results in flavor could be had by adding "too much sugar" and then neutralizing some of the sweetness by adding citric acid to the syrup. He supported his conclusions with questionnaires filled out by tasters at the California State Fair. The fruit so treated was said by samplers to taste even "fruitier" than when less sugar was present.

This was a typical example of the way our senses are being deceived by the yearning for sweets to which we've been educated. People want the sweetness, not the flavor of the fruit. If it is bathed in thick sugar syrup, fruit tastes better to them, not because the fruit flavor is made more intense, as the Sugar Research Foundation would have us believe, but merely because it's sweeter!

In the *Muskegon* (Michigan) *Chronicle,* February 3, 1960, the truth of this situation was emphasized in the findings of Mary Morr, of the Foods and Nutrition Department at Michigan State University. Dr. Morr found that fruits canned in light syrup usually have more true fruit flavor than those canned in heavy syrup. Too much sugar, she said, can mask the flavor of fruits.

There are two opposing viewpoints. Do you believe Dr. Morr, whose job it is to uncover objective facts, or the Sugar Research Foundation, whose job it is to sell sugar?

A Chance for Real Education

Education has its ups and downs in this country, but Chicago, Illinois, has taken an upswing in its concern for the youth in its schools and it's about time the rest of our cities follow suit. For the first time that we know of, a metropolitan school system has decided to "curtail" drastically the sale of sweets in the elementary schools and to test the withdrawal of candy and carbonated beverages from two of its larger high schools." This action is reported with no little admiration in the *Journal of the American Dental Association* (May, 1960).

We agree that such action is commendable, but it is puzzling that it should not be the normal action taken in all schools all over the country. It is not hard to imagine that a pupil who is exposed to an hour's instruction in the classroom on the nutritional evils of candy and soda should be confused upon entering the school cafeteria and being offered these very things as part of the wholesome lunches schools are always advocating. Whom do our educators think they're kidding? If a thing is true in the classroom, it is certainly no less true in the cafeteria.

Of course, economics is not a totally absent factor. Many a school board depends on candy and soda sales for new lights in the gymnasium or band uniforms. They are extremely reluctant to pass up a source of revenue that can yield many thousands of dollars in profits as candy sales do in some large cities. *Look at the Girl Scouts —their cookie sale is a yearly bonanza!* While the money is tempting and may be used to good advantage, certainly the end does not justify the means. It is basically, ethically, morally wrong for schools, or any other authority, to encourage those youngsters whom they influence to eat foods that are unhealthful for them. If money is a problem, surely there are other ways to get it. What is wrong with selling fruit and nuts instead of sweets? That would really be education!

What the "Authorities" on Sugar Say

A British health magazine, *Family Doctor* (the layman's organ of the British Medical Association), which seems to be akin to *Today's Health,* published by the American Medical Association, brought out a booklet entitled *All About Sugar.* In the booklet, one article after another, by medical doctors, gives sugar a wonderful build-up as a food of health—sugar water is recommended for babies who won't sleep, glucose drinks for hospital patients, plus statements that sugar isn't at all bad for the teeth.

Kenneth O. A. Vickery of the Health and Welfare Services Department, County Borough of Eastbourne, took out after *Family Doctor* hammer and tongs in a letter printed in the *British Medical Journal* (December 26, 1959). He refers to a memorandum drawn up by a panel of eminent dental surgeons which refers to "the grave national scourge of dental caries and underlines the close association between caries incidence and the consumption of fermentable carbohydrates, such as domestic sugar and glucose, noting also the absence of nutritionally protective factors in such commodities . . ."

The British Medical Association appears prominently in a list compiled by the British Dental Association of those organizations who "are urged to take note of and further by any means in their power the spread of knowledge regarding the dental health principles specified in the *Memorandum.*" Instead, the British Medical Association lines up with a high-powered advertising campaign for sugar, candy, syrup, ice cream, etc. What, asks Dr. Vickery, can the tiny budget of a local health authority do to counteract such a state of affairs?

Here is a deliberate about-face on the principles and facts of good nutrition and health by doctors whose business it is to know and spread the truth among those who have faith in them and have few other sources of information. It is appalling to think of a group of responsible physicians purposely offering false information to their readers for but one possible reason—financial gain. It is, at the same time, admirable to see a local health official take his political life in his hands, by protesting so vigorously a wrong being perpetrated on the public by his superiors.

We wonder how many of our local boards of health members would have the courage to protest to the American Medical Association about the sugar product ads which appear consistently in *Today's Health*—which leads us to wonder, too, if the *Journal of the American Medical Association* would ever print such a letter?

Hard Candy Ruins Teeth

Hard candy is a favorite with kids and adults. At Christmas, whole tins of it are gobbled up in no time. Cough lozenges act as an excellent excuse for school children to suck such candy during hours in which they would normally be forbidden to do so. But aside from this, stores offer vast assortments of sour balls, jaw breakers, rock candy, lollipops, etc., all the time.

Scientists researching the effects of sugar on teeth have found repeatedly that candies which are gooey or sticky or candies held close to the teeth for long periods of time, are the worst offenders when it comes to causing tooth decay. Evidence of this fact came in the *New York State Dental Journal* (March, 1961). In it, we read of a 50-year-old man whose entire remaining set of teeth on the lower jaw (he had an upper plate) showed severe erosion around their necks. Three years earlier, an X-ray had shown no evidence of this problem.

The patient said that, for the past year or so, he had been in the habit of sucking candy lozenges constantly, to relieve "nervous tension." All of the remaining teeth had to be extracted. Some were so bad that they broke during normal chewing before the extraction could be arranged.

Parents should not have to be warned about the logical outcome of the candy-sucking habit in their children. First teeth are considered expendable by some. However, it should be kept in mind that secondary teeth depend on the first teeth for alignment. Also, the candy habit started with baby teeth will not disappear merely because secondary teeth appear. It will persist until the second teeth are ruined by it. Teach your children to eat fruit when they must have something sweet.

Promoting the Candy Business

Is all fair in love and war—and business? We wonder where ethics comes into such a question. In August, 1961, we received a clipping in the mail which made us wonder if morality exists at all in business. Though we haven't the exact name of the paper, the clipping indicates that it is published in Portland, Oregon, and its name, or part of it, is the *Journal*. A staff writer, Tom Fershweiler, wrote one of the most disillusioning stories you are likely to hear of for a long time. As Mr. Fershweiler put it, the candy industry "abducted a registered nurse from the enemy camp and named her Miss Candy, 1961."

Can you imagine the meeting at which this cozy bit of promotion was hatched? We think it might have gone something like this:

IDEA MAN: You know, boss, the cigarette companies, the toothpaste people, the aspirin people, have all tried the medical angle, why don't we? People still believe almost anything if a doctor says it, or even somebody dressed like a doctor.

CANDY EXECUTIVE: Sure, but you know how doctors and nurses always tell kids to avoid sweets because they spoil the appetite for nourishing foods and cause cavities and that chocolate is a factor in acne.

IDEA MAN: I know what they *say,* but who gives the kids lollipops after they get their injections? Who allows the kids candy and ice cream when they're in the hospital? Who tells the parents that candy will give kids energy? Don't you see? The public is convinced that the medical profession is guarding the public's health by warning against candy, but just about every individual doctor eats candy, gives it to his children and allows his patients to have it, too. The nurses are the same! It should be easy to get someone in the medical profession to say he's on our side. He'll only have to say that *some* candy's good for everybody and that only radical crackpots and faddists are against candy for kids. And just think, he'll do for candy what the medical angle has done for cigarettes, aspirin and everything else it's been used for. "American Medicine knows what's good for Americans. It never makes mistakes and it's too honest to tell anything but the truth." Why parents will be *forcing* their kids to eat candy!

CANDY EXECUTIVE: I think you've got something there. But I like the nurse even better than the doctor. It's the mother image for the kids and someone for the real mothers to identify with. Let's get one about 25 years old, so that she'll give the impression of young motherhood herself. And if we can get a pretty one, as well, the men will be interested. It's a natural!

So the idea became a reality—"Nurse Helps Confectioners Fight Back," the headline reads. Lea Gallic of Chicago, a 25-year-old R.N. who is pretty in the quiet way that builds confidence, set out on a 55-city tour as Miss Candy, 1961. She says things like this, according to reporter Fershweiler: "Candy's dandy. It's a genuine food and often a dietary aid. It contains many dairy products and provides vitamins and minerals essential to health."

Can she be an R.N. and really believe that statement to be true? What dairy product, except for whatever little milk or butter fat there might be in milk chocolate or butter creams, can there be? As for the vitamins and minerals, they must come from the nuts sometimes found in candy bars and these food values are fast lost to the body through the other ingredients in the candy. We'd like to see some proof that a lollipop has some food value—any at all.

We think this promotion is one of the most infamous we've ever seen. We think it gives the entire nursing profession a black eye. We think it proves that the candy business will stop at nothing. Candy is a direct opponent to good health. Every bite you eat robs your body of nutrients it can ill afford to lose.

Understandable Confusion

It is interesting to read the "Letters to the Editor" section of the newspaper. You can learn a lot. For example, in the Toledo (Ohio) *Blade* (November 16, 1960), we found another voice crying in the wilderness against the sale of chocolate milk and candy in the public schools. A dentist wrote to deprecate the attitude taken by the *Blade* when the dental society attempted to eliminate these harmful products from the public schools. The paper apparently offered the same old wheeze about American kids needing the jaw breakers and colas to help them to grow up as well-rounded, regular guys. The dentist pointed out that well-rounded people need to be healthy and that good health includes good teeth. The writer also made several other points—and quite well, too—about preventive care and unscrupulous dental quacks and charlatans. And he didn't mention fluoridation once as a preventive! We agree with Dr. R. W. Cole in just about everything he said.

However, we can see the *Blade's* side of this thing, too. First of all, plenty of advertising comes from chocolate milk, soda and candy producers. Why cut the advertisers down—especially when most dentists don't seem to give a hang about it one way or the other? Consider the attitude most of them display when a nutritionist writes an article on candy or other sugar products. They smile tolerantly and stock up on lollipops to pass out to their young patrons after a successful session. They recommend sugar-laden toothpastes; their journals advertise sugar-rich chewing gum; they advise sugar-loaded ice cream as a source of calcium; they want to put fluorides into candies so the kids will take them more surely than if the chemical were only in water.

Sure there are dentists who don't believe in this kind of thing. There are dentists who won't keep soft drinks in the refrigerators at home for their children, whose children eat fruit for dessert and who aren't permitted to eat candy and ice cream. There are even dentists who don't eat these things themselves, but the count is mighty low. Would a ratio of one in a hundred be an exaggeration? One in a thousand? Think of the dentists that you know, the things you read that dentists write. Do you get the feeling that diet really means as much to them as it appears to mean to Dr. Cole?

No, one can't really blame the *Blade* for not knowing just what dentists want to see written about dental health. No wonder the *Blade* has a problem in forming a proper attitude: if it writes seriously about the dental dangers in sugar, it will be called radical by many dentists; if it writes breezily about dental problems, taking them as seriously as most of the public has been trained to take them by the example of the dental societies, the approach is criticized as too flip. Why has dentistry waited until now to throw up its hands in horrer at the sugar in Ma's apple pie and the ice cream cone? If the *Blade* is confused, so are millions of other Americans.

The Danger of Artificial Sweeteners

Why do we object to low-calorie sweeteners? Many think we are being unnecessarily strict in urging them to avoid saccharin and the other chemical substitutes, when we have already condemned the use of refined sugar. Our primary objection to sugarless sweeteners has been that they are strictly chemical compounds. They have no relation whatsoever to the natural foods with which the body can deal properly. They present problems to the body's organs which are bound to remain unsolved.

So much for that objection. In *Science News Letter* (April 29, 1961), Dr. Albert A. Branca, of the University of Delaware, calls our attention to another fault to be found with sugarless sweeteners. It does strange things to your blood sugar level. When one is accustomed to a sweet taste upon eating sugar, the sweet taste alone is enough to set in motion the bodily machinery that ordinarily operates when sugar is eaten. Insulin is released in the body, more glucose is used, glycogen is conserved. The result is a lowering of blood sugar. This also occurs when something sweet—even though it be something other than sugar—is eaten. Dr. Branca reported that 13 out of 14 normal students observed in a test had lowered blood sugar after drinking a solution of sugarless sweeteners.

If we had to choose between refined white sugar and an artificial sweetener, we would have to choose the refined sugar as being less harmful to the body. That is not to say that refined white sugar is healthful. Far from it. The only healthful sweet is that which occurs naturally in fruits and vegetables. The sugar that makes peas and corn, apples and peaches sweet is the only sugar one should eat if health is one's aim.

Sun

Don't Suffer for a Tan

In the summer months, many Americans are content, even anxious, to spend a good part of their recreational time jostling on a crowded beach for enough space to spread a beach towel. Why? To lie in the sun and bake. The hoped for result is a bronze tan that will give the one who acquires it psychological satisfaction and, somehow, a new social standing. Physically, the effect is often trouble.

The idea that long exposure to the sun is a healthful practice is a mistaken one. The sun's rays are powerful and can be very dangerous, especially when exposure is too long and too sudden. City dwellers who wait for a hot day and take their pallor to the beach for a one-shot tan are doing their skin a grave disservice. Every scrap of instinct and good sense tells the determined sun bather that he should retreat to a shaded spot. He is in torture as he tries to absorb enough sun to make himself tan. Actually, he absorbs enough sun to make himself sick. He may lose his appetite, feel headachey, feverish and nauseated and lose a couple of nights' sleep as the result of his day of fun at the beach. Wearing even the lightest shirt will be torture for him as it rests on his blazing-red back. How can anyone consider such a condition healthy?

Of course, the sun is a source of vitamin D, valuable to anyone, especially children. But the normal day offers many opportunities for the necessary exposure: a walk to the office or to the store, a quarter hour or a half hour (at first) in the garden, washing windows, hanging clothes. These are all opportunities for plenty of sun for most adults. Children need more because of growing bones, but they get more, too, because they spend more time out of doors playing. There is no need for the 4-hour baking sessions most people have in mind when they speak of getting "a little sun."

Some Consequences Not Apparent

G. P. magazine (June 1960) printed an article on sunlight by S. William Becker, Jr., M.D., of the Department of Dermatology at the University of Illinois. Dr. Becker has strong reservations about the value of sunlight, especially in light-skinned people, and points out that many of the results of prolonged exposure to strong sunlight are not apparent to the layman. For example, few are aware that, after a single, moderately severe sunburn, the blood vessels are so strongly affected that it takes 4 to 15 months for them to return to a normal state. Imagine the effects of repeated sunburn!

Sunburning over a period of years dries the skin to the point at which its elasticity is lost. The color darkens and becomes a blotchy brown or yellow. Definite skin cancers develop. In the *New York*

763

Herald Tribune (September 16, 1960), Science Editor, Earl Ubell told of the warning of Dr. Milton T. Edgerton of Johns Hopkins Hospital, Baltimore, that excess exposure to sunshine or sun lamps could cause hundreds of tiny cancers on the face or jaw. The therapy for such a condition is what Dr. Edgerton refers to as a resurfacing of the face. It is an operation which cuts off the thousands of little cancers and replaces the skin with grafts from the neck and chest.

Proves the Power of the Rays

Of course, such a serious condition is not the result of a simple exposure, or even a few exposures, to the harmful sun's rays or rays from sun lamps. The patients treated in this way by Dr. Edgerton have been well-to-do businessmen who nurse a year-round tan by means of a daily sun lamp exposure or a winter of real sun baths under the Florida sun. Also among likely victims are light-skinned farmers, ranchers and others whose trade or profession keeps them out of doors. After about 15 years or so of this frequent sunning, the trouble begins. Perhaps you know you never indulge in such persistent exposure to the sun. Maybe you only get one or two burns a year. You are tempted to disregard this warning. But remember, if the sun's rays are capable of such severe effects after prolonged exposure, they are having an unhealthful effect each time they burn your skin even mildly. If you're in the sun long enough to get a burn, you've been there too long.

An interesting theory was recorded in the correspondence section of the *Journal of the American Medical Association* (May 13, 1939), concerning the helpful effect of sunlight on bone. Dr. E. V. Wilcox went back to Herodotus' writings in 450 B.C. in which he told of a visit to a battlefield on which Persian and Egyptian soldiers had met 75 years previous. The skeletal remains of the fallen soldiers were still there. Herodotus was struck by the difference in the thicknesses of the Persian and Egyptian skulls. He wrote:

"The bones of the Persians lay in one part of the field and the bones of the Egyptians in another. The skulls of the Persians were so fragile that a mere pebble thrown at them would penetrate them. But those of the Egyptians were so strong that you could hardly break them with a stone. The cause of this, so the people said, and I readily agreed, is that from childhood, the Egyptians shave their heads and the bone is thickened by exposure to the sun. For the same reason, they do not become bald. Of all races of men, bald heads are rarest among the Egyptians. Such then is the reason for their strong skulls. And the reason why the Persians have weak skulls is that they cover their heads all their lives with felt hoods. . . ."

How accurate Herodotus' theory is, has never actually been resolved. We do know that sunshine is valuable in forming strong bone structure, but such formation takes place in childhood. It is

Sunflower Seeds

The Important Protein of Sunflower Seeds

It is understandable that, in many parts of the world where high-protein foods like meat are unavailable or scarce, food scientists are busy searching for foods of vegetable origin high in protein that can be substituted for the more expensive and scarce foods like meat and eggs. In countries like India and some of the African nations, food supplements and, indeed, entire meals made from some such food seem to be the only solution to the problem of continual hunger.

It is gratifying to find that sunflower seeds are being considered and studied more and more in this scientific search. The reason is plain to see. Sunflower seeds, in addition to being rich in the right kind of fats, minerals and vitamins, are an excellent source of protein. And now we find that the protein of sunflower seeds is especially valuable, because it is high in methionine, an important kind of protein which is usually lacking in vegetable foods.

An article from *Food Science,* published in Mysore, India, brought us this information. Written by 4 researchers of the Central Food Technology Research Institute of Mysore, the information appeared in Vol. 7, p. 326, of this publication. They tell us that the sunflower plant is believed to have originated in Mexico and was possibly introduced into Europe in the sixteenth century. It gradually became an important crop in eastern Europe, more especially, in Russia.

More recently, it has assumed great importance in Argentina, where the cultivation is said to have been developed by Russian immigrants. A chart giving the world production of sunflower seed shows that the U.S.S.R. leads in production, with Argentina a close second. Hungary and Yugoslavia are third and fourth, while the United States and Canada tail the list, producing about 1/200 as much as the leaders. These figures are for 1948. We hope and believe that production of sunflower seed in our country has increased greatly since then, for we are quite sure that there is considerably more interest in the seeds now than there was at that time.

Varieties and Content

Our Indian specialists tell us that there are numerous varieties of sunflowers, distinguished mostly by the height to which the plants grow. In general, they say, for producing good oil crops, the dwarf ones are best, because they have a lower and more uniform height, making them easier to harvest. The seeds of the dwarf varieties also have a higher oil content.

The hulls of sunflower seeds make up about half the content

767

—the other half being the kernel which is what we eat. The chemical content of the seeds, as these researchers quote, is indicated in Table 11.

Table 11: CONTENTS OF SUNFLOWER SEEDS

Constituent	Whole Seed	Kernel
Hulls	48 %	
Kernels	52 %	
Moisture	6.9%	4.5%
Fat	24.7%	41.5%
Protein	16.1%	27.7%
Crude fiber	17.9%	1.0%
Carbohydrates	21.3%	21.5%
Ash	3.1%	3.8%

From this breakdown, it appears to us that the hull of the sunflower seed is edible and nutritious, too, and we surely wish someone who is interested in feeding the world's hungry people would soon begin to find some dietary use for the hulls! Actually, hull and kernel together contain as much protein as many meats, more fat than any other vegetable food except for nuts and avocados and a high percentage of ash, which means that they are rich in minerals.

The Indian magazine goes on to tell us that many researchers have shown that the amino acid content of sunflower seeds is especially rich in methionine, meaning that, like sesame seeds, these could be used as substitutes for meat or other foods of animal origin. Other seed foods tend to be short in methionine. Table 12 gives the amino acid content of sunflower seeds as compared to that of several other seed foods. Methionine is the important protein to watch—note that sesame and sunflower seeds are high.

Table 12: AMINO ACID CONTENT OF SUNFLOWER AND OTHER SEEDS
(*Figures given are percentages.*)

Amino Acid	Sunflower Seed	Peanut	Soybean	Cottonseed	Sesame
Arginine	8.2	9.9	7.1	7.4	8.7
Histidine	1.7	2.1	2.3	7.4	8.7
Lysine	3.8	3.0	5.8	2.7	2.8
Tryptophan	1.3	1.0	1.2	1.3	1.8
Phenylalanine	5.0	5.4	5.7	6.8	8.0
Methionine	2.9	1.2	2.0	2.1	3.2
Threonine	3.9	1.5	4.0	3.0	4.0
Isoleucine	5.2	3.0	4.7	3.4	4.8
Valine	5.4	8.0	4.2	3.7	5.1

Facts about the Seed

We then learn that various researchers have discovered interesting things about sunflower seed protein: it is as valuable as animal protein in nourishing chicks; it is a good supplementary protein for corn (which is low in methionine); it is superior to the protein of peanuts, yeast or blood meal in nourishing rats; heating the seeds causes destruction of some of the value of the protein; and, finally, the digestibility of sunflower seed protein was found to be very good. Feeding sunflower seed to various animals, investigators have learned that you can use the seeds as the only source of B vitamins in a diet. In such a test, they showed up better than wheat germ or corn germ. As a source of pantothenic acid and niacin (two B vitamins), sunflower seeds turn out to be superior to soybean meal, wheat germ and corn germ.

Sunflower seed oil has been found, by various researchers, to be almost completely digested; it is high in the unsaturated fatty acids which make seed oils so valuable and it is especially high in linoleic acid, which is the one kind of fatty acid most esteemed by researchers in the chemistry of fats. This is, probably, the essential oil for preventing harmful deposits of cholesterol in arteries and kidneys and gall bladders of the human body.

Conclusion

In conclusion, the Indian authors say, "In view of the fact that protein malnutrition is widely prevalent among children belonging to the lower income groups of the population in several Asian countries, Africa and South America, attempts are being made in different countries to prepare concentrated protein foods from readily available sources to combat protein malnutrition. But many of these protein foods suffer from the drawback that they lack in the essential amino acid, methionine. As sunflower seed proteins are rich in methionine and contain adequate amounts of other essential amino acids, it will be desirable to cultivate sunflower seed on a large scale for preparing an edible meal rich in proteins. The meal can be incorporated with other more abundantly available meals like groundnuts (peanuts), soybean, etc., so as to obtain a blend which can provide high-quality protein rich in all essential amino acids."

We say amen to all these sentiments. And because our concern is more the American people, where many diets are deficient in protein, too—not because of lack of protein, but because of lack of attention to diet—we say let's all eat more sunflower seeds! Why not try incorporating them with peanuts, wheat germ and other foods of this kind to get our children and our senior citizens used to this very tasty and easily digested food! Any meat grinder or blender will reduce hulled sunflower seeds to a fine spread which can easily substitute for jelly, jam or hydrogenated peanut butter. Sunflower seeds as a between-meal snack will add lots of protein, vitamin and minerals to any day's diet.

Sunflower Seeds as a Laxative

Pumpkin and sunflower seeds made the *Journal of the American Medical Association* (December 17, 1960) in a letter from a doctor asking for an opinion of their laxative powers. He tells of several

Czech, Polish and Russian patients who have commented upon this property in the seeds.

The answer given is that there is no specific reason for laxative action in these seeds, except that they, like all seeds, have a high content of cellulose and hemicellulose, which act as roughage. These are elements which are not plentiful in the modern diet and which would certainly be an aid to elimination. Also, it is pointed out that sunflower seeds are a major source of cooking oil in Europe and act as a source of vegetable protein for animal feed.

We have always encouraged the use of these seeds as nutritious snacks and can think of no more pleasant way to get added doses of valuable protein, as well as vitamins and minerals. Our nutritionists and medical men rely too little on this type of snacking for energy and suggest, instead, candy bars and ice cream as between-meals pick-me-ups.

Get your children into the habit of eating nutritious nibblers if they must have something between meals. Sunflower seeds are tasty and nutritious, as well as satisfying. And if elimination is a problem, we think it is an excellent idea to add an extra intake of sunflower seeds to the diet, to see if they have a beneficial effect. Certainly, they are preferable to the harsh laxatives sold commercially for this purpose. Even if sunflower seeds should not have the desired laxative effect, the food value they contain makes them very worthwhile additions to anyone's diet.

Surgery

A Proposal to Control Unnecessary Surgery

The shocking exposure of unnecessary surgery, together with the conspiracy among medical men to "cover" for each other when the occasion demands, has often been discussed. Now and then, a courageous doctor will speak his mind on abuses within his profession, but his words often go unprinted or are shouted down until they become buried under a thousand denials and counter-accusations. Sometimes, the indictments against useless surgery come from men whose competence to judge cannot be denied. When this happens, the public has a weapon for self-defense. The advantage should be pursued and perhaps, now is the time.

Here are a few statements that cannot easily be laughed off or explained away:

1. After studying 246 cases in which hysterectomy (the removal of a woman's uterus) had been performed, Dr. Norman Miller, one of the foremost obstetricians in the United States, found that 33.1 per cent—one out of every three—were unnecessary. Microscopic

examination of the removed organs showed no sign of disease. In an article for the *American Journal of Obstetrics and Gynecology* (p. 804, 1946), Dr. Miller quotes a distinguished colleague, Bethel Salamons, as saying, "I would say a gynecologist is not a gynecologist until he ceases to perform unnecessary hysterectomies, for these operations have become nearly as overdone as the operation for tonsillectomy, appendectomy and curetage (scraping of the womb)."

"Routine" Removal of Appendix

2. Needless surgery is at an all time high, say the experts, and who could doubt them upon reading this: "Some gynecologists remove the appendix as a prophylactic measure at the time of pelvic surgery. At Wesley Memorial Hospital, prophylactic appendectomy is done almost routinely, providing the patient is in good condition . . ." So says W. W. Nelson, M.D., in the *American Journal of Obstetrics and Gynecology* (63: 905, 1952). Admittedly, these doctors remove a perfectly healthy organ, for no reason except that it might some day become infected and they call it "routine"! Followed to its logical conclusion, such thinking could lead to the "routine" removal of a lung or a kidney on the assumption that they might some day become diseased.

3. Dr. Robert J. Hawkins spoke of inadequate consultation in 95 per cent of obstetric cases in the *American Journal of Obstetrics and Gynecology* (63: 975, May, 1952). Of 88 cases in which fetal deaths occurred in a reported survey, only 21 had been properly explored and cared for by the attending physician.

Medical "Ethics"

4. Often, bungled or useless surgery gets by because no one will testify against the surgeon. The reason given is "medical ethics," and it is epitomized in the view expressed at an Ontario Medical Association convention whose members abide by the same code as do United States doctors. In discussing the question: Should a surgeon protect another if he found, during the operation, that the physician's diagnosis was incorrect? The medical association answered this for the record: "Never run down the other doctor's diagnosis and treatment." A newspaper editorial the following day ripped into this policy and ended with this: "If a second doctor is called in, the patient likes to think that he has come to save his life, not to cover up the error of the other physician." Replied a convention spokesman, "We doctors must stand together." This is small comfort to the patient who wonders about a diagnosis or the success of a completed operation and plans to consult another physician. What can he hope to gain?

5. In the *New York Herald Tribune* (March 8, 1956), columnist Earl Ubell quoted Dr. Kenneth B. Babcock, Director of the Joint

Committee on Accreditation of Hospitals, as reporting that in one hospital, a 21-year-old woman was sterilized "because she was moving to Wyoming"; in another hospital, ⅓ of the appendectomies were unnecessary; at one hospital, 600 out of 1,000 operations were abortions; denial of accreditation at still another hospital resulted from a report that 380 removals of the uterus were performed and 300 proved to be unnecessary.

"Errors" such as these are not confined to a few situations, they are quite common. The public is a victim, in many cases, of the "ethics" of doctors which forbid their criticizing, or informing on, the work of their colleagues. This same set of ethics permits surgeons to deliberately distort the facts of surgical fatality to absolve themselves of blame. This assertion was made by Dr. Joseph E. Campbell, Chief Pathologist of Cook County (Chicago, Illinois), in these words: "Too often, the surgical operative record . . . blithely ignores significant facts or even records complete untruths," (*Chicago Sunday Tribune*, March 6, 1960).

Check for More Careful Diagnosis

It can be reasonably assumed that if there were some check by an unbiased party on the work of the surgeon, he would diagnose more carefully and report more accurately on what happens in the operating room. If patients or their families could have access to such reports or to sworn reports by the surgeon, greater care would certainly be exercised in the knowledge that future consultants might be called upon to judge the prudence under which he acted. A surgeon who could defend his work by the principles of his craft would have nothing to fear from such checking. It is the incompetent, the careless physician, who, after an inordinate number of questions had been raised about his work, would be forced to mend his ways or choose another field of endeavor.

So-called tissue committees have been formed in many hospitals for just such a purpose. A group of physicians in a hospital examines each piece of tissue that is removed from patients in surgery. They check to see if their findings agree with those of the attending physician. Was the operation necessary? With such a system, when it is properly run, physicians who repeatedly recommend or perform useless surgery are bound to be shown up Unfortunately, committees such as this, formed from doctors who operate themselves or who are friendly with those who do, are bound to be biased in the actions they take. Once bias is a factor, the usefulness of such a group is ended.

Patients' Aid Society

In 1959, an independent group, Patients' Aid Society, Incorporated, was formed by Mr. James F. Donnelly, a former chief surgical technician with the United States Army in World War II. The group was to work for the adoption of the following points intended to help prevent unnecessary surgery and other medical abuses:

1. Independent Tissue Committee—all tissue or any part of the anatomy removed by surgery will be examined and reported on by one or more accredited pathologists who are independent of the surgeon and the hospital. The tissue would reach the pathologist identifiable only by a code number. He will have no knowledge as to the identity of the patient or the doctor, nor will he owe any particular allegiance to the hospital from which it came. He will have no reason to give anything but an accurate report.

2. Notarized Medical Records—the patient's medical record should bear the notarized signature of the accountable medical doctor or the hospital medical administrator who is responsible for the accuracy of the patient's medical record. Such a record would hold the doctor responsible for his work during the patient's hospitalization. He would think twice before allowing entries other than his own to be made by interns and nurses. If any mistakes are to appear over his notarized signature, he will make sure they are his mistakes.

3. Microfilm of Patient's Record—all medical records of each patient would be microfilmed as soon as possible after the patient's discharge, or photostated or copied by any other method that will prevent alteration or deletion or addition of material. The patient or next of kin should receive a copy of his own record on request. The patient's owning such a copy is in accord with the opinion of many medical authorities, including Dr. William J. Mayo, of the Mayo Clinic, who said, "How wonderful it will be some day when, every time a surgeon operates, he will give the patient or her husband or some responsible person a copy of the report which, in most hospitals, is dictated as soon as the operation is finished."

Who has a better right to such reports than the patient? Who would be more likely to need them in case of relapse or further hospital treatment in a new town or a different country? Why should medical men be so reluctant about giving these records to the patient? In any other business, if one pays for the consultation and then a further service, the complete record of the consultation, the materials used and the final result of the transaction, is available to the customer.

4. Hall of Medical Records—it is advocated that an agency be set up with a centralized headquarters, in which a permanent file, under code numbers, of all copies of patients' medical records will be kept—provided that the patient would agree to such a filing of his records. This would act as a safeguard against changes being

made in the records at the hospital at a later date. The original would be permanently recorded and no change would be possible.

The Society would also be interested in furthering new or improved safeguards in medical administrative procedure.

We are very much impressed with the aims of Patients' Aid Society, Incorporated. This group has really taken some positive steps toward the creation of an effective control over the medical empire.

Powdered Surgical Gloves Present a Problem

When a person is required to undergo surgery, probably the last thing he would think of is the way his surgeon gets into his sterile surgical gloves. Now we find (*Journal of the American Medical Association,* June 27, 1959) that this little detail might cost the patient an additional year of disability, if he should be unlucky. It seems that the powder used by the surgeon to facilitate slipping into the gloves, can cause serious complications. The talc which was commonly used until the late nineteen-forties has been replaced by starch-derivative powders.

Starch powders have been shown to be safer than the talc, but are not fool-proof, by any standards. Unfavorable reactions of the brain and spinal cord to these powders have been described in *Annals of Surgery* (December, 1955). The same issue of that periodical told of complications caused by the implantation of this starch in the surgical wounds of two patients. In *Surgery* (February, 1956), an article tells of 3 cases in which tumors were caused by starch powder after an operation, and the author goes on to say that such granules are identified daily in surgical specimens sent to the pathology laboratories.

The case described in the first-mentioned journal concerns a man who returned to the hospital 6 weeks after undergoing an operation for duodenal ulcers. His symptoms strongly suggested appendicitis and an operation to remove the appendix was immediately performed. His abdominal cavity, opened by surgery, released a liter of fluid. An examination of the removed tissue revealed cancer and further surgery was recommended. Removal of a large part of the colon and other intestinal parts was then accomplished. Examination of the removed tissue showed no actual cancer, but on close examination, starch particles were found to have caused the trouble. The patient, aside from a dangerous and useless operation, missed over a year's work. The article remarks that correct diagnosis could have avoided the third operation.

A more careful washing of surgical gloves before operations is advocated in the article, to be certain that starch powder has been removed from the exposed surfaces of the gloves. Glove changes during the operation should be effected at a safe distance from the operating table to avoid contamination due to the dust cloud which often results.

You can probably do little to supervise your doctor's use of such precautions if you should have an operation, but you can guard against infection by taking large amounts of vitamin C before the operation. Then, if some foreign matter should slip into the open wound, your body will have a better chance of preserving itself from serious complications.

Here is still another example of the problems doctors can cause when they employ modern methods of treatment carelessly.

Tallness

We're Getting Taller—Is That Good?

Tallness is considered a desirable asset in the United States. Mothers proudly stand beside their 16-year-old sons and brag about how "he just towers over me!" Young girls still like them tall, dark and handsome, and basketball players just don't get to be basketball players unless they're really tall. A commercial angle sneaks into the discussion when schools find that standard-size desks, sinks and toilets are not good enough anymore. They must be geared for taller users. College dormitories now buy their beds king-size—7 feet long. Purchasing agents for large hotel chains now order 80-inch beds instead of the standard 74-inch ones. Hotel towels have gone from 24 by 44 inches to 26 by 52 to accommodate taller guests, and even the 6-foot sofa has given way to monstrous couches of 8- to 12-foot lengths. The trend continues through dress sizes, shoe sizes and suit sizes. Lloyd Shearer, in noting some of these facts in *Parade* magazine (February 28, 1960), seemed mildly surprised at these increases, but hardly concerned. He seems to think that the advantage actually lies with the taller person and he is only reflecting the general consensus of opinion among Americans in this. As a matter of fact, the only problems faced by a tall man, as Mr. Shearer sees it, were these world-shakers: clothes may just hang; inconvenience in hotel beds; dating problems for the girl; "tall" jokes such as "How's the weather up there?" may cause embarrassment.

More Serious Problems Involved

We believe that there is more to be concerned about than this if our average height continues to increase. Serious problems of health are involved in excessive tallness. These problems seem to center about the circulatory system, especially. For example, in the *Journal of the American Medical Association* (April 5, 1952), a study appears which emphasizes the danger of blood clots in the legs of tall men. Meyer Naide, M.D., tells of 6 male patients over 6 feet tall, who experienced spontaneous blood clots of the leg. These conditions did not follow surgery or prolonged illness as in most cases. The other unusual point involved with these cases was their inability to take anticoagulant drugs without the good chance of blocking the pulmonary artery. Dr. Naide, therefore, considers clotting of this type in a tall person extremely dangerous.

Why this predisposition of tall persons to blood clots in the legs? The author makes a guess: he attributes part of the problem to the cramped positions that tall persons are frequently forced to assume when sitting. If clots form in the veins, strain resulting from severe activity or from unnatural leg positions could cause a separation of the clot from the vein wall and a closure of the pulmonary artery.

Blood Pressure and Height

In *Proceedings of Life Extension Examinees* (May-June, 1940), James J. Short, M.D., reported finding a relationship between the height of a subject and his blood pressure—directly proportional. This held true for men and women. Dr. Short remarks that it is entirely likely that the subjects included in the study, if they should increase in weight or height, would show a further rise in blood pressure. In such case, a greater amount of blood would have to be mobilized, resulting in increased friction and a greater force required for pumping. The force of gravity might also play a role in this, since, in a taller person, a longer—therefore, heavier— column of blood must be lifted to the circulation point, to be distributed to other parts of the body.

A more definitive study proving the same contention, was published in the *Journal of Laboratory and Clinical Medicine* (March, 1941) by Samuel Robinson, M.D. Basing his conclusions on the observation of 2,552 men and 2,021 women, he was able to state, positively, that the taller the person, the higher the blood pressure. He also found a steady decrease in tall persons as the age bracket increased, indicating that taller people do not live as long as shorter ones.

In *The Proceedings of the 40th Annual Meeting of the American Life Insurance Companies* (Vol. 23, 153-206, 1937), a report from the Metropolitan Life Insurance Company of New York, it is stated that tall men are considered exceptional risks where respiratory diseases are concerned.

At this same meeting, a paper by Dr. Charles B. Davenport was read. In it, he said that the following diseases are associated with tallness: varicose veins, varicocele (a varicose condition of the veins of the spermatic cord), pulmonary tuberculosis, goiter, hemorrhoids and valvular diseases of the heart. It is inherent in these facts that, as we as a nation are growing taller (and we certainly are), we as a nation will be more and more susceptible to these diseases.

Milk Is the Secret of Tallness

What is the cause of this dangerous trend to tallness? Heredity might be part of the answer, but only a small part. We're getting taller because our diet is saturated with milk and milk products such as ice cream, cheese and butter. Milk has a growth factor which is not to be found in any other food. We have found volumes of data from scientific experiments and observations which prove the relationship between milk and tallness.

For example, in *Medical Clinics of North America* (1939, New York number), an article told of a group of 240 male college students who were compared with their parents. (The parents were largely foreign-born and this accounted for the large difference in diet habits.) The young men were an average of 2.8 inches taller than their fathers and 4 inches taller than the average of the combined heights of both parents. They drank 125 per cent more milk than their parents.

Childhood is known to be the time for rapid growth, but it has been shown that milk consumption will add astounding impetus to the growth pattern. The *Lancet* (June 6, 1929) describes a study of school children in Scotland which illustrates this point. The youngsters were divided into 4 groups: the first was given a ration of whole milk daily; the second, separated milk; the third ate biscuit supplements containing the caloric value of separated milk; the fourth received no milk supplement at all. (All rations were in addition to what the children ate at home.) The milk drinkers, at the end of a 7-month period, showed an average height increase of 23.5 per cent over the non-milk drinkers.

In India, an experiment involving almost 700 boys proved the point once more, according to the *Journal of the American Medical Association* (October 20, 1956). A group of 337 boys were given skimmed milk powder rations each day, while a control group of 359 boys got no such ration. At the end of a 12-month observation period, results showed that even one ounce of skimmed milk powder per day would increase the height of the boys by 4 inches in a single year.

People often write us indignantly, asking how we can oppose the undisciplined use of milk by those who are past infancy. They say their doctors, the magazines they read and the teachers in their schools think the idea of limiting milk intake is preposterous. We believe that the facts speak for themselves and the relationship between tallness and increased physiological problems cannot be denied. Milk has been shown to influence growth. Milk is, then, one cause of the added troubles tall people face.

We are well aware of the nutritional advantages milk has to offer, but all of these nutrients can be gotten from other sources which do not expose one to the unexplained growth factor hidden in milk. We say avoid milk unless you cannot possibly get the nutritional elements it contains from some other food. The problem of tallness is one which will have to be reckoned with one of these days. Why expose yourself and your children to this unnecessary hazard?

Teeth and Tooth Decay

Between-Meal Snacks and Tooth Decay

Practically everybody knows today that foods high in refined sugar are one of the main causes of tooth decay. Most people have a general idea which of the sugary foods are most harmful from this point of view—of course, those which stay in the mouth for a long time, either because they are sucked or chewed, like hard candy and chewing gum, or because they are sticky and cling to crevices and angles in the teeth.

It is good to have the word of two dental researchers on exactly how these facts work out in everyday life. An article in the *American Journal of Public Health* for August, 1960, by Robert L. Weiss, D.D.S., and Albert H. Trithart, D.D.S., describes a study they did of the amount of tooth decay produced by various between-meal snacks. They were interested both in the kind of snack and how often it was eaten, two factors of great importance.

They studied between-meal snacks only, because, they say, most people in this country eat 3 meals a day and "the probability is very high that each of these meals will include substantial amounts of refined carbohydrates." So, since it might be assumed that all the children studied got plenty of refined sugars and starches at meals, the differences in tooth decay might be related only to the kind and amount of snacks they ate.

They studied 783 children in a West Tennessee region. About one-fourth of the children came from towns, the others were rural children. A list was prepared of all the food items known to be favorite snacks. About half of them can be classed as confections, the others are breads and cereal products, pastries, peanut butter and sweet spread. Parents were questioned as to which foods each child had eaten on the previous day and how often he had eaten it.

The list of snacks included: candies, chewing gum, soft drinks, fruit aides, Kool-Aid, ice cream, sherbet, popsicles, pastries, graham crackers, puddings, Jello, chocolate milk, cocoa, bread and sweet spreads (we assume they mean jellies, etc.), bread and peanut butter, dried fruits and other items which the parents were asked to specify.

Examination of the children's teeth was done in accordance with tests used often by dental researchers—the number of decayed, extracted and filled teeth. We need not go into the technique of the way in which the examinations were done and the figures compiled.

The Five Most Popular Snacks

Of the 5 most popular between-meal snacks, here is the order of popularity: chewing gum, candies, soft drinks, ice cream, pastries —that is, cookies, pies, cake and graham crackers. Gum was chewed by about one out of every three children. One out of every four drank soft drinks and/or ate pastry. One out of every five had ice cream, one out of every six had various combinations of bread, crackers, sweet spreads and peanut butter. The rest of the listed snacks were much less popular. Apparently, all of the foods were readily available for both the town and country children.

The average number of between-meal snacks of high sugar content or high degree of stickiness was 1.75 per day. Some of the children reported eating as many as 4 or more a day. Relating the condition of the children's teeth to the number of snacks they had per day, showed clearly that those who reported eating no sweet or sticky snacks had an average of 3.3 teeth per child that were decayed, extracted or filled. Those who reported eating 4 or more items had an average of 9.8 teeth per child marked with decay, extracted or eligible for extraction, or filled. Between these two extremes, the line goes steadily up—the more snacks, the more tooth decay. And the oftener the child snacks, the more tooth decay.

A Defeatist Attitude on Eliminating Sweets

The authors of this article, drawing a lesson for their readers in the Public Health Service, believe that the public has probably failed and in future will probably fail to learn the dangers of snacks that are high in sweets and sticky. Since the children seem to prefer, they say, snacks that are high in sweets, maybe the best plan would be to try to persuade the parents to cut down on the number of times these snacks are available. They aren't going to learn much about the harmfulness of sweets, anyway—it's too hard to understand, according to our authors. So better just concentrate on getting them to cut down on the number of times the kids get the sweets!

This report contrasts sharply with a study done in England and reported in the *British Dental Journal* for November 18, 1958. In this article, Geoffrey L. Slack, D.D.S., and W. J. Martin, D.Sc., describe the effects of giving a quick snack of a fresh apple every day to a group of children and comparing the condition of their teeth, later, with that of another similar group of children who did not get the apples. "One of the primary factors in dental caries is the retention of food particles in stagnation areas on and around the teeth. Thus, the removal of this debris can contribute much to the prevention of the disease. Immediate tooth brushing after eating has been shown to be effective. This ideal, difficult to achieve and maintain, is an unpopular chore for children of all ages. Tooth brushing twice a day is probably as much as can be expected of the average child," say our authors.

They gave apples to each child in their test groups with instructions that they were to be eaten at the end of each meal and after any between-meal snacks. "The unpeeled apples were cored and sliced horizontally to give apple rings about half an inch thick; this allowed the smallest number of apples to be used, freshly cut for each serving; the serving of whole apples would have been wasteful and uneconomical. The shape of the apple rings made it likely that the younger children, at least, would take a large enough bite to bring the posterior teeth into action." In addition, parents were urged to give the children apple slices to take to school for eating after lunch or snacks.

Ninety children who ate apples regularly and 81 who got no apples, formed the final group on which the study is based. Examinations for gum health were given as well as tooth health. It was found that the apple group showed a marked reduction in gum disorders within 6 months after the program began. The proportion of children with no gum disorders was also considerably higher in the apple group at the end of the test.

In the younger age group, the primary teeth (baby or milk teeth) of the children in the apple group had significantly less decay than those of the non-apple children. The same was true, in older groups, for permanent teeth. The authors feel that the number of children tested was so small that they can draw no broad conclusions, but they feel certain that more tests along these lines should be made.

Children Enjoyed Their Apple Snacks

We were interested in certain other comments they make. First of all, the "children were most enthusiastic in coöperating." Apparently it was no trouble at all to eat the apples.

Only certain apples were used, it was noted—those which have crisp, firm flesh. They say, "Very many types of apples were on the market, but were not of value for the purpose of this study. It was necessary for the flesh of the apple to be firm and crisp with a skin that was not too tough. . . . If it were possible to produce some material that had all the qualities of the ideal apple," they go on, they might have less trouble providing exactly the same thing for

be. Such teeth, concluded the researchers, as are submitted to high chewing loads, are structurally stronger, denser, more caries-resistant than teeth exposed to a low load. Such chewing also has a valuable detergent action.

Gum diseases respond favorably to a "hard" diet. For one thing, the exercise is a valuable aid to increased circulation of the gums. Calculus, or tartar deposit, which plays a local role in gum inflammation, is greatly reduced through the use of coarse fibrous foods.

Dr. Bastien's Suggestions

The German, French, Greek and Swiss peasants have good teeth and well-developed jaws, due, Dr. Bastien believes, to the crusty, crunchy, chewy foods they are used to eating. The type of foods Dr. Bastien has in mind may be seen by the suggested inclusions he offers for a day's menu: raw carrots, natural raw sugar cane (a fibrous, detergent, nondecay-causing stimulant to chewing exercise for the jaws and gums, readily available in Br. Bastien's Caribbean Islands,) ripened toasted corn, celery, dry apricots, whole grain cereal, whole grain bread, sugar-free chewing gum (we presume Dr. Bastien to mean plain chicle, not the commercial type sweetened with synthetic sweetners of which we completely disapprove) and cooked chicken bones (which are apparently meant to be chewed and eaten entirely—a usage of this food strikes Americans as unappetizing and odd). Most of these foods could easily be included in every day's menu.

Dr. Bastien closes with the remark that it is the duty of Dentistry to make the public aware of the problem of poor jaw strength and lack of exercise. There should be more positive action toward reversing the trend from the "puree" type of food to a dynamic, adequate, chewy diet.

More Toothbrushes and More Decay

In presenting his case, Dr. Bastien offers some very interesting material on the other known methods of controlling tooth decay. Oral hygiene, the first-known means of fighting decay of teeth, began in earliest civilization. However, M. K. Hine in *Dental Caries, Mechanisms and Present Control Techniques,* published in 1948, is quoted as saying, "Statistics show that, during the past generation, there has been an increase in dental caries *and* in the sale of toothbrushes . . ." We presume that the sale of toothbrushes is due to increased population and the rise in tooth decay is due to the same old sweet diet eaten by more people, plus the strong possibility that the toothbrushes being bought are not being properly used, if at all.

L. S. Fosdick, writing on the value of toothbrushing in the *Journal of the American Dental Association* (40, pp. 133-143, 1950), described his observations of two groups of students over a two-year period. One group of 523 students was instructed to brush its teeth within 10 minutes following each meal. A control group of 423 students brushed upon arising in the morning and retiring at night. The group who brushed after every meal experienced a 50 per cent reduction in caries attack over a two-year period, as compared with the controls. So it is not the number of toothbrushes in use that counts, but the time in relation to meals and manner in which they are used.

Does Balanced Diet Help?

Dr. Bastien tells us that theories on the value of diet as a control were shaken by observations made during World War II. European children living on what Dr. Bastien terms a substandard diet showed a decrease in dental caries. It should be recalled, however, that such World War II diets were especially low in the foods known to cause tooth decay. Refined sugars were almost unknown, as were other refined, processed foods. What foods were available for sustaining life were unprocessed and simple—the very best type for preserving the teeth. The conclusion that "caries is less common in malnourished than in well-nourished individuals" could hardly be proven if the *complete* diets of both groups were compared, not for quantity, but for quality.

Money Doesn't Guarantee Good Diet

Consider the results of another experiment to which Dr. Bastien refers: In 1957, 110 North American school children living in Port au Prince, Haiti, all from well-to-do families and "evidently on a nutritionally adequate diet," were compared for dental health with a similar group of native children from a poor and undernourished class. The well-to-do American children had a 40 per cent higher rate of dental disease than the natives.

This proves only one thing, and that is, that even children whose parents can afford to choose their diet with an eye to nutritious foods fail to do so. The wealthier children could afford candy, canned foods, desserts, sodas, etc. The native children were limited to raw sugar cane, fresh fruits and vegetables and bones—the very foods Dr. Bastien chooses as best for good dentition.

Another misleading conclusion is drawn when Dr. Bastien quotes P. Jay and others (University of Michigan, 1959) as saying, "Most patients know from personal experience that the inclusions in the diet of adequate amounts of milk, fruits, vegetable preparations will not prevent dental caries as is often claimed." The question of what is excluded from the diet is just as important as what is put into it. If one is eating candy between meals which consist of candied sweet potatoes, deep-fried, breaded pork chops and canned peas, topped off with a piece of cherry pie (for fruit) and a one-a-day vitamin capsule, one can't expect a decline in dental problems. Yet, this type of meal is considered nutritious by most people, especially with the supplement included, minimal as it is, and they will depend upon it for reducing decay. We believe it is important to be sure of getting vitamin and mineral-rich foods in the diet, but it is equally important to omit the carbohydrate-rich foods which are the sworn enemies of your teeth. Sugar, when it is refined, is pure carbohydrate, and wherever it is included in foods, that food is a means of encouraging decay.

Inconvenient to Eat Properly?

The trouble is that "Such a low-carbohydrate diet can be planned to meet the nutritional requirements of most individuals, but they are not consistent with contemporary eating habits and are, therefore, inconvenient to maintain." Public resistance to the use of such a diet, even for a few weeks, has limited its application as a preventive measure. Dr. Bastien laments that, unless public health education succeeds in promoting such eating habits, the low-carbohydrate diet will be little used as a caries control measure.

Of course, that is the answer. Little effort is made by public health officials and doctors or dentists to convince parents and children that sweets are the worst enemies of their teeth. Dentists give children a lollipop after a successful session of drilling; doctors do the same as a reward for a shot; bazaars, run by medical and dental societies to raise funds to back dental health projects, feature candy, cake, sodas and ice cream as big sellers. How can one expect people to be convinced of the dangers in such products, when they are being sold by the very persons who are warning against their use?

Dr. Bastien gives a vote to fluoridation, too, but we believe his plea for the use of hard textured "work-foods" is eminently more sensible and more likely to be effective in helping to maintain or regain dental health. The fluoridation experiment has hardly proved itself as the savior it's supposed to be and the potential dangers it carries would not be worth chancing, even if fluoridation's anti-caries effects were as definite as we are led to believe.

So we're back to the same old thing in preventing dental caries: keep your mouth clean and free from debris; eat a carefully selected diet low in carbohydrates (with a good supply of calcium-rich bone meal); and use Dr. Bastien's recommended work foods—raw carrots, celery, dried apricots, ripened toasted corn and other hard, natural foods, which you can easily incorporate into your daily diet.

Children Need Good Food, Not Fluoridation

Writing in the *Medical Journal of Australia* (February 20, 1960), Dr. N. E. Goldsworthy made an accurate but distressing observation. He said that his nation is so used to dental decay that it is considered inevitable and more or less normal. If that is true in Australia, it goes double for the United States. Parents are urged to bring their children with them to the dentist when the children are toddlers of 3 or 4 years. This is designed as a "practice" visit—to get the child accustomed to the dentist and his equipment. It is, you see, a foregone conclusion that the child is doomed to have plenty of professional contact with the dentist (fluoridation notwithstanding), so he might as well get used to the idea. These are the healthy children of America about whom we brag to the world. Yet, Dr. Goldsworthy points out the obvious truth that the human body is *not* healthy if teeth or other oral structures are diseased. Using that criterion, it would be surprising to find one child in ten who could be considered healthy.

One survey in New South Wales, Australia, revealed that, in an average group of children between 6 and 16 years of age, only 1.5 per cent showed teeth free from decay. Such surveys conducted in America have yielded equally discouraging results. Unfortunately, tooth decay is a nonhealing disease, and a progressive one as well. If 1.5 per cent are free from tooth decay this year, it is likely that even fewer will be free of decay by the time the subjects are one year older.

Unrealistic Weapons

In the United States, we have gone about combating this problem of decaying teeth in various ways. First of all, we spend a great deal of time and money urging our children to see the dentist twice a year and brush their teeth twice a day. New toothpastes are introduced periodically which contain new chemicals with unpronounceable names and which do nothing else but make their distributors rich. Fluoridation has been tried by many cities. None of these has had the advertised effect. Tooth decay has continued to be a problem, even for people who visit the dentist, brush their teeth often with toothpastes of the highest power and live in fluoridated communities. The answer, which is elaborately ignored by just about everyone with any real influence, lies in the diet we eat and feed our children. Scientific experts have pointed out this fact quite regularly through the years, and until our people are willing to act on it, we will continue to have tooth decay as a serious national problem.

An Astonishing Record

To show the possibilities involved in preventing tooth decay with good diet, let us go on with Dr. Goldsworthy as he reports on a home for children, Hopewood House in Bowral, New South Wales, Australia. A survey made there covered 10 years and included children 9 to 16 years of age. This was compared with observations on a similar group of children outside of Hopewood House.

The commonly used measure of decayed, missing or filled teeth was applied to 13 year olds of both groups. The children at Hopewood showed an average of 1.6 such teeth. Those living elsewhere had 10.7. Look at the record another way. The percentage of pupils at Hopewood House who had no tooth decay was 53 per cent; of those living elsewhere, only .4 per cent were without tooth decay.

The children at Hopewood were not specially picked. They had the same physical problems as their contemporaries outside the home —some had heart trouble from birth or had bad eyes, some were mentally slow. It was noticed, though, that there were considerably fewer colds and minor illnesses among the Hopewood children and, as a result, there was much better attendance at school for them.

How Expensive Is the Equipment?

The difference in tooth decay between those groups made Australian authorities gasp, as they have made authorities in every other country gasp. What had they discovered in this private home that nobody else had discovered? How much would the equipment cost to duplicate the conditions on a national scale? The heads of the school had a deceptively simple answer. They had only taken the advice of the serious scientists of the world who work with tooth decay. They had carefully controlled the diet of their charges. This was the only element of significant difference between the two groups.

The children at Hopewood House were given no white sugar or white flour products. Refined carbohydrates were virtually absent from their diet. Raw, fresh vegetables were used extensively. Nuts, dried fruits, fresh fruits, fruit juices and vitamin preparations made up a large part of the menu. Raw milk and other fresh dairy supplies were also supplied liberally. Meals were eaten at regular, specified times and there was no between-meal snacking, unless organized and controlled by the authorities of the Home.

Dr. Goldsworthy says this: ". . . . we can state unequivocally that abstention from refined carbohydrates is significantly associated with the maintenance of decay-free teeth. It will be objected that the white flour and sugar and their products are necessary, if not dietetically, then at least economically, because these items are the cheapest components of our food. However, the wealth of this favored nation (Australia), if wisely used, could easily provide the alternative types of diet. . . . Despite the laity's cherished belief that calories (or energy) can be obtained only from sugary food, there is no evidence that refined carbohydrates are essential to good health."

This statement is worth some comment. Isn't it interesting that, in spite of the superb results achieved with a diet free of refined carbohydrates, objections are anticipated because the refined carbohydrates were left out. We need these harmful foods because they are cheaper to buy! Then, later, comes the other false argument for eating refined carbohydrates: they are a source of necessary energy. What is not mentioned is that many natural foods are sources of energy as well. Any sweet food has sugar in it, a natural, healthful sugar. Pears, corn, apples, watermelons, peas, prunes, dates—all of these have energy—giving sugar that is safe and good for the body to use. It is an absolute lie to suggest that it is healthful for a child to eat candy for energy. Healthful energy is contained in sugar-rich natural foods such as those listed above. Refined sweets are a menace to health, and the energy they do give is bought at a very dear price. Tooth decay is only one of the undesirable consequences of eating refined carbohydrates.

Good Eating Habits Start Early

Dr. Goldsworthy's article closes with a plea to medical practitioners to advise the young mothers on nutrition. He says that, if a child is brought to a dentist with decay problems, the eating patterns have already been set and it is probably too late to change them without great difficulty. Advice on good feeding procedure should be given the pregnant woman or the young mother when her child is still an infant. This is the time for establishing good habits in a child's eating. If a child becomes used to eating fresh fruit when he wants a sweet, chances are very good that he will not turn to candy for a sweet when he grows older. Don't make the opportunity for your child's acquiring such a bad habit as eating refined carbohydrates. Simply don't have them around.

We think the policy followed by Hopewood House is an excellent one. We are not in accord with the use of milk and milk products to any great extent for any but infants. In extreme moderation, milk should not be harmful for children. However, the substitute of soya milk or another nutritional alternate, such as bone meal, can easily be made. For the rest, the program is an excellent one and one that any household can adopt. We think that the rule of regularity of meals with control of between-meals eating is a wise one. Smaller children seem to fall easily into a pattern or schedule, and their eating properly at mealtimes is more likely if they have not been filling up on snacks between meals. If your child must snack, make it easy for him to do so healthfully. Keep nuts and fruit handy so that candy and cookies won't even enter his mind. Your child's perfect teeth are not your dentist's responsibility, but yours.

Tooth Decay and Refined Foods

A 30-year study of the dental health of the residents of a South Sea Island, Tristan da Cunha, was ended in November, 1961, according to a report in the *New York Times* (December 3, 1961). A volcanic eruption caused the island to be evacuated, and the people have now been resettled in England, where, as the *Times* writer wryly puts it, "their bad teeth are being cared for by dentists of the British National Health Service."

In 1932, when the first dental survey was made on the island, conditions were considered ideal for the growth and preservation of healthy teeth. The islanders were entirely dependent for food on their own resources. Fish were abundant. There were some cattle, sheep, geese and hens. Eggs were collectd from sea birds. Some cabbages, onions and turnips were grown. The staple crop was potatoes. There was no bread because there was no flour. Sugar, tea and coffee were novelties, restricted to the occasional visits of ships.

With this simple diet, it was found that only 1.82 per cent of the teeth examined were decayed. Of the entire population, 83.32 per cent of the people were without tooth decay of any kind, past or present. The British Naval Dental Service said of this figure: " . . . no comparable immunity has been known to occur in any other population of predominantly European origin . . ."

By 1937, 5 years after the first dental survey was made, the islanders were making scones and bread twice during the week and almost every Sunday. Their caries rate rose proportionately; 4.2 per cent of the teeth examined showed decay and only 50.2 per cent of the mouths were free of caries.

By 1952, the natives were working for money at newly established canneries. The weekly food consumption for 230 persons on the island included 273 pounds of sugar, 413 pounds of flour and 102 pounds of jam. Decay was present then in 9.1 per cent of teeth examined and caries-free mouths numbered only 22 per cent of those seen. A 1955 survey showed consumption of granulated sugar to be 490 pounds a week and flour, 1164 pounds a week. In addition, the people were eating cookies, chocolate, icing, sugar, candies, etc. The dental state was, of course, worse than ever.

We believe this article is a valuable means of watching the scale of dental health tip directly with an increase in refined foods— especially sweets. It is clear, from these observations, that the longer one is able to avoid such foods, the longer one is likely to have teeth that will be free from caries. Careful diet is the answer to tooth decay, not fluoridation, nor toothpastes.

Television

The Eye, the Ear and TV Crime Programs

This article is reprinted with permission from the September, 1958, issue of the Eye, Ear, Nose and Throat Monthly.

The eye and ear are the most important organs which human beings—children and adults—use to learn what is going on in the world about them. Through the use of their eyes, they carry on nearly every activity of daily life, enjoying the printed word, fellow human beings, objects of beauty as well as the harsher aspects of being alive. The world human beings know is the world they see. And in almost as important a degree, the ear permits mankind, through hearing speech, to exchange ideas and opinions with others. The honking of a horn, for example, often implies danger, and it is the ear that makes a person aware of a threatening situation. The world human beings know is also the world they hear.

Television, the modern electronic wonder, brings the world into our homes in sight and sound. There are few things that happen in the real world of events, politics, science, education, or in the make-believe world of the movies, theatre, music and dance that cannot be projected on a TV screen. Television can influence our thoughts, our understanding, our likes and dislikes, our manner in speech, our deportment and morals, our ideas of right and wrong. For good or bad—and there is much to be said for the good—TV has become the unacknowledged legislator of the minds of millions of American children.

In some instances, TV makes children smart and cynical before their time. Seeing sophistication and violence paraded before them and having experienced neither, their imagination is excited but not nourished. At best, TV provides children with visual experiences at a rate faster than ever before in the history of mankind; at worst, it blunts the sensitivity of children and burdens them with anxieties not always comprehended. In the past, many children, of course, have been able to absorb the terror and sadism of some of the classic fairy tales, but how well TV is being assimilated at present, as it contributes to the violent world of some children's imaginations, has not been fully determined.

The caliber of crime programs—and these include the vastly popular "westerns"—seen by TV audiences adds little to a world of desired serenity. TV programs today portray innumerable saloon brawls, assaults, sluggings, murders, robberies, jailbreaks, attempted lynchings and dynamitings, to say nothing of other "minor" acts of violence. The overall impression gained from many of these TV programs, seen as they are by millions of children, is that life is cheap; death, suffering and brutality are often matters of callous indifference; and that many law officers, judges and lawyers are either dishonest, stupid or incompetent.

Unfortunately, relatively little research has been done on the medical and psychological impact of TV on children. Physicians are aware that, in some instances, terrifying crime scenes will produce such adverse effects as troublesome dreams, restless sleep, loss of appetite and scholastic difficulties. Certainly, it is difficult to dismiss the contention that habitual exposure to crime-and-horror TV programs frequently produces a callousness to the suffering of others and an atrophy of compassion and sympathy toward those in distress. The manner in which crime-and-horror are brought before the eyes and ears of American children—to this writer, at least—indicates a complete disregard for mental, physical and social consequences in our country.

What to do about correcting this situation is discussed periodically in the press—with no results. It may be presumed that, sooner or later, there will be a hue and cry for governmental regulation and all the associated evils of censorship. There is more to the problem of protecting the psyche and soma of American children than can be afforded by merely turning the TV set off.

TV Can Cause Epileptic Seizures

A pair of Swedish researchers reported in one of Sweden's medical journals on the possibility of epileptic seizures being induced by watching television. As seen in the *Journal of the American Medical Association* (January 30, 1960), the Swedes reported 3 cases of epileptic response to television in girls aged, respectively, 13, 12 and 14 years. This was one of several write-ups which have appeared recently remarking on the effect of television on those prone to epilepsy.

The *Roche Report* (May 1, 1961) told of 5 similar cases which were reported in the *Lancet* (January 28, 1961). The ages of those affected varied from childhood to middle age. In 1951, says the *Roche Report,* Dr. Samuel Livingston of Johns Hopkins Hospital told of 3 children "who had their first convulsive seizure while watching a television show."

There is a historic precedent for this reaction by epileptics to the light of a television screen. In ancient times, many prospective slave buyers insisted that the slaves be forced to look at the flickering of light that accompanied the spinning of a potter's wheel or a chariot wheel. It was presumed that any tendency toward epilepsy would quickly show itself during such a test.

No one appears able to answer the obvious question: why should such a violent reaction occur? However, that this is a genuine cause and effect relationship in some persons, cannot be denied.

The *Roche Report,* borrowing from the *Lancet,* told of a housewife, aged 42 years, who could be induced into seizures experimentally. There was no history of epilepsy and examinations showed her to be generally normal, even neurologically speaking. She described how she had been distressed while watching TV to see thick bars moving from top to bottom on her screen—a phenomenon most TV viewers have experienced. As she attempted to adjust the set, she lost consciousness and suffered what was termed "a major epileptic seizure."

Three other patients described in the *Lancet* article had similar stories to tell. Fits were provoked after fairly prolonged and close exposure to flickering TV screens. When tested later with a machine which approximated the flickering, all showed striking changes in their brain impulses and two of them had fits again.

They all described the flickering in the same terms: the picture disappeared from the screen and was succeeded by horizontal lines which seemed to move downward. It would certainly seem advisable for anyone who knows he is prone to epileptic seizures to avoid watching television. If that should be impossible, then special care should be exercised to look away when the picture becomes distorted or begins "flopping" over. Two other safeguards: do not stare at a well-lighted screen in a darkened room; wearing red eyeglasses will help filter out the long light waves which seem to be the ones which are most likely to provoke epileptic seizures.

Television Violence and Bed Wetting

The effects of television on Americans will probably make for wonderful discussions in the college classrooms of a hundred years from now. The trouble is that we must try to diagnose what this medium is doing to and for us right now! The violence which seems to be in vogue can certainly be held at least partly responsible for the delinquency which also seems to be in vogue.

Something that we hadn't considered, however, was the strong effect exposure to so much violence can have on the subconscious of a child while he is sleeping. In the *New York Herald Tribune* (May 26, 1960), there is a note in the television column telling of a Japanese doctor who blames bed wetting on television shows which depict excessive violence. He studied the habits of 70 bed wetting children and urged their parents to discourage their viewing violence shows as part of the cure.

If TV can inspire children to burn their playmates at the stake, to jump from windows in an attempt to fly, to hang themselves and to choke their friends—as it has done often enough—the idea that it can cause them to lose control over their bladders in sleep seems to be a very logical and acceptable conclusion. If we had such a problem with a child, we would certainly test the Japanese doctor's theory.

But even without any visible problems, parents must exercise firm supervision over the viewing habits of their children. Television can be a healthy influence, but it must be used with selectivity and judgment, especially where children are involved.

Temperature

Temperature and Diet Influence Infant Mentality

The hunt goes on and on to find the real cause of defective mentality which characterizes so many of our children at birth. What causes it to occur in this child and not in that one? Heredity accounts for a very few of such cases. It has long been our opinion that the mother's prenatal diet is one of the most important factors in producing a healthy child. This idea is certainly not unique with us, for there has been a tremendous amount of scientific evidence to back up this conclusion. Strangely enough, a large proportion of our doctors refuses to seize on this one demonstrated type of insurance, and seems almost indifferent to the prenatal diets of their patients. Oh, they may prescribe an all-in-one supplement to be taken once or twice a day, but it is done with no real concern. They advise that the mother not gain too much weight, but the way she does that is largely up to her. If she can stay within the weight limit on sodas and cake alone, well and good. If only she won't get fat, on one will ask her what she is eating. Of course, this is not enough. She must be getting the proper food throughout pregnancy if she is to minimize the risk of a child born with some abnormality.

Diet in the Summer Months

The ramifications of diet in pregnancy are explored with interesting results by Hilda Knobloch, M.D., and Benjamin Pasamanick, M.D., in the *American Journal of Public Health* (September, 1958). They are impressed by the fact that the diet of most of us seems to take a beating, for some reason, during the summer months. It could be due to the lack of appetite in most persons when the weather is really warm and it could be due, as well, to the sodas and ice cream which seem to take over the diets of many persons, almost exclusively, in the summer.

Now it has been conclusively shown that the development period of each organ and feature can be predicted in the human embryo. The period for development of the cerebral cortex—the seat of the infant's mental faculties—is the 8th to 12th weeks of gestation; that is, the third month. It was presumed by the authors that congenital mental defectiveness would occur in the fetus at this time in pregnancy, if it were to happen at all. They decided that if the mother's poor diet in hot weather is a factor, then those babies who were in their third month of gestation in hot weather would be more likely to be mentally defective than others.

An examination of the files of a home for mentally defective children disclosed birth dates of those admitted, and from this, it could easily be figured in which cases the third month of gestation occurred in the summer months of June, July and August.

The records of the Columbus (Ohio) State School, from 1913 to 1948 (excluding 1946), showed the number of admissions of those born in January to be 503, February 512 and March 520. July was next highest with 494 and October lowest with 463. Obviously, the number of mental defectives whose third fetal month occurred in the hot weather was highest. Further investigation of the yearly temperatures showed that the hotter summers resulted in more admissions than the cooler ones for children who had spent their third month in the womb at that time.

Results Follow Logically

There is a great deal of evidence to show that the results of this survey are logical, in the light of other findings. For example, the authors mention the work of Mills in which he showed that the thiamin requirement of rats doubles as the temperature changes from 65 degrees F. to 90 degrees F. Now, this B vitamin, as well as others, acts as a catalyst in the combustion of glucose, and this combustion plays a major part in the function of the brain. If the thiamin demand doubles in the expectant mother at such temperatures and for some reason is not met, how much thiamin can be left for the development of the fetal brain?

There have been many differences observed in the learning and retentive abilities of rat litter mates when, kept on uniform diets for three months, they are reared in separate cages kept at 55 degrees F., 75 degrees F. and 95 degrees F. The cooler the atmosphere, the more brain power they exhibited. This trait seems to carry over to humans. Students taking college entrance examinations during the summer achieve only about 60 per cent of the ratings obtained in the same examinations when taken in winter.

Going back to the Ohio scene, Dr. Mills reports that children in Cincinnati latitudes who are conceived in summer months have, statistically, only a 50 per cent chance of entering college, compared with those conceived in the winter months. He notes, incidentally, that only 4 out of 33 presidents were conceived in summer. Peterson's findings, also quoted in this paper, agree with Mills by noting that most feebleminded children are conceived in summer.

Protein Essential

We have seen that there is probably an added need for thiamin in warmer weather. Mills says that, as a rule, the total calorie intake is reduced in the summer months. This means that protein intake should be increased to meet even minimal requirements. In animals, he tells us, it is possible to control the depressive effects of heat by adequate diet, particularly with respect to vitamins and protein.

It has been demonstrated that infections during pregnancy can be prevented by adequate intake of proteins and vitamins by the mother-to-be. A shortage of protein is now almost generally accepted as the cause of prenatal infections such as rubella and other viral difficulties which can cause mental deficiency in the fetus. There might be a direct effect on the mentality of the fetus, due to a lack of protein in the mother, even without her ever having such a disease. There have been numerous studies showing the influence of the mother's prenatal diet on her child.

Two Types of Reaction

This kind of evidence usually brings two kinds of reactions. The first is from mothers who have had several children and who went through their months of pregnancy in the summer several times with no ill effect on the children. They say the theory is ridiculous, for they had absolutely no qualms about diet during pregnancy and yet, the outcome seems to be perfect. The second group is made up of young married women who are frightened at the findings we have presented here, and are sincerely concerned lest they conceive at a time when the third month of pregnancy would occur in the hot weather.

Neither of these views is a proper one, we feel. The mother who has been fortunate enough to have healthy babies up to now has no guarantee that her luck will hold without more careful attention to what she eats, for, in spite of what she believes, there is much evidence that diet is important. The new wife who is overly concerned, needs only to remember that some of the tragic births of feebleminded children result, according to Knobloch and Pasamanick, from poor diet induced by the normal lack of appetite in hot weather. If an expectant mother finds her appetite lagging, she can eat lightly, but eat only nourishing foods. Salads of all kinds are especially appealing and most nutritious. Lean meats and fish are not too filling and offer an excellent source of protein. All types of fruits and vegetables, so plentiful at this time of year, are easy to eat, require little or no preparation and make a strong contribution to good nutrition. Add to this the bone meal, rose hips, brewer's yeast, cod liver oil and other supplements a pregnant woman should be taking, and the temperature outdoors won't make a bit of difference to the health of the baby she's waiting for.

One strong warning: Stay away from sweets such as sodas and ice cream in the summer. Nothing can ruin your appetite faster and they will do you no good at all. On the contrary, these foods deprive you of the nutrients you already have and make you an excellent target for disease.

Toilet Training

When Is It Time for Toilet Training?

This article is reprinted from the book, Infant Care, *Children's Bureau, Publication No. 8, 1951, published by the United States Department of Health, Education and Welfare.*

When some neighbor tells you her baby was "trained" at a very early age, take it with several grains of salt. You can be sure it is really she who "trained" herself to recognize little signals that meant her baby was about to have a movement. Or, her baby happened to be one whose bowel movements came at quite regular times earlier than most babies' do.

Of course, it saves work if your baby doesn't soil his diapers. But don't fool yourself into thinking that a baby under a year old can learn to control either his bowels or his bladder. Antyhing that seems like "control" will be because you have remembered to put him on the toilet.

Why stress this so much? Because you can so easily make trouble for yourself and the baby if you start training too early. A child can get to feeling that his mother is his enemy if she urges on him things he is not ready for. His whole relationship with her can be injured by forcing and pressure.

A baby's body gets rid of its waste products without his having any say about it. His body works mechanically and automatically, from breathing and swallowing to emptying waste. Only very gradually does his nervous system develop enough so that he can consciously hold back, or push out, a bowel movement. He does not really "learn" to do this until his mind is mature enough so that he can make a connection between his feelings, and the special place where his mother wants him to relieve himself.

Bowel Control Comes First

If you consider all that must go into learning bowel control, you won't be in such a hurry to expect your baby to act "civilized." But how can you tell when he's ready to learn? Wait for these things:

1. When he is old enough to understand what the toilet is for. He learns this gradually by seeing others in the family use it.

2. When his bowel movements come at fairly regular times.

3. When you have learned the little signals (like staying very quiet for a minute or so, pushing or straining, with a reddening of his face) that tell you he is about to have a movement.

4. When he consents willingly to sit on the toilet.

Many babies are not ready to start learning bowel control by the end of the first year. One and a half or two years is a much more common time for them to learn willingly. If a child is not forced, control takes place very quickly when it does come. A few babies have unusual ease in adapting and have few accidents after they are a year old.

Make sure your baby feels easy about being put on the toilet. A low toilet seat over a pot is less likely to make a child fearful than one that is perched up on top of the family toilet. Some babies are not afraid on a high seat if it has a stout back, arms, foot rest and straps. But others resist being put on them. Whatever plan you use, be careful not to frighten the baby.

Let him sit on his toilet chair only a few moments the first few times—and then only if he is willing to go along with your idea. Take him off soon, even though he doesn't have a movement. As he gets used to his new seat, you can keep him on a little longer, but never more than about 5 minutes. A baby finds it very hard to sit still and you don't want him to get to hate this new routine.

Much of the trouble mothers have in helping their children learn bowel control (and later, bladder control) comes because the babies get the idea this is a battle. They may do this because their mothers feel it is so important for them to learn and are so insistent. This is once when a baby has the upper hand. No mother can *make* her child move his bowels. But a mother who refuses to have a battle over toilet training can be pretty sure that once he has caught on, her child will learn without much trouble.

A lot depends on her not letting him get to feel that this is a hateful bore. And on her not being in a hurry to get him "trained." Just keep in mind that your baby is an individual, and is different from every other baby in the time he is ready to learn bowel control. Occasionally a baby who is not yet a year old learns very quickly and responds well. Again, it may be just a matter of chance that a baby moves his bowels when he's on the seat.

If you act pleased when he happens to have a movement in the right place, he may get the idea and perform again the next time. But remember, for a long time to come, the *right* place and time for him to have a bowel movement will be when and where he needs to. You'll be lucky if he happens to feel like it when he's on the toilet.

So go slow. Being in a hurry to get a baby "trained" could cause a lot more trouble than dirty diapers. And keep in mind that even a slight illness may cause the baby to lose any control he has gained, so that you may have to start all over.

You can afford to feel that you "know better" if anyone acts surprised that your baby still soils his diaper. What you're after is not having fewer diapers to wash, but having a baby who feels like working with you instead of against you.

If you don't expect too much of your baby, you won't make him feel like saying or acting "No!" to everything you ask of him. To control his bowels is one of the first ways we begin to ask that a baby conform to our customs. We can make a good start, or a bad one. We can be so easy-going he wants to cooperate, or we can make him feel like objecting to almost everything we ask of him.

Another thing you'll want to be careful about is showing disgust if he happens sometime to play with his bowel movement. He has no idea of it as being dirty; it is merely something interesting that he has made.

If it happens that he dabbles in it simply clean him up, and say nothing. Be especially careful not to act shocked, or say he is naughty. If you have been praising him for moving his bowels and then turn around and tell him he is bad, how can he help being terribly confused?

Sometimes a baby handles his genitals when he is sitting on the toilet, or at other times when he is undressed. This is a common thing, and usually will not amount to anything if let alone. But sometimes it is disturbing to mothers, so if you feel uncomfortable about it you can try giving him a toy to hold while he's on the toilet seat. Don't confuse him by saying, "No, No." Save the "no's" for times you really need to use them.

How About Learning to Keep Dry?

Very few babies indeed are ready to start learning bladder control by the time they are a year old. In most cases, it is better to make no effort at all in this direction until well along in the second year, or even later. However, babies differ very much in the time when they are ready for different kinds of learning. If your baby stays dry for as long as two hours at a time during the day, and if there are times such as just after meals or naps, when you can be fairly sure of catching him in time, it's all right to try.

Just be sure not to put your baby on the toilet more than two or three times a day, and not to interrupt him at interesting play. And put him on only if he seems willing. If this tiresome interference with his freedom comes too often, he may resist learning.

Remember, try using the pot or the seat only very occasionally, and don't keep the baby sitting but a few moments. You will be more likely to have luck now and again if your baby is a little girl, as girls tend to learn a little earlier than boys.

Tonsillectomies

You Should Be Informed on Tonsillectomies

The tide has been turning in modern medicine's attitude toward tonsil removal. At its height of popularity, in the 1930's, the opinion that tonsils are no more than an actual, or a potential nuisance, had become the view of most practitioners. Gradually, the obvious concept that every part of the body has some function which may or may not be understood by our scientists, seems to have asserted itself. We hope so. Say what you will about the advances of modern surgery, an operation that has been avoided is the safest, most comfortable kind. The element of risk, in even the most minor operation, is always present. It seems only common sense to make sure that any risks we take with our health are necessary ones.

Quite aside from any danger involved in tonsil surgery, the difficulty of doing without an organ which has a definite function in preventing infection is not to be taken lightly. The tonsils are part of the body's lymph gland system, a system designed to act as a barrier to infections which would otherwise spread throughout the entire body. When an infection is present, the lymph gland closest to it becomes swollen and infected itself. This localizes the infection, keeps it in a single, less vulnerable spot, rather than permit its circulation to a place less likely to be able to cope with it. Antibodies to battle the infection also have their source here. If tonsils are to be removed because they are observed to be swollen at times, they are, so to speak, being punished for doing the job they are meant to do.

Two Sets of Tonsils

Actually, we have two sets of tonsils. One set is located at the opening of the throat, and the second set, the pharyngeal tonsils (called adenoids) are near the top of the nose cavity behind the nose. Since most of the germs we take in come to us through the nose and mouth, the tonsils and adenoids are ideally placed for doing their job of intercepting infectious elements. When they are removed, this very fertile avenue for infection is left unguarded.

It is apparent that, although physicians have come to recognize the folly of removing tonsils that do not have to be removed, operations which do just that continue to be performed in great numbers. In the *Journal of Pediatrics* (March, 1958), Harry Bakwin, M.D., wrote: "Contrary to the view of many discriminating physicians, the procedure (removal of tonsils and adenoids) is as popular now as it was 20 years ago, perhaps more so . . . The operation retains its vogue in the face of well-documented evidence that, in the overwhelming majority of cases, it is useless."

Dr. Bakwin lists several legitimate or reasonable indications for tonsillectomy, then he remarks that, "In actual practice, the overwhelming majority of children are operated upon for one or more of 3 reasons: parental pressure for the operation, large tonsils or adenoids and frequent upper respiratory infections (colds)."

Parents Still Insist

The author admits that he cannot explain the insistence of parents for tonsillectomies to be performed on their children. In spite of the publicity he says has been given the danger of indiscriminate removal of tonsils and adenoids, "There is still a widespread impression among the laity that it is, in some way, a desirable health measure and that it protects against colds." Also, Dr. Bakwin feels that health insurance plans have fostered the interest in tonsillectomies, since they remove the financial consideration of surgery.

The size of tonsils and adenoids is utterly unrelated to the need for their removal, says Dr. Bakwin. In a study reported in the *American Journal of the Diseases of Childhood* (53: 1503, 1937), I. M. Epstein followed 540 children, ranging in age from 2 to 13 years, before and at intervals of two years after the operation. He observed no relation between the size of the tonsils and the results of the operation. He also checked other visual aspects of the tonsils and concluded that the appearance of the tonsils should never influence one's judgment as to the wisdom of removing them to improve the child's health. Said Epstein: "The physician does not know an infected tonsil when he sees one."

Many people have sold themselves on the idea that to remove their children's tonsils will be to remove the reason for their children's colds. Writes Dr. Bakwin, "Yet, all available evidence shows that the operation neither prevents nor significantly reduces the incidence of these troublesome ailments. Gofafer, in 1932, observed no significant difference with respect to the frequency, severity or type of attack of disease of the upper respiratory tract in tonsillectomized and non-operated persons."

Illnesses Even More Frequent

A study in the *Quarterly Journal of Medicine* (12: 119, 1943) on the health of 909 girls from well-to-do families attending an English boarding school showed a similar fact. Sore throat was equally common among the operated and non-operated group. Common colds were more frequent in those who had had their tonsils removed. Pneumonia and pleurisy were rare in both groups, but still, the tonsillectomized group had more cases. Acute bronchitis was more frequent in this group, too. Removal of the tonsils, of course, protected those operated upon from tonsillitis, but the missing tonsils seemed to account for increased colds. The removal of adenoids increased the susceptibility to acute middle ear infections.

Dr. Bakwin lists further sources of studies and observations which show the futility of most tonsillectomies. Why is it, then, that parents persist in demanding that their children have their tonsils removed? Perhaps, they would be less anxious if they were aware of the dangers involved in the actual surgery.

In the 5 years, 1951 to 1955, 46 deaths from tonsillectomy in children under 15 years of age were recorded in New York City alone. While this figure might strike some as insignificant, it far outweighed the combined total deaths in the same period from diphtheria, mumps, rubella (German measles), scarlet fever, typhoid fever, varicella (chicken pox) and whooping cough. The main hazards at the time of surgery are anesthesia and hemorrhage. *Annals of Surgery* (140:2, 1954) carried evidence to show that, over a 5-year period in 10 university hospitals studied in the United States, the tonsillectomy mortality rate due to anesthesia was one in 1,560. What it was in lesser equipped and staffed hospitals we do not know. The problem presented is the difficult one of protecting the lower respiratory tract, while the upper respiratory tract is being worked on.

W. McKenzie, in the *Lancet* (2:958, 1953) wrote that he considers hemorrhage the greatest danger during the operation. This is especially true if the patient has now or has recently had a throat infection. Dr. McKenzie cautioned against operating on anyone whose temperature is 99 degrees F. on the eve of the operation.

Polio and Anesthesia

The relationship between bulbar polio and tonsillectomy has received plenty of publicity in recent years. In general, it is strongly advised that tonsillectomy be postponed to a time of the year during which polio is at its seasonal low. Siegel and co-workers published their findings on this point in the *Journal of Pediatrics* (38:548, 1951). Of 6,524 cases of polio in New York City over a 6-year period, the percentage of bulbar paralysis was significantly higher than expected in post-tonsillectomized persons within one month after the operation. The longer the time after the operation, the less the likelihood of infection.

A difficulty less frequently recognized than the anesthesia, the polio and the hemorrhages that occur, is the psychological trauma involved with a child who goes to the hospital for the first time— quite likely his first time away from home. He is suddenly surrounded by strangers in unfamiliar dress, when his parents might have led him to expect a pleasant vacation. He is often terrified and confused. He resents being lied to; he resents the pain; and he resents the enforced separation from his family. While most children get over this experience quickly enough, some, says Bakwin, show changes in their behavior—principally, fears, distrust and family antagonisms. One writer, Coleman, regards the psychic trauma sustained by some children from tonsillectomy to be as serious as post-operative hemorrhage or infection. W. S. Langford, in the *American Journal of Orthopsychiatry* (7:210, 1937) observed that, in 6 out of 20 children suffering from anxiety states, the condition was definitely related to tonsillectomies under ether anesthesia.

Ask Intelligent Questions

We have not amassed this sober evidence to create panic, nor are we unalterably opposed to all tonsillectomies. There are some cases in which the only sensible and safe answer is removal of tonsils that are responsible for serious illness. When confronted with such a situation, of course, remove them. Our point in reporting on the dangers involved in a tonsil operation is to convince parents that such a step is not to be taken lightly. Tonsillectomy is not inevitably followed by improved health. As we have shown, quite the opposite appears to be true. We believe these facts would lead parents away from insisting on tonsillectomies when their doctors haven't even mentioned the possibility. We hope this information will lead to intelligent questioning on the part of a parent when a doctor does suggest tonsillectomy as a therapeutic measure. Above all, we hope it will prevent useless operations.

How can one know when a tonsillectomy is really necessary? Several doctors have set out their criteria for deciding whether or not to operate.

Some Indications

Dr. I. Lopert wrote an article on that subject in the *Medical Journal of Australia* (August 26, 1958). In it, he remarked that, unless there is obvious presence of pus, with other general symptoms considered as evidence of chronic infection, enlargement of the tonsils is a vague and indefinite indication for surgery.

Frequent attacks of tonsillitis are an indication for surgery, says Dr. Lopert, but in children, frequent upper respiratory infections with sore throats are often mistaken by parents for tonsillitis. Colds, of course, are no specific cause for removal of tonsils.

If the lymph glands of the neck are chronically swollen, this can be a strong clue that there is a definite, deep-seated infection in the tonsils. Such swelling comes after the first or second attack of tonsillitis and will quickly disappear unless the above-mentioned infection is present. Then, the seat of the infection must be removed.

Recurrent attacks of earache without discharge and only slight changes in the drum are often used as an indication for operation. Such earaches in children two to eight are quite common, and can have many sources. If actual periodic deafness should occur, the nasal passage is often the source of infection and removal of adenoids is often the solution of the problem. However, in frequent attacks of otitis media, (inflammation of the inner ear), with high temperature, pain and bloodstained discharge, removal of tonsils and adenoids is to be considered. But the frequency of attacks and the severity of them should be factors in deciding to operate.

Dr. Lopert gave these two final indications for fixing the blame for ill health, fluctuating temperature, etc., on the tonsils: "First, evidence of chronic infection must be present in them. . . . Secondly, other organs must be excluded as possible sites of focal infection— namely, chronic infection of teeth and gums, the gall bladder, the appendix and last, but not least, the genitourinary system."

In conclusion, we urge that all parents of young children bear in mind the words of J. W. Lindahl, Assistant Surgeon to the Aural Department at London Hospital: Acute tonsillitis results from a combination of infection and lowered resistance, local and general. It has been suggested that one predisposing factor is an unbalanced diet with too much sugar and starch in relation to protein and green vegetables, and I believe there is much to be said for this theory (*Practitioner,* December, 1951).

Toothpaste, Fluoridated

What About Fluoridated Toothpaste?

A surprising reversal of customary professional procedure occurred when the American Dental Association broke a long-time official disapproval of toothpaste claims of decay prevention and gave its endorsement to Crest toothpaste. Full-page ads in newspapers all over the country announced to a long-suffering public that the American Dental Association had said that Crest is not a cure-all, but that "it has been shown to be an effective anti-decay dentrifice that can be of significant value when used in a conscientiously applied program of oral hygiene and regular professional care."

The photograph shows two packages of this ADA-approved toothpaste bought on the same day at different stores in Philadelphia, Pennsylvania. As you can see, one of the packages clearly warns:

CAUTION: CHILDREN UNDER 6 SHOULD NOT USE CREST

On the second package, clearly stated, we find the following:

REGULAR USE OF CREST IS ADVISED FOR EVERY MEMBER
OF THE FAMILY . . . INCLUDING CHILDREN OF ALL AGES

You will also note that Crest contains "fluoristan," which is a trade name for stannous fluoride.

This astonishing situation raises the following two very interesting questions:

1. How can Crest be both safe and unsafe for children under 6 at one and the same time?

2. How much confidence should we have in the advice of the ADA on fluoride when the ADA approves the mass use of a fluoridated product whose safety for children is obviously in such a confused state?

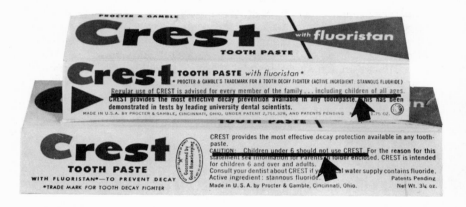

Which package do you use—and read? Note that the smaller one at top is safe for children, according to the printed message on the box. However, the larger box warns against its use for small children under 6 years of age. Both were purchased in the same city at the same time.

The story of fluoridated toothpaste is so incredible that we do not know where to begin telling it. Here are only some highlights in chronological order:

February 12, 1955: *Science News Letter* announces the expectation of a fluoride toothpaste and says, "Whether the fluoride toothpaste would provide too much fluoride for persons living in regions where the water has fluorine in it naturally or by controlled addition, is a question still to be decided." They opine that the Food and Drug Administration will require a special warning label.

February, 1955: *Chemical Week* quotes a spokesman of the American Dental Association as saying he "hopes that commercial interests will not jump the gun as they have done so frequently in the past," but will wait until exhaustive tests have proved the effectiveness and the safety of the new toothpaste.

In connection with this, it is worth noting the ADA statement of approval on Crest, published in the *Journal of the American Dental Association* for August, 1960. In this report, the Council on Dental Therapeutics of the ADA "wishes to point out that certain aspects of the potential usefulness of Crest have not yet been delineated by the studies thus far conducted." So it becomes apparent that the ADA, in August, 1960, acted in the *absence* of exhaustive tests which the ADA spokesman said, in February of 1955, that commercial interests should wait for. Thus, the ADA has itself not lived up to the standards it posed for industry. This is indeed something new for a self-proclaimed health agency.

February 26, 1955: *Business Week* reported that the Food and Drug Administration required a label on Crest stating, "Not to be used by children under 6 or in fluoridated areas."

November-December, 1955: *National Fluoridation News* reported Dr. F. F. Heyroth (one of the fathers of water fluoridation) as saying, at a hearing in Santa Fe, in answer to a question as to whether any dentifrice would suffice as an added measure against dental caries, "if you have in mind the stano-fluoride toothpaste, *we are not going to permit the sale of fluoride toothpaste in areas we fluoridate.*"

January 6, 1956: *Collier's* magazine ran a feature story on the development of fluoride toothpastes, showing unmistakable proof of the fact that tooth decay can now be a thing of the past. With a catch in its editorial throat and a tear in its advertising-hungry eye, *Collier's* concluded the article by saying, "It takes millions of dollars to launch a new dentifrice. It's fascinating that, in the course of one summer, all 5 of these firms—which already, as a group, were selling more than 75 per cent of the nation's toothpastes—should have decided, separately, that the fluoride idea is so good it cannot be ignored."

January 26, 1956: Proctor and Gamble took almost a full-page ad in the *New York Times* and probably in many other newspapers to announce "Triumph Over Tooth Decay." They announced that Crest is the only toothpaste that makes possible a major reduction in tooth decay *for people of all ages.* They called this an important milestone in medicine and likened it to Dr. Jenner's discovery of vaccination, Dr. Morton's discovery of ether and Dr. Fleming's discovery of penicillin. (In the 4 years since that time, you would naturally think that many people in the world immediately began to use this universal remedy and tooth decay disappeared overnight. But such, apparently, was not the case, because the story goes on.)

Contradictory Statements Begin to Appear

January 30, 1956: The Long Beach (California) *Independent* quoted Dr. Harold Hillenbrand, of the American Dental Association, as saying that there is as yet no adequate evidence that any fluoride dentifrice is effective in preventing tooth decay. The American Dental Association had no evidence, he said, that a fluoride dentifrice would be of any value to a person who, in early childhood, routinely drank water containing fluoride at the optimum level. He did not state (but it seems perfectly obvious to anyone of average intelligence) that using fluoride toothpaste might result in just enough added fluorine in the system to bring on chronic poisoning, since no one knows what the danger point is with each individual.

In August of 1960, the ADA approved Crest on the basis of 7 studies, 3 of which had already been published by January 30, 1956, when Dr. Hillenbrand of the ADA denied there was adequate evidence on behalf of any fluoridated toothpaste. What made these 3 reports, which were unsuitable evidence in 1956, acceptable evidence in 1960? We do live in an amazing world!

February 6, 1956: A letter to the editor of the St. Petersburg (Florida) *Independent* from Dr. William M. Holliday, Director of Professional Information at Proctor and Gamble, indicates that plenty of alarm has been roused by the label on Crest which warned against using it in fluoridated water areas. The company's trouble shooter assures the Floridians that they have nothing to fear from Crest. He says, in the areas where there is too much fluorine in water, "if a child under 6 were to swallow toothpaste repeatedly when brushing, the fluoride in Crest added to the fluoride from water or foods might increase the possibility of a stained appearance of the teeth, which sometimes occurs when excessive amounts of fluoride are swallowed. For this reason, people living in the areas where water contains large amounts of fluoride are advised to consult their dentists." What Dr. Holliday did *not* say is that the stained appearance of the teeth, to which he so *casually* referred, is one of the earliest symptoms of fluoride poisoning. Take it any way you like, this is the first time we know of that any advocate of fluorides to prevent tooth decay has admitted that one might get too much from a number of other sources, as well as water supply.

Dr. Holliday goes on to say that the safety of Crest toothpaste has been established beyond any doubt. Crest has been sold for more than a year in areas where the water has been fluoridated. It is now being sold throughout the United States, he goes on, and will cut down decay for everyone, of any age. These facts are approved by the Federal Drug Administration and the American Dental Association, he says.

No date on this one because the booklet does not carry a date. We refer to the attractive little booklet given out with Crest toothpaste which says: "Young children sometimes swallow toothpaste (so does everyone else who uses it, so far as we know). Additional fluoride taken in this way might add to the staining problem in the few communities where it already exists. . . . Young children in many communities now receive the benefits of medically approved, controlled water fluoridation. It never creates a staining problem." Apparently, the makers of Crest have not read any of the accounts of fluoridated areas where fluorosis or tooth mottling have appeared, so they can say simply that such a thing does not exist. It is not made clear by this pamphlet, as you can see, how the child in the heavily fluoridated areas, who, for example, may drink only two glasses of water a day and gets mottled teeth, differs from the child in the "scientifically" fluoridated area, who, for example, may drink much more water each day and gets the same amount of fluorine and the same amount of mottling. The first child might suffer from the additional fluorine in Crest, but the second won't, says the pamphlet. You figure it out. We can't. Here again, there is no comment about this mottling being one of the earliest signs of fluoride poisoning. Why do they try to keep this information so secret?

Ill Effects from Toothpaste

September, 1957: *Northwest Medicine* reported the observations of a Seattle doctor, Dr. T. E. Douglas, who found an increasing incidence of mouth irritations (called stomatitis) over a period of 15 months. Only one factor was common to all such patients. They all used a fluoride toothpaste. A controlled study showed that each time the patients stopped using the toothpaste, their mouth condition cleared. When they began to use it again, the condition returned. Each time the dentifrice was used again, the irritation became more difficult to get rid of.

October, 1957: An editorial in the *New York State Dental Journal* commented on the fact that Crest toothpaste is a highly acid product. The official position of the American Dental Association is that *tooth decay is caused by acid!* This puts the ADA in a peculiar position. It claims that acid causes tooth decay at the same time that it declares a definitely acidic dentifrice prevents tooth decay. This situation would be amusing if it weren't so serious. How much respect can one have for the scientific competence of the ADA? The course of action to be taken here is one recommended by Dr. E. B. Zeisler in the September, 1959, issue of the *Chicago Medical School Quarterly*. Dr. Zeisler wrote: "It is obvious that evidence which is self-contradictory cannot be valid and must be discarded at once." We repeat, "must be discarded at once."

But let us get back to the editorial in the October, 1957, issue of the *New York State Dental Journal*. This editorial stated: "It would be interesting to have a report of the (decay) inhibiting value of an acid dentifrice which contained no fluoride compound." Maybe the fluoride has nothing to do with it! Maybe it's the acid content of the rest of the toothpaste! But the American Dental Association has steadfastly said that acid *creates* decay! You figure it out. We can't. All we know is that the ADA article on Crest conveniently omitted any reference to the fact that it is an *acid* dentifrice.

January 18, 1958: the *Medical Journal of Australia* reprints the information uncovered by Dr. Douglas in Seattle about the mouth irritations caused by fluoride toothpastes. It seems strange that Australians on the other side of this planet know about this serious disadvantage, but the ADA, right here in Chicago, does not.

March, 1959: *Good Housekeeping* (which survives partly on advertising money from toothpaste manufacturers) answers a question about the Crest label ("Do not use for children under 6") by saying that the Food and Drug Administration has decided that this warning is not necessary and that all members of the family can now safely use fluoridated toothpaste. How do you suppose the Food and Drug Administration arrived at such a decision? Considering that it has taken more than 10 years for the highest dental authorities in the land to arrive at the highly controversial position that fluoridated water is safe, how could the FDA have possibly done any meaningful research in a matter of a few months to determine that the fluoride in toothpaste, of which one might swallow considerable amounts during a lifetime, is completely harmless, no matter how much other fluoride one is getting in water and in food! Such scientific antics stagger the imagination!

December, 1959: Dr. Thomas J. Hill writes in the *Journal of the American Dental Association* on fluoride toothpastes. He describes a number of tests done, including some he did himself. Some showed reduction in decay and some did not. Dr. Hill, who seems to be exceptionally clearheaded, with above average amount of common sense, points out that, in any experiment on dental decay, the tooth care that is bound to result with everybody concerned will certainly reduce a lot of decay, whether or not you use a special toothpaste. Furthermore, he says that the most important thing in such an experiment seems to be the individual differences in children and in the methods used by those who examine them. "It is evident," he says, "that one method which contributes to the control of caries is a regimented or carefully supervised oral hygiene program in school children. Regardless of the possible value of a dentifrice with therapeutic effect, methods of instruction and supervision in oral health contribute to the control of the dental caries rate."

April 15, 1960: According to the *New York Herald Tribune,* Dr. Francis A. Arnold of the National Institute of Dental Health wrote, in the *Archives of Industrial Health,* that the results of clinical trials made so far with fluoride toothpaste "are as controversial as those obtained by the use of other dentifrices." Now, Dr. Arnold is one of the distinguished sires of water fluoridation and one of the world's vaunted authorities on the subject of fluorine and teeth. His word is quoted by pro-fluoridationists throughout the world. It is strange that Dr. Arnold was unaware of the wonderful successes being achieved by Crest.

ADA's Statements

August, 1960: the *Journal of the American Dental Association,* in its "Evaluation of Crest Toothpaste," makes some of the most astounding statements we have ever seen. But, as we said earlier, their approval of the toothpaste has by now been announced in an ad campaign costing millions of dollars. Dealers are reputed to have run out of Crest and more full-page ads have appeared, apologizing for the delay and asking the American public to be patient.

We want to discuss just two of the astounding statements made by the ADA. It was found in the tests made, says the ADA spokesman, that brushing with Crest "under conditions normal in their homes" resulted in 12 per cent reduction in tooth decay in children tested. Brushing once a day (with Crest) *under supervision* brought about 34 per cent reduction. Brushing *3 times daily, under supervision brought* about 57 per cent reduction in tooth decay.

Now, to any sane and reasonable person, such a finding would indicate that brushing your teeth 3 times a day with or without toothpaste will result in less decay than brushing once a day, or possibly not at all. And up to quite recently, most dental authorities agreed that frequent brushing is a large part of the answer to tooth decay. But now, the ADA, so deeply in love with Proctor and Gamble that they can see nothing but Crest, Crest and more Crest, have decided that what the experiment shows is that, if you want to get 3 times as much reduction in decay, all you have to do is use 3 times as much Crest! This they call scientific!

The final "pay-off" is this admission of the ADA Council on Dental Therapeutics: "At the time of the Council's evaluation, complete reports of some of these studies (on Crest) were not yet published, but data not in the literature were made available to the Council."

This is really something new for science. This is one for the books. One of the essential requirements in any science is that information be published. Scientists routinely publish the data on which they base their conclusions. This is the commonly accepted procedure.

In their publications, they literally tell the world what was done, what results were obtained and what conclusions were drawn. Anyone can, therefore, check their data and agree or disagree.

But the ADA did not follow this procedure. It acted in part on the basis of secret information, not published and, therefore, not generally available. Here, as in many other instances involving fluoridation, the ADA attempts to compel us to trust its judgment and follow its advice. The necessary information is not published; we are not permitted to check on the ADA. *The ADA does not allow us to think for ourselves in this matter!*

Why has the ADA handled the situation in this way? It would take only a matter of a few months, at the most, for the complete reports to have been published. Since clinical trials of Crest have been going on over a period of years, why couldn't the ADA wait those few more months, so that its action on Crest could come under full public scrutiny as is the usual procedure in scientific matters? What was the urgency? Why was this decision made *before* all reports were published?

Such aspects of this pseudoscientific proceeding merit a Congressional investigation of the dentifrice industry, the fluoridation farce and the ADA. Perhaps an investigation would reveal that the answer to such questions as the above is *payola*. Who knows? Anything is possible. It has happened with antibiotics in the United States Public Health Service, and it can happen in other situations.

Tourniquets

Dangers in Tourniquet Application

Anyone who has ever had a course in first aid knows what a tourniquet is and how it is applied. The application of a tourniquet is one of the more dramatic things a layman can accomplish while waiting for the doctor, and people are most anxious to try their hand at it.

The *Medical Journal of Australia* (February 20, 1960) carries a letter signed M. J. M. Lapin who asks that overenthusiastic use of the tourniquet be discouraged. Says Dr. Lapin, "While I have never seen a life or limb saved by indirect pressure, I have, on many occasions treated tissue completely devitalized by the use of a tourniquet—tissue which could probably have been saved if either no first aid had been given or if a simple pressure bandage had been applied directly to the wound. . . . The use of the tourniquet should be abolished in accident cases, except perhaps for traumatic amputation or snake bite."

It is to be hoped that the information contained in this letter achieves a wider circulation among medical authorities in this and other countries. When last we heard, the application of a tourniquet was being taught in first aid classes as though it were only slightly less important than vital brain surgery, and the impression was that it should be used for everything but nosebleed.

lem. Dr. Otis R. Farley, Director of the Medical and Surgical Branch of St. Elizabeth's Hospital, Washington, D. C., stated (*Science News Letter,* March 5, 1960) that many of these popular drugs can alter the body's ability to fight infections. Others can cause skin rash, affect the function of the adrenal glands and of the entire enzyme system. Moreover, Dr. Farley emphasized, there is no specific antidote for many of the tranquilizing drugs, *and many of them have proven fatal when given in seemingly small dosages.*

Properly used, tranquilizers can be valuable tools in treating serious mental or nervous-system disorders. The big trouble is that they haven't been restricted to their proper limitations.

Tests Show Harm

In general, the group of drugs called tranquilizers are muscle-relaxers. They depress the central nervous system, causing the body to relax.

Mildest of the 3 principal types of tranquilizers are those made from a chemical known as meprobamate (Miltown, Equanil). Continued or excessive use of these has been "associated with drowsiness, ataxia (failure of muscular coördination), coma, hypotension (low blood pressure), convulsions and muscular flaccidity (weakness)," according to a report on tranquilizer poisoning in the British medical journal, *Lancet,* for February 4, 1961. Stronger than the meprobamates or the reserpines (Serpasil, etc.) extracted from the Indian snake root plant, *Rauwolfia serpentina.* "One of the most serious complications of administration of *Rauwolfia serpentina* is duodenal ulcer." (*World Wide Abstracts,* October, 1958.) In 18 months at a 250-bed general hospital, there were 42 cases with intestinal perforation and hemorrhage in patients taking reserpine for hypertension (high blood pressure), reported the *Annals of Internal Medicine* (May, 1958). In addition, this class of drugs can cause clogging of the nasal passages and swelling of the glottis (throat box) to the point of strangulation. Most potent of the tranquilizers are the chloropromazine or phenothiazine compounds (Thorazine, Phenergan). These "may depress so greatly as to produce a shock-like reaction. Jaundice has been reported in a small percentage of patients on Thorazine; so has often-fatal agranulocytosis," a lowering of the body's white blood cells, needed in fighting off disease and, without enough of which, an individual can succumb to the slightest infection. (*Pageant,* April, 1961.)

From Skin Rashes to Accidents

What about some of the other side effects of tranquilizers—some of the physical and psychological hazards the drug makers conveniently omit in their promotional leaflets? Here are just a few choice examples.

"Women who routinely resort to tranquilizers should know there is evidence that these drugs can upset the menstrual cycle. The latest report to that effect—the work of Dr. M. James Whitelaw of San Jose, California—deals with 17 women who were observed for a minimum of 5 months while taking tranquilizers. Only 5 retained their normal cycles during the tests." (*Good Housekeeping,* May, 1961.)

"Outside the central nervous system, reserpine has been shown to increase gastric acidity. Quiescent (latent) peptic ulcers may be activated, and massive hemorrhage has occurred. Agranulocytosis (the deadly blood disorder previously described) is uncommon, but one review . . . cites 22 cases, 8 of them fatal, in chloropromazine-treated patients." (*Journal of the Canadian Medical Association,* January 15, 1958.)

"While many reports have appeared which stress the production of jaundice after chloropromazine has been used for a period of time in large doses, the authors of this paper noted that jaundice may appear even after small amounts have been taken. A survey of the literature revealed two other reports stressing the relation of jaundice to small doses of chloropromazine." (*Journal of the American Medical Association,* September 28, 1957.)

"The belief of many doctors that Miltown and Equanil can never be fatal no matter what the dosage was contradicted today by the *Medical Letter,* an independent drug-evaluation publication, in a blunt warning to doctors. 'Medical literature records at least 4 suicides with meprobamate (scientific name for the mild tranquilizer) and the number is doubtless far greater,' the paper said, citing 8 documented cases in Philadelphia." (*New York Post,* December 14, 1960.) The nonprofit medical publication—which has many highly respected physicians on its staff—went on to emphasize that experimenters have found that as little as a 16-grain overdose might prove fatal, and that the drug may lower blood pressure hazardously or depress breathing.

Addicts and Alcohol

In this and other investigations, the use of all 3 main classes of tranquilizers has been shown to be extremely dangerous when combined with alcohol, frequently causing irrational behavior, unconsciousness and sometimes death. Moreover, addiction comparable to that of narcotics has been reported frequently, including the same type of withdrawal symptoms as with narcotics, often with tremors and convulsions resulting.

Dr. Neville Murray reported, in the *Journal of the American Medical Association,* that 68 auto drivers taking a newly introduced tranquilizer in average doses were involved in 6 major road accidents and 10 minor ones.

Faulty Nutrition Common Cause

Where does all the testimony on tranquilizers and the "magic-pill" fad lead us? First and foremost, they should be used only when mature medical judgment can offer no alternative treatment for a serious disorder. They are *not* to be taken every time some tension or strain of ordinary daily life makes someone "nervous." Essentially, happiness and tranquillity are reflections of health. Our nerves, like every other part and organ of our bodies, are made up only of what we eat. When, over a period of months or years, we eat little or nothing to nourish our nerves, there's no question but that we are going to suffer from a weakened nervous system—from excessive anxiety, irritability, depression and all the other symptoms for which millions now take tranquilizers.

If tranquilizers won't nourish our nerves, what will? Most important of the nerve nutriments are the B complex vitamins and calcium. American diets are short on both of these! Any wonder that there are so many nerve-jangled people today or that the tranquilizer craze is booming?

Instead of taking tranquilizers, put the things your nerves need on your dinner plate. Include generous portions of foods rich in all the B vitamins and in calcium—and stay away from any and all "foodless foods," such as sodas and other sweets, which rob you (and your nerves) of the nutritional elements you need. Also, don't hesitate to add natural supplements high in vitamin B complex (brewer's yeast, wheat germ, desiccated liver) to your diet. Agriculture and food processing being what it is today, your diet is very likely to be much less sound than you'd like it to be.

Furthermore, normal anxiety and tension are essential to creative activity, to human accomplishment. If you just don't care, you're never going to do much. The progress of civilization has come about through men and women who *were* concerned, anxious, dissatisfied and, most of all, alert. Let's be sensible about nerves and nervousness. The therapy most nervous people need is sound diet.

Vaccinations

Experts Warn: Vaccinations Are Risky

Some time ago, information was published on the danger of encephalitis, or inflammation of the brain, as the result of vaccination. The likelihood of such a consequence was shown to be greatly increased if the first vaccination were administered after the age of two. Therefore, parents in one European country were advised that special notes of permission, stating that they are aware of the danger involved, would be required of them if an initial injection were to be given a child who is older than two years.

We were somewhat surprised to find that an entire book, *Postvaccinal Perivenous Encephalitis,* by E. DeVries, devoted to this very problem of injections, vaccinations and their results, was published in 1960, under the auspices of The Netherlands Society of Psychiatry and Neurology. The book is largely a collection of case histories seen by the author and others, with descriptions of symptoms and response to treatment detailed. It is always made perfectly clear that vaccination is largely, if not entirely, responsible for the onset of the illness.

Just what happens to such a victim is best described in quotes from the book: "Case No. 48. This girl . . . was healthy before vaccination . . . Pustules developed slowly, but were quite distinct on the ninth day without, however, redness of the surrounding skin . . . she developed some fever, vomited at night, then became soporous (sleepy) and died on the eleventh day after vaccination.

"Case No. 33. A boy . . . had been healthy before vaccination . . . General malaise (illness) ensued 8 days after vaccination . . . headache and dizziness with vomiting were reported. This was progressive and stiffness of the neck was noted on the next day. . . . On the fifteenth day, paralysis of both legs and abdominal muscles was noted, with retention of urine and feces. At the same time, swallowing became difficult and speech defective. He died with high fever on the twentieth day after vaccination." He was 10 years old.

The value of this book, we think, lies in its clinical, objective reporting of dozens of such cases in which vaccination figured as a factor in sudden death. We take vaccination very calmly in the United States. Doctors give injections to children routinely, often without even consulting the parents. We believe that the value of what is hoped to be gained should be weighed against possible serious consequences.

More and More Shots

The *International Medical Digest* (February, 1961) carried the latest listing of the schedule of suggested vaccinations for children taken from the *Pediatric Herald* (August, 1960). It is quite a staggering course for a child to face. Injections begin at 1½ months and end at 16 years. Included are eight polio vaccine shots, two small-pox shots, five DPT's (diphtheria, whooping cough and tetanus) and three adult-type DT's (diphtheria, tetanus).

We are strongly opposed to this whole cult of vaccination therapy. We believe that the person who eats properly and, in general, takes proper care of his body, is prepared by nature to fight the invasion of virus infection. We know that there is much serious harm that could result from the injections themselves and the introduction of foreign elements into the blood stream.

We would like to point out the fantastic increase in suggested polio vaccine dosages since the vaccine first appeared in 1954. When it was introduced, one shot was practically guaranteed to immunize your child from polio. Later, it was suggested—just to be on the safe side—that two shots would do the trick. Then, we were told that 3 shots were needed, not suggested now, but *needed*. This dosage was held as sufficient for several years; then, we were told, 4 shots should be given; then, some doctors advocated a booster every year. Now, the official recommendation is 8 shots.

Did Not Really Buy Immunity

The parents who took their children to the doctor for the accepted two injections of one cubic centimeter of polio vaccine a month apart followed by a third after about 7 months, did not really buy immunity at all. *International Medical Digest* puts it this way: "Preliminary evidence indicates that a considerable proportion of infants have a less than optimal or relatively shortlived antibody response when immunized in this fashion." The new schedule calls for 3 injections a month apart, then a fourth 8 to 12 months later, then a fifth in about 3 years. Then, at 2 years, 12 years, and 16 years.

Now where do all of the people who are going on the earlier information fit in? We have seen no warnings in the daily papers telling these people their children are not properly immunized. All of these children who are poorly immunized have no way of knowing it, unless they or their doctors have seen either of the two publications mentioned here. (Of course, if they don't see a doctor before the next polio season, they're out of luck.)

Then we must consider the carefree attitude of the people who thought their children were immune all this time. They stopped observing all of the anti-polio precautions. They let their children go to crowded swimming pools, movies, dances, fairs and circuses during the height of the polio season with no fear, because they presumed them to be immune. How many who had been injected contracted polio? Quite a few.

The promised immunization through Salk vaccine is an absolute fiction; still, every communications medium warns us to get the 3 minimal shots for them if we would have our children escape polio. The implication is that the 3 shots, ipso facto, give immunity. However, none of the professional journals dares to suggest this anymore. Even a 70 per cent rate of protection is hedged now.

Then there are things such as the article from a Swiss medical journal *Schweizerische medizinische Wochenschrift* (June 4, 1960) which tells of Salk vaccine complications. The author cites side effects from this vaccine, as reported by 4 authors whom he names, among others, but his paper is concerned with facial paralysis resulting from injections of the vaccine. Dr. Bauman says that, "After 138,526 first and second vaccinations and 69,000 third vaccinations with the Salk vaccine had been given at the Cantonal Pediatric Clinic in Aarau, Switzerland, an increase in the incidence of facial paralysis . . . and of periodontal (gum) disease . . . has been observed and could be considered as complications or side effects of the Salk vaccination." In one case, the facial paralysis occurred "immediately after vaccination."

In *Dental Abstracts* (October, 1960), we saw an article which described the use of smallpox vaccine injections for the treatment of—are you ready?—*herpes simplex,* or cold sores! This is a problem which is characterized by the author, S. L. Rosenthal, as "more uncomfortable than dangerous . . . The ulcers heal without scar formation in from 7 to 10 days." To combat this, 100 patients (people chronically subject to these sores) received weekly smallpox vaccinations for an average of 9 weeks. A good percentage reported cure. But such sores are a simple manifestation of nutritional deficiency. Many experiments have shown vitamin C and the bioflavonoids to be effective in treating them. Why resort to smallpox vaccine, a dangerous substance, especially in such large doses? It would have been as easy, as effective and much safer to inject vitamin C for 9 weeks, if injections had to be used. But a check into the diets of these patients would probably have accomplished as much, if they had been willing to make some changes in their eating habits. Why are injections always looked to as the first answer?

A Dangerous, Valueless Treatment

A technique for injecting a hardening substance into the sacroiliac region has been in use recently as a measure against low back pain. The theory is that some low back pain is caused by relaxed supporting ligaments which allow instability in the area of the sacroiliac. The idea, then, is to harden, or firm up, these ligaments by injections of "vegetable oil and anesthetic."

The *Journal of the American Medical Association* (July 23, 1960) printed a report by J. E. Kepplinger and P. C. Bucy on the dangers involved in this procedure, or in any intraspinal injections, for that matter. The authors relate the case of a 53-year-old woman who suffered from a dull pain in the lower part of the back. The doctor she consulted administered 7 injections of the type described between March and May of 1957. From the beginning of the treatment, she experienced great pain in her lower extremities, with periods of numbness over her whole body. She had trouble walking, severe headaches, stiff neck and shoulder pains. By July 1, she required a cane for walking. By August, she was in the hospital for spinal fluid tests. By September 1, 1957, the lady was unable to walk, and by October 1, the patient had complete spastic paraplegia (paralysis of the lower limbs due to spinal cord injury). She is still the same and recovery is unlikely.

The authors say: "Intraspinal injections, for whatever purpose —anesthesia, localization of intraspinal lesions, intrathecal (spinal sheath) therapy—sometimes cause serious neurologic complications. Intrathecal injections of streptomycin and sulfonamides are apt to cause severe reactions in the spinal cord . . . Treating pain in the lower part of the back with injections of sclerosing (hardening) agents is inadvisable. There is no clear-cut evidence that this method of therapy is of value . . . The risk of permanent, disabling neurologic defects is too great to justify the use of sclerosing agents for treating back pain, particularly in view of the uncertain anatomic basis on which the treatment rests and the inadequate evidence that the treatment is of any value."

"Show Cause" Urged

The editor of *International Medical Digest,* in which the article was summarized, noted that, "Hayne has pointed out for years the contraindications to spinal therapy for many and probably all conditions. Spinal puncture should be reserved for diagnosis."

Think of the serious disablement which must be caused in many cases similar to the one described above, only because this advice to avoid spinal puncture is ignored. Would it be too much of an infringement upon the professional rights of our doctors to require them to show cause to a committee before instituting such dangerous therapy? It would at least force doctors to consider carefully before starting a treatment which can be crippling, if not fatal.

While we are discussing the subject of vaccinations, may we ask where does your physician inject your children? It is most likely that he uses the well-padded buttocks as his target. Most doctors do.

In the *Journal of the American Medical Association* (July 23, 1960)—later condensed in *International Medical Digest*—there appeared this startling passage: "Anyone concerned with infants and children must be aware that injection into the buttock may cause paralysis in the lower extremity. It is not often recognized that serious sciatic nerve injury can result from intragluteal (buttocks injection) administration of therapeutic and prophylactic agents. Injection injury of the sciatic nerve is more common than supposed and may be responsible for paralytic deformities which may be misdiagnosed as congenital club feet or the sequelae (aftermath) of poliomyelitis. The newborn infant, and especially the small premature infant, is more likely to suffer from this complication. Any age group is vulnerable and injury may result from a solitary injection. By abandoning the intragluteal site and choosing another area for intramuscular injections, physicians may spare their patients unnecessary handicaps."

It is surprising that, in the light of so prevalent a danger, doctors are not taught in medical school to avoid such sites of injection or that they personally do not choose to inject a child elsewhere, rather than risk injuring him. To the contrary, the buttock is still the favorite site for injections and, though this information has appeared in at least two public professional journals since July, 1960, chances are that your doctor has not yet changed his procedure. Demand that he change it, at least where your children are concerned. If your child is to get injections—and we still say avoid them whenever possible—at least don't run any risks that are unnecessary.

Here we are calmly informed of yet a new danger inherent in the use of injections, a danger about which apparently little was known before now. It is another of the consequences of medicine's "treat-now-investigate-later" attitude. We wonder how many more problems brought on by injections will be showing themselves in the next 10 or 20 years. Be careful about injections for yourself and your children; this terrifying series of new difficulties certainly shows that their full potential for harm is not known. Maintaining good health in your children through use of proper foods, is the safest and most effective way to avoid disease. In our opinion, a parent who is sure his child's nutrition is top grade, can feel safe in refusing protective injections of any kind for him. As for therapeutic injections, perhaps if you request it, the medication your doctor wants to give can be had in pill or capsule form. It would certainly be safer.

Vaccine—A Two-Week Life Span

We came across an interesting letter in the correspondence section of the *British Medical Journal* (June 24, 1961). It was written by a doctor who wished to share his method of storing vaccines with his colleagues. He noted that many physicians are not able to maintain a refrigerator in their offices, for one reason or another, and vaccines must be kept at a low temperature. His solution is a large thermos jug three-quarters filled with ice, with the vaccines in their original containers lying on top of the ice.

The next sentence is what caught our eye—"Smallpox vaccine kept this way also retains its potency for two weeks instead of the usual one." Does that mean that a doctor must replenish his smallpox vaccine every two weeks? Does any doctor do so? Are other vaccines that perishable? We know the new Sabin polio vaccine must be used within two or three weeks or it will spoil. We do not know if the Salk vaccine has better keeping qualities, but have no reason to assume that it would be more lasting than the newer Sabin product.

It is difficult for us to believe that the average practicing physician has his eye on the calendar with each shipment of vaccine he receives. Does he destroy or return each vial that is in his office more than two or three weeks? The packing, unpacking and scheduling of arrivals and departures would take a good part of his office hours. We are more inclined to believe that most physicians are not aware that a vaccine deteriorates so quickly, or if they do know it, they take a chance on the preparation's retaining its potency. Actually, we believe that the physician has no idea of just how potent the vaccine he gives really is. This means that many people who have had their recent smallpox shot before a foreign trip are likely to be no more equipped with antibodies than those who have had no injection at all. And what of the youngsters who have lined up for their fourth or fifth Salk shot? Suppose this "unstandardized product of an unstandardized process" (so-called in the *Journal of the American Medical Association,* February 25, 1961) has been standing around the doctor's office for more than two weeks, or even a month? How can its results, or the results attributed to it, be depended upon?

Of course, the problem of the manufacturer who must put out a product which will be useless after more than two weeks, from vat to syringe, is a tough one. The transportation takes that long in many cases. What company would survive with such a deadline and such risks?

If you do decide to get injections of any type of vaccine, ask your doctor how long the vial has been in his office. Insist on his using the newest he has.

Varicose Veins

Varicose Veins and Alcohol

When we speak of the dangers involved in using alcoholic beverages, we cannot ignore the problems drinking presents to the circulatory system. Frequent use of any stimulant causes the heart to work harder than it should and this strain results, eventually, in weakening that organ. Attendant to diseases of the heart itself are the diseases of the arteries which carry the blood through the body. If they become clogged or narrowed, the consequence can be fatal. That alcohol affects the blood passages can readily be seen by the red noses and vein-streaked cheeks of many who overindulge in the use of liquor.

People who will smile with amusement at the possibility of acquiring a red nose from drinking alcohol, will become deadly serious if presented with the likelihood that this same habit can cause varicose veins. They have friends who have experienced the pain and enforced inactivity brought about by this ailment, and they are determined to avoid being similarly afflicted.

Angiology (12/8: 382-84) does indeed link varicose veins with alcoholism. H. Tanyol and H. Menduke reported in that periodical on observations of 206 male subjects, 136 of whom had major varicose veins in the legs and 70 who acted as controls and who had no varicose symptoms. Patients were asked questions on their consumption of alcoholic beverages in terms of number of "shots" of whiskey, glasses or bottles of beer and glasses of wine per day or per week.

Of the varicose patients, only 16 (or 12 per cent) were complete abstainers; of the controls, 30 (or 43 per cent) were. Average alcohol consumption in the first group was 68 grams per day; in the control group, it was one gram.

The authors did not present any more absolute conclusion from these facts than to say, "These observations suggest that alcohol is an important factor in varicose veins." They do not say why this is so, but offer this guess: the consumption of alcohol in excess results in a widening of the arteries and the formation of new capillaries. The resultant circulation of more blood, faster, might force a simultaneous widening of the veins.

If alcohol is to be in the picture for you, in spite of the dangers it presents, we suggest special care to insure a sufficient intake of vitamin C to strengthen the blood vessels and vitamin E to maintain maximum efficiency in the work of the heart. The B vitamins, of course, will be needed to replace those destroyed by the alcohol itself.

Vegetable

Blanch Vegetables before Freezing

To a health seeker, eager to preserve every possible trace of vitamins and minerals in his food, blanching vegetables when you freeze them may seem to be a waste of the most valuable elements the foods contain. Why heat your good garden vegetables in steam, then drain off the water and plunge them into ice water, then drain again before freezing?

An article from *Illniois Research* for summer, 1959, gives us the answer straight from a laboratory. And the answer is a clear and unhesitating "blanch." There is not the slightest doubt about it. All vegetables *must* be blanched before freezing, if you want to preserve vitamins, taste, flavor and palatability.

Frances O. Van Duyne and Virginia R. Charles of the Department of Home Economics of the University of Illinois, who wrote the article, tell us they conducted their research on several lots of freshly harvested broccoli, corn, peas, snap beans and spinach. They processed the vegetables on the same morning they were harvested.

Part of each lot was blanched, cooled, packaged and frozen in accordance with accepted methods—that is, steaming for a given length of time, then plunging into ice cold water to cool and packaging as free from all water as possible. The other half of each food was packaged and frozen raw, without blanching.

The two experts then checked on the vitamin C content of the various foods after certain lengths of time in the freezer. They tell us that, even after two weeks in the freezer, the blanched and unblanched samples differed in the amounts of vitamin C retained.

Blanched beans retained 79 per cent of vitamin C; unblanched, only 62 per cent. Blanched spinach retained 52 per cent of its original vitamin C, whereas unblanched retained only 28 per cent. After 8 months of freezer storage, the unblanched spinach contained only one per cent of the original amount of vitamin C.

Table 13 shows the results on beans, peas and broccoli of all tests made at intervals of 1, 3, 6 and 9 months.

The matter of palatability showed even more clearly the wisdom of blanching all vegetables. Color, texture, flavor, absence of off-flavor and general acceptability were rated. During the entire 9 months, the blanched vegetables were tasty and attractive. They were bright green and tender and had a good flavor, with no off-flavors reported.

But vegetables that had been frozen unblanched, which had been stored only one month, developed off-flavor and lost color. After 3 months of storage, frozen peas were faded, snap beans were slightly gray. Broccoli was tough in texture and strong in flavor. Further deterioration took place as storage time increased, so much so, that the vegetables soon became inedible. The skin of the peas became tough, the stems of broccoli fibrous. Flavor was very poor and a strong off-flavor which was described as hay-like became noticeable. The same thing happened with corn which, unblanched, developed a very disagreeable flavor and deteriorated in texture.

Table 13: VITAMIN C RETENTION IN BLANCHED AND UNBLANCHED VEGETABLES

Vegetable	Months in Freezer	Retention of Vitamin C Blanched	Unblanched
Broccoli	1	66%	66%
	3	64	57
	6	60	40
	9	54	36
Peas	1	70	63
	3	75	55
	6	71	36
	9	70	37
Snap beans	1	85	58
	3	83	44
	6	64	15
	9	43	3

Reason for Blanching

There is a very good reason why vegetables need to be blanched before freezing. All of them contain certain enzymes, which are chemical substances whose function is to bring about chemical changes. Enzymes begin to make changes in vegetables as soon as they are picked from the garden. If these enzymes are not inactivated by heat, they will continue to function in the frozen food bringing deterioration in color, texture and taste. The high heat achieved by steaming the vegetables for a specified period of time inactivates the enzymes and permits the food to remain unspoiled. So actually, you are not "spoiling" vegetables from the health viewpoint, when you blanch. You are making them more healthful.

The reason for dunking the blanched vegetables in ice water as soon as they have finished steaming is to halt immediately the action of the heat, so that vitamins will not be lost. Of course, some vitamins, especially vitamin C, are bound to be lost in the steaming and cooling process. But, as you can see from the figures given above, you are saving vitamins in the long run when you blanch vegetables.

We do not advise cooking or blanching fruit before freezing. It can go into the freezer just as it comes from the vines, trees or bushes. If you are freezing your own berries, for instance, there is no necessity to even wash them. You know that they are clean enough to eat, for you have been eating them from the vines. With peaches and other fruits that discolor rapidly after they are cut, we recommend using a mixture of lemon juice and honey. Mix it through the cut fruit before freezing and you will find that the fruit will not darken when you thaw it before eating.

Frozen fruits, especially those you freeze yourself, are better for you than the canned and processed fruits that are available during winter months. We think that your own frozen fruits and vegetables, picked at the peak of their goodness and frozen within minutes of the picking, are far preferable to fresh vegetables and fruits available in the stores during the winter. This market produce has been stored for perhaps weeks or months and may have lost most of its goodness.

Vegetable Juices

Vegetable Juices in Your Health Program

What is our viewpoint on vegetable juices? Do we recommend drinking raw vegetable juices? Do we claim for them that they will cure certain conditions or that health-conscious persons should take them every day just as a further aid to good health? We have always soft-pedaled the question of taking vegetable juices, mostly because there seems to be no way whereby one can demonstrate experimentally what benefits they might bring. Using large amounts of vegetable juice means leaving out considerable quantities of other food. Is any benefit due to the inclusion of the juice or the exclusion of the other, less nutritious food?

A serious consideration of the pros and cons of vegetable juice appeared in a British publication, the *Monthly Bulletin of the Minister of Health Laboratories,* Vol. 12, p. 78, 1953. Written by H. E. Magee, D.Sc., MRCP, the article seems to be quite fair to both sides. Dr. Magee reviews the material that has appeared on the subject in medical and scientific literature. There have been reports, he says, of successful therapy for a number of conditions. Two Russian scientists used vegetable juices for treating high blood pressure, with good results. Obesity has been treated successfully. Heart and blood vessel diseases, as well as gout, were treated successfully in 1936 by an M.D. using fruit and vegetable juices. Nephritis (inflammation of the kidney) was treated successfully in several experiments. Another researcher claims that juices helped in the treatment of gall bladder trouble, high blood pressure and other heart and blood vessel disorders. Seven patients fasted for 3 days or more, then were given fruit and vegetable juices and, gradually, other foods which resulted in a good, well-balanced diet were added, with vegetable juices still playing a large part in the diet. Symptoms such as breathlessness, headaches and insomnia disappeared so long as the patients kept to their diet.

Vegetable juices have been used, too, for disorders of the digestive tract. Take, for example, Dr. Cheyney's experiments with cabbage juice for ulcer patients. This California M.D. treated 13 cases of stomach or duodenal ulcer with the usual bland ulcer diet, all cooked, plus about one quart of raw cabbage juice per day. In all cases, symptoms subsided in about a week and the average healing time (controlled by X-rays) was 7.3 days for the stomach ulcers and 10.4 for the duodenal ulcers, compared to 42 and 37 days, respectively, for cases who got the ulcer diet, but no cabbage juice. Cheyney also cured stomach ulcers in guinea pigs with cabbage juice.

Two other researchers have used raw cabbage juice successfully on ulcer patients. There are also, says Dr. Magee, numerous references in the medical literature to beneficial effects of vegetable juices on infant diarrhea, gastroenteritis (inflammation of the stomach and bowel), colitis, dyspepsia and toxic states of the intestine. It seems, he goes on, that the pectin in the raw juices absorbs toxic substances and harmful bacteria from the bowel so that they are harmlessly excreted. Then, the mucous membrane can recover its health. There is nowhere any indication that juices which have been heated or cooked will produce any of these benefits. In all the cases described above, fresh, raw juices were used.

What Is the Food Value of Juices?

Dr. Magee did some investigations on the nutritive content of fruit juices. These are the only such figures we have ever been able to find and we wish they were more complete. However, they do throw considerable light on just what amount of some food elements one can expect to find in certain vegetable juices.

The juices which were tested were held in a refrigerator for about 12 hours before they were tested. This accounts for the fact that there is no listing of the vitamin C present. There was no vitamin C in any of the juices but kale. It had been oxidized during the time of storage. This is one of the most important facts for all of us to remember—the highly perishable quality of vitamin C. Once a fruit or vegetable has been cut, chopped, squeezed or otherwise exposed to large amounts of air, you can be pretty sure that there is little or no vitamin C left. This is why we urge readers to eat fresh foods just as soon as they are prepared—don't peel fruit or juice it, don't chop vegetables or juice them until just before you are going to eat or drink them.

In Table 14, the amount of sugar is given in grams per 100 milliliters, which is about ½ cup. It is worthy of note that the spinach juice is not very high in calcium compared with the amount in the fresh vegetable, which seems to indicate that the calcium is simply not released into the juice, possibly because of the oxalic acid content of spinach. None of the vegetable juices contained any significant amount of carotene (vitamin A) except carrots and water cress. So it seems that the other vegetables hold on to their vitamin A, for we know that the whole vegetable contains considerable amounts.

Table 14: COMPOSITION OF FRESH VEGETABLE JUICES COMPARED TO THE VEGETABLE ITSELF

Vegetable	Total Sugars (as glucose) in grams per 100 ml. (gm.)	Iron in mg. per 100 ml. (gm.)	Calcium in mg. per 100 ml. (mg.)	Vitamin B₁ in mg. per 100 ml. (gm.)
Broccoli Leaves	3.00(0.4)	0.60(1.52)	18.70(160)	15.0
Cabbage	4.17(8.3)	1.02(1.0)	16.90(65)	75.0(75)
Carrots	7.11(5.4)	0.30(10.6)	0.49(48)	30.0(60)
Celery	2.06(1.2)	0.43(0.6)	0.62(52)	15.0(30)
Kale	3.71	1.60(2.5)	11.60(200)	15.0(120)
Melon	4.33	0.42	0.40	30.0
Parsley	0.44(8.8)	1.12(8.0)	6.30(325)	30.0(120)
Spinach	1.85(1.2)	1.02(4.0)	0.75(595)	Nil (100)
Tomato	3.06(2.8)	0.08(0.4)	4.05(13)	15.0(60)
Water Cress	0.20(0.6)	2.12(1.6)	2.90(222)	30.0(120)

(*The content of the vegetable appears in parentheses beside the juice figure.*)

Potassium Content Is Higher in Juice

Dr. Magee tells us that former investigations have shown that the raw whole vegetable contains more nitrogen, pectin, sodium, calcium, sulfur and phosphorus than the juices. But the potassium content of the juice is higher than that of the whole vegetables. This seems to indicate that these substances are retained by the pulp and do not find their way into the raw juice.

Searching for an explanation of Dr. Cheyney's reports on using vegetable juices for ulcer treatment, Dr. Magee investigated the "buffering" capacity of each juice and compared it to that of milk, which is the standard ingredient of ulcer diets. He tested by adding hydrochloric acid to each juice and then tested its acidity. He found that most of the juices have a reaction or pH just about as alkaline as milk. Spinach juice could take even more hydrochloric acid than milk before it became highly acid. Cabbage, kale and parsley juice were not far behind. So it seems that the reason why vegetable juices may make such a difference in ulcer cases is just that they protect the stomach lining against the acid which is present there in too large a quantity. Dr. Magee gives some credit for this "buffering" action to the minerals, such as potassium, magnesium and so forth, that also pass into the juice.

Amino Acids or Proteins Are also Present

There are, too, certain amino acids, or forms of protein, in vegetable juices. Cabbage juice, for instance, contains relatively large amounts of lysine, tryptophan and methionine. What other food elements are present in vegetable juices, we can only guess, he says, since tests have not been done on the less important vitamins and the trace minerals.

It is well to keep in mind that the very qualities which make juices valuable render them dangerous if they are kept for long in a state where bacteria could grow in them. Dr. Magee mentions especially *botulinus*, which is one of the deadliest poisons known. Juicing fresh vegetables and letting the juice stand unrefrigerated can thus present a grave risk. The main reason why canned and bottled foods must be heated to such high temperatures is to prevent the growth of such bacteria. So, if one plans to use raw vegetable (or fruit) juices, they should be prepared immediately before eating and consumed at once, *not stored*. Vitamins and enzymes are lost during storage and toxic bacteria may easily spoil the juice if it stands any length of time.

Why Drink Juices?

Why should one juice vegetables or fruits rather than eating them whole? In general, we believe that the average healthy person, wanting simply to preserve good health and prevent illness, will get more benefit from eating his fruits and vegetables whole rather than juicing them. As we have shown above, considerable amounts of the minerals and vitamins are lost in juicing. In addition, as Dr. Magee points out, "the whole vegetable has the advantage of the indigestible material, which, besides its stimulating action on peristalsis, provides a medium in the large intestine for the microbiological syntheses which are coming to be recognized as important in nutrition." In other words, constipation is prevented and helpful bacteria are encouraged in the intestine which will produce vitamins, if one eats the whole vegetable or fruit rather than juicing it.

It is well to keep in mind that everything we have said about the healthful properties of juices refers only to raw, freshly made juice. In canned, bottled, cooked or otherwise processed juice, all, or nearly all, the vitamin C will be destroyed, enzymes will be nonexistent and the quality of other ingredients will be so changed that one cannot expect the same results one gets from raw juice.

Remember that any kind of juice is a concentrated food. Don't drink as much of it as you would of water. It's a lot more than just water. We know of cases where drinking enormous amounts of carrot juice caused hands to turn yellow. This indicated that the individual was getting too much carotene which was not immediately harmful. But moderation should be used in all things.

If you possibly can, get organically grown vegetables, or grow your own. The chemicals and insecticides which pollute all foods today contaminate the vegetables you plan to juice. You cannot wash them away, no matter how hard you scrub. Although we have never seen any tests that prove this, it seems obvious to us, that, in the raw juice from such vegetables, the chemicals and insecticides would be concentrated.

Vegetarianism

Not All "Natural" Products Are Harmless

Vegetarians sometimes remonstrate with us, telling us that we are recommending meat and eggs, which may contain possibly harmful substances, whereas they eat only harmless foods like vegetables and fruits. We have been surprised how much information has come our way indicating that foods of the vegetable family can be harmful, too. We present here some evidence along these lines.

An article in the *British Medical Journal* (August 27, 1960), tells of a disease called fasciolopsis which occurs as a result of eating food contaminated with the larvae of a certain fluke, or worm. In the outbreak described, 5 people in one section of England were stricken as a result of the wet summer of 1958. In districts where cattle and sheep are infected with these worms, the excreta of the animals may carry the eggs which, during a rainy season, are deposited on vegetation growing in the neighborhood. Anyone eating the growing things is infected with the eggs of the worm which later mature in the body of the person and eventually inhabit the liver where they cause great distress.

The 5 persons described in this article suffered from excruciating pain, fever, rash, tenderness of the liver and such weakness and disability that they were confined to bed for quite long periods of time. Strong drugs given to all of them resulted in killing some of the worms. However, the aftereffects of the drugs were so unpleasant that several of the patients refused to take more of them and are still, according to the article, infected with the worms.

In this case, all of the patients habitually ate quite large quantities of water cress. This is an excellent food, rich in minerals, chlorophyll and vitamins. But, in this particular instance, the water cress was growing naturally in an area heavily infested with the eggs of the liver fluke. Apparently, it was impossible to remove these by a casual washing or perhaps the patients did not wash their water cress at all. At any rate, after long and painful interludes, the proper diagnosis was made and the water cress was pinpointed as the cause of the trouble.

Does this mean that the health-conscious person should not eat water cress or any other greens? Certainly not, for they are fine foods. It means simply that one should be especially careful to know the source of the greens one eats. We do not know what the incidence is of infestation with this worm in America. In any area where it is known to prevail, greens meant to be served raw should not be eaten.

The *Journal* makes this recommendation: "ideally, water cress should be grown under artificial conditions . . . in practice, it is often cut from natural beds fed by streams running through pastures." If you have your own water cress, fine. You know the safety of your own community terrain. If you buy commercially grown water cress, it might be well to check on where it comes from. It doesn't seem to be advisable to pick water cress indiscriminately anywhere you chance to find it. It may be infected and dangerous.

Oxalic Acid and Calcium

Rhubarb, spinach and members of the spinach family contain oxalic acid. This is a natural food acid just as citric acid, malic acid, etc., are. It was not put there by processors. In the usual amounts in which we eat rhubarb or greens, of the spinach family, there is no danger to anyone.

But oxalic acid has an affinity for calcium. It ties up calcium in the digestive tract so that it is unavailable for the body to use. Someone forced to live for considerable periods of time on diets which include rhubarb or spinach every day, would certainly run into difficulty from lack of calcium which might show itself as muscle cramps, heart difficulty, etc.

Life magazine for January 15, 1951, carried a terrifying story about a weed which has been taking over much pasture land in the west—a weed which is fatal to sheep that eat it. The leaves are rich in oxalic acid and sheep which eat the weeds exclusively during seasons when other food is not available, may die within hours because the oxalic acid has combined with the calcium in their blood, making it unavailable for use by the body.

Again we say—don't shun foods like spinach and rhubarb. Eat them in moderation and include plenty of calcium-rich foods at the same meal. It seems to us that the food which poses the greatest threat to modern Americans because of its oxalic acid content, is chocolate. Many children eat chocolate every day of their lives—in chocolate milk, in sodas and sundaes, in puddings, in chocolate bars. The amount of oxalic acid consumed must undoubtedly have a lot to do with tooth decay, bones that break easily and heart trouble.

Contain Toxic Substances

Medical literature has published several articles on goiter which apparently resulted from feeding infants on soybean milk rather than cow's milk. Such a circumstance usually involves children who are allergic to cow's milk. In these conditions, the entire diet of the child may consist of soybean milk. It seems very easy to correct the disorder, for the thyroid gland becomes normal again within a few weeks after the soy milk is discontinued.

There is a substance in soybeans which may prove toxic if the beans are eaten raw. For this reason, we always advise cooking the beans. They are not very appetizing raw anyway, so it seems only reasonable that most people would cook them.

Turnips and members of the turnip family of vegetables, as well as cabbage, Brussels sprouts, cauliflower, soybeans, peanuts, radishes, kale, mangels, red cabbage, lentils and peas, have a tendency to promote goiter, especially when they are eaten raw or in large quantities. There is, it seems, a substance in such vegetables which is anti-thyroid. That is, it is to some extent poisonous to the thyroid gland. Cooking such vegetables destroys this substance.

It seems unlikely that anyone in present-day America would have such a fondness for one of these or such a limited selection of food that there could be any danger to health from these vegetables. And it is true that most observations on their toxicity have been made either under abnormal conditions in a laboratory or in some area where food was scarce during a famine, blockade or war. In some European countries during the last war, for instance, turnips formed the staple food for many families who were cut off from their usual food supplies. Such conditions can cause harm.

But there are people in every kind of society who, for one reason or another, have peculiar food patterns. Instead of eating a variety of foods, selected especially for their variety and their nutritive value, such people may confine themselves to one or two foods. If one of these vegetables should happen to be one of the foods used in such a case, trouble might result, especially if it were eaten raw.

What About Potatoes?

Potatoes come originally from a plant called nightshade, which is a plant whose fruits are poisonous. Originally, the fruits of the potato were above ground and apparently, their poison content helped preserve the plant from herb eating animals. Farmers developed the potato so that the fruits, or vegetables as we call them, grow underground, away from the sunlight. So the original poison is not present in the potatoes we eat. However, it develops in sprouts of potatoes and sometimes in potatoes whose green color indicates that they have grown partially out of the ground and hence, in sunlight.

The *Medical Press* for August 31, 1960, reported that some potatoes imported into England contained exceptionally large amounts of solanin, the poisonous compound—some 20 times the normal and harmless amount. One family, which had eaten the potatoes roasted in their skins, became ill. The solanin lies directly under the skin and consumers who had peeled their potatoes before eating them had suffered no harm.

What is the lesson? Never eat potatoes? If you do, always peel them? Certainly not. Potatoes are a fine food which should be regularly included in meals. But you should avoid eating potatoes and skins of those that have sprouted or ones that have a greenish color. If you peel these, you're safe. And don't eat the sprouts.

These Can Be Harmful

Here are some miscellaneous notes on other vegetable foods which, under certain circumstances, might prove dangerous: Eating a kind of bean called the fava bean produces a condition called favism in susceptible persons. Lathyrism is a disease produced by overeating a pea of the genus *Lathyrus sativus*.

Cassava, which we know as tapioca, contains, in its native state, a poison which is known as linamarin, which is destroyed by heating or drying the root, after which it becomes the product with which we are familiar. Honey has been known to contain poisons if the bees have fed on plants which are poisonous to us but not to them.

An example of a plant poison which was used until recently as a chemical additive in food is coumarin. This substance, which is widely distributed in food, was used as a flavoring in many foods. It was generally added to vanilla in ice cream and chocolate because it seemed to "round off" the vanilla flavor. During a routine toxicity investigation carried out by a commercial laboratory, it was found that coumarin is toxic. It had always been regarded as completely safe because it is a "natural component of food." The Food and Drug Administration ruled that it must not be used in food from that date on. (One cannot help but wonder about all the other "natural" additives that the Food and Drug Administration now casually permits in food!)

There is no reason for anyone to become alarmed over the information given above. We are merely trying to show our vegetarian friends that they cannot accuse us of recommending foods which may be harmful under some circumstances, while they recommend only completely harmless, wholesome fruits and vegetables. As we have shown above, foods of the vegetable kingdom also have a potential for harm under certain circumstances. Your best bet is a well-rounded, widely varied diet that includes, in moderation, all good, unprocessed foods—meat, eggs, nuts, seeds, vegetables and fruits in good proportions.

Vital Organs

The Partners of the Blood Stream

When we think of the miraculous manner in which the blood stream nourishes and defends the body, it is with an awed sense of how dependent we are on the stream of vital fluid within us. Yet, far from being the helpless dependents of our blood, we are the ones who determine whether our blood itself will be strong or weak, healthy or sickly. We have an entire network of organs to circulate, renew, purify and nourish the blood.

The chief organ of the circulatory system, of course, is the heart. This remarkably efficient pump, made of the toughest muscle fibres in the entire body, is a roughly pear-shaped organ located in the center of the chest, with its bottom inclined toward the left side. According to Peter Pineo Chase, M.D., in his book, *Your Wonderful Body,* when the body is unexcited and in repose, the heart pumps about 5 pints of blood a minute. It is this strong pumping action that forces the blood through the arteries into smaller vessels and capillaries, carrying oxygen, food and various protective organisms to every cell of the body. Having done its work, the blood, still moved by nothing but the pumping strength of the heart, enters the veins loaded with waste products and returns to the heart, most of it moving directly against the force of gravity.

When you consider that this incredibly vigorous pumping is carried on every moment of your life—that if the heart were to stop beating and rest for just a few minutes, it would mean certain death—then you begin to get a picture of the enormous burden on this one organ and the vital importance of its health.

This tough muscular organ is divided into 4 chambers, with valves permitting blood in the proper amounts to enter and leave them. The two upper chambers are called the right and left auricles. The lower chambers are the right and left ventricles.

Blood freshly oxygenated in the lungs moves through the pulmonary vein into the left auricle. From there, it flows through the mitral valve into the left ventricle. When the ventricle is full, the valve closes until the heart, with a powerful contraction, squeezes the blood upward through the aortic valve into the aorta, the principal artery of the body. As soon as the left ventricle relaxes and opens, the mitral valve reopens and admits more blood. This process takes place about 70 to 80 times a minute. When you take your pulse, what you feel is the successive surges of blood pumped by the left ventricle.

At the same time, blood that has exchanged its oxygen and other nutritional products for the wastes of cellular activity, is being returned through the vena cava, the greatest vein of the body, into the right auricle. It passes through the tricuspid valve into the right ventricle which, when the heart contracts, forces the waste-laden blood into the pulmonary artery and thence into the lungs.

In the lungs, carbon dioxide is exchanged for oxygen from the air that has just been breathed in. The carbon dioxide is exhaled. The freshly oxygenated blood enters the pulmonary vein and once more flows into the left auricle, completing the cycle.

The Health of the Heart

It is perfectly obvious that anything that interferes with the health of the heart is going to keep the blood from doing its work properly. Too weak a heart action will not send enough blood to the extremities. Pumping that is too strong and fast will endanger the blood vessels. A healthy heart is precious and irreplaceable.

Yet, you may be endangering the health of your heart this minute, if, while you are reading this, you happen to be smoking a cigarette or drinking a glass of chlorinated water.

Editor Rodale has often expressed his well-founded belief that chlorine, used to "purify" drinking water, is responsible for a great deal of the heart disease in the United States. In his book, THE PREVENTION METHOD FOR BETTER HEALTH, he cited medical evidence that chlorine may cause injury to the mitral valve, palpitations and irregular heartbeat.

Why take a chance with such a dangerous substance? Irresponsible authorities may decide to chlorinate your city's water supply, but you don't have to risk the health of your heart by drinking chlorine. If you must drink treated water, boil it first. This will evaporate the chlorine and make the water far safer. Better still, drink bottled pure spring water, which is available almost everywhere these days.

The harmful effects of smoking on the heart are so well known there is no disputing them. Nicotine is one of the deadliest poisons known to man. A stimulant, it speeds the heart action, narrows the blood vessels, raises the blood pressure. *Science News Letter* (February 26, 1955) said: "Smoking affects your heart whether you are a normal person or one with heart disease." Your family doctor will tell you that, whether or not he gets lung cancer, the habitual smoker is weakening his heart and consequently, shortening his life.

Other common diet items to be avoided, for the best health of your heart, are excessive coffee and tea and all animal fats, especially whole milk, cream and butter.

On the positive side, there are many delicious foods you can eat with positive benefit to your heart. These are the foods that contain substantial amounts of vitamin E.

Vitamin E has been used in the treatment of heart disease with outstanding success at the Shute Clinic of London, Ontario. Its physiological effect seems to be to help the tissues throughout the body to use and store oxygen effectively. Since the primary work of the heart is to drive oxygen to the tissues by pumping the blood, there is no difficulty in understanding that a food substance that reduces the demand for oxygen will proportionately reduce the burden on the heart.

The foods richest in vitamin E are the unsaturated vegetable oils—sunflower, safflower, corn, wheat germ, soybean, cottonseed —and the plants from which they are derived. A breakfast bowl of wheat germ, a between-meals munch of sunflower seeds, use of corn oil as a salad dressing—such dietary habits, regularly pursued, can do much to relieve your heart of strain.

We do not advise any of our readers to attempt self-doctoring for any kind of heart condition or difficulty. An ailing heart *must* be cared for by a qualified doctor. But for those with healthy hearts who have the good sense to want to stay that way, we believe vitamin E will provide invaluable help.

If you are overweight, you are putting incessant extra strain on your heart and should reduce. A high protein diet, rich in vitamins and including substantial amounts of the unsaturated vegetable oils, is the type of gradual weight reduction we recommend.

The Lungs

The largest internal organs we have, the lungs are a spongy tissue that fills most of the chest cavity. Upon their health depends our ability to take oxygen into the body, to transfer it to the blood and to get rid of carbon dioxide, a gaseous waste product of cell oxidation that could kill us if too much of it accumulated in our bodies.

The ability of the lungs to function properly has two great enemies—polluted air, whether polluted with tobacco smoke or with industrial smoke and chemicals, and infections of the respiratory tract, such as tuberculosis, pneumonia, influenza and the common cold.

If you live in a city, you are, in all probability, breathing polluted air all the time. For the health of your lungs and your body in general, it is vital that you get out into the open country as often as you possibly can. On week ends and on holidays, get far away from factories, auto traffic and closed rooms where suicidally inclined people smoke. Go into a forest or to a producing farmland—someplace where there are many plants growing. Plants breathe in carbon dioxide and exhale oxygen. The air in the vicinity of growing things is richer in oxygen and a delightful tonic.

The lungs have a remarkable ability to clear themselves of foreign irritants of all sorts, given half a chance. What destroys them, via lung cancer and other diseases, is the continual, day-by-day piling up of irritants faster than they can be removed. But even a few days of breathing pure, high-oxygen air can work wonders.

To avoid respiratory infections, eat lots of vitamin C combined with citrus bioflavonoids. The bioflavonoids, contained in large quantities in the white underskin and pulp of citrus fruits, in combination with vitamin C, have been proven to reduce the incidence of colds. They have also been reported by many doctors, including the well-known Morton S. Biskind, M.D., to bring about faster recovery from all types of respiratory infections.

Since citric acid is a known cause of tooth erosion and has other destructive effects on the system, we do not recommend the eating of many oranges or grapefruit. This is one case where we believe the food supplements are better than the food from which they are derived. What we endorse is the regular taking of supplements of vitamin C and bioflavonoids, to help protect the health of your lungs and respiratory system. Good, healthy lungs will not fail you in your need for properly oxygenated blood.

The Kidneys

In its passage through the body, the blood flows through two bean-shaped organs located at the small of the back, on either side of the spine. These are the kidneys, made of spongy tissue very similar to that of the lung. Scavengers of the blood stream, the kidneys extract urea, a waste product of the cells, and other impurities from the blood, along with enough water to keep them dissolved as they are passed into the bladder, to be periodically excreted as urine. Should the kidneys fail in their action, urea accumulating in the blood would very quickly cause a fatal disease named uremia.

Fortunately, the kidneys are very tough little organs. If one is removed, the other will usually do the work of two. The greatest danger to the effective action of the kidneys seems to be an excess of salt. As pointed out by Isaac Asimov, Ph.D., a leading biochemist, in his book, *The Living River,* "if the body has an excess of sodium ion, this must be carried off through the kidneys. For every milligram of sodium ion removed, a certain quantity of water is necessary to transport it and is used, even though the body may be short of water."

Dr. Asimov points out that excessive consumption of salt, even while it holds water in the body tissues, causes the kidneys to remove too much water from the blood stream. An insufficiency of water in the blood permits urea and other wastes to solidify and crystallize and leads to the formation of kidney stones. These are agonizingly painful. So do your kidneys a favor, as well as the rest of your system—give up table salt. As much salt as your body requires occurs naturally in the foods you eat. Drink plenty of pure spring water and eat a wholesome, salt-free diet, and you will never have to worry about your kidneys.

Bone Marrow

In partnership with the spleen, the bone marrow is responsible for the supply of healthy, active red cells in the blood. According to Isaac Asimov in *The Living River,* 200 billion red cells break down daily and need replacement. The bone marrow—particularly that of the long bones of the arms and legs—is usually quite up to the job of manufacturing that many red cells every day. Occasionally, for reasons that have not yet been determined, the bone marrow fails to perform this work fast enough. Then, the condition develops that is known as pernicious (*not* iron-deficiency) anemia. It is a disease that, once contracted, cannot be cured. It can be controlled with little trouble, however. This was formerly done with liver extract injections. More recently, vitamin B_{12} (cobalamin), in minute quantities, has been found to be almost invariably successful in the control of this illness.

Eat plenty of liver, which is the best dietary source of vitamin B_{12}, to protect yourself against all types of anemia. The liver contains large amounts of iron and the B complex vitamins. Desiccated liver tablets, as a dietary supplement every day, will give you the very best assurance.

The Liver

The liver, itself, is an all-important partner of the blood in its work. It is through the liver that most of our digested food is carried up from the intestines (via the portal vein), processed and brought to the heart, for arterial distribution to the entire body. The liver organizes the amino acids from our food into the proper proportions that will best nourish the body tissues, and then releases them into the blood plasma. The liver stores the surplus B vitamins (including vitamin B_{12}) in our diet, and releases them into the blood stream as needed.

But the liver has two great enemies—alcohol and salt. Avoid these two poisons, and the chances are excellent that you will never have trouble with your liver—or with the health of your blood— as long as you live. Provided, of course, that you also give yourself the proper nourishment required for general good health.

Vitamins

The Superiority of Natural Vitamins

"Prove it!"

How many times do we hear that challenge—particularly when we tell our friends that natural food supplements are more valuable to good health than the synthetic variety. None of us carries a file for ready reference with him, so that he can whip it out and quote chapter and verse when called upon, but we would like to offer some ammunition for your next encounter with someone who thinks "health nuts" are the only ones who subscribe to the theory behind natural supplements. Serious scientists are well aware of the obvious fact that a synthetic vitamin can't possibly have with it the surrounding components of a vitamin as it occurs naturally. Many of these components have yet to be discovered. How many different B vitamins does one get in brewer's yeast—12, 15, 25? No one really knows, but taking a synthetically produced vitamin B complex capsule can hardly be expected to give one elements of which the makers of the capsule are not even aware. Persons using desiccated liver, for example, were getting valuable vitamin B_{12} long before it was isolated and manufactured synthetically. Yet, the synthetic B complex supplements being used until then were considered complete, and those who urged the use of synthetic over natural supplements were insisting that one is as good as the other.

The Bioflavonoids Are a Case in Point

The next time you are confronted with that argument, you might mention the work of St. Rusznyak and A. Szent-Gyorgi, who discovered the bioflavonoids. In their experiments, they were able to show that ascorbic acid (vitamin C) is accompanied in the cell by a substance of similar importance and related activity. If both substances are absent, the symptoms of a vitamin C shortage are obvious (scurvy) and the symptoms of an absence of the second substance are obscured. However, in certain types of disease, those characterized by increased fragility of the capillaries, ascorbic acid alone is not effective. Yet, such a condition can readily be cured by the administration of extracts of lemon juice or Hungarian red pepper. The extracts were found to be equally effective in strengthening the capillaries against hemorrhage and against the invasion of the blood stream by infectious organisms. But the point is that vitamin C, of itself, would have been completely ineffective in these instances, no matter how pure or how carefully manufactured it might be. It had to work in its natural setting, with the flavonoids.

Vitamin C Action Is 3 Times Stronger

In 1960, in a German periodical, *Sportartztliche Praxis,* Ludwig Prokop, M.D., wrote that, "The superior quality of nature's vitamin C in orange juice shows especially in the fact that it has a 3 times stronger action on the oxygen deficiency and recovery quotient. . . . Apart from the juice, which contains small amounts of vitamins A, B and different salts, the cause of this frequently established fact may be found first of all in the stabilization of ascorbic acid by rutin (vitamin P) which guarantees a far better utilization of vitamin C."

The doctor reached these conclusions after endurance tests with athletes, in which the loss of oxygen through stress was measured, and then the speed with which it was regained in those getting vitamin C from orange juice, those getting it in a synthetic vitamin C preparation and those getting placebos, who acted as controls.

Synthetic B Vitamins Shown Inferior

A booklet published by Anheuser-Busch, Incorporated, in June, 1943, listed a series of experiments involving the use of B vitamins which had appeared in medical and chemical journals from all over the world. In each, it was demonstrated that the synthetic vitamin B supplements simply did not do the job of maintaining normal body functions. For example, in the *Proceedings of the American Society of Biological Chemistry* (April 15-19, 1941), there was a report which showed that large daily supplements of synthetically produced thiamin, riboflavin, pyridoxine, choline chloride, calcium pantothenate, nicotinic acid and Factor "W" resulted in the complete failure of lactation of an albino rat, the infant mortality being 95 to 100 per cent. The missing factor was tentatively labeled B_x and appeared in rice polishings, wheat germ, dried grass, liver extract and brewer's yeast.

Another experiment, written up in the *Journal of Experimental Medicine* (76, 1-14, 1942), led to the conclusion that a deficiency in the B complex vitamins could be one of the causative factors in high blood pressure. Rats deprived of B complex exhibited a rise in blood pressure, followed by a fall. Use of thiamin, without accompanying B vitamins, caused the blood pressure to rise above normal in a week's time. However, when B complex-rich yeast or liver extract was added to the diet, the blood pressure returned to normal.

The liver and kidneys rely on a supply of B vitamins for good health. In the *Journal of Clinical Investigation* (21, 385, 1942), it was reported that, when rats fed a low-protein, high-fat diet developed fatty degeneration, decay and cirrhosis of the liver, and hemorrhagic and decaying kidneys, the situation could be prevented from further deterioration by the daily addition of two grams of brewer's yeast to the diet. The addition of the two valuable B vitamins, thiamin and riboflavin, alone, did not have any beneficial effect.

Foxes and Humans Respond to Brewer's Yeast

Kingstad and Lunde, in *Skand. Vet.* (30, 1121-43, 1940), told of silver foxes fed a synthetic diet consisting of known ingredients plus cod liver oil, salt mixture and various components of B complex. "When all known synthetic members of the B complex were given, the animals failed to grow, their coats became depigmented (lost color), the fur quality deteriorated and the animals died. These changes could be prevented by the inclusion of such natural or complete sources of the vitamin B complex as yeast or liver."

Fifteen persons suffering from lichen planus (a skin disease) were treated with injections of vitamin B (*Journal of the Canadian Medical Association,* 44, 120, 1941). No improvement was obtained until brewer's yeast or liver extract was administered orally. With this measure, a generally beneficial effect was obtained.

Another article in the *Journal of the Canadian Medical Association* (46, 413, 1942) summed up the case for naturally occurring B complex vitamins: "Deficiencies of the B complex usually occur together and no simple synthetic vitamin will control these deficiencies adequately. High potency of one or more factors in B vitamin complex preparations is not necessarily a true index of their therapeutic value, since all of the various B complex factors must be present in properly balanced amounts, such as in yeast."

Natural Vitamin K for Hemorrhages

Vitamin K, in its natural form, has been shown to be effective against hemorrhages which result from the administration of bishydroxycoumarin dicoumarol (an anticoagulant drug). In the *Journal of the American Medical Association* (February 14, 1953), M. Verstraete wrote that, "Once hemorrhage has started, blood transfusions and vitamin K preparations are usually given. However, the practical value of various types of commercial vitamin K seems to exert little or no influence on hypothrombinemia (slow blood clotting) induced by bishydroxycoumarin. The natural, oil-soluble vitamin K or its oxidized form, on the contrary, is capable of acting as an antidote against bishydroxycoumarin. . . ."

We believe that the most concise conclusion on the whole question of natural versus synthetic supplements appeared in *Science 97* (April 30 and May 7, 1943), when A. J. Carlson wrote: "On the whole, we can trust nature further than the chemist and his synthetic vitamins." That statement is the cornerstone of our system for healthful living. We have yet to see nature, in all of her subtleties, duplicated by science. We refuse to depend upon attempts at such duplication in foods or food supplements. We believe that those who do depend upon such duplication are deluding themselves and asking for trouble.

Medicine's Attitude toward Nutrients

The time lag between an important discovery and its acceptance and general use is a frustrating thing. We can only imagine how Lister felt when he heard of the deaths in surgery before his theories on infection through unfriendly bacteria became accepted, or how Semmelweis hated seeing so many mothers die needlessly in childbirth when he had the answer to childbed fever. The vitamin story has bred similar frustrations in those of us who have been aware of it for many years and yet see so little done with this life-saving information. Strange to say, those who are least inclined, as a group, to make use of the value of nutrients, medical doctors, were enthusiastically informed of the potential by their own journal 20 years ago. They were also told that the real danger does not lie so much in obvious deficiencies, but in deficiencies which manifest themselves in vague symptoms which seem to be indefinable in any other context but a shortage of nutrients.

Dr. Julian M. Ruffin, M.D., defined these symptoms in the *Journal of the American Medical Association* (November 1, 1941): "Among the early symptoms of vitamin deficiencies are anorexia (loss of appetite) with ensuing loss of weight, weakness, lassitude (laziness) and easy fatigability, insomnia, increased nervousness and irritability, headache, palpitation, precordial (diaphragm) distress, vague gastrointestinal disturbances such as flatulence, indigestion, constipation or mild diarrhea, nausea and indefinite abdominal pain. The patient usually just does not feel well without being able to state exactly what is wrong. One realized at once that the symptoms of the so-called gastric neuroses, psychoneuroses and neurasthenias are essentially those mentioned. . . ."

The Usual Treatment

Who of us has not had a friend who suffered from just such symptoms? Many of us have experienced them ourselves. When one sees a doctor about such problems, the treatment is seldom a nutritional one: if the complaint is tiredness and laziness, the prescription is likely to be a pep pill; if nervousness and irritability are the problem, tranquilizers will probably be the doctor's answer. Anything in between is usually handled with some form of aspirin.

It's a rare doctor who will ask you what types of foods you eat (not just if you *do* eat), except in cases of ulcer, heart disease, gout, etc. The pills will probably make you move faster or slower (whichever you asked for) so long as you keep taking them, but actually, the problem will be worsening though it is disguised. The pep pills will make you work faster and harder on the same energy which was barely enough to let you move around before; the tranquilizers will make you oblivious to the warnings of your nerves that tell you they need help. When you stop taking the pills, the tiredness or the nervousness will set in with new intensity, your body will be in worse shape after such treatment than it was before, due to months of fighting the added burdens of increased activity when it was physically tired, or to sustaining ticking nerves which had no expression of relief because of a drugged personality.

The deficiencies in nutrients, which are not at once evident the way scurvy is for a lack of vitamin C or pellagra for thiamin, are the ones our doctors seem to ignore. Before drastic treatment with drugs which can have serious side effects, doctors should prescribe a period of vitamin intake along with improvement of the diet. It won't take long for improvement to show itself if a vitamin shortage has been the cause of the illness. If this proves ineffective, then more rigorous therapy might be indicated, but why not try to right the basic wrong rather than to disguise it? To ignore this approach is to chance the health of many. Dr. Ruffin wrote: "It is highly probable that, for every patient having an advanced vitamin deficiency, there are many patients having a subclinical or mild deficiency case. . . ."

Changing Habits of Diet

What throws many doctors off in tracing deficiencies is the notion that a diet which is filling is nutritionally sufficient. This simply is not so. Dr. Ruffin cites the diet of the tenant farmer in the South during fall, winter and spring. It consists generally of white bread, corn bread, hominy grits, potatoes (usually fried), fatback and other pork products, cowpeas and molasses. This diet is definitely deficient, but the farmer thinks it's fine and would probably not change it, even if he could. The case is not unlike the man whose day begins with black coffee and a bun. You can tell him it is a breakfast utterly barren of nutrition, but he will probably continue to eat it—and will probably tell any doctor who asks him that his diet is a good one.

In 1941, Dr. Ruffin was already aware of the mistake of using synthetic vitamins. He put it this way: "The fact that single deficiencies are rarely, if ever, encountered, is an excellent argument against the treatment of deficiency states with chemically pure substances. There are probably other vitamins as yet unknown which are essential to health." He went on to illustrate with a case history of a man, 26, admitted to Duke Hospital complaining of loss of weight, diarrhea, weakness, sore tongue and tingling and numbness of the extremities of 6 months duration. Examination showed deficiencies of at least 3 vitamins: pyridoxine, riboflavin and ascorbic acid. He was given pyridoxine (50 milligrams) intravenously for 10 days, with no improvement. Then, large intravenous doses of riboflavin, niacin and ascorbic acid failed to produce any effect. Finally, a 3 cubic centimeter daily dosage of liver extract (a natural source of all the B vitamins, as are brewer's yeast, wheat germ and desiccated liver) was followed by rapid improvement, then complete recovery. The natural source provided the necessary combination, or the unknown nutrients that were needed. Synthetically, it simply couldn't be done. It still can't be done. Most researchers will readily admit that a complete catalogue of the nutrients contained in foods is far from being done and to approximate their natural relationship as it occurs in food, is impossible.

Times Have Changed

This was the thinking in the official organ of the American Medical Association in 1941. Since then, there has been no proof that the facts are different; yet, the attitude of official medicine certainly has changed. We see statements that there is no such thing as a subclinical vitamin deficiency, that Americans eat a good diet which makes deficiencies in them highly unlikely, if not impossible. We are told that anyone who stresses the need for natural vitamins is a quack. Where does this put Dr. Ruffin and the magazine that printed his views so respectfully in 1941. Is he a quack? Is the magazine a quack sheet? It is strange how attitudes change—bees are good when they are making honey and bad when they sting. Vitamins as they occur naturally are helpful and respectable therapeutic agents, when the American Medical Association says they are, but needless expense, useless, wasteful, faddish, when we recommend them. Good diet is sadly lacking in our population and is vital to good health when the American Medical Association says so, but when we use the same argument, we are exaggerating the importance of diet, we are viciously attacking the miraculous food industry of our country, we are alarmists, faddists and crackpots. The inconsistency of organized medicine's position on the question of diet and nutritional supplements is becoming more and more obvious. The medical journals print records of authoritative experiments and observations which show the general lack of nutrition in Americans, and which describe deficiency symptoms we see every day. Yet, the newspapers carry feature articles which insist that we are all perfectly well, eat the best diet one could hope for and need no nutrients. Doctors take the same attitude in their offices. If the journals aren't printing the truth, why are they published? If they are accurate, then why are their findings ignored? Can it be because there is more profit in drugs than in prescribing good nutrition and natural food supplements? We would appreciate seeing a feature column which explains the shift in attitude from a recognition of subclinical nutritional deficiency symptoms to a denial by some of our best known syndicated medical and nutritional columnists that such symptoms or conditions exist at all.

The Vanishing Vitamins

By Robert Rodale

The amount of vitamins available to Americans in their food has declined steadily for the past 15 years.

Here are the figures which show the decrease in nutrients:

VITAMIN A	—26.3%	NIACIN	— 6.5%
THIAMIN	—13.5%	FOLIC ACID	—14.2%
RIBOFLAVIN	— 8.5%	ASCORBIC ACID	—19.2%

Source of this information is the comprehensive Department of Agriculture record of the total amount of food consumed year by year by Americans and published in the annual report entitled *Consumption of Food in the United States.* Running to over 50 pages of tightly crammed tables, the *Consumption of Food* report tells how much of each different item of food the average American eats. To make the figures as accurate as possible, the Department of Agriculture even checks the quantities of food produced in home gardens and includes those amounts in the report. Thousands upon thousands of Department of Agriculture workers stationed at every phase of the food production and importing chain, tabulate the flow of foods into stores, restaurants and homes. In addition, food pro-ducers and processors report their volume of business to the govern-ment in an annual census. All of this statistical activity provides a detailed picture of our eating habits that is of great value in esti-mating our national nutritional health.

One of the first things that is noticeable in these figures is that we are buying fewer pounds of food than ever before. While in the years 1947 to 1949 each person used a retail weight equivalent of 1549 pounds of food, in 1960, he used only 1465 pounds. That is a decline of 5.4 per cent. However, according to the government figures, the number of calories we consume each year has declined much less—from 3250 to 3190 per day. That is a decline of only

1.8 per cent. Why should it be that we are coming home from the store with fewer pounds of food, yet end up eating almost the same total amount of calories? The answer, I believe, is the dramatic trend to "convenience" foods that has mushroomed in the postwar period. Back in 1947 to 1949, as I will show later, we bought greater quantities of foods that required peeling, washing, trimming and home cooking. Now, we leave the store with packages of instant mashed potatoes, dehydrated soups and frozen TV dinners. These items of food weigh less per calorie supplied. The most important effect of these convenience foods is on our food preparation habits. Women no longer want to take the time necessary to prepare fresh foods in the home. The number of hours that the average woman spends in preparing meals has dropped greatly in the past 15 years. What effect has this trend had on our intake of vitamins? A close look at the *Consumption of Food* report will provide the answer:

First, let's look at vitamin A. The amount of this vitamin "available for consumption" by Americans has dropped more than any other—from 8,200 International Units in 1947-49 to 7,000 in 1960. What foods are rich in vitamin A? Butter, enriched margarine, some vegetables and fruits, liver and some fish. Butter and margarine consumption has stayed about the same. We used 16.9 pounds of the two products combined in 1956 and the same amount in 1960. Meat, fish and poultry consumption has gone up slightly from an average of 156 pounds a year for the 1947-49 period to 179 pounds in 1960, so we won't find the answer there. The answer is found, I believe, in the large decline in leafy green and yellow vegetables. Our consumption in this category for the years 1947-49 was 98 pounds, and by 1960, it had dropped all the way to 80 pounds. When you realize that the average portion of spinach, for example, contains 10,680 units of vitamin A, you can see how a decline of almost 20 per cent in our consumption of green and yellow vegetables can have a drastic effect on the amount of vitamin A we get.

Drop in Consumption of Vitamin-Rich Foods

The *Consumption of Food* report gives individual figures for specific vegetables and all kinds of foods, in fact, so we are able to look deeper into this enigma of the vanishing vitamins. Let's review what has happened to our preference for a few vegetables. Cabbage consumption has gone from 10.4 pounds in 1956 to 9.4 pounds per person in 1960. In the same period, carrots went from 6.8 pounds down to 5.3 pounds. While we used 16.5 pounds of lettuce and escarole in 1956, the amount dropped to 15 pounds in 1960. The fact that even the salad craze has not been able to stem the decline in the use of lettuce, carrots and cabbage is significant indeed.

Now let's look at some other vegetables. Celery is down from 7.3 pounds per capita in 1956 to only 6.7 pounds in 1960. Sweet potatoes—extremely rich in vitamin A—have taken an alarming drop in favor from 7.6 pounds in 1956 to 6.2 pounds in 1960. Dry edible beans and peas have gone from 8.7 pounds in 1956 to 7.8 pounds in 1960. And bear in mind that I am not comparing one good year with one bad year. In almost every case, there has been a steady and distinct decline in consumption of these foods.

Several other highly important food groups have shown moderate to serious drops in favor. We are eating 37 fewer eggs a year. While in 1955, we ate 371 eggs on the average, in 1960, we ate only 334. Consumption of fish is down from 11.4 pounds in 1953 to 10.5 pounds in 1960. All fruits are down slightly, from 145.2 pounds in 1956 to 143.5 pounds in 1960.

The drop in our average vitamin C ration from 117 milligrams a day in 1947-49 to 105 in 1960 is also the result of the decline in favor of vegetables. White potatoes are a fairly good source of vitamin C, but since our use of that food has gone up slightly (from 99 pounds in 1956 to 102 pounds in 1960) the blame for the drop can be attributed only to the green leafy vegetables and, to a lesser extent, to fruits.

Flour and Cereals Decline

One other important category of food that has shown a large decline in popularity is flour and cereal products. In the 1947-49 period, we ate 170 pounds of flour and cereal products, while by 1960, usage had declined to 146 pounds. The smaller amounts of thiamin, riboflavin and niacin that are available to us in our food can be traced in part to this decline in the popularity of grains.

So far, I have reported primarily the foods that have gone *down* in consumption. You are probably wondering what we are eating *more* of to make up for the things we have cut down on. There are two food categories that show significant increases—meats and poultry and fats and oils. While the figures for these foods have not changed much since 1956, if we go back to the 1947-49 period, we find that meat, fish and poultry have gone from 156 pounds a year per person to 179. And fats and oils have gone from 65 to 67 pounds a year per person. These increases are reflected to a degree in our protein consumption, which is up slightly from 94 grams a day in 1947-49 to 95 grams in 1960. And our fat consumption has gone from 142 to 146 grams a day in the same period.

Why Our Eating Habits Change

While it is no doubt true that most of us eat the things we like, there are several factors other than taste and our appetites that govern what is served at our tables. Cost is important. When a food comes on the market in large quantity and at low cost, we take advantage of the bargain. Convenience of preparation is also important, as I mentioned earlier. Even convenience of purchase is a factor. Neat, plastic-wrapped packages stimulate super market sales of all kinds of items—luncheon meat, cheese, onions, fish. The old days of corner store merchandising are gone, and with them, went some of our old food-buying habits.

In my opinion, though, modern advertising and merchandising methods can bear most of the responsibility for the changes in our food-buying pattern—and, yes, even the decline in the amount of vitamins available for consumption. The housewife today is bombarded with food advertising morning, noon and night from radio, TV, magazines and newspapers. Over 61 million dollars were spent in 1960 for food advertising, and a look at how that figure is broken down by food categories is extremely revealing. Here is the report, compiled by Media Records, Incorporated:

BAKING PRODUCTS	$18,603,000	CONDIMENTS	$10,103,000
CEREALS AND BREAK-		DAIRY PRODUCTS	18,207,000
FAST FOODS	5,027,000	MEATS AND FISH	9,512,000

Note that the amount of money spent for advertising fruits and vegetables is so small that it is not even reported. In view of the tremendous pressure being put on the housewife to buy other foods, is it any wonder that she spends less money on the unglamorous green and yellow leafy vegetables, even though they are loaded with vitamins?

Price cutting by stores also encourages housewives to buy certain foods. Meat items, particularly poultry, are continually being sold at cost or even below cost to lure customers. The idea is that a woman who comes to a store to buy chicken at a bargain will buy other foods, too. Fruits and vegetables are hardly ever featured in such merchandising schemes, because they don't have the appetite appeal of inch-thick sirloin steaks or pan-ready fryers.

Feed Additives and Meat-Buying Habits

Chemical feed additives also have had their effect on our meat-buying habits. In the past 15 years, it has become common practice to add antibiotics, arsenic and hormones to animal and poultry feed rations, making it possible for the farmer to produce more meat with smaller amounts of grain. Where it used to take 12 weeks to raise a chick to broiler stage, now it is common practice to butcher at 9 weeks. Chemicals have cut poultry raising costs so much that the average retail price of chicken has dropped from 59.5 cents in 1950 to 42.5 cents in 1961. So you can see that animal feed additives are having an important influence on what foods Americans select in the super markets. An interesting sidelight on the use of antibiotics to stimulate poultry growth is the fact that the amounts of antibiotics used in the feed formulae have to be increased every year, as the birds are developing resistance to their power.

Returning to the subject of the vanishing vitamins in our food, we have not even considered any changes that are occurring in the basic composition of food. We are eating more fruit out of cold storage, more processed foods of all kinds and more food grown on depleted soils. Those facts are not considered in the government statistics on our lower intake of vitamins. And, most alarming, the bottom has not been reached. Our consumption of vitamin A dropped 200 units from 1959 to 1960 and there is no assurance that it won't drop more in future years. These facts should be convincing evidence of the false logic behind the official pronouncements that "America is the best fed nation on earth."

What About Applying Vitamins to the Skin?

For a long time, we have been interested in the subject of the topical application of vitamins—that is, rubbing them in and absorbing them through the skin. Our search through scientific literature yielded almost nothing except some accounts of using vitamin E ointment for various blood vessel ailments.

In their book, *Alpha Tocopherol in Cardiovascular Disease,* W. E. Shute and E. V. Shute tell of using the ointment on patients suffering from indolent ulcers. In one case, the ulcer was caused by radiation for cancer. Vitamin E ointment applied locally was the only treatment given and healing was complete within 60 days.

Reaction Not Identical in All Cases

On the other hand, the Shutes indicate that not everyone has the same reaction to the ointment. A woman patient who had phlebitis developed ulcers on her legs and was unable to tolerate the vitamin E ointment, even though she was taking 400 units of vitamin E orally at the time. But, for patients who have no difficulty with the ointment, the Shutes recommend vitamin E both orally and locally for ulcers. They begin by using the ointment on only a very small area of the ulcer until they see how the patient responds. If there is no adverse reaction, the ointment can be used over the whole ulcer.

We discovered an article in the *Journal of Nutrition* for June, 1956, which started us off on another search for material on locally applied vitamins. This article by 4 researchers at the Squibb Institute for Medical Research tells of research with laboratory animals which indicates, without a shadow of a doubt, that certain vitamins can indeed be successfully absorbed through the skin.

How Experiments Were Done

Just how do you suppose such a discovery is made? If it were your assignment, how would you go about discovering whether or not the vitamins in question had been absorbed? The methods used were so interesting that we want to describe them in some detail.

Rats were used, since they will easily develop vitamin deficiencies if they are deprived of the various vitamins. The rats were given this basal diet: casein (the protein from milk), sucrose (for carbohydrate), a mineral mixture (containing all the important minerals and trace minerals, we suppose, since no minerals were involved in the test), cod liver oil (to guarantee against any deficiency of vitamins A and D) and vegetable oil (to supply fat). Synthetic B vitamins and vitamin E were added. Then, in a test for one vitamin, that particular vitamin was omitted from the diet.

The vitamin being tested was applied to a shaved area on the animal's neck, after which careful precautions were taken so that the rat did not lick off any of the vitamin preparation. Measurements were then made of the amount of that particular vitamin excreted. In this way, the experimenters knew that the vitamin had been absorbed, for otherwise, there would be no excess to eliminate.

Test Periods Lasted Two Hours

These were the vitamins tested: thiamin, riboflavin, pantothenic acid and pyridoxine—all vitamins of the B complex—and vitamin D. The test period was for only two hours—that is, the vitamins had to be absorbed in that length of time, for they were carefully removed after that.

It seemed that there was a possibility that vitamins might be absorbed through skin that had been irritated by shaving. To show that irritation was not present, a violent poison which cannot be absorbed through the skin, but can be absorbed through an open cut was rubbed into the spot. It was not absorbed. So the researchers knew from this that their test was a real test of normal, unbroken skin absorption of vitamins.

The absorption of the first B vitamin, thiamin, was considered "highly efficient." The rats used in this test had been without the vitamin for so long that they were beginning to show signs of deficiency—a neuritis which results from lack of thiamin. The rats recovered from the neuritis and began to gain at a normal rate soon *after the vitamin was absorbed through the skin.*

With riboflavin, another B vitamin, absorption through the skin was not as effective as absorption of the vitamin given orally. But it was absorbed—no doubt of it.

Hair Color Restored

In the case of pantothenic acid, another B vitamin, a very interesting thing happened. The rats deprived of pantothenic acid stopped growing *and their dark hair turned gray within two to five weeks.* Adding pantothenic acid to the diet prevented this or cured it after it had taken place. Applying the vitamin locally brought about the same result—the rats began to grow again at the normal rate and their gray hair once again turned black. This demonstrated that enough of the vitamin was absorbed through the skin to bring about this change.

Rats' Feet Affected

Depriving a group of rats of pyridoxine (another B vitamin) produced a typically scaly breaking-out on the rats' feet. Applying the vitamin locally resulted in a disappearance of the symptoms within two weeks. Our researchers refer to earlier experiments in another laboratory in which human patients with seborrhea of the "sicca" type failed to respond to quite large doses of pyridoxine daily over a 4-week period. The vitamin was injected or given by mouth. The patients then stopped taking the vitamin by mouth or by injection and instead, applied it in the form of an ointment. With this type of therapy, the skin disorder disappeared within 5 to 21 days. These results indicated, it is believed, that in certain diseases, there may be some kind of defect in the cells of the skin so that the vitamin fails to reach the affected site if it is given by mouth or injection.

The results obtained with vitamin D were just as satisfactory. The conclusion arrived at by the researchers from the Squibb Institute is that, "in view of the small doses of the vitamins administered and the limited time allowed for absorption, the utilization of the vitamins studied is considered highly efficient."

It seems to us that the local application of vitamins might turn out to be extremely valuable for all of us who are suffering from some condition which makes it impossible for us to absorb vitamins taken in the regular way. The patients suffering from seborrhea are a good example. Apparently, something in the make-up of the cells of their skins prevented them from using the pyridoxine they got in their food. But when it was applied directly to the skin cells, it was absorbed.

Vitamins Are Necessary as One Grows Older

An M.D. who believes that some of the symptoms of aging can be reversed with large doses of vitamins wrote an article about his theory in the *Journal of the American Geriatrics Association* for November, 1955.

"Perhaps the saddest fact that every human being must face is that, if he lives long enough, he will eventually undergo progressively increasing deteriorative changes in the structure and function of the body, until these become so severe, that he can no longer survive," says Dr. William Kaufman. "The so-called 'normal' aging process makes his joints less flexible, decreases his muscular working capacity and strength, impairs his coördination and sense of balance, brings about mental changes and increases capillary fragility—in addition to causing many other obvious or subtle changes in the bodily structure and function."

How right he is! And how cheering the news that, in an actual controlled test, he showed that certain of these disagreeable traits of old age can be reversed. Dr. Kaufman concentrated first on mobility of joints for his test. He has developed a method for measuring how supple one's joints are—wrists, fingers, shoulders, thigh and knee can be manipulated in such a way that one's physician can get an estimate of just how much movement is hindered and how much freedom of movement is left. So, Dr. Kaufman used this method with his patients—663 of them—to test the effectiveness of vitamins in decreasing stiffness and increasing flexibility.

He concentrated on one of the B vitamins, niacin (in the form of niacinamide), and gave enormous doses of this vitamin to his patient every couple of hours for several doses, then measured the joint function again. He found, without any exception, that the joint mobility in every patient taking large amounts of this one B vitamin alone, or in combination with other vitamins, improved to a clinically significant degree. He tells us that, in individual cases, taking this one B vitamin raises the measurement of mobility from 6 to 12 units during the first month and from one-half to one unit each month that therapy is continued thereafter. He points out that not all joints improve equally well. Some almost immovable joints improve not at all, but others recover full or partial range of movement. In all cases, however, the improvement generally is quite considerably above that to be found in untreated patients.

In addition to the huge doses of niacinamide, he also gave large doses of vitamin C and several other B vitamins and fairly high doses of vitamins A and D. He also used injections of vitamin B_{12} in some instances. He did not notice, he said, that any or all of these added to the improvement, although he is quite sure that they did not hinder it in any way.

Along with increased movability of joints, Dr. Kaufman found that patients' muscles functioned better after they had been taking vitamins for some months. He discovered this by measuring the strength of their handgrips, using a machine for this purpose, and another test in which the patient makes strokes on a tally. In every case, the proficiency of the patients improved. Dr. Kaufman did not create any supermen or women, he tells us. But the patients, by taking vitamins, improved to such an extent, that they could go about their daily work without undue fatigue, whereas before, they had not been able to.

They also found, almost without exception, that their sense of balance improved. "Many patients with subjective and objective evidence of impaired balance sense, recover their ability to balance themselves normally during the first 3 months of niacinamide therapy and this benefit continues for as long as they take this vitamin." Those who did not notice any benefit from taking just the one B vitamin sometimes found that there was improvement when they took, as well, other B vitamins, including vitamin B_{12}.

Checking on the mental state of his aging patients, Dr. Kaufman found that a considerable number of them noticed an improved state of mind. Depression and nervousness, over-reacting to noise and other stimuli—these were symptoms that seemed to be improved while they were taking the B vitamin. Some patients did not have this experience and Dr. Kaufman says there is no way of knowing who will and who will not. In many cases, adding the other B vitamins helped in alleviating mental symptoms.

Vitamin C in Massive Doses

Dr. Kaufman used vitamin C to improve the condition of blood vessels (especially the small vessels, or capillaries) of his patients. He tells us that, "After the age of 50, with increasing age, there was a significant trend toward increased capillary fragility, *even in those patients who had from 50 to 75 milligrams of ascorbic acid (vitamin C) in their average daily diet.* Decreased blood levels of vitamin C have been reported in older people."

He gave them large doses of vitamin C (1500 to 2000 milligrams a day, divided into doses of 250 milligrams each) and found that, after 3 to 6 months of treatment, the capillaries become much less fragile. What would this mean to the patients? Capillary fragility seems to be one certain forerunner of "strokes," because the fragile blood vessel wall can easily collapse, causing hemorrhage. When such a hemorrhage occurs in the brain, the heart or an important artery, the result can be permanent crippling or death.

Why do you suppose, with evidence like this available, all doctors do not advise their older patients to take large doses of vitamin C daily? Think of the suffering and heartache that could be avoided!

In addition to helping the tone of the blood vessel walls, the large doses of vitamin C improved the condition of the patients' teeth and gums. Those who still had their own teeth reported that loose ones were tightening. Dentists reported that there was an improvement in gum structure. One dentist, who carefully followed 8 of these older patients who took both the B vitamins and vitamin C for more than 6 years, noticed that he did not find the anticipated resorption of alveolar tissue so often seen as part of aging. This refers to the shrinking of gums and the bone structure beneath them which results in loose teeth, bleeding and eventual gradual drying up of the gum tissue.

Vitamin B₁₂ for Mental Symptoms

Dr. Kaufman's work with vitamin B_{12} is exciting. He describes the following symptoms for which this vitamin provided constant relief: fatigue, increased nervous irritability, mild impairment in memory and ability to concentrate, mental depression, insomnia and lack of balance. Sometimes, the following symptoms were also relieved: dyspepsia, sensations of numbness, difficulty in bladder control, breathlessness associated with impaired heart muscle sounds. None of these patients had anemia or the brilliantly red tongue which is associated with pernicious anemia.

None of the vitamins helped at all, *except vitamin B₁₂*. Dr. Kaufman gave it in injections—100 micrograms once a week. Less than this did not seem to bring improvement. Omitting the vitamin B_{12} injections caused all the symptoms to recur slowly.

Dr. Kaufman's conclusions are as follows: "Vitamins used in doses which are far in excess of quantities available from food as it is ordinarily prepared and eaten, may be considered to act as pharmacologic agents (that is, drugs). The prolonged continuous oral administration of niacinamide (alone or in combination with other vitamins) can effect remarkable changes in bodily function and structure of an aging population which subsists on a diet adequate in calories and protein."

It seems to us that Dr. Kaufman's experience with his 663 patients is living proof that aging is a stress situation necessitating far more of all the food elements than are needed for a non-stressful situation. The older person should be taking much larger doses of vitamins and minerals than the younger person. In addition to his much greater need, the older person tends to eat less healthfully, thus depriving himself of even more desperately needed food elements. It's so much easier to live on toast and tea or cereal or pleasant-tasting cakes; the tendency is always to avoid healthful foods rich in protein and fresh fruits and vegetables rich in vitamins and minerals. But Dr. Kaufman tells us that even when one is getting enough protein and calories, he can still benefit, as he becomes older, by taking extremely large doses of vitamins. We would, of course, add mineral supplements as a most important part of the treatment, since minerals and vitamins work together for the body's welfare.

Inadvisable to Take Isolated B Vitamins

As you know, we do not believe you should take isolated B vitamins such as Dr. Kaufman prescribed. He found, if you recall, that many patients did better when they got large amounts of all the B vitamins. The best sources of these are brewer's yeast, liver (fresh or desiccated), wheat germ, fresh fruits and vegetables, meats and seed foods of all kinds. For very high potencies of B vitamins, you can get special preparations made from yeast and liver. And, of course, natural vitamin C preparations (from rose hips, green peppers and so forth) are the best source of this vitamin. Bone meal provides calcium, phosphorus and other badly needed minerals. Fish liver oil is important for vitamins A and D.

Vitamins Win Wars against Infections

With each cold season comes the argument about whether or not vitamins can be used effectively to combat infection. In spite of the mountains of convincing experiments which scientists have offered, many still refuse to credit nutrients with greater powers against infection than the sugar-water patent medicines laced with aspirin compounds, which have absolutely no healing effect whatsoever.

We are offering a small selection from hundreds of recorded experiments in which the actions of vitamins against various infections are shown. Perhaps, one or the other of these will prompt you or one of your friends to try vitamins and diet as a treatment next time you get a cold or other infection. If these results were achieved by others, they can be achieved by you.

B Vitamins and Protein for Vital Antibodies

Antibodies which are built up in the blood stream to fight against infection are less readily formed or more rapidly lost in the badly nourished individual. The depletion of these antibodies has been repeatedly demonstrated in persons whose diets are deficient in either amino acids, pantothenic acid, pyridoxine or phenylglutamic acid. (Rene J. Dubos, M.D., and Russell Schaedler, M.D., *Journal of Pediatrics,* July, 1959.)

Protection for Antibodies

In tests using albino rats as subjects, it was shown that the production of antibodies to combat injected diphtheria toxins was markedly impaired in cases of deficiency of pantothenic acid, pyridoxine (both B vitamins) and phenylglutamic acid (an amino acid). Moderate impairment in the production of these antibodies was also noted where deficiencies of thiamin, biotin, riboflavin, niacin (all B vitamins), tryptophan (an amino acid) and vitamin A existed. (A. E. Axelrod and J. Pruzansky, *Annals of the New York Academy of Science,* 63, 202, 1953.)

Typhus Severe When Deficiency Signs Developed

In 1931, Zinsser and associates found that a diet lacking all of the known vitamins, carried to the point at which deficiency signs developed, increased the severity of typhus infection in guinea pigs and rats, as well as manifestations of rickets.

In 1939, Pinkerton and Bessey reported that a riboflavin deficiency in rats so lowered their resistance to the typhus infection that the rats died within 3 or 4 days, when they appeared to be lightly stricken enough to live for 3 or 4 weeks. The administration of riboflavin to these rats, even when they were at the point of death, caused a complete recovery in 24 hours.

In a complete series of tests, Fitzpatrick found that rats showed an increased susceptibility to typhus when their diets showed the following deficiencies: low protein, one-tenth of the optimum requirement of all B vitamins missing (pantothenic acid, riboflavin and thiamin proved to be the most vital). It was also discovered that rats kept on a natural laboratory diet, including fresh vegetables, were less susceptible to infection than those on a synthetic diet, which, incidentally, caused a weight increase. (P. F. Clark and others, *Bacteriological Review,* 13, p. 99, 1959.)

Pyridoxine Anti-Infection Aid

The need for the B vitamin pyridoxine in acquiring protection from disease, is emphasized in experiments done by Stoerk and Eisen of Columbia University. Three groups of rats were used, one of which was fed a diet deficient only in pyridoxine. Of the other two groups—one was fed on restricted amounts of a complete diet, the other received a complete diet and ate at will. Only the rats on a complete and adequate diet did not lose weight. But it is more interesting to note that of the group of 9 that was fed a pyridoxine-deficient diet, 6 showed absolutely no infection-fighting antibodies presence in the blood stream, and the other 3 had very low numbers of antibodies. In the other two groups (16 animals in all), all had measurable numbers of antibodies, and 13 were comparatively high. It was concluded that the B vitamin pyridoxine is obviously vital in encouraging anti-infection organisms in the blood stream. (H. C. Stoerk and H. N. Eisen, *Proceedings of the Society of Experimental Biology and Medicine,* Vol. 62, p. 88, 1946.)

Better Health with Vitamin A

Fifty school children were divided into two groups. They were given vitamin A in the form of halibut liver oil or foods high in vitamin A and compared with a group of 25 control children whose histories, compared with the experimental group, showed a high resistance to colds.

The 50 children on vitamin A showed an increase in general health, a gain in weight and a decrease in the incidence and severity of colds. (W. L. Aycock and G. E. Lutman, *American Journal of Medical Science,* Vol. 208, p. 389, 1944.)

Vitamin-Poor Diets Fatal

During an epidemic of grippe in central Europe, it was found (Niemann and Foth) that 3 out of 12 infants on a carbohydrate-rich, vitamin-poor ration succumbed.

An epidemic of a type of pneumonia broke out at an industrial school near Edinburgh, Scotland. It was discovered that the food was poorly cooked and low in vitamins A and D. When cod liver oil and raw fruit juice were given, along with a properly cooked diet, the epidemic cleared up rapidly.

Holmes and co-workers gave 185 industrial workers a tablespoonful of cod liver oil (rich in vitamins A and D) daily, and compared their number of colds and time off with 128 persons who received no treatment. Fifty-two per cent of the cod liver oil group had no colds during the 4 winter months of the experiment, and only 33 per cent of the controls showed this freedom. Fifty-two per cent of the cod liver oil group and 41 per cent of the controls lost no time from their work during the 4 months.

Forty-two tuberculosis patients were paired, with similarities in age and sex as well as degree of illness and prognosis. The sanitorium was in an isolated region where the supply of vegetables and fruit was limited. Twenty-one of the patients were given a supplementary orange once each day for extra vitamin C, and their 21 partners were given supplementary carbohydrates in the form of a pastry. Of the cases fed the extra vitamin C, 17 became better, 3 remained the same and one became worse. The clinicians in charge of examining were of the opinion that the vitamin C helped in curing the tuberculosis infections. (E. R. Robertson, *Medicine,* Vol. 13, p. 123, 1934.)

Ascorbic Acid Fights Colds

Activity of antibodies against common cold germs has been known to be increased by ascorbic acid (vitamin C) in the tissues. In one experiment intended to prove this activity, Cowan, Diehl and Baker (*Journal of the American Medical Association,* 120: 1268, 1942) gave college students 200 milligrams of ascorbic acid daily and found that they averaged 1.9 colds per year, while controls averaged 2.2 colds. Chances of this difference occurring by coincidence were reported to be 3 or 4 in 100.

In the *Medical Journal of Australia* (2: 777, 1947), the dosage recommended at the onset of a cold is 750 milligrams or more with 500 milligrams or more 3 or 4 hours later. (Herbert D. Brody, *Journal of the American Dietetic Association,* June, 1953.)

Vitamin A

The Uncommon Services Vitamin A Performs

Vitamin E is the specific nutrient most often mentioned in connection with the heart and the rest of the circulatory system. We do not mean to imply by this attention to vitamin E that other nutrients are not important to circulation. *All* nutrients are vital to good health and each contributes directly or indirectly to the health of every organ of the body. We were pleased, therefore, to see an article in the *Medical Journal of Australia* (August 19, 1961) in which other nutrients, vitamins A and D, were discussed in connection with their value to the circulatory system.

F. C. H. Ross and A. H. Campbell became aware of the incomplete and inconclusive information on the effects of vitamins A and D on the heart. For 10 years previous, Dr. Ross had used vitamins A and D in the treatment of certain patients. On studying the records of these patients, it became apparent that the group of patients treated with these nutrients had shown reduced incidence of heart disease. In trying to understand the reason for this effect, various explanations were suggested. One of the most obvious was the possibility that the vitamins influenced the body's use of cholesterol.

In order to check this, the effect of vitamin A and vitamin D capsules upon the incidence of coronary heart disease was observed over 5½ years in 136 patients, with 271 patients serving as controls. (That is, they received ordinary medication with no vitamins A and D added.) Each capsule used contained 6,000 units of vitamin A and 1,000 units of vitamin D suspended in 0.1 milliliter of peanut oil. They were given 3 times a day for a period of at least 6 months from 2 to 5 years in most cases. Tests were set up to determine whether, in fact, the patients could objectively be considered as victims of heart disease.

Of the 407 patients observed, those in the treated group of 136 who developed coronary heart disease were only 8 (5.8 per cent), while the number in the untreated group of 271 who became afflicted was 43 (15.8 per cent).

Cholesterol Level Reduced

It was seen that the vitamin preparation had a definite effect on the serum cholesterol level when the level was above 250 milligrams per 100 milliliters. In 13 subjects, the serum cholesterol level was reduced an average of 30 milligrams per 100 milliliters after 2 to 4 weeks, a figure considered statistically significant. In contrast, the untreated controls showed no significant alteration in their average cholesterol levels after a similar length of time.

As the data came in and the authors consulted other researchers, they became convinced that the vitamin A was really the active ingredient in the capsules, with the vitamin D contribution uncertain. The authors then voiced some misgivings as to the amount of vitamin A being consumed by the average person. They noted that it is likely to be 15 per cent below the amount actually available in common foods and that this is dangerously close to the recommended allowance of vitamin A. ". . . the minimal requirements of vitamin A are not known with certainty and the recommended figure may be too low to prevent a disordered cholesterol metabolism in older persons on a diet of high fat . . . it can be presumed that many individuals consume less than the estimated requirements."

Good Income No Guarantee of Good Nutrition

The writers further concerned themselves with the fact that high economic status does not guarantee an optimum intake of the proper nutrients. Furthermore, the authors write, "In Australia and America, owing to changing food habits, there has been a definite fall in vitamin A consumption per head in the last 20 or 30 years. . . . It is of interest also that, in underdeveloped countries such as New Guinea, with a low incidence of coronary heart disease, the vitamin A intake is high. . . . Of course, the fat-poor diet may be equally important in such groups. But the Eskimos, who are reputed to have a fat-rich diet with a low incidence of coronary heart disease, have a high vitamin A intake from fish and marine animal livers."

There are other areas of health in which vitamin A figures importantly and which are no more publicized than the coronary heart disease relationship. For example, *Science News Letter,* September 27, 1953, printed a brief summation of the discovery of Dr. Albert Sobel and Dr. Abraham Rosenberg, as reported to the American Chemical Society, that vitamin A could be used to protect the arteries of diabetics. These researchers discovered that rats with diabetes cannot convert carotene into vitamin A as efficiently as normal, non-diabetic rats can. "If diabetics cannot convert the yellow pigment into the vitamin," said the article, "this may have something to do with the hardening of arteries, which comes on prematurely in diabetics. . . . The discovery that the conversion of carotene to vitamin A is impaired in experimental diabetes, can be regarded as the first step toward the discovery of an agent to control the premature aging of the arteries (arteriosclerosis) found in individuals suffering from diabetes mellitus."

We wonder if doctors who habitually treat diabetics with insulin, and only that, are aware of the work of these two men. We have seen no more about vitamin A and diabetes, nor do we see the vitamin recommended as a regular adjunct to other therapeutic measures for diabetics. It could certainly do no harm for any diabetic to make certain that his diet is rich in foods that have a high vitamin A content.

Oral Cancer

Nutrition Reviews (August, 1959) tells of vitamin A in relation to oral cancer, the cancer that constitutes 8 or 10 per cent of all cancer observed in the United States. N. H. Rowe and R. J. Corlin constructed a study to explore the possible relationship between a shortage of vitamin A and precancerous sores. Five groups of hamsters were set up; all were given cancer-causing agents, some were given uniform vitamin A supplementation. The incidence of clinically observable tumors was so much greater in the unsupplemented group that, "These data suggest that vitamin A deficiency increased the susceptibility of hamsters to carcinogen-induced benign and malignant tumors."

The removal of the stomach due to cancer or some very serious ulcer condition is likely to result in a strong vitamin A deficiency. The *Lancet* (February 20, 1960) carried a report on 4 men and a woman who had undergone such surgery. All showed vitamin A deficiency afterwards. The authors decided that, "vitamin A should be administered prophylactically (as a preventive measure) to patients who have undergone gastrectomy. A course of 100,000 International Units of vitamin A given daily for 2 weeks every 6 months, seems advisable." Patients who have undergone such serious surgery can ill afford to miss the valuable aid vitamin A can give in bringing the body back to good health.

There are, of course, many references in the literature to vitamin A as a treatment for acne and other skin diseases, as well as its happy effect on poor vision and its value as an infection fighter. We intended here to cover the lesser known aspects of this vitamin's value in preserving health. In this connection, it might be of interest to mention the fact that drinking alcohol causes a rise in the vitamin A content of the blood stream, provided there is a normal store of it in the liver to draw from. So reliable is this reaction in animal experiments, that it can be used by a blood specialist to tell if the liver does have a good vitamin A supply. (So says an ad in *Food Technology,* August, 1954, placed by Distillation Products Industries.) If the vitamin is present, a drink of liquor will bring it into the blood and, if it does not show up in the blood, it can be assumed that the body is suffering from a basic shortage of vitamin A. If it is true that vitamin A shortage is related to heart disease, is it not possible that alcoholism and heart diseases have a connection through the vitamin A factor? If each drink demands more vitamin A from the liver's reserve, then a habitual drinker whose vitamin A intake is not what it should be, could easily fall prey to heart disease brought on by a vitamin A shortage.

Vitamin A Helps You to Taste

On July 30, 1960, the Long Island Jewish Hospital, through the Nutrition Foundation, reported on tests that showed vitamin A to be of great importance in the sensitivity of our taste buds. The tests were conducted with laboratory animals who were deprived of vitamin A and seemed to lose their sense of taste as a result. They were apparently unable to distinguish between regular tap water and ultra-sour quinine water and would drink either with equal indifference or thirst when they were presented.

Does the lack of vitamin A explain that often-heard phrase: "Nothing tastes right to me anymore." Is it this lack that makes people lose their appetite? Could it be a shortage of vitamin A that causes the common perversions in appetite that make kids "hate" vegetables and go for purple popsicles, or turn their noses up at a sweet apple and pick, instead, a gooey piece of candy? Maybe America is really not tasting anything! We sugar and salt everything to make it taste like something it is not, because, possibly, our taste buds are not acute enough to detect a good, subtle flavor.

The vitamin A-rich foods can be identified by their deep yellow (yams, sweet potatoes, squash) or green (spinach, kale, cabbage) color; sea food also offers a good supply. Be sure to include them in the diet for good health, and we believe one should take a vitamin A supplement (such as halibut liver oil) daily, to be sure of a sufficient intake of the vitamin.

Vitamin B

Therapeutic Uses of Thiamin

After about 20 to 35 days, the normal patient develops the first symptoms: easy fatigue, loss of appetite, irritability and emotional instability. This describes the first days of a deficiency of vitamin B_1 (thiamin), according to the *Pennsylvania Medical Journal* (June, 1943). Sounds familiar, doesn't it? Probably everyone reading these pages can think of several acquaintances who have exhibited these very traits and wondered what was wrong.

As the deficiency progresses, confusion and loss of memory appear, followed closely by gastric distress, abdominal pains and constipation. Heart irregularities crop up and finally, prickling sensations in the lower extremities, impaired vibratory sense and tenderness over the calf muscles.

The article goes on to say that to secure a beneficial therapeutic result, a constant intake of vitamin B_1 must be maintained. This vitamin cannot be stored in the body in significant amounts, for most of it is excreted. An individual who was receiving 100 milligrams of vitamin B$_1$ a day, by mouth, was found to excrete 86 milligrams in the feces and 11 milligrams in the urine. It is obvious, from this, that close watch must be maintained on one's thiamin intake, for a single day without it could wipe out even a healthy person's supply. Where illness or stress of any kind is involved and the vitamins are called upon to help in repairing damage, the vigil against shortage becomes even more necessary.

The value of thiamin in treating certain physical and mental disorders has been illustrated through articles in the medical journals of the world. Here are some of the reports filed by scientists on their experience with this nutrient.

Adequate Thiamin Essential to Pregnant Women

In the *Journal of Pediatrics* (September, 1944), D. W. Van Gelder and F. U. Darby told of beriberi occurring in infants and even being present at birth. The authors blame this condition on the diet of the mother, either in pregnancy or during lactation. An adequate intake of all the B vitamins is essential at these times. For infants with large heart (a symptom of beriberi), in whom no other reason for this condition is apparent, large doses of thiamin hydrochloride are recommended. Also, in the case of a nursing mother whose diet is nutritionally lacking, the child should receive additional vitamin B$_1$ until foods containing this vitamin are added to his diet.

In the *Texas State Medical Journal* (May, 1943), L. P. Hightower advocates the administration of vitamin B$_1$ to all patients with indefinite heart symptoms, particularly if there is a history of dietary deficiency. He recommends injections of 100 milligrams of thiamin per day, accompanied by a diet high in vitamin B-rich foods. We are told that this is usually followed by prompt improvement. The size of the heart is reduced and encouraging alterations appear in the electrocardiogram.

An article in the *British Heart Journal* (January, 1944) by A. Schott, describes 3 cases of circulatory disturbances due to vitamin B$_1$ deficiency. Two of the patients had taken excessive amounts of alcohol (known to take a toll of the B vitamins in the body) and the third patient's condition was caused by deficient diet only. Each of the 3 responded favorably to treatment with thiamin.

In reviewing the possible causes of vitamin B$_1$ deficiency, C. J. O'Sullivan, in the *Journal of the Irish Medical Association* (April, 1952), lists insufficient dietary intake, defective utilization, inadequate absorption, interference from antibiotics in the intestines and increased demand in illness, fever and pregnancy.

Heart Failure a Common Symptom

Dr. O'Sullivan tells of a 72-year-old man who seemed to be suffering from bronchitis and failure of the right side of the heart.

Antibiotics and cardiac therapy were begun, but response was poor. The patient worsened slightly during 6 days of this treatment.

Attending doctors decided to review his nutritional history and found him suffering from an inadequate B vitamin intake. The diagnosis was changed to right heart failure on a thiamin deficiency basis. Dramatic and early response followed treatment with 100-milligram injections of thiamin, plus thiamin tablets. The heart disease symptoms ceased and the patient was soon walking.

The doctor commented that the unusual feature of this case was the complete absence, apart from heart failure, of the usual classical signs of vitamin B_1 deficiency. It may be, he goes on, that the fatal right heart failure of some illnesses is due to a thiamin deficiency developed during such an illness, due to poor storage capacity in the body for vitamin B_1 and partly to the inadequate diet of such individuals. Any increased demand, then, coupled with lack of appetite, usual in such cases, could conspire to such a consequence.

We wonder how many heart patients are told to include a good intake of B vitamin-rich foods, such as brewer's yeast and the organ meats in their diet? Even well persons need this fortification; certainly a heart patient needs anything in the way of good nutrition that he can get. Desiccated liver is a good source of B vitamins and is especially valuable for low-fat diets because the fat has been removed.

Alcohol Can Cause Thiamin Deficiency

Alcoholism and the deficiency of B vitamins are often mentioned together, and rightfully so. A letter to the *British Medical Journal* (December 4, 1945) stated the situation exactly. It explained that alcohol does not inhibit the action of vitamin B_1, but that the high caloric value of alcohol increases the patient's requirement for all the B vitamins. At the same time, the alcoholic, from lack of appetite, reduces his dietary intake. Alcoholic psychoses probably are due, says the correspondent, to a lack of vitamin B_1 and niacin, both of which are needed to process carbohydrates such as alcohol. These vitamins are being used much faster than they are replaced, if they are replaced at all. The signs of vitamin B_1 deficiency are usually the first to appear, though an alcoholic suffers from many nutritional deficiencies.

It has been suggested that a shortage of vitamin B_1 is what makes an alcoholic turn to drink in the first place. He feels a hunger for some lack and tries to satisfy this craving with alcohol. Of course, this only aggravates the craving and increases the lack, and a vicious cycle is soon operating.

Sciatica and Herpes Zoster

Victims of sciatica, the painful inflammation of the sciatic nerve which runs down the back of the thigh and leg, can take some hope from a letter by E. Braner, which appeared in the *British Medical Journal* (April 15, 1944). He told of obtaining good results from the use of vitamin B₁ injections in treating this disease. For quick results, Dr. Braner used ampules containing 25 milligrams of thiamin per cubic centimeter. Three to 6 injections on consecutive, or alternate, days were given.

Herpes zoster, that stubborn and painful clustering of small blisters near the ear (sometimes called shingles), was effectively treated with thiamin by A. L. Oriz (*Medical World,* November, 1958) in 25 cases. The patients were given intramuscular injections of 200 milligrams of thiamin hydrochloride daily, but the doctor expressed the opinion that even a lesser dosage would have been equally effective.

S. Waldman and L. Pelner told of similar results (*New York State Medical Journal,* September 15, 1947). Twenty-three cases of herpes zoster were treated with a combination injection consisting of one cubic centimeter of thiamin (100 milligrams per cubic centimeter) and one cubic centimeter of neostigmine methylsulfate (1:2000). The injection was repeated every other day until the severe pain was relieved. In 7 cases, two injections were enough to bring results; and in 13 others 6 injections or less were required. Of the remaining 3 patients, two did not continue the treatment and one got relief from vertebral injections. These results strike us as remarkable, considering that many physicians tell their patients they have no cure for this ailment.

Impairment of the field of vision, as well as the ability to focus, known as amblyopia, is usually connected with the consumption of alcohol and tobacco. F. D. Carroll, in the *American Journal of Ophthalmology* (June, 1945), tells of a case in which about half of the patient's calories came from alcohol, with his consumption of B vitamins considered inadequate. Without decreasing tobacco or alcohol consumption or improving diet, normal vision was restored by administration of 40 milligrams of thiamin per day by mouth and 20 by vein. Improvement was maintained after the hospital stay as long as the patient took two 10-milligram tablets of thiamin a day; without them, vision became impaired.

Taking Some of the Pain Out of Dentistry

In dentistry, the use of vitamin B₁ has shown itself to be beneficial in a number of ways, as witness the article by J. L. E. Bock (*U. S. Armed Forces Medical Journal,* March, 1953). Dr. Bock says that dental postoperative pain is promptly and completely relieved in most patients by the administration of thiamin and much pain can be prevented by using thiamin before the operation. The healing time of drying tooth sockets is greatly reduced by thiamin therapy.

The low pain threshold which is peculiar to many dental patients may be indicative of thiamin deficiency. In most cases, dental pain is relieved promptly by the oral infiltration of 10 milligrams of thiamin hydrochloride, the results being equal to 100 milligrams injected intramuscularly.

It is quite possible, says Bock, that the loss of thiamin from the nerves is one of the major chemical factors in the production of pain. There is ample evidence that replacement of free thiamin to injured and diseased nerves not only restores proper functioning, but relieves pain. Perhaps thiamin is not the sole factor in producing pain, but, says Bock, it is of prime importance in nerve physiology and should be given whenever a problem concerning the nerves arises, or is suspected.

Morning Sickness Responds to Vitamin B₁

As we have seen earlier, in pregnancy, a thiamin deficiency in the mother can result in the same condition in the child, when he is born, or can show itself in a nursing baby as the result of thiamin-poor milk from the mother. In tests of 50 patients, 16 of whom were pregnant women, Lockhart, Kirkwood and Harris (*American Journal of Obstetrics and Gynecology,* September, 1943) found that, in the late pregnancy and early post-delivery, the thiamin requirement is 3 times that of a nonpregnant woman.

Many expectant mothers suffer from almost constant nausea and vomiting. In the *American Journal of Obstetrics and Gynecology* (August, 1942), an article tells of complete relief from this condition by the administration of vitamins B₁ and B₆ intramuscularly or intravenously. The dosage of vitamin B₁ was 25 to 100 milligrams, of vitamin B₆ usually 50 milligrams. The number of injections and the intervals between them varied with individual patients. Of 44 patients treated with thiamin, 6 showed excellent results, 33 improved to varying degrees and 5 showed no improvement. Vitamin B₆ gave even better results, completely relieving nausea in 12 of 36 cases and providing varying improvement in the rest. Two of the patients were relieved of accompanying migraine. None had any undesirable side reactions.

Even better results for vitamin B₁ were recorded in the correspondence section of the *Journal of the American Medical Association* (July 22, 1944). M. M. Marbel tells of an English study of constant vomiting among pregnant women. Each patient was given an intramuscular injection of 100 milligrams of thiamin hydrochloride every other day. Fifty per cent improvement was noted after the first injection, and the vomiting ceased after the fourth or fifth injection in every case. All the patients gained weight within a week, and went on a general diet, after a week, without any recurrence of vomiting.

These are but a few of the findings on the therapeutic effectiveness of vitamin B₁ as contained in a compilation published by Merck and Company, Incorporated. Why doctors don't make more use of this information we do not know. Perhaps they haven't the time to read the necessary literature. If this is the case, any doctor should be grateful to have these facts brought to his attention. We can think of no other legitimate reason a doctor would have for ignoring these authoritative findings, when they might be effective in treating a patient. In every case, researchers pointed out that there were no dangerous side effects from the therapeutic use of thiamin. How many of the popularly used drugs can claim as much?

We do not recommend the use of any of the B vitamins separately, except as therapy. We believe that everyone should have a regular intake of vitamin B-rich foods every day. All of these vitamins interact on one another for maximum beneficial effect. A daily inclusion of such foods as brewer's yeast or liver in the diet will eliminate any possibility of thiamin deficiency diseases, as well as act favorably in the healing of any already present.

Versatile Vitamin B₁₂

A letter to the editor of the *British Medical Journal* for April 22, 1950, reveals an encouraging experience in treating shingles with vitamin B_{12} injections. Says Dr. K. E. Jolles, "After reading last year of the treatment of herpes zoster (shingles), I decided to try the new form of vitamin B_{12} concentrate." He goes on to say that he treated 6 patients with injections and had excellent results. He used the vitamin at all stages of the disease—the first early stage at which the skin redness has just appeared and in a case of secondary infection with a great deal of underlying inflammation. Dr. Jolles gave, in every instance, an injection of two milliliters of the vitamin preparation on the first, second and fourth days of treatment. The injection was painless. No further complications appeared after the first injection and by the end of a week, the patient was well.

Using Vitamin B₁₂ Injections for Psoriasis

An M.D. in Albany, New York, discovered that injections of vitamin B_{12} are useful in treating psoriasis. After experimenting with smaller doses, he decided on giving injections of 1000 micrograms of vitamin B_{12}. The injection was given intramuscularly daily for 10 days, followed by what doctors call a "maintenance dose." In severe cases, the regular dosage was given for as long as 15 or 20 days or longer. In some cases, he says, no results were noticed until 20 or more injections were given.

There were 34 patients; of these, 11 showed complete improvement, 10 improved 75 per cent to 80 per cent, 6 patients improved slowly, 2 patients showed no results, 5 patients had slight recurrence, indicating that, apparently, the treatment had been stopped too soon. The patients improved once again when it was resumed.

Noncooperative Patients Showed No Improvement

The two patients who showed no improvement, incidentally, were noncoöperative, according to Dr. Ruedemann. One of them weighed 280 pounds, the other 220, indicating, it seems to us, that they could not have been much concerned about their health.

Dr. Ruedemann says, in the summary of his article in the *American Medical Association Archives of Dermatology and Syphilology* for June, 1954, that the injections were easy to give, had absolutely no ill side effects on patients, stimulated coöperation by the patients and bolstered their morale. "The rapid response," he says, "on patients with long-standing, recalcitrant psoriasis would be difficult to attribute to spontaneous involution."

Seborrhea Yields to Vitamin B$_{12}$

The *New York State Medical Journal* (August, 1950) carried the results of experiments by Drs. Andrews, Post and Domonkos in treating various skin disorders with B vitamins. The most remarkable results were shown in the use of vitamin B$_{12}$ against seborrhea (a disturbance of the sebaceous glands marked by an excessive flow of sebum, forming white or yellowing greasy scales on the body—usually marked by itching). Thirty-seven cases of this type of dermatitis were studied in detail. The patients were given injections of 10 to 30 milligrams of vitamin B$_{12}$ once a week or, in some cases, once every two or three weeks. Of the 37 cases, 16 were greatly improved or completely cured, 16 were somewhat improved, 3 were slightly improved and 2 patients noticed no change. These results were superior to those of any other local treatment with ointment, X-ray or antibiotics.

More on Shingles and Vitamin B$_{12}$

The use of vitamin B$_{12}$ as a treatment for shingles was responsible for remarkable recoveries of 6 victims of this disease, according to Gordon B. Leitch, M.D. (*Northwest Medicine,* April, 1953). Dr. Leitch injected his patients with 1,000 micrograms of vitamin B$_{12}$ intramuscularly. The dosage was repeated daily for 4 or 5 days, and lowered to 500 micrograms for continued treatment for a few days.

In each case, the pain, which had been so intense as to require the use of sedation, subsided or ceased entirely within 24 hours of the initial 1,000-microgram injection. Retrogression and healing of the herpatic sores began in from 36 to 48 hours.

In none of the cases described by Dr. Leitch was there the least unfavorable reaction to the daily use of vitamin B$_{12}$.

Vitamin B$_{12}$ and Lupus Erythematosus

The effective treatment of a skin disease, known clinically as lupus erythematosus (characterized by disc-like patches with raised reddish patches, depressed centers and covered with scales or crusts), has baffled doctors for years. Samuel Goldblatt, in *Acta Dermato-Venereologica* (33: 216-235, 1953), reported on results he achieved in treating this disorder with vitamin B$_{12}$.

Seventeen patients were included in the report, and all were successfully treated. It was noted that, aside from the manifestation of the disease on the skin, lassitude, fatigability, a type of anemia and a lowered keenness of vibratory sense appreciation were common to all patients.

Small doses of vitamin B$_{12}$ (15 micrograms at weekly intervals) were effective in healing the disc-like skin breaks. Increased dosage (100 micrograms daily, or 3 times per week) would probably speed the recovery, says Dr. Goldblatt. For severe and extensive cases, doses of 100 to 1,000 micrograms daily for 1 to 2 weeks are suggested. Maintenance therapy should be continued for several months after complete healing of the skin lesions. Doctor Goldblatt concluded that vitamin B$_{12}$ is an effective and nonhazardous treatment for all phases of lupus erythematosus.

One reason why the injection of vitamin B$_{12}$ appears to be so successful is that this vitamin is not easily assimilated, especially by older digestive tracts. It seems there is a factor in the stomach, called the "intrinsic factor," which is necessary for assimilation of the vitamin and may not be present. Hence, in emergencies like those outlined above, doctors give injections to make certain the vitamin reaches its goal.

Don't Ignore These Lesser-Known Vitamins

Anyone who can read and who is the least bit aware of nutritional elements in the diet, knows about the more common vitamins and minerals. He sees lists of added synthetic nutrients on cereal boxes, white bread wrappers and patent medicine bottles—thiamine, vitamin C, iron, vitamin B$_{12}$, riboflavin, vitamin A, vitamin D are all familiar names. There are other vitamins, just as important to good health, which have not had the public relations job they deserve. This creates a danger, because people tend to ignore them in their daily diets and in the supplements they use. We would like to sketch a few of the less prominent B vitamins here to make our readers aware of their value.

The Value of Inositol

Inositol's modern claim to fame is its action against cholesterol. In *Newsweek* magazine (September 11, 1950), there appeared the report of a paper read to the 118th National Meeting of the American Chemical Society which offered evidence of inositol's power in lowering cholesterol levels in the blood.

The experiment was simple. Two groups of rabbits received one gram of cholesterol daily, while one of the groups got, in addition, half a gram of inositol. The animals were kept on a controlled diet. At the end of the experiment, the rabbits who were fed cholesterol alone showed a cholesterol increase of 337 per cent, while those fed inositol with their cholesterol dosage showed a much smaller increase, 181 per cent. The results were considered to be indicative of—though not directly comparable to—the effect inositol has on cholesterol readings in man.

Because inositol's status as a full-fledged B vitamin has been established only recently, there is much that is still to be learned of its activity in the human body. *Science News Letter* (May 19, 1956) reported that human blood serum can be replaced by inositol. It is needed for the growth and survival of cells in bone marrow, eye membranes, embryo, intestines, etc. The fact that inositol occurs in large amounts in tissues of the human brain, stomach, kidney, spleen, liver and the heart muscle, gives some clue as to its value in the diet. Inositol also appears in desiccated thyroid gland and in human hair—a fact which has led to much speculation as to its value in restoring color to gray hair or even restoring hair to bald heads!

Preoperative Measure

In a booklet, *Inositol,* published by Corn Products Sales Company (Chemical Division), the observed physiological values of inositol are listed. For example, inositol given to those about to be operated on for stomach cancer, is considered to be a valuable preoperative procedure because it cuts down on total liver fats. It also seems to have a mild inhibitory action on certain types of cancer cells. In *Science* (97, 515, 1943), it was reported that intravenous injection of inositol into mice with transplanted cancers retards the growth of the tumors to a degree directly proportional to the dosage of the inositol.

Herbst and Bagley (*Journal of Urology,* 59, 505, 1948) administered inositol to 6 patients with cancer of the bladder, and concluded that it had a favorable effect. The original tumors were found to have lessened in size due to the treatment.

In the *American Journal of Digestive Diseases* (8, 290, 1941), inositol was pointed out as an agent against constipation. It was found by Martin, et al, to have a marked effect on peristaltic action of the stomach and small intestine (that is, the muscular action which moves fecal waste through the alimentary canal).

Principal dietary sources for inositol are dried lima beans, beef brains, beef heart, desiccated liver, cantaloupe, grapefruit, peaches, peanuts, oranges, peas, raisins, wheat germ, cabbage, brewer's yeast and many other vegetables, meats and fruits in lesser amounts.

Benefits from Choline

The value of choline in human existence is exemplified by the fact that it is richly contained in colostrum, the name given to the extra-rich milk mothers give in the first days of nursing—the milk nature provides to give the infant a good start in his weakest days. This has been enough to prod scientists on to finding what other services toward maintaining or regaining good health in later years choline could perform. The list is impressive.

Choline has been identified by University of Toronto researchers to be essential to the health of the heart and blood vessel system of young rats (*Science,* June 11, 1954). Young rats, after short periods on a diet low in choline and high in fat, as well as older rats on choline-deficient diets for longer periods, develop damaged heart arteries and aorta (the main artery of the heart). The walls of these important blood vessels get fat deposits and show hardening. The doctors also stated that choline is needed for healthy livers and kidneys. These findings were intended for further testing on higher species until their relationship to man could be established.

Favorable Action on Heart Disease

Choline's ability to act favorably in cases of heart disease was demonstrated by L. M. Morrison and W. F. Gonzales and recorded in the *Proceedings of the Society of Experimental Biology and Medicine* (January, 1950). A group of 230 acute heart disease patients were studied. One hundred and fifteen of these served as controls. They were discharged from the hospital on recovery after about 6 weeks. They were then observed for a 3-year-period. The other 115 patients, when they were released from the hospital on the same basis as the first group, were also observed for 3 years. But during this time, they were given a choline supplement for varying lengths of time—one, two or three years.

Of the 115 patients who did not receive choline, 35 patients, or 30 per cent, had died after 3 years. Only 6 of these died of a cause other than heart disease. In the choline-treated group of 115 patients, 14 patients, or 12 per cent, had died after 3 years. Five of these deaths were due to some cause other than heart disease.

In a German journal, *Deutsche Medizinische Wochenschrift* (February 16, 1951), choline was named as a successful agent in the treatment of hepatitis. Thirty-seven patients were involved in this experiment. Ten of the 37 served as controls; then, 13 patients were treated only with choline; another group of 8 patients was given dextrose into the stomach in addition to the choline; 2 patients were given methionine in addition to the choline; and finally, 4 patients were treated with injections of a choline compound. It was found that treatment with choline reduced the duration of virus hepatitis to about half.

An experiment written up in an Italian journal was excerpted by the *Journal of the American Medical Association* (September 16, 1950). In this case, the action of choline against hyperthyroid conditions was examined. Choline hydrochloride was administered to 14 women and one adolescent girl for two weeks—one gram by mouth daily. Eight patients took the medication, half strength, for another two weeks. By the 4th day to the 12th day the patients experienced a feeling of well-being. The circumference of the neck diminished by one centimeter. When the medication was stopped, the subjective symptoms reappeared in the majority of the patients. They were again controlled by reintroduction of the treatment. In 3 patients with acute hyperthyroidism, combined treatment with choline hydrochloride and 150,000 units of vitamin A every 5 days for two or three weeks gave good results.

Foods especially rich in choline are snap beans, soybeans, egg yolk, lamb kidney, beef liver, calves' liver, pork liver, peas, pork kidney, spinach, brewer's yeast, wheat germ and other vegetables in lesser amounts.

The Potency of Biotin

The B vitamin, biotin, according to an article in *Scientific American* (June, 1961), is so potent that no human cell contains more than a trace of it. Liver, one of the richest sources, contains less than one part per billion. Still, it is an essential constituent. Earl Ubell, Science Editor of the *New York Herald Tribune,* explained the valuable function of biotin this way, in his column of April 16, 1959: "The biotin molecule . . . grabs a big protein molecule composed of thousands of atoms. . . . This new protein is capable of sweeping an atom of carbon dioxide and hooking it onto a number of other molecules which are important in the production of fat and other body substances. But here's the important step: the protein that does this cannot function without biotin. So, without biotin the body's fat production is impaired."

Avidin and Biotin

Researchers have found a poisonous substance, avidin, in raw egg white. If fed large doses of egg white, humans and animals develop skin rashes, loss of hair and muscular incoördination. Biotin acts as an antidote for this reaction, but the avidin removes biotin from whatever other important chemical work biotin performs. So, when biotin is busy counteracting avidin in egg white, it can't do its regular job, and this accounts for the rashes, hair loss, etc.

A severe rash, seborrheic dermatitis, and Leiner's disease, a condition which manifests itself in a burned-lobster appearance of the skin, are described, in the *Journal of Pediatrics* (November, 1957), as due to a biotin deficiency. Nine cases of seborrheic dermatitis and two cases of Leiner's disease in infants are described as showing marked improvement when treated with biotin. The doses given were 5 milligrams of biotin injected intramuscularly daily for 7 to 14 days. Milder cases are affected well by two to four milligrams orally for two to three weeks.

Such a lack of biotin is a rarity. Biotin, as was seen above, is needed by the body in only minute amounts, but it *must be there.* You can be sure your quota is being met if these foods are frequently in your diet: beef liver, lamb liver, unpolished rice, soybeans, soy flour, salmon, sardines, cauliflower, cowpeas, brewer's yeast.

Natural Occurrence Important

It should be remembered that, as with all vitamins, we approve only of those which occur naturally. This is especially true of the B complex. They are safest and most effective when taken with their natural components. It is true that synthetic vitamins are used therapeutically or experimentally by doctors, but when this is done, it is done under controlled conditions, and the doctors are presumed to be on the lookout for nutritional imbalances which can create real problems.

We are impressed once more, as we go through the information on the more obscure B vitamins, that they are all contained in abundance in the foods and natural food supplements that we continually recommend—brewer's yeast, wheat germ, desiccated liver, all of the organ meats. If you are eating the natural way, if you are supplementing your diet to make up for the stresses caused by poisons you can't avoid in our modern environment, your B vitamin problems are solved. You are getting what you need to keep healthy.

Vitamin C

Poultices Made of Vitamin C

Sores which will not heal are one of the most unpleasant and dangerous phenomena of ill health. Those of us who are apparently healthy often suffer from such sores. Bedfast individuals, as well as people in wheel chairs, are closely acquainted with the perils of bedsores—those stubborn, painful areas which arise chiefly because free movement is impossible for the patient. People who are afflicted with ulcers of any kind know well the prolonged, painful and disagreeable course such sores may take, with dressings that must be changed frequently, with unpleasant odors from the sores, as well as from the drugs used to treat them.

How fine it would be if someone might discover a simple, quick and effective salve or poultice that would close such sores or wounds with healthy new tissue, thus giving the patient an opportunity to return to good health and preventing any possibility of the open sore or wound becoming more serious—perhaps eventually becoming malignant.

An English physician, working with elderly bedridden patients in a London hospital, has been experimenting with vitamin C applications. In the *Lancet* for February 11, 1961, Dr. A. J. Mester of the Geriatric Unit, St. Alfege's Hospital, London, writes of his experiments.

In cases of ulcers, says Dr. Mester, there is usually an impaired blood supply to the skin and tissue around the ulcer. There is also, usually, infection at these spots. So it seems reasonable to give such a patient large amounts of vitamin C by mouth to strengthen the tissues and to fight the infection. However, he goes on, "this rarely meets with much success." Perhaps, as two other investigators have suggested, the work vitamin C does in regenerating healthy tissue is a purely local one. So, why not apply the vitamin C directly to the ulcer?

Accordingly, he says, "since the beginning of this year, I have used local ascorbic acid (vitamin C) in the treatment of pressure bedsores and chronic ulcers, particularly in bedfast geriatric patients who usually have arteriosclerosis and often some concurrent low-grade infection."

He treated indolent ulcers and pressure sores in the usual ways first, he says. He gave antibacterial drugs and drugs to dilate the patient's arteries. He relieved the pressure on the sores.

Treated Ulcer with Vitamin C Dressing

If all this effort were unsuccessful, he tried vitamin C. He irrigated the ulcer with "a sterile isotonic solution containing 15 milligrams of ascorbic acid (vitamin C) at pH 6, after which the wound was dressed with gauze soaked in 5 milliliters of the same solution. This procedure was repeated daily for a week."

Pharmacists and doctors will readily understand the terms used here. For the rest of us, suffice it to say that "irrigating" a wound means simply to perfuse or wash it with the solution. The word isotonic means simply that the solution must be such that the character of the ascorbic acid is not destroyed. The phrase pH refers to the acidity of the mixture. Vitamin C is an acid and an effort was made here to reduce its acidity somewhat, probably so that its application would not be painful on an open sore.

How Ulcers React to Vitamin C

Here, in Dr. Mester's own words, are the results of his experiment. "Twenty-two patients have now completed this course of treatment; 3 have shown little improvement, but in the remaining 19, there has been a dramatic change with development of fresh granulations. Many of these elderly patients had had extremely indolent (painless) ulcers that had shown no improvement for months, and even years. It is, therefore, unlikely that the sudden change with the formation of granulation tissue could have been part of the natural course of the lesion (sore).

"Once these fresh granulations had formed, after 7 days' topical ascorbic acid treatment, the vitamin C was omitted and the wound left to heal spontaneously. In 17 patients, healing has been complete and 11 have been discharged from hospital; the others, started more recently, are progressing satisfactorily." Dr. Mester believes that other physicians should make use of his experience in order to investigate more thoroughly the use of vitamin C locally at the sore point. We are in complete agreement with his point of view and hope sincerely that all practitioners, medical and nonmedical, will do whatever they can along these lines and publish their findings.

What use can we others make of this information? First of all, it should be a lesson to all of us of the extreme importance of enough vitamin C for all the body tissues. You can't get too much vitamin C; many chemicals and poisons destroy this vitamin, so that most of us "civilized" people are almost bound to be short in it. Drinking a bit of orange juice at breakfast isn't enough. You should eat as much fresh, raw fruit and raw vegetable food as you possibly can and take a natural vitamin C food supplement in addition.

If you are already suffering from a sore that won't heal—an ulcer, a bedsore, a wound—can you use such a solution on it as Dr. Mester did? We see no reason why you should not and we suggest that you ask your physician to write Dr. Mester for further information.

John Wyeth and Brother, Limited, London, the pharmacists who made up the solution for Dr. Mester, tell us that it is not stable (that is, will not keep its potency) for longer than several weeks, so it cannot be stocked in a drug store, but must be made fresh for use. So, until someone develops a process for retaining its potency, there seems little hope that such a product will be available in drug stores.

Using Vitamin C Poultices at Home

However, a poultice of vitamin C can easily be made at home. Vitamin C pills dipped in water and rubbed on poison ivy, insect bites, skin disorders, burns, cuts and wounds of all kinds have been most successful in bringing about rapid healing and in causing healthy new tissue to form.

However, we must remind you that vitamin C oxidizes rapidly, so solutions cannot be made and stored for future use, even in the refrigerator. That is, as soon as the water touches the vitamin pill, the vitamin is destroyed rapidly. As you can see, even the synthetic ascorbic acid cannot be made into a solution that will retain its potency. The natural vitamin C is even more difficult to hold on to, once it has been mixed with water.

Do you know how long it takes for an apple or a peach to darken where you have sliced it with a knife? This means the vitamin C has been destroyed, almost as soon as the air hits it. This is how fast the vitamin C may disappear from the rose hip powder or the natural vitamin C tablet that you dip in water and apply to a sore spot.

So, if you use a natural vitamin C tablet for applying to the skin, work fast. And, if it is at all possible, keep a wet dressing saturated with the vitamin on the wound. We are speaking here of minor wounds—cuts, burns, insect bites, minor skin irritations. It has been our experience that vitamin C applied to such wounds goes to work immediately, bringing healing to the injured tissues and, simultaneously, counteracting any infection that may be present.

We know that vitamin C is intimately concerned in the repair of body tissues. It must be present for the formation of collagen to take place. This is the cement which unites individual cells. If, for some reason, the tissue around the wound is deficient in vitamin C and in such condition that the vitamin C in the blood cannot reach it, perhaps the direct application of the vitamin may accomplish a near miracle.

We firmly believe that long-established, serious ulcers or other wounds or sores should be treated by a physician, although there seems no evidence that vitamin C could be harmful in any way.

We believe that vitamin C may be responsible for many of the cures recorded in herb medicine. Fresh leaves, fruit and flowers are rich in vitamin C. So it seems quite possible that using one of these as a dressing on a wound may liberate enough vitamin C to heal the wound.

We are concerned chiefly with prevention of illness, not cure. But we feel that Dr. Mester's use of vitamin C topically is, in a very real sense, prevention. Open sores that do not heal, cuts and burns which are irritated day after day may become malignant. They are also a constant drain on health and a threat to future health. If the application of vitamin C can prevent such an occurrence, then it is surely one of our most worthwhile weapons against disease.

Vitamin D

Importance of a Vitamin D Supplement

Probably the least obvious of all the vitamins in its activity is vitamin D. By this, we mean to say that, unlike vitamin B_{12} or vitamins C or E, one can rarely take an injection or an oral dose of vitamin D alone and expect to see a significant change in a specific disease. Vitamin D is a substance whose prime reason for existence is that it is necessary to help the body to use calcium. As everyone is well aware, calcium is vital to the growth and development of young bones (without it, rickets, a children's disease of weak, demineralized bones, occurs) and the maintenance of firmness and strength in bones already formed. But usually, the credit for good bones goes to calcium and the value of vitamin D is quietly ignored.

In order that calcium be retained in the body long enough to do some good, it must combine there with phosphorus. But phosphorus depends upon the presence of vitamin D for its proper absorption into the blood stream. So it is apparent that vitamin D is the first essential factor in the process of calcium assimilation.

There is another phase of the relationship between healthy bones and vitamin D which points up this nutrient's great value. Vitamin D is believed to control the workings of the enzyme, phosphatase. This enzyme acts to release phosphorus from the bones so that the previously mentioned marriage between it and calcium can take place. Again, the interaction of these elements, so essential to normal growth, is shown to be dependent upon vitamin D.

Can Vitamin D Be By-Passed?

Perhaps it has occurred to you to wonder if one could simply combine one's phosphorus-calcium intake in foods and by-pass the need of vitamin D to help combine them in the system. Apparently not. H. Steenback and D. C. Herting (*Nutrition Reviews,* 14, 191, 1956) showed in their work that the proper *rate* of bone growth is also controlled by vitamin D. Experiments in which the calcium intake of laboratory rats was varied showed that vitamin D was responsible for suppressing growth when dietary calcium levels were high and for stimulating growth when dietary calcium intake was low.

These same researchers reported that the acidity of the gastric juices is affected by the amount of vitamin D in the diet (*Journal of Nutrition,* 57, 649, 1955). These juices are named as a cause of stomach ulcers when they have too high an acidity. One might logically conclude from this that the diet of an ulcer patient should be checked to determine whether or not it contains sufficient vitamin

D-rich foods. This vitamin might be considered a preventive as well as a part of the treatment where ulcers are involved.

Vitamin D's Bad Publicity

Writers of popular science columns in newspapers and magazines throughout the country have found vitamin D to be good copy. A typical headline reads, "Doctors Say Vitamins Can Be Harmful." The reader goes on to see that the first paragraph warns of serious consequences due to vitamin D intake. If he stops there, he will not discover that the writer qualifies this warning as he goes on. *United Press International* columnist, Delos Smith, who wrote the headline above some time ago, went on to say that vitamin D intoxication can be caused in most cases only by "large doses taken for a long period of time."

Dr. Colin B. Holman of the Mayo Clinic is given as the source of Mr. Smith's information. Upon being asked to define the dosage required to produce ill effects from vitamin D, Dr. Holman had to decline, "since many persons apparently tolerate huge amounts of vitamin D without any obvious ill effects." The column described the possible ill effects as nausea, abdominal pain, headache, drowsiness, dizziness and haziness of memory.

These side effects can be attributed to many of the modern drugs now on the market, as the least of their undesirable consequences. One does not have to take large doses of tranquilizers or pep pills to chance dizziness or nausea. Drowsiness is almost certain after the use of antihistamines.

As Dr. Holman noted, high dosages of vitamin D over long periods of time are required to produce any untoward effects, and this only in rare cases. This cannot be said for most drugs. Side effects are frequent and occur even with the most conservative dosage.

No Two People the Same

With this in mind, there can be no question about whether or not one will choose to include vitamin D in one's diet. It *must* be included. The question can only be: how much vitamin D shall I take? Again, we must go into the problem presented by individuality. No one expends exactly the same amount of energy, has the same metabolism, eats exactly the same kinds and amounts of food as everyone else. This means that the need for any nutrient, including vitamin D, by any individual will vary.

There is this to consider in deciding on the amount of vitamin D required by the individual: the amount of exposure to sunlight. The sun's ultraviolet rays act upon a substance secreted by the oil glands of the skin to make vitamin D. The vitamin is then absorbed through the skin and available for use in its job of processing calcium and neutralizing the gastric juices. It is not known just how long it takes for this absorption to occur, so it is quite possible that swimmers and others who might rinse their skins shortly after being exposed to sunlight, could be washing their vitamin D away before it can do them any good.

It should also be borne in mind by sun worshippers that suntan interferes with absorption of the vitamin D. Tan is nature's way of protecting one against ultraviolet light. The deeper the tan, the less vitamin D can be manufactured by the body. For some people who have outdoor occupations, a deep tan by June is not unusual. That means that, through the entire summer, they will manufacture a minimal amount, if any, of vitamin D. Then, when winter comes, there is no vitamin D stored to meet the need created by sunless days and winter clothes which leave little skin surface exposed. Furthermore, the values of winter sun for transforming vitamin D are negligible.

Today, mothers give their children supplementary fish liver oil, richest of all sources of vitamin D. Most doctors advise this procedure almost from birth. Unfortunately, mothers often discontinue using it soon after the children have been put on regular table food. They forget that the children are growing until they are fully mature— usually until about 18 years of age. During all of this time, bone development is continuing and the growth is no less important now than in the infant years. It is now that the narrow chest which lends itself to respiratory diseases and the narrow pelvic structure which creates difficulty for a woman in childbirth, can be formed. Now is the time that a tendency to osteomalacia (an adult disease that corresponds to rickets) is instituted. The bones become weak and soft because they have been robbed of their mineral content in earlier years. Lack of vitamin D in the diet can be the cause of such a condition.

We believe that an intake of at least 300 to 600 units of vitamin D per day is best for maintaining the proper growth and development of a child. For adults, the question of vitamin D's need is pushed aside by the National Research Council. For vigorous adults leading normal lives, they say, the need is minimal. Who is a vigorous adult? Can you think of 5 middle-aged friends offhand who aren't plagued with high blood pressure, frequent headache, varicose veins, backaches, etc.? They all think they're healthy. They think they're normal, too. They are sure they don't need vitamin D. But are they assimilating the calcium they need to make strong bones and healthy blood? Do they have the phosphorus in their systems that will help to burn their body sugars at a proper rate? (Phosphorus pulls sugars through the intestinal wall into the blood stream to be stored for energy as it is required. Without vitamin D, the phosphorus needed for this job isn't present and the tired feeling many adults complain of might be traced to this very thing.)

Preserve Two Essential Minerals

Many adults pay little attention to their diets. They might be very short of calcium and phosphorus. The less they have of these two essential minerals, the more they need of vitamin D, to conserve as much as possible of these minerals.

More than 400,000 units of vitamin D per day is considered a toxic dose for adults. For children, 50,000 units is considered undesirable if taken over long periods daily. In babies, 30,000 units daily can create a problem. However, it is not likely that anyone taking his vitamin D in a natural supplement such as fish liver oil and following the suggested dosage on the label, will get an overdose of vitamin D. We believe that everyone should supplement his vitamin D intake with fish liver oil, especially during winter months.

It is difficult to get a good vitamin D intake from everyday foods. Aside from fish, eggs and liver, few foods offer an appreciable amount. Dairy products (though we do not approve of their frequent use for many reasons) do have a respectable vitamin D content. Sometimes they are "fortified" with synthetic vitamin D. Many milk suppliers sell what they call "irradiated vitamin D" milk. This means that the ergosteral, the raw substance occurring in foods which is transformed into vitamin D by sunlight, has been exposed to artificial ultraviolet rays and is already vitamin D in the milk.

Taken in a natural form such as fish liver oils, in the amount suggested on the container, few things could be more necessary to good health than vitamin D. Most nutritionists tell us we are woefully short on calcium in our systems. Let us at least make use of what we do get by keeping a good vitamin D supply at all times.

Vitamin E

Doctors—Just Try Vitamin E!

Dr. Evan Shute, in the *Summary* (December, 1960), begs, literally begs, that physicians give vitamin E (alpha tocopherol) a trial in treating cardiac disease, as well as other disabilities. He reminds physicians that, in the treatment of acute phlebitis alone, 37 groups of workers in 14 countries have found themselves in agreement with Dr. Shute's conclusions that vitamin E is as safe and effective, or more so, than the more commonly employed treatments. The same is true with chronic phlebitis, a disease in which there is little else to be done, but try to maintain the painful status quo. Dr. Shute says, ". . . try a high dose of alpha tocopherol and discover how frequently these painful crippling legs are eased. There is no alternative suggestion of any value. And the trial would be simple,

safe and scientific. What else can one do?" Before one resorts to
surgery for intermittent claudication, Buerger's disease, Raynaud's
disease, skin grafting in burn cases, etc., he urges the trial of vitamin E first.

Curative Value of Vitamin E

Dr. Shute describes a speech to professionals in Venice, Italy,
in 1955. "I asked my audience to add up what was wanted in a
cardiac drug and see what the sum would be. Curiously, such an
equation always produces alpha tocopherol, which is able, as is no
other physiological agent, to oxygenate tissues, prevent thrombosis,
or the embolism of established thrombi-dilate capillaries and other
vessels, stimulate collateral circulation, decrease damaged capillary
permeability, resolve scar, resemble digitalis in its action on the
hypoxic heart and so forth. All these properties of alpha tocopherol
have long been demonstrated in a host of animal and human experiments and are known to every worker in this field. They cannot be
controverted. No other therapeutic agent used for heart disease has
more than a fraction of these properties. None is safer, including
digitalis. . . ."

Convincing Qualifications

One is forced to wonder, after such qualifications, why anyone
would have to be prodded and begged to use vitamin E. The famous
detail men, the salesmen who visit American doctors on behalf of
any one of the hundreds of new drugs introduced each year, have
only the barest fraction of Dr. Shute's experience and knowledge,
yet they talk for 10 minutes on a new heart drug and the doctor
they visit is willing to try it. Sometimes the drug has one or two
experimental tests in its favor; there has been no time for side effects
to show; its effect on patients with other diseases is not known. But
the drug gets a friendly, hopeful reception. The doctor might use
a sample on the next appropriate patient. Now vitamin E has at
least 20 years of successful experimentation behind it. Over 300
papers attesting to its worth have appeared in medical literature
all over the world. Still, your doctor is likely to look at you pityingly
if you should suggest that he use vitamin E in treating you or someone in your family. He may tell you it's useless, not proven, not
effective in your case—but ask him if *he* has tried using it for anything. Ask him how he can be so certain that the authors of these
300 papers are wrong or incompetent in their methods of research.
How does he get that impression? If it is the medical society who
fosters this idea, why is it done? Why is only vitamin E chosen for
disapproval, when sulfas and hormones—to name just two types of
dangerous and still mysterious drugs—are freely employed with the
full blessing of organized medicine?

As is its purpose, the *Summary* carries reports on the most recent work done with vitamin E, both experimental and clinical. The versatility of this nutrient is evident in the instances which we will describe below.

Burn Cases

What is usually done about serious burns, for example? If the patient manages to survive at all, skin grafts are attempted often with small success.

In one case treated by Dr. Shute, the patient was a 6-year-old boy who had spilled scalding water over his chest and back 9 weeks before the examination. Attempted skin grafts had not been successful and when seen by the Shutes, ". . . his body was bathed in pus, and one could smell him 6 feet away." After 13 weeks of treatment by Dr. Shute, complete healing occurred. The procedure was to give 300 milligrams of alpha tocopherol orally and to apply tocopherol ointment locally (each day, we presume). Nothing else was used except for penicillin ointment applied to the infected wounds on alternative days of the first 10 days. None of the scars thickened or contracted, i.e., pinched together, as they formed. This seems to be a characteristic of alpha tocopherol-treated wounds and should prove especially valuable where scars of the face, neck or arms are involved.

Clears Up Second Degree Burns

There is also the case of a 6-year-old boy who let a hot iron fall on the back of his hand. The ensuing second degree burn of the back of the hand and 4 fingers made his parents consider taking him to the best clinics for skin grafts. They first allowed the Shutes to give 300 milligrams of alpha tocopherol orally, as well as to apply sulfa ointment locally for the first 8 days, after which tocopherol ointment was applied to the fingers. In 15 days' time, the hand was clean and scabbed. In 31 days' time, it was healed completely and flexibility of the fingers was perfect.

Two cases of radiation burns caused by X-ray treatment for cancer and eczema are outlined. In the one instance, the physician used only tocopherol ointment applied locally and complete healing occurred in 91 days' time. In the second, the patient's doctor could do nothing, so the patient began the use of alpha tocopherol on his own. The area was healed in 6 weeks.

Strong Effort Rewarded

Another case involved a boy of 14 years, who spent 17 months in the hospital, where skin had been grafted to severe wounds of his legs 5 times without success. His abdomen, from which the skin had been taken, had also not healed. He was emaciated and despondent. He had been sent home to die when Dr. Shute entered the case. Hopelessness made the patient uncoöperative. The boy was given

450 milligrams of alpha tocopherol a day, tocopherol ointment was applied to the wounds and pressure areas and tocopherol was also sprayed on them. In the next 24 months, his wounds were all healed and now he lives a normal life which includes participation in all sports, including swimming.

Then there was the 70-year-old man with a leg ulcer, due to arteriosclerosis, which measured 15 by 7 centimeters in size. The stench from it was so bad that his co-workers refused to work with him. After 57 weeks on a daily oral dose of alpha tocopherol (400 milligrams), the sore was healed and remained healed thereafter, though it is generally known that such ulcers tend to recur.

Osteomyelitis, an ailment which frequently occurs in middle-aged people as a companion to diabetes, manifests itself in unhealing ulcers or sores frequently found on the lower extremities. The *Summary* for December, 1960, describes 3 such cases successfully treated. Wouldn't vitamin E be an excellent preventive measure against such a consequence in diabetic patients?

A Civil Defense Measure

Dr. Shute notes that the application of vitamin E in healing superficial wounds is unusually effective and very quickly relieves the accompanying pain. The resultant scar remains flexible and desirably thin. This is especially important if the scar is at a joint.

Dr. Shute brings up a very interesting point which we never considered before now. He remarks upon the great value of a treatment such as alpha tocopherol—cheap, self-applicable, easy to use, can be widely distributed when danger threatens, in the event of war. In nuclear war, for example, the majority of injuries would be of the very kind alpha tocopherol handles best—burns, scars, open wounds, ulcerations, etc. Dr. Shute says that, in spite of an effort to call the value of vitamin E to the attention of civilian defense 11 years ago, nothing has been done about investigating its possibilities. In that time, nothing else has been developed that would be as effective and certainly the need to take such a precaution grows greater each day.

The value of vitamin E in fertility has had a good bit of study in animals and humans over the last decade. One of the most ambitious projects along this line was a 5-year follow-up by F. G. Darlington and J. B. Chassels, D. V. M. (National Stud Farm, Oshawa, Ontario), on a group of thoroughbred horses who had vitamin E included in their diet. The result was that a group of mares aged 17 (equivalent in age to a woman of 40) maintained a fertility rate higher than the national average for all fertile mares regardless of age. The only change in their care was the vitamin E added to the diet.

As to the quality of the mares' offspring, sired by stud horses also taking vitamin E, one racing day at Toronto's Woodbine Track, 6 of the 8 winners were such horses. One of the acknowledged best horses ever bred in Canada, Victoria Park, was also one of these horses.

While breeding horses may not be the same thing as breeding humans, studies of this type do have a suggestive value as to the place of alpha tocopherol in the management of human fertility. It should also be borne in mind that vitamin E therapy in humans has shown a power to increase fertility and to reduce the incidence of miscarriages in women who are prone to this difficulty.

The *Summary* goes on for many pages to give abstracts of papers on the use of vitamin E in treating fibroid tumors, irregular menstrual periods, avoidance of congenital malformations, improvement of myocardial infarction survival rate, changes in the nervous system, control of incontinence of urine, varicose veins relief, gum disease relief, etc. The application of vitamin E to relieve disease is apparently only touched by science up to now. Its value in so many directions leads one to wonder how many other ways it can be used and why experimentation is not being carried on with the greatest haste and enthusiasm.

Here are just a few of the many therapeutic uses for vitamin E which are not generally known.

Vitamin E in the treatment of skin diseases is discussed in the Russian journal, *Vestnik Dermatologii i. Venerologii* (32: 31, 1958) by Dr. M. E. Barabasch. Twenty-eight patients were involved in the study. Eight had chronic ulcers of the leg and one had leg ulcers caused by X-ray. For these, he used the preparation both internally and externally. For the other 19 patients, only external application was involved. This was accomplished by soaking a piece of cheesecloth in vitamin E concentrate and applying it to the sore part.

Psoriasis and Leg Ulcers

Of 11 psoriasis patients, 9 experienced complete disappearance of the rash and in the other two, there was a considerable degree of improvement. The patients had been psoriasis victims for from 5 to 33 years. The vitamin E had shown complete or partial (in two cases) effectiveness within 3 months.

The patients suffering with leg ulcers experienced similar results. Some of these 10 patients had been treating their leg ulcers for as long as 12 years. The patients, using vitamin E internally as well as externally, took an average of about 1,000 milligrams per day. All were healed within two months, some in 30 days.

Two patients with X-ray ulcers started improving after almost 2 months on vitamin E, as was evidenced by a decrease in the size of the ulcer and a lessening of pain. Tuberculosis ulcers also started healing much faster than they had without vitamin E. The one scleroderma victim also showed definite improvement.

That vitamin E is a factor in the health of the reproductive system is indicated in an article by E. Linder (Czechoslovakia) in *Internationale Zeitschrift für Vitamin Forschung.* He treated 55 men with poor sperm count by administering 150 to 200 milligrams of alpha tocopherol (vitamin E) by mouth daily for 4-week periods. Of the 55, 36 per cent became normal and 38 per cent improved, while in the rest, there was no change. The doctor noted that patients who do not benefit from 3 courses of vitamin E treatment, each of 8 weeks duration, are not justified in continuing the treatment.

At the 3rd World Congress on Fertility and Sterility in Amsterdam, Holland, 1959, Dr. R. Bayer bolstered the case for treating the habitual failure of pregnancy, due to abortions, stillbirths and premature births, with vitamin E. By giving the wife two tablets of 100 milligrams of vitamin E daily for 3 months, and the husband one tablet of 100 milligrams daily for one month, the failure of their pregnancies was reduced to 8 per cent in 103 cases.

Aid in Withdrawal Symptoms of Drug Addicts

In these days of increased drug addiction, the report in the *Acta Medica Iran* (1: 215, 1956-1957) should be of great interest to city governments as well as medical men. Ten cases of opium addiction, of 4 to 14 years duration, were given 200 to 1,000 milligrams daily for 3 to 19 days. Abstinence symptoms improved along with ability to sleep and lessening of pain. The period of withdrawal treatment was shortened. The author suggests a maintenance dose of 100 to 200 milligrams daily for several weeks after recovery.

Perhaps such treatment would aid addicts to other drugs in getting through the horrible period of withdrawal more easily and speedily. We have seen no literature on such experiments conducted with vitamin E in the United States, where the addiction problem is becoming acute. In *La Presse Medicale* (68: 855, 1959), the most common cause of myopia, an elongation of the front-to-back diameter of the eye, due to a looseness of certain fibres of the coating of the eye, is discussed. C. and G. Desusclade have treated this affliction with vitamin E—100 milligrams each morning for 3 months of each year. This treatment is said not only to arrest the progress of this myopia, but has improved the condition in 15 per cent of the cases treated.

We join Dr. Shute in begging organized medicine in the United States to try—only try—vitamin E in the many types of disease which have no other real cure and in which Dr. Shute and others have demonstrated this vitamin's effectiveness. We urge our readers to talk to their doctors about vitamin E. Ask them to write to the Shute Foundation of London, Ontario, Canada, for a copy of the

Summary. We are convinced that the doctor who once tries vitamin E in his practice will never work without it thereafter.

Answer to Critics of Vitamin E

A medical doctor who writes a widely syndicated column took up the question of vitamin E. Dr. Walter Alvarez, whose column is printed in, we suppose, hundreds of American newspapers, wrote:

"Many people write me asking if they should mortgage their home or borrow money and travel far to the institute they have heard about which advertises to cure some disease. I certainly would never think of going to such a place. Today, a woman writes asking if she should take her very sick child to a place where marvelous cures are supposed to be worked with vitamin E. All I know is that a while ago, I read a big book on the world's experience with vitamin E and the conclusion of the editors was that it was of no value on any known disease of man. We, all of us, get large amounts of vitamin E in all our foods. I know that there are many enthusiasts who have reported marvelous results from using vitamin E, but I know that other men, who have tried to confirm these results, have failed completely. It is very hard to decide if a drug is of value, especially if one is an enthusiast."

Dr. Evan Shute, of the Shute Clinic, London, Ontario, Canada, took up Dr. Alvarez' challenge and wrote him the following letter. We think it is a masterpiece, both for the information it contains and for its moderate, restrained and reasonable tone. This is the tone we think is most effective for letters to editors, Congressmen or public health officials. Be sure you have all the facts, then write with good humor, but firmness, as Dr. Shute has. For those readers who regularly follow Dr. Alvarez' column—here, we think, is the best answer to his statements about vitamin E.

"DEAR DR. ALVAREZ:

"I often read your very wise and humane column which is carried by so many papers, but I must admit that both you and your column sank very low in my estimation today when I read your notes on vitamin E. They show so much bias, so much misinformation and so little appreciation of current literature, that I was astonished.

"There are now about 300 teams of medical 'enthusiasts' who have written papers emphasizing the therapeutic effectiveness of alpha tocopherol (vitamin E) in cardiovascular disease, not to mention the numerous papers on reproductive difficulties. These include some of the great names in the profession, people whom you would be proud to have on the staff of the Mayo Clinic, for example. Their papers are what matters, of course, not any 'big book' of 'other men's pearls' (which, by the way, you gave no date for; it could have been 20 years old).

"I count myself among these 'enthusiasts' and I know you will be interested to hear that I was asked to describe our studies on 'Vitamin E in Obstetrics and Vascular Disease' at the Pan-American Fertility Conference in Miami Beach two months ago (their suggestion as to title, not mine) and am being asked to describe them to the doctors of Saskatchewan in a refresher course being sponsored by the Saskatchewan Board of Health a month from now. You know, surely, that I am listed in American Men of Science, belong to many international medical societies and have served as president of a national society in one of my specialties.

"There are many overwhelming references which I could cite which would change your viewpoint, I am sure, but let me mention just 3:

"1.   The study of Livingston, P.D., and Jones, C. (England)— *Lancet* 2:602, 1958—on intermittent claudication.

"2.   The study of Kawahara on Venous Thrombosis—*Surgery,* Vol. 46, p. 768, 1959.

"3.   The study of Tolgyes, S., and Shute, E. V.—*Canadian Medical Association Journal,* 76:730, 1957—giving colored photographs of our results in treating early gangrene. I would ask you to look particularly at figures 1, 2, 3 and 10, 11, 12 and 13, and ask yourself if any inert substance could produce a result like that.

"Surely you are aware that the last paper in the literature to cast doubt on our findings appeared fully 10 years ago!

"You point out in your column that we get 'large quantities of vitamin E' in our food. Dear Dr. Alvarez, surely you know better. This and all its relevant details were discussed by me in the last issue of the *Summary,* which I am sending you, from page 51 onwards. I will mention just one item in it to you now because I hope you will read the whole article at your first opportunity. It points out that the diets suggested by the National Research Council of the United States contain 6 International Units of alpha tocopherol per day. What anyone absorbs may be *much less* than this, but this is what is laid on his plate. It has recently been proven by Horwitt and others that the daily requirement is 30 International Units of alpha tocopherol per day. What must your conclusion be?

"Finally, I am sending you a reprint which appeared a few weeks ago in the *Canadian Medical Association Journal* describing the intensive studies being undertaken in Russia at this moment on the value of this agent in cardiovascular disease. The Russians surveyed all the medical literature first, including any adverse opinion you could have uncovered, but looked at our evidence, too. Then they decided to undertake this definitive study. You know how excellent

Russian medicine is, as well as Russian nuclear physics. Didn't you speak too soon, Dr. Alvarez? Their results can make your country look foolish once again.

"I think and hope that you are an honest man as well as an able physician. I sincerely hope and expect that you will consider the points that I have brought to your attention, as well as the many others which are discussed in the *Summary*. Upon changing your views I will expect you to relate your change of heart in your column. If you fail to do so, I shall know where you stand both by the ethical standards of our profession and by the still older standards of honesty to which all men subscribe.

"Yours sincerely,

EVAN V. SHUTE,
F.R.C.S. (C)"

Do Doctors Study Vitamin E's Record?

Evidently, Dr. Alvarez didn't follow the advice so ably given to him by Dr. Shute in the letter above, for, in another of Dr. Alvarez' columns, which appeared in syndication on October 15, 1961, the question of the value of vitamin E as a therapeutic measure is revived once again. Under a subhead, "Vitamin E Has No Value in Treating Illness," Dr. Alvarez writes: "Beside me as I write is a big book on vitamin E. And the editor of it concludes by saying that, after reading the literature on this substance, his impresssion is that it has no value in the treatment of disease. . . . It (vitamin E) is found in so many foods that it is almost impossible to make up a diet that does not contain all the vitamin E that an animal needs."

Does it all sound familiar? For over a year, Dr. Alvarez has sat with one big book on vitamin E which can tell him nothing new. How old is the book? He doesn't say. Could it have been written 20 years ago, when there was little experimentation and evidence on the powers of vitamin E? Surely no authority on vitamin E could have read through the hundreds of reports on successful treatment of humans and animals with vitamin E since the 1940's and still contend that there is no evidence on the value of the vitamin in the treatment of disease. The evidence is overwhelming!

Furthermore, in spite of the information conveyed to him by Dr. Shute, Dr. Alvarez persists in keeping alive the myth that no one could possibly need more vitamin E than one gets in the average diet. If intake of vitamin E can reverse a disease condition in the body—and it most certainly can!—then it is obvious that that body was not getting the amount of vitamin E needed to prevent the disease. It is hard to believe that Dr. Alvarez has gone beyond the "big book" he keeps referring to, to do any serious research on the current standing of vitamin E. We have, however, and we know that, to say the least, Dr. Alvarez' conclusions on vitamin E are mistaken.

A Big Joke

Another columnist, Burton H. Fern, M.D., played vitamin E for laughs. In a copy of his column sent to us, he answered these questions: "Does vitamin E help varicose veins? How much should I take?" with this answer:

"Filled with vitamin E, varicose veins merely bulge more. So far, no one can prove that humans need vitamin E. In vitamin pills, it merely calms 'worry-warts'!"

We wonder if the "joke" got a good laugh in Dr. Fern's home town. Would the folks still be laughing if they knew that, in spite of Dr. Fern's assertion that there is no proof for the need of vitamin E in humans, the United States government ruled that such a need had definitely been established.

We would like to cite a few experiments with vitamin E, conducted by the world's scientists, which show that it does more, much more, than Dr. Fern says it can.

The basic disorder which causes varicose veins is circulatory. In the *American Journal of Physiology* (153:127, 1948), Zierler, Grob and Lilienthal asserted their belief that alpha tocopherol is vigorously antithrombic (fights clotting). This suggests to them that it may help prevent intravascular blood clotting. Alpha tocopherol is recognized as an oxidative agent.

A Danish journal, *Acta Pathologica* (29: 73, 1951), carried a report on 8 patients with venous disease of the legs. The authors concluded that "a local deficiency of vitamin E" exists in certain types of chronic venous disease.

A study of 25 cases, most of whom had leg varices and who were given 100 to 150 milligrams daily of a special vitamin E preparation, plus a coumarin (anticoagulant) preparation was reported in *Lekarske listy* (7:549, 1952), a Czechoslovakian journal. The results were compared with similar cases of thrombosis seen in their clinic since 1946. It was found that the average number of days necessary before the patient was able to walk was cut in half. The combined treatment was preferable to the use of the coumarin derivative alone. The author, O. Bruchner, later used vtiamin E as a preventive for similar disorders with success.

A Nine-Year Review

A review of 9 years' experience with alpha tocopherol appeared in the *Canadian Medical Association Journal* (74: 715, 1956). There were 327 cases of thrombophlebitis and phlebothrombosis treated. All were treated with nothing but alpha tocopherol. Provided the dosage was adequate, the results were classed as dramatic and gratifying. Inflammation promptly subsided and the clotting dissolved. The heat, swelling and tenderness quickly disappeared.

Arizona Medicine (16: 100, 1959) carried an article by R. F. Bock in which he concluded that postoperative and postpartum thrombophlebitis respond well to 1,100 International Units of alpha tocopherol per day. The results often show themselves within 12 hours, and pain is relieved in 24 hours. Clinical results are apparent in 24 to 48 hours.

Varicose ulcers are also cured by alpha tocopherol, says Bock. It can be used prior to surgery as a preventive against dangerous blood clots. It is characterized as safer and just as effective as dicumerol and heparin and never accompanied with hemorrhage complications. Bock saw no side effects from alpha tocopherol use.

These are but a few of the many reports on the value of vitamin E in treating vascular disorders. If Dr. Fern has done any research on the question, he must have come across some evidence that is inexplicable, if vitamin E has no value and if he still insists that no one has shown that it is necessary to human life.

A Clue to Vitamin E Shortage

The obvious importance of vitamin E and the mysteries which have yet to be solved before vitamin E is fully explained, are emphasized by a report in *Gastroenterology* (February, 1961). It told of the appearance of brownish-yellow coloring on the smooth muscle fibers due to deposit of certain granules when a vitamin E deficiency is induced in animals. What is interesting about this discovery is that 61 per cent of the subjects in this study who suffered from an inflammation of the pancreas and 27 per cent of those who suffered from nutritional cirrhosis of the liver, showed the same colored granule deposit. It was also present in the small intestine in nearly all the cases. Furthermore, 17 per cent of the patients with pancreatitis and 65 per cent with nutritional cirrhosis showed the coloring in the stomach, prostate gland, urinary bladder, bronchi, esophagus, gall bladder, colon and uterus. These findings raise the possibility that some of the gastrointestinal motor disturbances encountered in cases of inflammation of the pancreas and cirrhosis, may be due to deposits of these granules caused by vitamin E deficiency.

Vitamin E in the treatment of diabetes was being used effectively in 1947, according to *Medical Record* (160: 667, 1947). M. B. Mololchick told of a 55-year-old man with diabetes mellitus and angina pectoris. He was put on 200 milligrams of mixed tocopherols and the angina was gone in 3 weeks. Also, after 3 months of treatment with mixed tocopherols, the patient's blood sugar was normal.

An Italian journal (*Gionale di Clinica Medica,* 31:1, 1950) carried U. Butturini's article telling of 50 diabetics treated with alpha tocopherol. For 10 per cent, there was no help from the treatment, 26 per cent were able to reduce their insulin intake somewhat and 64 per cent were taken off insulin entirely.

E. C. Gargollo and M. A. Merlo wrote in the Spanish journal, *Revista Clinica Espanola* (69: 25, 1958) of treating 20 patients with moderately severe diabetes for 80 days with daily doses of 200 International Units of alpha tocopherol, plus tolbutamide. Very favorable results were obtained. The authors believed the alpha tocopherol and tolbutamide act upon each to the benefit of the patients.

We believe vitamin E is important to maintaining good health. We believe that the average modern diet offers far less than the minimal amount needed by the body to function properly. It is quite understandable to us that so many common diseases of modern America respond to treatment with vitamin E. Obviously, they occur because of a vitamin E shortage in the daily diet. Modern food processing has reduced the daily vitamin E intake by 100 International Units. We believe it is essential that the diet be supplemented, to that extent, at least.

Vitamin K

Why We Need Full Nutrition

If you or someone you know has a hard time with the repair of bone fractures, they may be lacking in vitamin K. *Medical News* (April 6, 1960) tells of the experiments of a Belgian physician who administered the vitamin to a series of adult rats and rabbits with complete fractures of the tibia. The diets were completely identical for all the experimental animals, except that some received a vitamin K supplement and some did not.

X-rays of the fractured bones of the treated animals showed well-developed callus and primary bone formation at the site of the break. The untreated animals did not have nearly so much new bone formation. As a matter of fact, the space between the bone ends seemed to have no mineral deposit and the fracture was still apparent.

Walking

Walking for Health

By J. I. Rodale

I once visited H. A. Schweigart, M.D., a famous research physician, in Hannover, Germany, who has been doing medical research under German government grants. He is a great believer that malnutrition is the cause of many diseases. He described to me researches he had performed which indicated that cancerous tissue always showed a deficiency of oxygen. As a result, he always walks several miles every day to insure a thorough oxygenation of the body.

Our system of good health basically comprises two things—exercise and nutrition. But by exercise, I don't mean hours of back-breaking work that produces bulging muscles. All that's required is a few minutes each day of setting-up exercises plus at least one hour of walking. You might say, "I do so much walking in my kitchen," or at work, but in my opinion, there's no substitute for the steady, swinging gait of a spirited walk.

What does walking do for you? Many things! It speeds up the circulation. It sends oxygen to all parts of the body. It improves one's spirits. It's a stimulus to the brain and encourages thinking. But most important of all, it starts the various glands to secrete their hormones. For example, at rest, the adrenal gland is more or less inactive, but after 10 minutes of exercise, the adrenals begin to secrete cortisone.

What happpens to people who sit around too much, who ride when they should walk? Their adrenal glands make practically no cortisone at all. This deficiency could be one of the causes of arthritis. Then, the doctors prescribe cortisone, but it is an artificially made cortisone that can't be the same as the kind your body makes. This leads to side effects. Regular taking of cortisone can lead to softening of the body's bone structure and easy fracturing from simple falls. It also seems to lead to mental trouble in some persons. So, isn't it better to insure against disease by keeping your own adrenal glands functioning and producing your own cortisone?

And so it is with the other glands of the body. They need stimulation to be active. The thyroid gland, the pituitary, the pancreas, the prostate—all must be kept active by exercise. Many men get prostate gland trouble and go through the torture of mutilating surgery because, for one thing, they lead inactive lives physically. There are other causes, but the lack of physical exercise is an important one.

Walking and regular exercise are factors in preventing the

891

blood pressure from going up unduly and keeping the pulse from going above normal. For many years, I suffered from a high pulse, and at that time, rarely exercised or walked. Then I began to walk an hour every day, and in a few months, my pulse went down about 7 to 8 beats a minute.

Incidentally, the late Dr. Raymond Pearl, of Johns Hopkins University, made a study of the pulse records of thousands of persons who had died and found that, the higher the pulse, the shorter the life. This is pure mathematics. If the pump runs too fast, it will soon run down. The heart is a pump and each beat of the pulse means one pump action of the heart, one squeeze. But if the pump that's made to run at a certain speed runs too fast, what's going to happen to it? You'll find the answer in the mortality statistics.

Another advantage of walking and exercise is that they help keep down the cholesterol level in the blood. Cholesterol, as you know, is a fat compound that coats the artery walls, contributing to hardening of the arteries. It narrows them down so that the blood cannot circulate freely. Walking is one of the best medicines for the health of the arteries. It gives flexibility to all the tissues of the body, it tones up the muscles and takes the starch out of the joints. It speeds up all the processes of the body that are slowed down by inactivity. As a German doctor once said, "Ach, valking. . . . Dot iss goot meditzeen. But you cannot find it in a meditzeen cabinet."

Another important effect of exercise is to induce perspiration. "By the sweat of thy brow shalt thou earn thy daily bread," and I would add, "By the sweat of thy sweat glands canst thou avert disease and medical disasters."

By means of the sweat glands, the body gets rid of many toxins, or poisons, that man takes in through his chemicalized foods and through the poisons in the atmosphere. If he doesn't get rid of a lot of this by perspiration, if he sits around inactively, these poisons accumulate in his system and make him ripe for many disease conditions, possibly even including cancer. Yes, an inactive life may be one of the causes of cancer.

As I said before, I used to lead a very inactive life, rarely walking, always riding, even if it was only for 3 or 4 blocks. I suddenly woke up to its dangers when I read a certain anecdote involving Dr. Thomas Sydenham, known as the father of English medicine who lived in the 1600's. It seems he had a patient with the gout, but all his remedies proved ineffective. So he sent him to see a certain doctor about a hundred miles from London, who he said was the world's greatest authority on the gout.

The patient soon found that there was no stagecoach that went to this town so he had to ride a hundred miles on horseback to see the doctor. But when he got there, nobody had ever heard of the doctor he had come to see. So he rode the hundred miles back to London, called on Dr. Sydenham, and asked him, "On what kind of wild-goose chase did you send me?" Sydenham replied by asking him, "How's your gout?"

"What gout?" replied the patient.

The physical action of 200 miles on a horse's back, the perspiration it produced, the oxygen it sent into all the obscure parts of his body, the hormones that his glands made, all contributed to clearing up the symptoms of the man's gout.

Someone asked a Dr. Abernethy of those times, what was a good cure for the gout? He replied, "Live on 6 pence a day, and earn it." This meant lots of bodily movement and exercise.

In those days, people knew the value of walking. Samuel Pepys, who was contemporary with Dr. Sydenham, did a lot of walking. I shall quote from his diary. May 12, 1662: "Mr. Townsend called on us by 4 o'clock and by 5, the 3 ladies, my wife and I, and Mr. Townsend, his son and daughter, were got to the barge and set out.

Wasserman, August von

August von Wasserman, famous for his test for diagnosing syphilis, was born in Bamberg, Bavaria, February 21, 1868. His medical training was received at the Universities of Strasbourg,

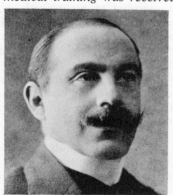

Vienna and Berlin. Upon completion of this study, Wasserman entered private practice as a physician in Strasbourg. During this period, he also worked under Robert Koch at his Institute for Infectious Diseases at Berlin where he learned new research techniques which were to help him later in his studies on syphilis. In 1913 he became director of the Kaiser Wilhelm Institute in Berlin-Dahlem and it was here that he, together with Albert Neisser and Carl Bruck developed a serum which could be used to detect the presence of antibodies formed to thwart the invasion of syphilis germs in the blood or spinal fluid. The procedure for use of this serum developed into what is known as the Wasserman test, considered to be the most reliable method for determining whether or not a patient is syphilitic. Wasserman died in Berlin on March 16, 1925.

We walked from Mortlake to Richmond and so to boat again. And from Teddington to Hampton Court Mr. Townsend and I walked again."

What I like about it is to see whole families walking together. This practice should be revived.

The English historian, Trevelyan, who lived in the 1800's, must have thought a lot of the value of walking, for he once said, "I have two good doctors—my right leg and my left leg."

Harry Golden, in his book, *Only in America* speaks about a *New York Times* reporter's interview with Mr. Roebuck of Sears Roebuck, on his 90th birthday. He asked him to what he attributed his good health and longevity. The following was Mr. Roebuck's reply:

"Son, I sold out to Mr. Sears. Mr. Sears made 10 million dollars and now he's dead. Mr. Sears sold out to Julius Rosenwold, who made 300 million dollars, and now he's dead. All I want you to tell your readers is that on his 90th birthday Mr. Roebuck took his usual walk in Central Park."

As you can see, it was his usual walk—he walked every day and it kept him alive and happy.

I have checked newspaper accounts of hundreds of cases of extreme old age, and on the average, they were great walkers. There was the case of one old man, 115 years old, short, thin and wizened. When asked his formula, he said that for years he had walked all day long . . . this man walked from morning to night, with, no doubt, stops for eating, visiting with friends, strangers and such things.

Many years ago, Dr. John Finley, editor of the *New York Times,* himself an ardent walker, used to present a medal to those of his friends who walked 3 miles or more a day.

It was estimated that William Wordsworth, the great English poet, had walked 180,000 miles during his lifetime. He claimed this accounted for much that was excellent in his writings, and he lived to be 80 in a time when people died young. Wordsworth was a very happy man.

In studying the effects of exercise on the human body, I made a rather startling observation. I noticed that most of the conductors of famous symphony orchestras lived to ripe old ages. Pierre Monteux, still alive, is 86, Toscanini died at the age of 88, Vaughan Williams at 86, Sibelius at 90, Weingartner, Mengelberg, Richard Strauss and Koussevitzky, all over 80. Sir Thomas Beecham at 80 took a bride of 27. I figured there must be one common denominator for it. And this is what I came up with:

The orchestra conductor stands for hours moving his arms vigorously in the act of conducting his orchestra. And he does this not only when making public appearances, but for days and days during the endless rehearsals required to perfect the performance. Some of these leaders perspire so much that many of them have to make complete changes of garments during intermission. This is why musical conductors never go to Turkish baths.

Now . . . if this is true, if these famous conductors live long because of this exercise, why don't jazz conductors live as long . . . In the first place, jazz music being what it is, the jazz leader usually doesn't lead his band as vigorously. He stands crunched up with little movement. Besides, he moves in an environment of people who lead dissipated lives.

In many occupations there is much brisk arm movement. I once met an old window cleaner whom I knew, who was 73 years old. After chatting a bit, I asked him, "How's your heart?" "What heart?" he replied. Here was a man who, for 20 or 40 years, had spent much of his days moving his hands briskly over windowpanes. Who knows, perhaps moving his hands, which are nearer the heart, has a beneficial effect on the heart tissues and on the lungs? All these years his work made him breathe more fully, drawing in oxygen and supplying it to every organ of the body. This could be a wonderful longevity factor.

Carpenters spend much time moving their hands, hammering nails, sawing, etc., but they do not do it quite as briskly nor cover the range of distance as do the hands of the symphony orchestra conductors and window cleaners.

Chiropractors and osteopaths spend a good part of their time moving their arms while giving adjustments to people. Do chiropractors live longer? Nobody has ever thought to check.

There can be no question that exercise and movement are factors in living long. In my section of Pennsylvania, Allentown, there was a man who, for 40 years, was a track-walker for a railroad. For 8 hours each day, he walked the track to check for imperfections and other trouble. A few years ago, he retired and said, "Now I will rest." He sat on his porch all day long. He was a healthy man, but within a year, they laid him away to eternal rest. He suffered a heart attack. His heart was not used to his body being at rest. He was killed by inactivity.

Professional athletes have the same problem. They are all right while they are engaged in their particular form of athletics. But when they retire from this activity and fall into sedentary habits, it shortens their lives. There are records of athletes who remained active till the end of their days and lived into ripe old age. It isn't the exercise that shortens athlete's lives. It is the later inactivity.

Nature protects the athlete by reducing his pulse below normal and increasing the size of his heart above normal. A Dr. Bramwell made studies of the pulse of animals and found that animals which are very active have low pulses. "For example," he says, "the pulse rate of the hare, an exceedingly athletic animal, is under 70, while

that of its cousin, the rabbit, a sedentary creature, who never strays
far from his burrow, is over 200. To compensate for the difference
in pulse rate, the hare's heart, relative to its body weight, is 3 times
as large as the rabbit's."

It is possible, therefore, that people who begin to walk every
day will benefit by a gradual increase in the size of their heart.

The idea that what is known as "Athlete's Heart" is dangerous
is purely a myth. Just the reverse is true. It is a protection and a
help to the athlete in his athletic work.

There is a dangerous modern trend towards inactivity—the
desire to live in houses that are all on one floor. Some call them
ranch houses. But apartments are also culprits in this respect. Dr.
Joseph Freeman of Philadelphia, at a recent AMA meeting deplored
this tendency. He speculated that those who do not climb stairs
regularly may have bone defects that people don't usually have if
they live in double level homes. He says that the legs of people
who don't climb stairs tend to lose tone. He says, "Steps are demanding and are an ideal method of exercise, of inciting bone
reactions, of maintaining muscle tone, of sharpening attention by the
requirements for coördinated effort of eye, muscle and bones and
by instituting beneficial strains which contribute to a sound bone
structure. It could even prevent bone fractures."

I would suggest that people who live in apartment houses
walk up and down the stairs of their apartment houses as much as
possible.

No discussion these days is complete without some quotation
from Benjamin Franklin, and this is especially true about exercise.
It is amazing how modern he was. He once wrote to his son, "There
is more exercise in one mile's riding on horseback than in 5 in a
coach, and more in one mile's walking on foot than in 5 on horseback, to which I may add," said Franklin, "that there is more in
walking one mile up and down stairs than in 5 miles on a level floor."

Franklin once remarked that the amount of exercise is not to be
measured by time or by distance but by the degree of warmth it
produces in the body. He didn't know it, but that warmth which
comes after some exercise is a sign that the glands are beginning
to make thyroxin and so on. What a man this Franklin was!

Oh yes, the doctors are getting over the idea of prohibiting stair
climbing in most types of heart cases.

So . . . when are *you* going to start to put walking into your
daily health program, along with your other routine health measures?
Come now, don't give me any excuses. You can find the time. I will
not take "no" for an answer. My friend, you will never regret it.
I guarantee it. Just try it for a little while and see if it doesn't drive
away depression and make you feel a thousand per cent better.

To men and women in business, to people who have problems,

to poets, to politicians who wish to become honest, to grocers and butchers and candlestick makers, I urge you to walk . . . and you will be amazed at what will happen. It might even help you to stop taking aspirin. Who knows?

A friend of mine, who lives at 72nd Street in New York and used to take taxicabs to and from his office on 44th Street, now walks to work every day and he says he'll never give up this practice. Besides, think of the money he saves.

You might find walking a good method to prevent overeating. If you have a weight problem and get hungry at wrong times, get out and walk. Perhaps it might curb your appetite.

Walking is a great medicine. One old man told me recently, "When I don't walk, my feet hurt." Walking is excellent exercise for the health of the feet.

So don't stack the health cards against yourself. Sick people can sometimes walk themselves back to health and by walking, well people can prevent themselves from getting sick. Doesn't it make sense?

Warts

Plantar Warts Respond to Vitamin A

Painful and persistent plantar warts, which grow on the sole of the foot, have been treated with X-ray, acid and surgery. All of these treatments have been almost as painful as the warts themselves and the rate of recurrence has been annoyingly high—almost the rule. In *Clinical Medicine* (July, 1959), Robert A. Lehman, Ph.D., and Manning M. Melton, M.D., reported on a survey of 119 physicians who collectively treated 228 cases of plantar warts with an aqueous solution of vitamin A palmitate, which effected substantial benefits or complete cures in 208 cases (88 per cent). Of those which were completely cured, only one case of recurrence was noted.

It is hoped that the word on the effectiveness of this vitamin A treatment will be spread among all of our doctors, for many are prone to use X-ray or surgery without a second thought. The treatment with vitamin A is considered to be relatively painless and allows a complete ambulation immediately after the injection. An average of 4.2 injections is required, each about a week apart, and only a band-aid is necessary as a dressing.

By the way, chances are that a diet rich in vitamin A foods will keep you free from the problem of plantar warts. If the body has enough of this vitamin, there should be no disease caused by a shortage of it.

Water

Who Polices Your Water Supply?

Apparently, the United States Public Health Service is so busy urging cities to fluoridate their water supplies, that little things such as keeping the water free from disease germs and dangerous chemical dumpings have been left alone for the time being. It is to be hoped that the legislative and executive powers in Washington will take note of a paper by Walter A. Lyons, Director, Division of Sanitary Engineering, Pennsylvania Department of Health, as it appeared in the January, 1961, issue of the *Journal of the American Water Works Association*. His two basic questions about the country's water supply are: Is it safe? Is it adequate?

As to the adequacy, it is easily dealt with when Dr. Lyons quotes Walter Picton, of the United States Department of Commerce, who said that 25 per cent of our water supplies are inadequate. It is not the water you lack to wash the car or sprinkle the lawn that matters, but, says Mr. Lyons, "A water shortage is a health problem in itself, because the quantity of water which is available has a great deal to do with personal hygiene, removal of fecal material and the simple fact that, when there is not enough safe water, people are forced to use water from unsafe sources. Many experiences during time of war and in underdeveloped countries have shown that water shortages affect the health of the people." It would be reassuring to know that all possible steps have been taken to insure us against this problem, at least, but apparently they have not been taken.

Two Basic Categories of Contaminants

Now to the safety of our water supply. The two basic categories of contaminants are biological and chemical. That the biological contaminants are not yet eliminated can be seen in the typhoid fever epidemic in November, 1959, at Keene, New Hampshire. Typhoid is a water-borne disease. We have had other recent water-borne disease outbreaks—Curwensville, Pennsylvania, and Ravenna, New York, to name just two. The filtration plants and chlorination stations are intended to take care of this problem. Mr. Lyons admits that these are not foolproof. Sampling of the water supply does not tell the whole story. It is an examination of only a small part of the water that goes to all consumers. As a method of checking the water, an "indicator organism" is used to determine the presence of contamination by microörganisms, but, as the term implies, it is only an indication of contamination, only a warning signal. Just how serious the contamination is no sampling like this can tell.

The other safeguards are also subject to misinterpretation or mechanical failure. If your community water supply is chlorinated, the condition of the chlorinator is vitally important. Does it have adequate capacity and is the water allowed sufficient time in contact with the chlorine to be fully treated before reaching the consumer? Unless it is, the process is wasted and the product untrustworthy. The facilities for sedimentation, filtration and storage are all potential hazards unless they are properly maintained. Indeed, the very suggestion by a person of Mr. Lyon's stature that poor maintenance is a possibility in such a sensitive and vital area, is appalling.

Mr. Lyons then went on to talk of chemical contaminants in the water, due to wastes carelessly deposited in the source (usually a river) by large industrial plants and agricultural insecticides and pesticides, which are washed into rivers, reservoirs and other water sources by rain. The industrial wastes are often highly toxic and many cases of poisoning of animals drinking these untreated waters have occurred, before the cause was discovered and the industry forced to find other means of disposing of its waste products. Some poison wastes require special equipment for removal. Ordinary filtration and sedimentation procedures simply do not handle the job. This means that extra precautions should be taken, especially by communities close to large industrial plants, to maintain a careful check on the chemical make-up of the water, both as it enters the purifying facilities and after it has been processed.

Carcinogenic Water

In *International Medical Digest* (February, 1961), there is a report of a paper read before the Society of Legal Medicine in France, in which it was stated that shellfish and ordinary fish are commonly found to contain carcinogenic (cancer-causing) hydrocarbons. The source is the sand and mud of rivers, due to pitch from coal- and gas-consuming factories and furnaces in the area. This mud is quite an active medium, rich in bacterial flora, algae and certain animal organisms. Mixed in with this living matter are very fine grains of free hydrocarbons. This mixture constantly enters the water of the rivers and the sea, either by natural processes or by dredging. In the spring, billions of microscopic animals, upon entering the river and sea waters, are filtered by mussels and oysters. In this manner, it is presumed, the benzpyrene is absorbed by edible fish, shellfish and bivalves (clams, mussels and oysters). These are the fish we are eating, taken from the water we are drinking.

The problem of insecticides and pesticides is more subtle and, therefore, much more dangerous. These chemicals are intended to kill living things. It is continually surprising to find that many people appear to think the insecticide has some feeler or intelligence device which permits it to know it should kill insects, but nothing else. They let it wash into their water supply and are surprised to find that it kills fish, too. They will drink water which contains this poison and be amazed when it makes them ill. These poisons are so deadly, that even breathing the fumes of them as they are applied, can be fatal. Why would they be less so when consumed in water?

These problems do not even touch on the difficulty we face in the pollution of our water supplies—especially rivers—by household detergents. They are insoluble poisons and are spewed into our rivers as waste in one community, only to turn up in the drinking water of the next town downstream. Foolproof control of them has not yet been perfected and the result is a dangerous threat to all of us who must consume river water.

We are, of course, opposed to the use of such substances in the first place. However, if they are to be used, their proximity to a water supply should be carefully noted and the water avoided, or at least treated to eliminate any trace of them.

Well Water Safer

These situations have made it clear to us that the source of water least likely to be contaminated is a well. Lucky is the community whose source is the clear water of deep underground streams which are, at least, safe from the surface contamination of pesticides and industrial wastes. There are many communities throughout the country which derive their water from wells—Schenectady, New York, for one—and they are more and more to be envied. Indeed, if one is relocating and can choose, a community whose water comes from wells rather than a river or lake, would be one worthwhile inducement for a health-conscious citizen.

The problem of pure drinking water is not completely solved with a reliable source or the efficiency of the purification processes used. (Bottled spring water or a private deep well is the only truly safe type.) The distribution system—the network of pipes that take the water from the reservoir to your home—can seriously affect the quality of your water. The thousands of cross connections which exist in every community go to work when the system does not have adequate pressure in any of its parts. If a sewer and drain are stopped and a low pressure situation should exist all at once, the water in the pipes can become dangerously polluted. A sample of the water taken at the source of supply cannot tell the engineer of such a danger. Spot checks of the water as it comes from the taps in various parts of the city should be constantly run.

Not Safe, Says Official

It is quite shocking to find that Mr. Lyons admits: "There are many purveyors of water in our state (Pennsylvania) who could not answer with satisfaction, 'Is it safe?' About 5 per cent of our public water supplies do not meet the United States Public Health Service drinking water standards, which is our standard for quality. We also

INDEX

Accident proneness
  age and, 7, 10, 11-13
  as a disease, 5
  background and, 5
  chemicals in food and, 18
  nutrition and, 7-10, 17
  overweight and, 621
  tranquilizers and, 816
Accidents
  age and, 7, 10, 11-13
  emotional instability and, 5, 6-8
  nutrition and, 7-10, 12-13
  see also Automobile accidents
Acne
  drug combination for, 34-35
  effect on personality, 31
  fat metabolism and, 33-34
  foods and, 32-33
  hormones and, 31-32
  in history, 30
  prevalent theory on, 31
  sulfur and, 32
  sunlight and, 32
  tetracycline and, 32
  topical liver applications, 500-501
  vegetable oils and, 36
  X-ray treatments and, 32
Adrenal gland, 432, 580
Aging
  accidents and, 7, 10, 11-13
  anemia and, 43-44
  bones and, 10-11
  changes in, 851-852
  factor in, 588-589
  glands and, 596
  nutritional deficiencies and, 297-298
  relativity of, 589
  vitamin C level and, 853
  see also Old age
Alcohol
  automobile accidents and, 6
  blood vessels and, 823
  thiamin and, 863
  varicose veins and, 823-824
  vitamin A and, 860
Alcoholism
  need for nutritional research on, 37
  tryptophan metabolism and, 37-38
  vitamin C deficiency and, 36
Algae, 38-39
Allergy
  defined, 566-567
  foods commonly causing, 701
  in multiple sclerosis, 562
Aluminum, 39-41
Amblyopia
  smoking and, 737
  symptoms of, 290
  thiamin and, 9, 864
  vitamin B_{12} and, 290, 737

American Dental Association
  approval of fluoridated toothpaste, 805, 807, 811-812
  opinion on fluoridation, 313-315
Anemia
  among elderly, 43-44
  among teen-agers, 48
  anti-convulsant drugs and, 46-47
  causes of, 42, 45, 246
  heart and, 46
  intestinal bleeding and, 44
  pernicious, and bone marrow, 838
  prevalence of, 42
  protective foods, 47
  protein deficiency and, 47
  vitamins and, 47
  see also Iron-deficiency anemia
Anesthesia
  conduction, in childbirth, 167
  dangers of general, in childbirth, 166-167
  side effects, 248
Antibiotics
  deafness and, 249, 427
  in animal feeds, 366 (table), 367 (table), 368
  in meat, dangerous, 69
  output of, 367 (table)
  side effects of, 242, 244-245, 246, 248-249
Antibodies
  deficiencies affecting production, 855
  immunity and, 83-84
  milk and, 548
  production of, 83
  pyridoxine and, 856
Anticoagulants
  during pregnancy, 51
  gangrene of the breast and, 51-52
  in the body, 49-50
  side effects of synthetic, 50-52
Antiperspirants, 227
Appendix
  postradiation infection and, 52-53
  removal and inguinal hernia, 53
  unnecessary removal of, 52, 53, 771
Appetite, 581, 617
Apples, 397-398
Arsenic
  cancer and, 56, 57
  case of poisoning, 483
  in the atmosphere, 56-57
  mass poisoning case, 55-56
Arteriosclerosis. *See* Hardening of the arteries.
Arthritis, 91, 265
Aspirin
  effects in the body, 59-61

Harvey, William, 411
Hassall, Dr. Arthur H., 145
Hay fever, 493-494
Health
  average attitude towards, 419
  light and, 496-497
  organic vs. chemical foods and,
    603-604
  pleasure in good, 420-421
  soil and, 550-551, 745, 747-750
Health consciousness
  hypochondria and, 418
  patriotism of, 422-423
  value of, 418
  view of, in U.S., 418-420
Hearing
  antibiotics and, 249, 427
  aspirin and, 424-425
  helping older people's, 428
  protecting, 427-428
  streptomycin and, 425-426, 427
  terramycin and, 427
  vitamin A and, 9-10, 380
  vitamin B_{12} and, 380
  see also Deafness
Heart
  anemia and, 46
  attacks, 186-187
  chlorinated water and, 835-836
  choline and, 870
  description of, 834, 835
  overweight and, 836
  salt and, 721, 722, 724
  size, and exercise, 896
  smoking and, 836
  stoppage, and raised limbs, 308
  symptoms, and ointments, 467
  thiamin and, 862-863
  vitamin E and, 836
  work of, 834-835
Heart disease
  among children, 172
  cholesterol and, 187-188
  dietary fat and, 266
  eggs and, 266
  in old age, 589-590
  softened water and, 906
  vitamin E and, 880
  vitamins A and D and, 858, 859
Heat
  itch and, 469
  multiple sclerosis and, 564
Hemopericardium, 51
Heparin, 50
Hepatitis
  choline and, 870-871
  polluted water and, 645, 646, 652
Hernia, 53
Herpes zoster
  description of, 864
  thiamin and, 864, 867
  vitamin B_{12} and, 866
Hiccups
  causes of, 428-429
  common remedies for, 430

extended, and weight loss, 429
  fetal, 430
  medical treatments of, 430
  surgery and, 429
High blood pressure
  among Eskimos, 278
  in old age, 589
  kidney disorders and, 481-482
  side effects of drugs for, 243
  tallness and, 776
  vitamin B and, 840-841
  walking and, 891, 892
Hippocrates, 415
Hiroshima effect, 100-101
Hodgkin's disease, 453
Homeopathy, 339
Hormone
  acne and, 31-32
  functions in the body, 437, 579
  in menstruation, 512
  treatment for leukemia, 486-487
Hormone drugs
  during pregnancy, 666
  harmful effects of, 34, 239
  in meats, 153
  misuse of, 436-437
  uses, 239
  see also Corticosteroids, Sex hor-
    mone drugs
Hospitals
  detergent problems in, 903-904
  expenditure comparison, mental and
    general, 522 (table)
  expenditures of mental, 520-521
  experiences with disinfectants, 70
  major problems of, 440
  menus in mental, 521-522
  Pickerills' plan, 440-443
  shortcomings of mental, 523
Hot dogs, 632
Hunger, 616-617, 618-619
Hydralazine, 245
Hydrogenation, 153
Hypertension. See High blood pressure.
Hypnotism, 64-65

Infections
  difficulty in transferring, 70
  resistance to, and smoking, 737
  respiratory, and kidneys, 482
  respiratory, and sudden infant
    deaths, 549
  spread of, and injections, 443
  transmission of, and polluted water,
    645-646, 652
Injections
  buttocks, and sciatic palsy, 444,
    821-822
  complications of intraspinal, 820-
    821
  preferred site for, 444
  spread of infections and, 443

[917]